# Techniques in
# Hip Arthroscopy and
# Joint Preservation
# SURGERY

# Techniques in
# Hip Arthroscopy and Joint Preservation
# SURGERY
# With EXPERT CONSULT Access

## Jon K. Sekiya, MD
Associate Professor and Team Physician
MedSport
Department of Orthopaedic Surgery
University of Michigan
Ann Arbor, Michigan

## Anil S. Ranawat, MD
Assistant Professor
Orthopaedic Surgery
Weill Medical College of Cornell University

Assistant Attending
Orthopaedic Surgery
Hospital for Special Surgery
New York, New York

## Marc R. Safran, MD
Professor and Associate Director
Sports Medicine
Department of Orthopaedic Surgery
Stanford University
Redwood City, California

## Michael Leunig, MD
PD Dr. Med.,
Department of Orthopaedic Surgery
University of Bern
Bern, Switzerland

Head of Orthopaedics
Department of Orthopaedics
Schulthess Clinic
Zürich, Switzerland

ELSEVIER
SAUNDERS

**ELSEVIER**
SAUNDERS

1600 John F. Kennedy Blvd.
Ste. 1800
Philadelphia, PA 19103-2899

TECHNIQUES IN HIP ARTHROSCOPY AND
JOINT PRESERVATION SURGERY

ISBN: 978-1-4160-5642-3

**Copyright © 2011 by Saunders, an imprint of Elsevier Inc.**

---

**Notice**

Knowledge and best practice in this field are constantly changing. As new research and experience
broaden our knowledge, changes in practice, treatment and drug therapy may become necessary or
appropriate. Readers are advised to check the most current information provided (i) on procedures
featured or (ii) by the manufacturer of each product to be administered, to verify the recommended
dose or formula, the method and duration of administration, and contraindications. It is the
responsibility of the practitioner, relying on his or her own experience and knowledge of the patient,
to make diagnoses, to determine dosages and the best treatment for each individual patient, and to take
all appropriate safety precautions. To the fullest extent of the law, neither the Publisher nor the Editors
assume any liability for any injury and/or damage to persons or property arising out of or related to
any use of the material contained in this book.

The Publisher

---

**Library of Congress Cataloging-in-Publication Data**

Techniques in hip arthroscopy and joint preservation surgery / [edited by] Jon K. Sekiya, Marc R. Safran,
Michael Leunig, Anil S. Ranawat. – 1st ed.
    p. ; cm.
  Includes bibliographical references.
  ISBN 978-1-4160-5642-3
  1. Hip joint–Surgery.   2. Hip joint–Endoscopic surgery.   I. Sekiya, Jon K.   II. Safran, Marc R.
    III. Leunig, Michael.   IV. Ranawat, Anil S.
  [DNLM: 1. Hip Injuries–surgery. 2. Arthroscopy–methods. 3. Hip Joint–surgery.  WE 855 T255 2011]
  RD772.T43 2011
  617.5'81059–dc22

                                                                                    2009039236

*Acquisitions Editor:* Daniel Pepper
*Developmental Editor:* Julie Goolsby
*Publishing Services Manager:* Anitha Raj
*Project Manager:* Beula Christopher/Sara Alsup
*Cover Designer:* Ellen Zanolle

Working together to grow
libraries in developing countries

www.elsevier.com | www.bookaid.org | www.sabre.org

ELSEVIER | BOOK AID International | Sabre Foundation

Printed in the United States of America

Last digit is the print number: 9  8  7  6  5  4  3  2  1

# Contents

# Video Table of Contents

# Foreword to "Arthroscopic Management of Hip Diseases"

Today, surgeons routinely use the arthroscope for the diagnosis and treatment of joint problems. However, few surgeons apply the arthroscope to the hip joint. The reasons for the lack of interest in this procedure are because the deep position of the hip joint which makes it difficult to reach and there is small number of indications. In order for the surgeon to be adept at a difficult operation, he must perform the surgery frequently. Because of the lack of indications for hip arthroscopy, it is almost impossible to perfect the technique. The surgeon will often discard the procedure or refer it to someone who has experience in it.

Unlike the knee, the hip joint is made up of two opposing joint surfaces. It is a well-contained and stable joint, so it is protected from trauma. Therefore, many of the problems that occur in the hip joint are chronic and result in conditions that are difficult to diagnose and treat. Although the arthroscope is invasive, it has a low potential for complications and its low morbidity make it very useful for these chronic hip conditions. For instance, what is a better way to remove a symptomatic loose body from the hip than with the assistance of the arthroscope? The alternative method would involve a large incision and dislocation of the hip.

I first performed hip arthroscopy in 1977 to evaluate a painful hip that had been nailed for a subtrochanteric fracture. Roentgenograms and laboratory studies were normal. I suspected that the problem was due to arthritis. At that time, I was using the arthroscope in other joints mainly as a diagnostic tool, so why not the hip? Since there were no procedural publications on the subject at that time, I performed a technique that Dr. Lanny Johnson[i] described to me. His method was first published in 1981.[ii] The procedure was performed with the patient supine on a fracture table. I visualized the hip through an anterior portal and arthritis was found. A hip replacement was carried out shortly thereafter.

Between 1977 and 1984, I performed a total of ten cases using the supine position. On occasion, it was difficult to enter the hip joint with this method, especially in obese individuals, because the instruments that were available were the same short instruments that were used in the knee. Therefore, I felt that a change was necessary. It all came about in the fall of 1983 when I was unsuccessful in the removal of loose bodies from a hip in a heavy woman placed in the supine position. Following the case, my partner, Dr. Tom Sampson, and I discussed the problem, and at his suggestion came to the conclusion that since the lateral approach permits the fat to drop downward, away from the operative sight, better access to the hip joint would be achieved. We started by supporting the patient's leg in a wrap around the calf, which was connected to overhead weights by a rope placed through pulleys hung from the ceiling. After performing the procedure successfully in several patients placed on their sides, including a 5 ft. 5 in. tall, 270 lb person, I contacted the woman who had loose bodies that I earlier failed to remove using the supine approach and scheduled her for another surgery in which I now successfully extracted five loose bodies by the lateral approach.[iii]

After using the overhead traction device in a dozen patients we found that more distraction was needed to adequately examine the joint and to keep from damaging the joint surfaces. The distraction necessary to achieve this could not be obtained with overhead traction. I then utilized a fracture table with the attachments adjusted for patients placed on their sides. Satisfactory distraction was achieved in every case with this device. However, there were drawbacks, which included difficulty in rearranging the table for the lateral approach, the inability to adjust the perineal post to prevent excessive pressure on the pudendal nerve, and the absence of a device to measure the amount of traction for safety reasons. In individuals with stiff joints, or in patients with hip contractures, a large amount of traction might be necessary to adequately distract the hip. In this situation a dangerous amount of pressure may be placed on the nerves of the limb and the perineum and if applied too long could cause paralysis.

Once publications on the subject began to appear, a few more surgeons began to perform the procedure and finally specific instruments and traction devices were developed, which made the procedure easier and safer. Drs. Thomas Byrd,[iv] Joseph McCarthy,[v] Henri Dorfmann,[vi] Eijner Eriksson,[vii] and Richard Villar[viii] led this early charge and were instrumental in refining the procedure to the extent that made it more feasible. Instruments exclusive for the hip were developed. These included longer arthroscopes and instruments that were essential to maintain the portals and reach the depths of the joint and curved instruments that helped in reaching the corners of the joint and made it possible to operate on the curved acetabulum. Despite these advancements, the procedure only gained a little of the popularity that arthroscopy of the other joints had gained. The reasons, at that time, appeared to be from a lack of indications and to poor outcomes due to the association of degeneration in so many of the cases. In the meantime, the few of us who were performing the procedure gained more experience.

In 2003, the work of Professor Reinhold Ganz[ix] and his associates in Switzerland regarding hip impingement brought new light on the cause of degeneration in the hip joint. His

---

[i]Johnson LL: Personal Communication.

[ii]Johnson LL: Diagnostic and Surgical Arthroscopy: The Knee and Other Joints, 2nd Ed. St. Louis: CV Mosby, 1981, pp. 405-411. 292-6804.

[iii]Glick JM, Sampson TG, Gordon RB, Behr JT, Schmidt E: Hip Arthroscopy by the Lateral Approach. Arthroscopy 1987; 3: 4-12.

[iv]Byrd JWT: Hip Arthroscopy Utilizing the Supine Position. Arthroscopy. 1994; 10: 275-280.

[v]McCarthy JC, Day B, Busconi B: Hip Arthroscopy: Applications and Technique. J Am Acad Orthop Surg. 1995; 3: 115-122.

[vi]Dorfmann H, Boyer T, Henry P, de Bie B: A Simple Approach to Hip Arthroscopy. Arthroscopy. 1988; 4: 141-142.

[vii]Eriksson E, Arvidsson I, Arvidsson H. Diagnostic and Operative Arthroscopy of the Hip. Orthopedics. 1986; 9: 169-176.

[viii]Villar RN: Hip Arthroscopy. Oxford: Butterworth-Heinemann, 1992.

[ix]Ganz R, Parvizi J, Beck M, Leunig M, Nötzli H, Siebenrock K: Femoroacetabular Impingement: A Cause for Osteoarthritis of the Hip: Clinical Orthop. 2003; 417: 112-120.

procedure to correct this was found to be adaptable to arthroscopy. The hip surgeons took notice and found arthroscopy to be beneficial in their practice and started to perform the procedure, greatly increasing the numbers that used it. As more arthroscopies were carried out, more refinements were made, more information about the anatomy of the hip was attained, and the outcomes of the procedure improved. This brings us to today where hip arthroscopy has become an integral part of the diagnosis and treatment of hip diseases. More advances will come in the future. Already there have been trials of the use of polymers for resurfacing knee joints in patients and hip joints in cadaver specimens.

The hip is the largest joint in the body and is the site of major diseases in patients of all ages from childhood to the elderly. Therefore, it is imperative for the surgeons who treat the hip to know all the treatment options available including arthroscopy. The significant features of arthroscopic surgery are not only the fact that it uses minimal incisions and reduces morbidity, but also is designed to preserve the joint as much as possible. This book is valuable in that it combines both arthroscopy and the more established open techniques in the diagnosis and treatment of these hip conditions. It is not easy for surgeons to grasp the challenge of arthroscopy of the hip when it was hardly used just a decade or so ago. This text, with its combination of open and arthroscopic methods, should certainly expand surgeons' knowledge and give them more alternatives in the treatment of some of the most difficult conditions of the hip joint. It should also spark interest for traditional surgeons to attempt this procedure. Furthermore, the section on arthroscopy will help surgeons in their endeavor to learn the principles of arthroscopy as they relate to the more conventional open procedures and to hone the arthroscopic skills necessary to diagnose and treat the various hip diseases that they will encounter.

JAMES M. GLICK, M.D.

# Foreword to "Open Management in Joint Preservation Surgery"

The timing of this textbook consisting of chapters on the diagnosis and nonprosthetic surgical management of difficult yet common problems of the hip is propitious. Conservative management of hip arthosis, usually through dropping the pressure in the joint, was widely written about in the seventies and early eighties has not been updated with a dedicated volume in the last fifteen years.

This is true, despite significant new observations about the etiology of hip arthrosis, new high-tech imaging techniques, new surgical approaches, and new procedures which have evolved to improve the outcome of treatment in this special group of patients.

The majority of these patients suffer from irritable hips and early arthosis. Most have deformities and morphological abnormalities that are secondary to congenital or acquired disturbances of normal hip development.

Most of the innovations in diagnosis and treatment can be directly attributed to those that studied with or were influenced by the orthopedic department at the University of Bern, Switzerland. The chairman of the department during this time, Reinhold Ganz, was a master surgeon and successor to world-famous hip surgeon Professor Maurice Mueller.

Bern, always an active academic center, provided a fertile environment for further refinement of "the conservative approaches" to the problems of the young adult with painful hip joints.

In 1984, Professor Ganz with the collaboration of his team, focused on the problem of the residuals of hip dysplasia and developed a new "Periactabular Osteotomy" that allowed unrestricted correction of the associated deformities. In addition, the procedure could be carried out through a single exposure.

Although there are many different surgical procedures for the correction of dysplastic hips, "the Bernese" periacetabular osteotomy became a popular and well-accepted procedure for the treatment of hip dysplasia in the patient with closed physeal plates.

The long-term follow up of the patients who had undergone PAOs actually contributed to the identification of femoroacetabular impingement, the next major discovery in Bern during the Ganz tenure.

In Orthopedic Surgery, the sixties and seventies were dominated by teaching and studying outcomes of total hip arthroplasty. There was change in the focus of a majority of orthopedic surgeons from classical operations such as osteotomies, as postulated by Pauwels and his students, to the complicated subject of hip replacement with synthetic materials. These materials were studied to understand their behavior under conditions of motion and load.

Indeed, study of factors producing accelerated wear in artificial hip joints or causes of their frequent dislocations identified the phenomenon of motion-induced impingement caused by mechanical conflict between the components of the hip joint replacement. This observation led to design modifications of both femoral and acetabular components to avoid this occurrence. Understanding of this problem in the setting of total hip arthroplasty strongly suggested the possibility of the existence of this problem in the natural hip and in hips treated with osteotomy.

Indeed in the relatively small group of patients with dysplastic hips who had pain following periacetabular osteotomy, physical findings on examination, and radiographic evidence identified impingement between the femur and the acetabulum as the cause of these residual symptoms. Many had classical findings of impingement on the femoral head and characteristic acetabular labral damage at the time of re-operation.

The paramount contribution that expanded the understanding of the pathological findings of hip impingement came with the study of the anatomical course of the medial femoral circumflex vessels. This doctoral thesis, by Katharina Ganz and Nathalie Kruegel, offered objective evidence that it was possible to dislocate the human hip joint without the complication of avascular necrosis.

This finding opened the door to surgical exploration of symptomatic hips in patients with what had been thought previously to be negative x-ray images. Quite rapidly the concepts of "cam" and "pincer" impingement became accepted as the cause of symptoms in these hips and the subtle radiographic and MRI findings were defined.

Finally, the interest in joint-preserving surgery continued at the Inselspital in Bern, but with a major difference. The goal of surgery was no longer to increase congruency and the relative area of the articular surface, but rather the elimination of the conflict between the femur and acetabulum during the functional motion of the joint.

This book is a much awaited reference on the details of these new concepts, including the very important subject of the role of arthroscopy in the management of these difficult cases.

JEFFREY W. MAST, M.D.
RENO, NEVADA
AUGUST, 2009

# Acknowledgments

I would like to thank the many people who have helped me develop into a hip arthroscopist from the very beginning in medical school, where my interest was first sparked by Evan Ekman, Dave Ruch, and Gary Poehling. Ed Wojtys furthered this interest in hip arthroscopy in my residency and has been a mentor to me since in all aspects of my career. Ron Delanois helped me when I was just starting out in the Navy with my first hip scopes teaching me his tricks. Freddie Fu gave me the opportunity to come back to Pittsburgh and join his outstanding group (my fellowship alma mater!) and develop a really busy hip arthroscopy practice. And of course Marc Philippon who was gracious enough to let me come to Vail and scrub with him and really teach me the art of hip arthroscopy of which he has been such a tremendous pioneer in developing many of these techniques and really pushing our field forward. I would like to thank my co-editors, Marc Safran, who has also been a real mentor to me in the hip surgery realm and in many other aspects of my career, and he is a good friend as well; and Michael Leunig, who lends such tremendous expertise to this book with his pioneering work in femoroacetabular impingement and so much other groundbreaking hip research; and Anil Ranawat, who has done a lion's share of work toward getting this book completed and without his tremendous effort and his insight, ability, and energy, this book never would have been completed. I also want to thank the love of my life, my best friend, and ever supportive wife, Jennie: thanks for everything. And to my sons, 3-year-old Kimo and 1-year-old Koa, I love you guys more than you know.

JON K. SEKIYA

I would like to thank Jon Sekiya and Anil Ranawat for bringing me in to their vision (and doing the bulk of the work), and to Michael Leunig for bringing his knowledge, experience, and expertise to help round out this wonderful work. I am very thankful for and appreciate the friendship, expertise, professionalism, and efforts of my co-editors. I would also like to thank the many authors who contributed their knowledge and expertise to this compilation that I hope will serve as a reference and guide for many surgeons, experienced and novice, around the world as we embark on this new era of understanding and treating the non-arthritic hip. I also thank our development editors who have allowed us to put together a book that is first class.

I am particularly indebted to my many mentors for their help in my education as a clinician, surgeon, and researcher and the many sports medicine experts who have taken me under their wing over the years and helped guide me in my early years of hip arthroscopy. I am also very appreciative of my friends and colleagues in the MAHORN group who have shared the vision of trying to collaborate and cooperate to solve the problems of understanding the non-arthritic hip. I think all hip arthroscopists owe a debt of gratitude for the foresight of Jim Glick as well as Reinhold Ganz for his contributions to the understanding of the pathophysiology of the non-arthritic hip.

And lastly, but most importantly, I want to thank my wonderful, saintly wife, Lee, for her unwavering support and her sacrifices to allow me to chase my professional dreams. And for my children, Janna, Nathan, and Clark, who have always supported me, no matter how late I come home or how many weekends I spend on these pursuits, with their unconditional love—thank you for your support and love. I love you with all my heart.

MARC R. SAFRAN

I would like to thank my mentors who have shaped my young surgical career and who have all been instrumental in unique ways in helping me with this book. I have been exposed to and trained by true giants in orthopedics. At my residency at the Hospital for Special Surgery, Drs. Russell Warren, Tom Wickiewicz and David Altchek first exposed me to arthroscopy and Sports Medicine. I first learned open hip surgery from Drs. Thomas Sculco, Paul Pellicci, Eduardo Salvati, and David Helfet. During my Sports fellowship at the University of Pittsburgh, Drs. Freddie Fu and Christopher Harner furthered my interest in joint preservation, arthroscopy, and Sports Medicine. It was there that I first met Jon Sekiya, who has been a great source of inspiration, teaching, and support for this book as a co-editor. After Pittsburgh, Dr. Robert L. Buly encouraged me to apply to the prestigious Maurice Mueller Hip Fellowship in Switzerland. My experience in Zurich and Bern was inspiring. It was here where I was introduced to Dr. Michael Leunig and Professor Reinhold Ganz. Michael Leunig has provided guidance, friendship, and tremendous support of this book and my career. After Switzerland, I traveled to the United Kingdom, where I met Mr. Derek McMinn and Mr. Richard Villar. When I returned to HSS, my friends and mentors have been Drs. Dean Lorich and Bryan Kelly, who have both supported, guided, and trained me throughout my entire career. There have been other notables like my co-editor, Marc Safran, who has been extremely supportive throughout this entire process as well as Larry Dorr, who has been a family friend for many years.

Lastly, I would like to thank my family. My oldest brother, Amar Ranawat, has been a friend, mentor, and a great curbside consult, even if he is a total joint surgeon. Most importantly, I thank the greatest anatomist, scientist, friend, and surgical mentor anyone could have, my father, Dr. C.S. Ranawat. My father never pushed me to be an orthopedist but rather provided lessons for success in life. His "Ranawat Rules" govern my approach to my own family as well as my work life. He has always supported me, even my interest in this field, which at times he questioned. Thank you, Dad. I love you and you have no idea how much I respect you. Last but not least, I have to thank my wife, Dana, whose support and love have been unwavering, as well as my son, Cooper, and my little one on the way. I love you guys and this book is for you.

ANIL S. RANAWAT

The continuous questioning of the pre existing dogma concerning primary osteoarthritis has led to the novel concept of femoroacetabular impingement and its role in native hip osteoarthritis. All of us are indebted to Professor Reinhold Ganz for his contributions to our current comprehension of hip anatomy, pathology, and joint-preserving surgery.

MICHAEL LEUNIG

# List of Contributors

**J. Mack Aldridge, III, MD**
Fellowship Director
Triangle Research Associates, P.A.
Orthopaedic Surgery
Durham, North Carolina

**Champ L. Baker III, MD**
Fellow
Division of Sports Medicine
Department of Orthopaedic Surgery
Rush University Medical Center
Chicago, Illinois

**Champ L. Baker, Jr., MD**
Clinical Assistant Professor
Department of Orthopaedics
Medical College of Georgia
Augusta, Georgia

Staff Physician
The Hughston Clinic
Columbus, Georgia

**Nikolaos V. Bardakos, MD**
Consultant Orthopaedic Surgeon
The South West London Elective Orthopaedic Center
Epsom, Surrey, UK

**Paul E. Beaulé, MD, FRCSC**
Associate Professor
Surgery, University of Ottawa

Head
Adult Reconstruction Orthopaedics
The Ottawa Hospital
Ottawa, Ontario, Canada

**Martin Beck, MD, PD**
Head
Clinic for Orthopaedic Surgery
Luzerner Kantonsspital
Luzern, Switzerland

**Michel P. J. v/d Bekerom, MD**
Department of Orthopaedic Surgery
Academic Medical Center
Amsterdam, The Netherlands

**Benoit Benoit, MD, FRCS**
Division of Orthopaedics
Ottawa Hospital General Campus
Ottawa, Ontario, Canada

**Karen K. Briggs, MPH**
Director of Clinical Research
Steadman Philippon Research Institute
Vail, Colorado

**Robert L. Buly, MD**
Associate Professor
Orthopaedic Surgery
Weill Cornell Medical College

Associate Attending
Orthopaedic Surgery
Hospital for Special Surgery
New York, New York

**Denise Chan, BSc, MBT**
Orthopaedic Research Coordinator
Sport Medicine Centre
University of Calgary
Calgary, Alberta, Canada

**Lorenzo Childress, MD**
Rubin Institute for Advanced Orthopedics
Center for Joint Preservation and Replacement
Sinai Hospital of Baltimore
Baltimore, Maryland

**John C. Clohisy, MD**
Professor, Orthopaedic Surgery
Co-Chief, Adult Reconstructive Surgery
Director, Adolescent and Young Adult Hip Service
Department of Orthopaedic Surgery
Washington University School of Medicine
St. Louis, Missouri

**Ronald E. Delanois, MD**
Fellowship Director
Rubin Institute for Advanced Orthopedics
Center for Joint Preservation and Replacement
Sinai Hospital of Baltimore
Baltimore, Maryland

**Octavia Devon, MD**
Resident
Urology, University of Florida

Shands at the University of Florida
Urology, University of Florida

Malcolm Randall VA Medical Center
Urology
Gainesville, Florida

**Michael Dienst, MD**
OCM Orthopaedic Surgery Munich
Munich, Germany

**Keelan R. Enseki, MS, PT, ATC, OCS, SCS, CSCS**
Adjunct Instructor
Physical Therapy
Sports Medicine and Nutrition
University of Pittsburgh
Pittsburgh, Pennsylvania

**Teresa M. Ferguson, MD**
Department of Orthopaedic Surgery
University of Iowa Hospitals and Clinics
Iowa City, Iowa

**Reinhold Ganz, MD**
Professor and Chairman Emeritus
Department of Orthopaedic Surgery
University of Bern
Bern, Switzerland

**Michael B. Gerhardt, MD**
Director, Center for Athletic Hip and Groin Disorders
Santa Monica Orthopaedic and Sports Medicine Group
Team Physician, CD Chiva USA
Team Physician, US Soccer
Santa Monica, California

**James A. Goulet, MD**
Professor
Department of Orthopaedic Surgery
University of Michigan Medical School

Director
Division of Orthopaedic Trauma
Department of Orthopaedic Surgery
University of Michigan Hospitals
Ann Arbor, Michigan

**Carlos A. Guanche, MD**
Southern California Orthopedic Institute
Van Nuys, California

**Daniël Haverkamp, MD, PhD**
Academic Medical Center
University of Amsterdam
Department of Orthopaedic Surgery
Amsterdam, The Netherlands

**Marcia A. Horner, BA**
Office Manager for William C. Meyers, MD
Department of Surgery
Drexel University College of Medicine
Philadelphia, Pennsylvania

**Victor M. Ilizaliturri, Jr., MD**
Professor of Hip and Knee Surgery
Universidad Nacional Autónoma de México
National Rehabilitation Institute of Mexico

Chief
Adult Hip and Knee Reconstruction
National Rehabilitation Institute of Mexico
Mexico City, Mexico

**Jon A. Jacobson, MD**
Professor
Department of Radiology
University of Michigan

Director
Division of Musculoskeletal Radiology
Department of Radiology
University of Michigan
Ann Arbor, Michigan

**David Kahan**
Department of Surgery
Drexel University College of Medicine
Philadelphia, Pennsylvania

**Bryan T. Kelly, MD**
Assistant Professor
Orthopaedic Surgery
Weill Cornell Medical College

Assistant Attending
Orthopaedic Surgery
Co-Director, Center for Hip Pain and Preservation
Hospital for Special Surgery
New York, New York

**Vikas Khanduja, MRCS(G), MSc, FRCS(Tr and Orth)**
Consultant Orthopaedic Surgeon
Department of Trauma and Orthopaedics
Addenbrooke's—Cambridge University
Hospitals NHS Trust

Consultant Orthopaedic Surgeon
Department of Trauma and Orthopaedics
Cambridge Nuffield Hospital
Cambridge, UK

**Mininder S. Kocher, MD, MPH**
Associate Professor
Department of Orthopaedic Surgery
Harvard Medical School

Associate Director
Division of Sports Medicine
Children's Hospital Boston

Department of Orthopaedic Surgery
Children's Hospital Boston
Boston, Massachusetts

**Jason Koh, MD**
Clinical Associate Professor
Surgery, University of Chicago
Pritzker School of Medicine
Chicago, Illinois

Vice-Chairman
Orthopaedic Surgery
NorthShore University HealthSystem
Evanston, Illinois

**David A. Kuppersmith, BS**
Clinical Research
Steadman Philippon Research Institute
Vail, Colorado

**Christopher M. Larson, MD**
Director of Education
Minnesota Sports Medicine Fellowship Program
Minnesota Sports Medicine
Twin Cities Orthopedics
Eden Prairie, Minnesota

**Jo-Ann Lee, MS**
Nurse Practitioner
Research Assistant, Orthopaedics
Massachusetts General Hospital
Boston, Massachusetts

**Michael Leunig, MD**
PD Dr. Med.,
Department of Orthopaedic Surgery
University of Bern
Bern, Switzerland

Head of Orthopaedics
Department of Orthopaedics
Schulthess Clinic
Zürich, Switzerland

**Kartik Logishetty, MD**
Guy's, King's and St. Thomas' Medical School
King's College London
London, UK

**Dean G. Lorich, MD**
Associate Professor
Orthopaedic Surgery
Weill Cornell Medical College

Associate Director
Orthopaedic Trauma Service
Hospital for Special Surgery
New York, New York

**Travis Maak, MD**
Chief Resident
Orthopaedic Surgery
Hospital for Special Surgery
New York, New York

**Tallal Charles Mamisch, MD**
Research Instructor
Clinical Research
MR Methodology and Spectroscopy Unit

Research Instructor
Orthopaedic Surgery
Inselspital, University of Bern
Bern, Switzerland

Visiting Research Instructor
Orthopaedic Surgery
Children's Hospital, Harvard Medical School
Boston, Massachusetts

**Aditya V. Maheshwari, MD**
Clinical Fellow
Ranawat Orthopaedic Center
Hospital for Special Surgery
New York, New York

**David R. Marker, BS**
Rubin Institute for Advanced Orthopedics
Center for Joint Preservation and Replacement
Sinai Hospital of Baltimore
Baltimore, Maryland

**René K. Marti, MD, PhD**
Professor Emeritus
Orthopedics, University of Amsterdam

Professor Dr.
Orthopedic Department
Academical Medical Center
Amsterdam, The Netherlands

Prof. Dr. Med.
Klinik Gut
St. Moritz, Switzerland

**Hal David Martin, DO**
Doctor of Osteopathy
Sports Medicine/Hip Disorders
Oklahoma Sports Science and Orthopaedics

Northwest Surgical Hospital
Oklahoma City, Oklahoma

**RobRoy L. Martin, PhD, PT, CSCS**
Associate Professor
Physical Therapy, Duquesne University
Pittsburgh, Pennsylvania ·

Staff Physical Therapist
Centers for Rehab Services/Center for Sports Medicine
University of Pittsburgh Medical Center
Pittsburgh, Pennsylvania

**Joseph C. McCarthy, MD**
Clinical Associate in Orthopaedic Surgery
Department of Arthroplasty
Harvard University
Cambridge, Massachusetts

Vice Chairman
Orthopaedic Surgery
Department of Orthopaedics
Massachusetts General Hospital
Boston, Massachusetts

Director
Center for Joint Reconstructive Surgery
Department of Orthopaedics
Newton-Wellesley Hospital
Newton, Massachusetts

**Mike S. McGrath, MD**
Rubin Institute for Advanced Orthopedics
Center for Joint Preservation and Replacement
Sinai Hospital of Baltimore
Baltimore, Maryland

**Morteza Meftah, MD**
Orthopaedic Fellow
Ranawat Orthopaedic Center
Hospital for Special Surgery
New York, New York

**William C. Meyers, MD**
Chairman
Department of Surgery
Drexel University College of Medicine
Philadelphia, Pennsylvania

**Nick G. Mohtadi, MD, MSc, FRCSC**
Clinical Professor
Sports Medicine Centre
University of Calgary
Calgary, Alberta, Canada

**Michael A. Mont, MD**
Director
Rubin Institute for Advanced Orthopedics
Center for Joint Preservation and Replacement
Sinai Hospital of Baltimore
Baltimore, Maryland

**Ryan M. Nunley, MD**
Assistant Professor
Department of Orthopaedic Surgery
Washington University
St. Louis, Missouri

**M. Elizabeth Pedersen, MD**
Orthopaedic Resident, R5
Sport Medicine Centre
University of Calgary
Calgary, Alberta, Canada

**Murat Pekmezci, MD**
Assistant Clinical Professor
Orthopaedic Surgery
University of California
San Francisco, California

**Aaron Perdue, MD**
Assistant Professor
Department of Orthopaedic Surgery
Vanderbilt University
Nashville, Tennessee

**Marc J. Philippon, MD**
Associate Clinical Professor
Department of Surgery
Faculty of Health Sciences
McMaster University
Hamilton, Ontario, Canada

Managing Partner, Orthopaedic Surgeon
The Steadman Clinic

Steadman Philippon Research Institute
Vail, Colorado

**Mario Quesada, MD**
Rubin Institute for Advanced Orthopedics
Center for Joint Preservation and Replacement
Sinai Hospital of Baltimore
Baltimore, Maryland

**Amar S. Ranawat, MD**
Assistant Professor of Orthopaedic Surgery
Weill Cornell Medical College
Hospital for Special Surgery
New York, New York

**Anil S. Ranawat, MD**
Assistant Professor
Orthopaedic Surgery
Weill Medical College of Cornell University

Assistant Attending
Orthopaedic Surgery
Hospital for Special Surgery
New York, New York

**Chitranjan S. Ranawat, MD**
Professor of Orthopaedic Surgery
Hospital for Special Surgery
New York, New York

**Margaret M. Rich, MD, PhD**
Assistant Chief of Staff
Pediatric Orthopaedics
Shriners Hospitals for Children
St. Louis, Missouri

**Hassan Sadri, MD**
Consultant Orthopaedic Surgeon
Clinic of Orthopaedic Surgery
Geneva University Hospital
Geneva, Switzerland

Head
Department of Orthopaedic Surgery
Hospital of Fribourg—Riaz
Riaz, Fribourg, Switzerland

**Marc R. Safran, MD**
Professor and Associate Director
Sports Medicine
Department of Orthopaedic Surgery
Stanford University
Redwood City, California

**Thomas G. Sampson, MD**
Director of Hip Arthroscopy
Post Street Surgery Center

Medical Director
Total Joint Center
Saint Francis Memorial Hospital
San Francisco, California

**Perry L. Schoenecker, MD**
Professor
Orthopaedic Surgery
Washington University School of Medicine

Interm Chair
Pediatric Orthopaedics
St. Louis Children's Hospital

Chief of Staff
Shriners Hospital for Children
St. Louis, Missouri

**Karl F. Schultz, MD**
Clinical Instructor
Orthopaedic Surgery
University of Michigan

Attending Physician
Orthopaedics, Veterans Hospital of Ann Arbor
Ann Arbor, Michigan

**Jon K. Sekiya, MD**
Associate Professor and Team Physician
MedSport
Department of Orthopaedic Surgery
University of Michigan
Ann Arbor, Michigan

**Michael K. Shindle, MD**
Fellow
Orthopaedic Surgery
Hospital for Special Surgery
New York, New York

**Klaus A. Siebenrock, MD**
Professor and Chairman
Department of Orthopaedic Surgery
Inselspital, University of Bern
Bern, Switzerland

**Moritz Tannast, MD**
Department of Orthopaedic Surgery
Inselspital, University of Bern
Bern, Switzerland

**Mehul M. Taylor, MD**
Fellow
Minnesota Sports Medicine Fellowship Program
Minnesota Sports Medicine
Twin Cities Orthopedics
Eden Prairie, Minnesota

**James R. Urbaniak, MD**
Virginia Flowers Baker Professor of
   Orthopaedic Surgery
Orthopaedic Surgery
Duke University Medical Center
Durham, North Carolina

**Zackary D. Vaughn, MD**
Fellow
Orthopaedic Sports Medicine
Stanford University
Redwood City, California

**Richard N. Villar, BSc, MA, MS, FRCS**
Consultant Orthopaedic Surgeon
The Richard Villar Practice
The Wellington Hospital
London, UK

**James E. Voos, MD**
Fellow
Orthopaedic Surgery
Hospital for Special Surgery
New York, New York

**Stuart L. Weinstein, MD**
Ignacio V. Ponseti Chair and Professor of Orthopaedic
   Surgery
Department of Orthopaedic Surgery
University of Iowa
Iowa City, Iowa

**Stefan Werlen, Dr. Med., MD**
Head
Department of Radiology
Klinik Sonnenhof
Bern, Switzerland

**Yi-Meng Yen, MD, PhD**
Clinical Instructor
Orthopaedics, Harvard Medical School,
Children's Hospital Boston
Boston, Massachusetts

**Chad T. Zehms, MD**
Staff Orthopaedic Surgeon
Orthopaedic Surgery
Naval Hospital Great Lakes
Great Lakes, Illinois

Staff Orthopaedic Surgeon
Orthopaedic Surgery
Prevea Health
Green Bay, Wisconsin

# General Topics

# CHAPTER 1

# History and Evolution of Hip Surgery

*Nikolaos V. Bardakos and Richard N. Villar*

## INTRODUCTION

The history of hip surgery dates back to the eighteenth century, but it was the introduction of the antiseptic method by Lister in 1865 that marked a series of innovations that, over the years, decreased postoperative infection rates and encouraged surgeons to embark on increasingly complex operations around the hip joint. Until the middle of the twentieth century, when Sir John Charnley introduced the clean air operating enclosure (1964), the development of hip surgery paralleled that of the treatment of tuberculosis. However, with the development of antibiotics and the continued increase in life expectancy, the immense impact of two other hip diseases on patients' quality of life drew the attention of surgeons: congenital dislocation and osteoarthritis.

Surgical techniques around the hip joint have come a long way. Procedures that are now considered obsolete (e.g., the hanging hip procedure) kept evolving until the advent of low-friction arthroplasty, which was also introduced by Sir John Charnley; this procedure revolutionized the treatment of arthritis of the hip joint. Although the results of hip arthroplasty among older adult and middle-aged patients have generally been excellent, the limitations of this procedure for younger patients (up to the age of 55 years) were soon realized. This led to marked improvements in the techniques and biomaterials used for arthroplasty as well as to the revival of hip-joint–preserving procedures. In the absence of severe degenerative changes, younger, active patients with symptomatic structural abnormalities are increasingly managed with joint-preserving operations, with the goals of improving function in the short term and preserving bone stock in the long term. This chapter will provide an overview of the historical development of these procedures and their current status.

## OVERVIEW OF THE EVOLUTION OF HIP SURGERY

### Amputation

With the exception of trauma and acute hematogenous arthritis, tuberculous joint disease was the single most common indication for operative intervention at the hip until the advent of effective antibiotics after World War II. During the eighteenth and nineteenth centuries, amputation of the hip joint was sometimes performed for severe wounds and infections. Successful cases of hip disarticulation were reported by Larrey (1812) and Astley Cooper (1824) for trauma and chronic infection, respectively. By 1867, the reported mortality rate for this operation was 57%; this rate steadily improved and reached an acceptable level only after World War II. Hip disarticulation is used today mainly for cases of malignant tumors. The basic technique was described by Boyd in 1947.

### Resection Arthroplasty

The mutilating nature of amputation through the hip joint encouraged surgeons to develop a limb-sparing procedure. The British are credited with the first application and popularization of hip joint resection. After successfully performing a similar procedure on the shoulder of a 14-year-old boy, Charles White carried out such an operation on a cadaver and was convinced of its successful potential. In 1822, Anthony White performed the first successful hip joint resection at Westminster Hospital in London on a patient with a chronic abscess and a dislocated hip. In the United States, this operation was first performed by Lewis Sayre in 1854 on a 9-year-old girl, who had what appeared to be tuberculosis. Sayre reported about 59 such operations, with 39 survivors. In 1940, Gathorne Robert Girdlestone described the five essential steps of the surgical technique; his name has since been closely identified with the procedure (i.e., Girdlestone resection arthroplasty). Girdlestone applied this procedure mainly to patients with tuberculosis, but he also used it with patients with bilateral osteoarthritis to restore mobility. The use of antibiotics has now limited the use of hip joint resection only to cases that involve unsalvageable periprosthetic infections.

It is of note that joint resection is the first orthopedic operation for which special instrumentation was developed. Moreau used a flexible saw that was constructed by an instrument maker in London in 1790; Heine, who was from Würzburg, Germany, developed his "chain osteotome" in 1832, for which he was awarded the Monthyon Prize in Paris in 1835.

### Arthrodesis

Arthrodesis of the hip joint was first reported separately by Heusner and Lampugnani, both in 1885. They were inspired by Eduard Albert, who 3 years earlier had performed an ankle fusion. Although Heusner and Lampugnani performed their first operations for old congenital dislocations of the hip, arthrodesis was widely used for the treatment of tuberculosis after Russell Hibbs from New York first reported about its use for that indication in 1911. For this reason, a large number of extra-articular techniques were developed. Trumble (1932) first designed an ischiofemoral fusion that put the graft under compression, and Brittain (1941) added a concomitant intertrochanteric osteotomy for better deformity correction.

Watson-Jones (1939) and Charnley (1953) refined the techniques of intra-articular arthrodesis used in the absence of sepsis (e.g., osteoarthritis, congenital deformities). The former, with his transarticular nail arthrodesis, was the first to describe an effective means of internal fixation for this operation; the latter, with his central dislocation and internal compression arthrodesis, led Schneider to introduce the Cobra-head plate in 1966, which has since been the most popular technique of fixation. Hip arthrodesis remains in the armamentarium of the orthopedic surgeon for the treatment of the young or middle-aged manual laborer with unilateral arthritis of the hip, although it is probably not the first choice.

## Other Procedures

Lesser procedures of the past for the treatment of osteoarthritis are now considered obsolete and have been abandoned. In 1956, Voss described the hanging hip procedure, which rested on the principle of reducing the joint reaction force by tenotomizing the muscles around a congruent hip joint. Although this was considered effective for providing pain relief and, by some, even for reversing the degenerative process, its results were less dependable and enduring than those of the simultaneously evolving osteotomies. Drilling operations (e.g., forage, medullostomy) and neurectomies are also of purely historical value today.

The modern use of hip-joint–preserving techniques is justified by the less-than-optimal results of total hip arthroplasty among younger patients and the improved understanding of the mechanical basis of osteoarthritis of the hip. In addition to age and activity level, the ideal candidate for a hip-joint–preserving operation must have a mechanically identifiable cause of his or her symptoms. In addition, new surgical approaches have been developed, with the safe surgical dislocation of the hip having gained wide acceptance. The most commonly used techniques will be covered in more detail in the following paragraphs.

### Proximal femoral osteotomy

The proximal femur has historically been the site of choice for the realignment of the hip. Intertrochanteric osteotomy (ITO) is the most established hip-joint–preserving procedure. In 1826, John Rhea Barton of Philadelphia performed the first osteotomy on a patient with posttraumatic ankylosis and successfully produced a painless pseudarthrosis. He and Kirmission (1894) were the first to describe proximal femoral osteotomy.

Early on, adult sequelae of developmental hip dysplasia were the most common indications for an ITO (Table 1-1). Early reports of realignment osteotomies of the proximal femur involved either displacement or angulation. Hip dysplasia was the first application of this procedure, although now it rarely constitutes an indication, at least for an isolated femoral osteotomy. Adolf Lorenz (1919) described his "bifurkation" operation, and Schanz (1922)—among others—also introduced a variation of Kirmission's procedure, mainly for unreduced congenital dislocation of the hip. Both of these procedures were of the pelvic support osteotomy type. Lorenz outlined ten indications for his procedure, with advanced osteoarthritis being the eighth. In his report in 1935, McMurray from Liverpool adopted Lorenz's procedure, and he is the one who popularized proximal femoral osteotomy for the treatment of osteoarthritis. The so-called Lorenz-McMurray procedure was described—but not performed in reality—as an excessively oblique cut (Figure 1-1). Although it was originally described as a purely displacement osteotomy, it did secondarily employ valgus angulation. McMurray believed that the primary mechanism of pain relief

## Table 1-1 LANDMARKS IN THE EVOLUTION OF PROXIMAL FEMORAL OSTEOTOMY

| Surgeon | Year | Contribution | Comments |
| --- | --- | --- | --- |
| Barton | 1826 | First osteotomy performed | Intentional creation of pseudarthrosis |
| Lorenz | 1919 | "Bifurkation" operation | Used to treat congenital dislocation |
| Schanz | 1924 | First skeletal fixation system for osteotomies | Did not obviate the need for a cast |
| McMurray | 1935 | Lorenz-McMurray procedure | Femoral osteotomy applied for osteoarthritis |
| Blount | 1943 | Blade plate | First internal fixation device |
| Pauwels | 1950 | Varus osteotomy | Originally described as purely angulation osteotomy |
| Pauwels | 1956 | Valgus osteotomy | Originally described as purely angulation osteotomy |
| Imhäuser | 1965 | Triplane osteotomy | Used for slipped capital femoral epiphysis |
| Sugioka | 1972 | Rotational osteotomy | Used for osteonecrosis of the femoral head |
| Bombelli | 1983 | Extension concept added to Pauwels's osteotomy | Used for dysplasia |
| Ilizarov | 1992 | Pelvic support osteotomy | Addition of second osteotomy for axial realignment and lengthening |

was the bypass of the proximal femur during the transmission of loads from the pelvis to the distal fragment. Displacement osteotomies were widely used in England, with Malkin (earlier) and Nissen (later) being their most eminent proponents.

The prototype angulation osteotomy was described in 1950 by Pauwels, who designed a varus osteotomy above the lesser trochanter without displacement; he initially applied this procedure to young adults with hip dysplasia associated with the subluxation of a spherical femoral head. In 1956, he introduced valgus osteotomy for those hips that obtained improved congruity in adduction and for nonunited fractures of the femoral neck. About 10 years after the original description by Pauwels, the procedure came to include the medial displacement of the distal fragment (Figure 1-2).

Early on, Pauwels realized the importance of medial displacement for relieving tension from the iliopsoas and adductor muscles. He was also aware of the necessity of maintaining the overall alignment of the hip. Pauwels's contribution to the current understanding of hip biomechanics cannot be overemphasized. He was the first to explore the concept of reducing muscle moment arms by changing the orientation of the proximal femur, and he stated that a horizontal sourcil denotes biomechanical equilibrium.

His ideas were taken a step further by Bombelli, who reached the same conclusions through a modified consideration of the primary hip forces. In addition to his theoretical model, Bombelli also modified Pauwels's valgus osteotomy by adding extension in the sagittal plane for improved femoral head coverage in dysplasia, for the relief of flexion contracture, and for the correction of hyperlordosis. He also suggested that, in the

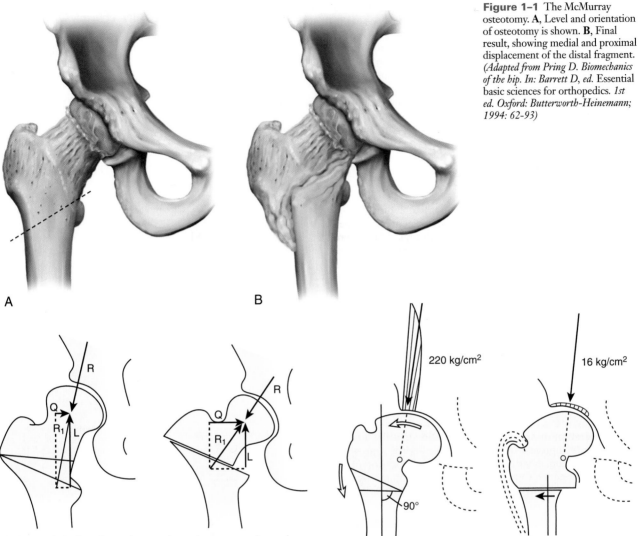

A                                    B

**Figure 1–1** The McMurray osteotomy. **A,** Level and orientation of osteotomy is shown. **B,** Final result, showing medial and proximal displacement of the distal fragment. *(Adapted from Pring D. Biomechanics of the hip. In: Barrett D, ed. Essential basic sciences for orthopedics. 1st ed. Oxford: Butterworth-Heinemann; 1994: 62-93)*

**Figure 1–2** Action of varus intertrochanteric osteotomy, increasing transverse component Q and decreasing longitudinal component L. *R,* The resultant compressive force. $R_1$, The joint reaction force. *(Adapted from Pring D. Biomechanics of the hip. In: Barrett D, ed. Essential basic sciences for orthopedics. 1st ed. Oxford: Butterworth-Heinemann; 1994: 62-93)*

**Figure 1–3** The effect of the capital drop osteophyte for increasing the weight-bearing area of the hip joint and decreasing the joint reaction force after a valgus intertrochanteric osteotomy. *(Adapted from Pring D. Biomechanics of the hip. In: Barrett D, ed. Essential basic sciences for orthopedics. 1st ed. Oxford: Butterworth-Heinemann; 1994: 62-93)*

case of a valgus osteotomy, one should exploit the inferomedial capital drop osteophyte (Figure 1-3) and put the lateral capsule to enough stretch to stimulate the formation of the roof osteophyte, both for the purpose of increasing the weight-bearing area of the joint.

The skeletal fixation of femoral osteotomies was first described by Schanz in 1924, who devised a simple external fixation system composed of one screw on either fragment. Because of the obvious biomechanical instability of his device, Schanz's patients still relied on a plaster-of-Paris spica cast. Blount of Milwaukee popularized the use of internal fixation in 1943 with the use of the "V" blade plate. Interestingly, McMurray used two casts for fixation, whereas Pauwels used a short intramedullary nail until the application of the cast. In 1955, Müller introduced fixed-angle blade plates; the 95- and 110-degree versions are still the ones that are most commonly used for the fixation of varus and valgus ITOs, respectively, although a dynamic hip screw is now also used. The advantage of today's blade plates is inherent in their design, which allows for the appropriate translation of the distal fragment. Pauwels, Müller, and Bombelli are the surgeons who set forth the principles of femoral osteotomy.

Recent refinements of the varus osteotomy have focused on the amelioration of abductor weakness, which is the major drawback of this procedure. Müller (1984) recommended a simultaneous distal transfer of the greater trochanter, and Nishio (1984) described a dome osteotomy of the femoral neck, which leads to distalization and lateralization of the greater trochanter. The Morscher osteotomy (1999) combines the distal transfer of the greater trochanter and the lengthening of the femoral neck without reorienting the femoral head.

Salvage femoral osteotomies include hip joint resection, Colonna's trochanteric reconstruction (1960), and pelvic support osteotomies. These osteotomies were originally described by Lorenz and Schanz, and they were popularized by Milch and Bachelor. However, they fell into disfavor because of the significant shortening and valgus malalignment that they produced. Ilizarov (1992) modified the procedure by adding extension in the sagittal plane and a second more distal femoral osteotomy for lengthening and realignment. The best indication for this operation today is the sequela of neonatal hip sepsis in the older child or adolescent.

With the development of so many different types of osteotomies, it is easy to forget the principle stated in 1964 by Blount in his article published in the *Journal of Bone and Joint Surgery:* "... all of them are in fact variations of one procedure which must be modified according to the clinical and roentgenographic findings." Depending on the underlying pathology, a number of combined corrections in the frontal and sagittal planes may be implemented and may even be coupled with derotation.

Thus, it is imperative that the surgeon be familiar with the basic tenets of deformity correction. When the osteotomy is at a level that is different from the center of rotation or angulation, the secondary translation of the fragments at the level of the osteotomy will occur (this is the second osteotomy rule, according to Paley and colleagues). When one considers the proximal femur, this corresponds with the medial or lateral displacement of the shaft in the case of a varus or valgus osteotomy, respectively (i.e., displacement–angulation osteotomy). This ensures the optimal alignment of the entire lower extremity, provided that no other deformity is present. Despite the clinical and geometric documentation of the beneficial effect of femoral translation, some surgeons do not advocate this principle, because there are concerns about the technical feasibility of a future total hip replacement.

### Acetabular Osteotomy

Much like femoral osteotomies, acetabular osteotomies are divided into reconstructive (e.g., redirectional, reshaping) procedures and salvage procedures. These operations are intended for patients whose main pathology is on the acetabular side; congruously dysplastic hips comprise the prototype indication for these osteotomies. Unlike osteoarthritis, for which improved congruence is the goal, dysplastic hips require improved coverage to reduce contact pressure within the joint. Numerous reconstructive pelvic osteotomies were devised during the twentieth century, with each trying to address the problems of the previously described procedures (Table 1-2).

Salter introduced his single innominate osteotomy in 1961. Among other drawbacks, this osteotomy pivots on the symphysis pubis, thus severely limiting the degree of correction that can be obtained in adult patients. The Pemberton acetabuloplasty (1965) hinges at the triradiate cartilage, thereby allowing for a change in both the volume and orientation of the acetabulum. The Dega osteotomy (1965) resembles the Pemberton procedure but leaves a posterior portion of the iliac cortex intact, thereby forming the hinge. The double pelvic osteotomy was introduced by Sutherland and Greenfield in 1977, who added to Salter's technique a cut of the pubis medial to the obturator foramen; this bone cut is the pivot point of this osteotomy. The use of single and double pelvic osteotomies in adult patients has now been abandoned.

Triple pelvic osteotomies were described in an effort to overcome the drawbacks of single and double osteotomies, especially the lateralization of the hip. The operations described by LeCoeur (1965), Hopf (1966), and Steel (1973) are all slight variations on this theme, with the ischial bone cuts made close to the symphysis pubis. Steel popularized the triple osteotomy in the United States. The problem that these procedures share is the significant deformity that is created after large corrections; Tönnis (1977) and Carlioz (1982) addressed this problem by describing juxta-articular triple pelvic osteotomies. Although these procedures avoid the strong sacropelvic ligaments, thereby enhancing the mobility of the acetabular fragment, they may create a considerable gap between the ischium and the acetabular fragment that will necessitate special measures for stabilization.

### Table 1-2 THE EVOLUTION OF PELVIC OSTEOTOMIES

| Type | Surgeon | Year | Principal Drawbacks |
|---|---|---|---|
| **Reconstructive** | | | |
| Single | Salter | 1961 | Lateralization of joint; not for skeletally mature patients |
| | Pemberton | 1965 | |
| | Dega | 1965 | |
| Double | Sutherland and Greenfield | 1977 | Lateralization of joint; not for skeletally mature patients |
| Triple | LeCoeur | 1965 | External rotation deformity after large corrections caused by attached sacrospinal ligaments |
| | Hopf | 1966 | |
| | Steel | 1973 | |
| Triple juxta-articular | Tönnis | 1977 | Violation of posterior column; large gap between ischium and acetabular fragment |
| | Carlioz | 1982 | |
| Periacetabular spherical (rotational) | Wagner | 1965 | Limited anterior coverage and medialization; blood supply jeopardized; technically difficult |
| | Eppright | 1975 | |
| | Ninomiya and Tagawa | 1984 | |
| Bernese periacetabular | Ganz | 1983 | Reorientation of acetabular fragment difficult |
| **Salvage** | | | |
| Shelf | Albee | 1915 | No medialization; unchanged relationship between head and acetabulum |
| Medial displacement | Chiari | 1953 | Articulation with fibrocartilage |

Periacetabular spherical osteotomies include those described by Wagner (1965), Eppright (1975), and Ninomiya and Tagawa (1984). These operations are technically demanding, and, because they are partly intra-articular, they jeopardize the vascular supply to the acetabular fragment. A concomitant arthrotomy for intra-articular pathology is therefore not recommended when these procedures are undertaken.

The Bernese periacetabular osteotomy, which was developed in 1983 by Swiss and American surgeons and described in 1988 by Ganz and colleagues, addresses many of the problems described previously, and it is currently the acetabular osteotomy of choice in most centers worldwide. Purported advantages include (but are not limited to) the retention of vascularity, the integrity of the posterior column, the reproducibility of technique, and the need for minimal internal fixation. The most serious complication is considered by Ganz himself to be the intra-articular extension of the osteotomy, with a reported rate of 2.7%. The main difficulty of this procedure is to determine intraoperatively the desired degree of reorientation of the acetabular fragment. To this end, computer navigation may be a valuable aid in the future.

Salvage acetabular osteotomies are indicated for patients with acetabular pathology and incongruous joints, with no more than moderate degenerative changes. Shelf operations, which are designed to increase coverage by laterally extending the roof of the acetabulum, were first described by König (1891) and performed by Albee (1915) in patients with dislocated hips. They were subsequently popularized by Gill (1926) from the University of Pennsylvania. Their sole indication today may be for the adult patient in need of a salvage osteotomy whose hip is not deformed enough for a Chiari procedure.

The medial displacement iliac osteotomy was developed by Karl Chiari from Vienna in 1953, but it was only reported in the English-speaking literature in 1974. This procedure is essentially a capsular arthroplasty. Abduction is increased, and, although head coverage by the true acetabulum is decreased, total coverage is augmented by part of the femoral head articulating with newly formed fibrocartilage.

### Hip Arthroscopy

Michael S. Burman (1931) is credited with the first recorded attempts of hip arthroscopy on cadavers. His technique encompassed the distention of the joint with fluid and the use of a 4-mm arthroscope. He described an anterior paratrochanteric portal that was not dissimilar to today's anterolateral portal. Because of the lack of distraction, he was unable to visualize the acetabular fossa and the ligamentum teres.

Takagi (1939) first reported about the clinical application of hip arthroscopy in four patients: two patients with Charcot joints, one tuberculous patient, and one patient with septic arthritis. It took more than 30 years from the time of Takagi's report for another report to emerge. In 1976, Aigman described an attempt at diagnostic arthroscopy and biopsy. Richard Gross was the first to report about hip arthroscopy in the North American literature in 1977. Subsequently, it was James Glick and his partner, Thomas Sampson, who pioneered hip arthroscopy in North America and who modified the surgical technique by positioning the patient in the lateral decubitus position rather than the supine position. Further key technical refinements took place during the mid-1980s and are attributed to Ejnar Eriksson and colleagues, who estimated the distraction forces needed, and to Lanny Johnson, who described anatomic landmarks and techniques of needle placement. Although the conventional technique involves the use of distraction, Dorfmann and Boyer (1988), who were both rheumatologists in Paris, developed a technique without distraction for entry into the peripheral compartment. In Great Britain, hip arthroscopy was first attempted by the senior author (RNV) in 1988, and its use has been increasing ever since. Technical suggestions for the optimal use of supine patient positioning were made by J.W. Thomas Byrd during the 1990s, and Marc Phillipon recently modified supine positioning by placing the extremity in 15 degrees of internal rotation, 10 degrees of flexion, neutral abduction, and 10 degrees of lateral tilt.

A common indication for hip arthroscopy has been the presence of loose bodies causing mechanical symptoms. In the absence of associated major structural abnormalities, hip arthroscopy is the preferred treatment for intra-articular disorders, with labral lesions being the most common. Other indications include extra-articular disorders that affect the iliopsoas tendon and bursa and the tensor fasciae latae and its adjacent trochanteric bursa (Figure 1-4). An endoscopically assisted technique for triple innominate osteotomy has also been described by Wall and colleagues. Clearly, the technique and applications of hip arthroscopy are still evolving.

## EVOLUTION OF HIP SURGERY IN RELATION TO SPECIFIC CONDITIONS

### Hip Dysplasia

Traditionally, arthritic changes in dysplastic hips were thought to be initiated in the cartilage as a result of the axial overload of a maloriented acetabulum. The classic description of the acetabular rim syndrome by Klaue and colleagues (1991) indicated that a partial

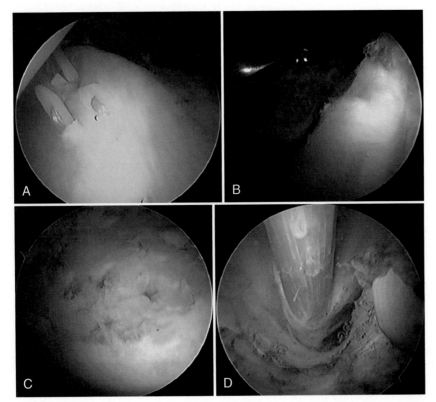

**Figure 1–4** Some of the modern uses of hip arthroscopy. **A,** Labral repair. **B,** Osteoplasty of femoral head–neck junction. **C,** Microfractures. **D,** Release of iliopsoas tendon.

detachment of the labrum or a fatigue fracture of the acetabular rim (i.e., os acetabuli) may be the first insult to the joint.

Femoral osteotomies were historically the first surgical treatment for hip dysplasia. Varus osteotomy and the transfer of the greater trochanter were established for varus deformities, whereas valgus-extension ITO was popularized for the treatment of impingement.

Acetabular osteotomies are now the procedure of choice for congruously dysplastic hips. Today, a femoral osteotomy is rarely indicated in isolation, but it may be needed in conjunction with a pelvic osteotomy in about 10% of patients. A reorientation pelvic osteotomy improves both femoral head coverage and joint congruency. The Bernese periacetabular osteotomy allows for a concomitant arthrotomy to treat intra-articular pathology. Alternatively, intra-articular pathology may be addressed arthroscopically in the same sitting. In mild cases (i.e., center-edge angle >16 degrees, acetabular inclination <15 degrees) and in the presence of mechanical symptoms, hip arthroscopy alone may be a viable option for the treatment of labral pathology.

## Femoroacetabular Impingement

The concept of the proximal femur abutting the acetabular rim was described as early as 1936 by Smith-Petersen, who theorized that the impingement "will give rise to congestion of the synovia, synovitis, and, because of periosteal irritation, hypertrophic changes." He described his technique of excision of the acetabular rim (i.e., "acetabuloplasty") and presented its application in 11 cases.

The principle of "primary" osteoarthritis is now considered obsolete. In the nondysplastic hip, current thinking holds that mild developmental abnormalities (e.g., "silent slip epiphysis," abnormal epiphyseal extension) during childhood cause aberrant morphologic alterations of the proximal femur or the acetabulum during adult life, thereby resulting in cam, pincer, or, most commonly, mixed femoroacetabular impingement. These conditions are, in turn, established as precursors to osteoarthritis.

Current treatment options include safe surgical dislocation, osteoplasty of the femoral head–neck junction, recession of the acetabular rim, and reverse periacetabular osteotomy. Femoral osteoplasty and acetabular recession may also be performed arthroscopically. Some surgeons prefer a combined treatment during which they address soft-tissue intra-articular pathology arthroscopically and excise the bony abnormalities through a limited anterior approach. In general, however, the optimal treatment for pincer impingement is still debated.

## Perthes Disease

Containment is the primary goal of both conservative and surgical treatment for Perthes disease. Surgical containment has traditionally been obtained with femoral varus derotation osteotomies, acetabular reorientation, or augmentation procedures. For patients with established disease with hinge abduction, a valgus-extension femoral osteotomy will lengthen the extremity, restore the abductor lever arm, and relieve the flexion contracture that is present.

For late-onset disease, mechanical articulated distraction has emerged as a new alternative. Arthrodiastasis minimizes loads across the joint while maintaining movement. Reported results have been promising and have expanded the use of articulated hip distraction to other conditions (e.g., osteonecrosis, idiopathic chondrolysis).

Pain in the young adult with a history of Perthes disease and a congruent hip joint is likely related to impingement, thus requiring a femoral head–neck junction osteoplasty or acetabular rim trimming. Among patients with severe Perthes disease,

if there is an intact posteromedial portion of the femoral head, a flexion-valgus femoral osteotomy will position this in the weight-bearing region of the joint.

## Osteonecrosis of the Femoral Head

Osteotomies for osteonecrosis must protect the femoral head from shear forces and, in cases of subluxation, realign the head in the acetabulum. A valgus-flexion ITO will serve those purposes for a patient with a typical anterolateral lesion, with or without collapse. The flexion component will bring the healthy posterior portion of the head into the weight-bearing area. For the rare patient with a necrotic lesion in the medial aspect of the femoral head, a varus ITO is indicated. The combined necrotic angle of Kerboul and colleagues has been shown to be a critical factor for outcome. Ideally, this angle should be less than 200 degrees before an osteotomy is performed.

In 1972, Sugioka devised a rotational transtrochanteric osteotomy that is essentially a rotational flap of the proximal femur based on the vascular pedicle of the medial circumflex vessels. Subsequently, Wagner and Zeiler reported their results in 1980. Sugioka's good results (79% good or excellent at 11 years) have not been reproduced by other surgeons, and the high potential for nonunion has been recognized.

Core decompression, which was developed by Ficat and Arlet during the early 1960s for diagnostic purposes, remains the most commonly performed operation for early-stage disease. Several modifications of the original technique are now used, and it is also performed along with other procedures, such as electrical stimulation and the placement of vascularized or nonvascularized grafts. The approach of safe surgical dislocation of the hip has also allowed for grafting the femoral head through a trapdoor, as described by Meyers in 1983, rather than through the femoral neck (i.e., the "lightbulb" procedure described by Rosenwasser and colleagues in 1994) or the lateral cortex. Additional joint-preserving treatment methods for advanced stages include the sequestrectomy followed by the cementation of the head, as described by Hernigou (1993), and the augmentation of other procedures with pluripotential stem cells. Hip arthroscopy also has a place in the staging of lesions and the relief of mechanical symptoms. Cortical strut grafting (i.e., the Bonfiglio procedure), which was described by Phemister (1949) and popularized by Bonfiglio and colleagues (1958), is rarely if ever performed today.

## Slipped Capital Femoral Epiphysis

Sturrock reported the first case of internal fixation for slipped capital femoral epiphysis (SCFE) in 1894. His case was complicated by an acute infection that required the removal of the nail 2 days after surgery. Open reduction and bone graft epiphysiodesis was developed by Dunn in 1964, but it was only used by a few; the currently widely accepted percutaneous fixation for stable SCFE was popularized by Morrissy in the 1980s and reported by him in 1990.

The deformity of SCFE is one of extension and external rotation with an element of apparent varus. Before the era of safe surgical dislocation, the triplane (flexion/internal rotation/varus) intertrochanteric osteotomy, which was introduced by Imhäuser (1965), was the procedure of choice to correct impingement and possibly to avoid osteoarthritis.

In 1997, Ganz refined Dunn's technique for open reduction. With the use of the surgical dislocation, an intracapsular correction through the physis is now possible, both acutely and at a later stage. With this technique, Leunig and colleagues reported about 30 patients who had their slips reduced and fixed with screws. In three of these patients, the screws sustained mechanical failure; in one patient, heterotopic ossification developed. There were no cases of osteonecrosis postoperatively.

## Acetabular Retroversion

Acetabular retroversion was unknown until Reynolds and colleagues described it in 1999; those authors also described the crossover sign as a means for diagnosing the condition. Acetabular retroversion is seen in isolation, but it is also seen in about one in six cases of dysplasia (17%) and in patients with other conditions. Clinically, it should be suspected in patients with limited internal rotation of the hip. Since the original description of this condition, several authors have reported about its relation with osteoarthritis. The principal treatment option is an acetabular reorientation procedure, but trimming of the rim—either open or arthroscopic—may be implemented when a positive crossover sign is associated with sufficient posterior coverage of the femoral head, as indicated by a negative posterior wall sign.

## SUMMARY: FUTURE DIRECTIONS

Hip-joint–preserving surgery is mechanically based. Recent advances in hip surgery have dramatically enlightened the current understanding of the pathoanatomy and pathomechanics of hip disorders and improved their treatment, thereby effectively postponing or obviating the need for total hip replacement in young adults. The limited reparative response of the associated cartilage is now the main obstacle to further improving outcomes.

Possible future directions include the use of patient-specific computational modeling and finite element analysis for preoperative planning and postoperative assessment; the more widespread use of hip arthroscopy; and the use of computer navigation for osteotomies, especially on the pelvic side. A novel magnetic resonance imaging technique that makes use of a negatively charged gadolinium contrast detects early osteoarthritis by recognizing the reduction of proteoglycans in affected cartilage. Biologic agents are being investigated for use in patients with osteonecrosis, and recombinant factors offer promise for bone and cartilage regeneration.

## ANNOTATED REFERENCES AND SUGGESTED READINGS

Blount WP. Blade-plate internal fixation for high femoral osteotomies. *J Bone Joint Surg.* 1943;25:319–339.

Bombelli R, Santore RF, Poss R. Mechanics of the normal and osteoarthritic hip: a new perspective. *Clin Orthop.* 1984;182:69–78.

Brand RA. Hip osteotomies: a biomechanical consideration. *J Am Acad Orthop Surg.* 1997;5:282–291.

The rationale of osteotomies from a biomechanical standpoint is presented. The author discusses the limitations of osteotomies and emphasizes the fact that three-dimensional congruence cannot be achieved in all human activities; this might explain the variable results of these procedures.

Byrd JWT, ed. *Operative hip arthroscopy.* 2nd ed. New York: Springer-Verlag; 2005.

Ezoe M, Naito M, Inoue T. The prevalence of acetabular retroversion among various disorders of the hip. *J Bone Joint Surg Am.* 2006;88:372–379.

The authors retrospectively reviewed anteroposterior pelvic radiographs of 250 patients (342 hips). The prevalence of acetabular retroversion was 6% (7 of 112) in the normal group, 20% (14 of 70) in the osteoarthritis group, 18% (13 of 74) in the developmental dysplasia group, 6% (2 of 36) in the group with osteonecrosis of the femoral head, and 42% (21 of 50) in the Perthes disease group. The authors conclude that acetabular retroversion occurs more commonly in association with various hip diseases in which the prevalence of arthritis is increased (Level of Evidence: Diagnostic III).

Ganz R, Gill TJ, Gautier E, et al. Surgical dislocation of the adult hip: a technique with full access to the femoral head and acetabulum without the risk of avascular necrosis. *J Bone Joint Surg Br.* 2001;83:1119–1124.

Ganz R, Klaue K, Vinh TS, et al. A new periacetabular osteotomy for the treatment of hip dysplasias: technique and preliminary results. *Clin Orthop.* 1988;232:26–36.

Harris WH. Etiology of osteoarthritis of the hip. *Clin Orthop.* 1986;213:20–33.

When summarizing his and other investigators' experience with hip osteoarthritis, the author theorizes that subtle developmental structural abnormalities lead to the formation of the so-called pistol-grip deformity and account for what was previously called *primary osteoarthritis.* He also suggests the existence of a new developmental disease that is characterized by the presence of an intra-acetabular or inverted labrum (Level of Evidence: Prognostic V).

Jones R. The Classic: British Orthopaedic Association Symposium on the treatment of osteoarthritis of the hip 1920. *Clin Orthop.* 2005;441:4–6.

A reproduction of the speech delivered in 1920 by Sir Robert Jones, President of the British Orthopaedic Association, this is a succinct description of the options that orthopedic surgeons had for the treatment of osteoarthritis of the hip during the years after World War I. Treatment methods such as manipulation, cheilectomy, and arthrodesis are discussed.

Klaue K, Durnin CW, Ganz R. The acetabular rim syndrome: a clinical presentation of dysplasia of the hip. *J Bone Joint Surg Br.* 1991;73:423–429.

Millis MB, Kim Y-J. Rationale of osteotomy and related procedures for hip preservation: a review. *Clin Orthop.* 2002;405:108–121.

This is a solid review article about the mechanical theory of hip osteoarthrosis and its significance for selecting the appropriate joint-preserving technique; an excellent bibliography is provided.

Parvizi J, Campfield A, Clohisy JC, et al. Management of arthritis of the hip in the young adult. *J Bone Joint Surg Br.* 2006;88:1279–1285.

This is a concise review of the surgical options available today for the young adult with osteoarthritis of the hip. Procedures that involve joint-preserving surgery and prosthetic replacement are discussed.

Peltier LF. A history of hip surgery. In: Callaghan JJ, Rosenberg AG, Rubash HE, eds. *The adult hip.* 1st ed. Philadelphia: Lippincott-Raven Publishers; 1998:3–36.

This is a dedicated chapter about the history of hip surgery, and it is accompanied by a thorough bibliography. Additional historic information may be found in the chapters for each specific procedure of this reference textbook.

Smith-Petersen MN. Treatment of malum coxae senilis, old slipped upper femoral epiphysis, intrapelvic protrusion of the acetabulum, and coxa plana by means of acetabuloplasty. *J Bone Joint Surg.* 1936;18:869–880.

Trousdale RT. Acetabular osteotomy: indications and results. *Clin Orthop.* 2004;429:182–187.

The author presents a historical background and a very nice outline of the current indications of acetabular osteotomy. Suboptimal results are to be expected among patients with significant degenerative changes after Bernese periacetabular osteotomy. The diagnosis and management of acetabular retroversion are also discussed (Level of Evidence: Therapeutic V).

# CHAPTER 2

# Arthroscopic and Open Anatomy of the Hip

*Michael B. Gerhardt, Kartik Logishetty, Morteza Meftah, and Anil S. Ranawat*

## INTRODUCTION

The hip joint is defined by the articulation between the head of the femur and the acetabulum of the pelvis. It is covered by a large soft-tissue envelope and a complex array of neurovascular and musculotendinous structures. The joint's morphology and orientation are complex, and there are wide anatomic variations seen among individuals. The joint's deep location makes both arthroscopic and open access challenging. To avoid iatrogenic injury while establishing functional and efficient access, the hip surgeon should possess a sound anatomic knowledge of the hip.

The human "hip" can be subdivided into three categories: 1) the superficial surface anatomy; 2) the deep femoroacetabular joint and capsule; and 3) the associated structures, including the muscles, nerves, and vasculature, all of which directly affect its function.

Several bony landmarks define the surface anatomy of the hip. The anterosuperior iliac spine (ASIS) and anteroinferior iliac spine (AIIS) are located anteriorly, with the former being palpable. These structures serve as the insertion points for the sartorius and the direct head of the rectus femoris, respectively. Posterolaterally, two bony landmarks are palpable: the greater trochanter and the posterosuperior iliac spine. The greater trochanter serves as the insertion point of the tendon of the gluteus medius, the gluteus minimus, the obturator externus, the obturator internus, the gemelli, and piriformis. The posterosuperior iliac spine serves as the attachment point of the oblique portion of the posterior sacroiliac ligaments and the multifidus. During arthroscopic and open access to the joint, both of these landmarks are useful tools for incision planning, and, in combination with the anterior bony prominences, for initial orientation (Figure 2-1, *A*).

The hip is a synovial, diarthrodial, ball-and-socket joint that is comprised of the bony articulation between the proximal femur and the acetabulum. The acetabulum is formed at the cartilaginous confluence of the three bones of the pelvis: the ilium, the ischium, and the pubis. When aligned with the anterior pelvis plane, the acetabulum is inclined at approximately 55 degrees and anteverted at approximately 20 degrees, although there are gender variations. The acetabular cup is roughly hemispheric in shape. It covers 70% of the femoral head, and it has a wave-like profile of three peaks and three troughs, including the acetabular notch. The proximal femur consists of a femoral head, which articulates with the acetabulum, and a tapered neck, which is angled onto the femoral shaft. A normal femur has a neck–shaft angle of approximately 130 degrees.

There are a total of 27 muscles that cross the hip joint. They can be categorized into six groups according to the functional movements that they induce at the joint: 1) flexors; 2) extensors; 3) abductors; 4) adductors; 5) external rotators; and 6) internal rotators. Although some muscles have dual roles, their primary functions define their group placement, and they all have unique neurovascular supplies (Table 2-1).

The vascular supply of the hip stems from the external and internal iliac arteries. An understanding of the course of these vessels is critical for avoiding catastrophic vascular injury. In addition, the blood supply to the femoral head is vulnerable to both traumatic and iatrogenic injury; the disruption of this supply can result in avascular necrosis (Figure 2-2).

## HIP MUSCULATURE

### Hip Flexors

The primary hip flexors are the rectus femoris, iliacus, psoas, iliocapsularis, and sartorius muscles. The rectus femoris muscle has two distinct origins proximally: the direct head and the reflected head. They originate at the AIIS and the anterior acetabular rim (in close proximity to the anterior hip capsule), respectively. The tendinous fibers of the rectus femoris coalesce distally and become confluent with the other quadriceps musculature in the thigh. The quadriceps consists of four distinct muscles: 1) the vastus intermedius; 2) the vastus lateralis; 3) the vastus medialis; and 4) the rectus femoris. The rectus femoris is the only quadriceps muscle that traverses both the hip and the knee joint. The rectus femoris is a powerful hip flexor, but it is largely dependent on the position of the knee and hip to assert its influence. It is most powerful when the knee is flexed, whereas significant power is lost when the knee is extended. The rectus femoris is innervated by the femoral nerve (i.e., the posterior division of L2 to L4).

The iliopsoas is another powerful hip flexor that begins in two distinct regions proximally. The iliacus has a broad origin, arising from the inner table of the iliac wing, the sacral alae, and the iliolumbar and sacroiliac ligaments. The psoas originates at the lumbar transverse processes, the intervertebral discs, and the adjacent bodies from T12 to L5, in addition to the tendinous arches between these points. Distally, the two large muscular bodies converge to become one distinct structure—the iliopsoas—and subsequently jointly insert at the lesser trochanter of the proximal femur. The nerve to the iliopsoas (i.e., the anterior division of L1 to L3) supplies the iliopsoas muscle.

The sartorius originates at the ASIS and proceeds to traverse obliquely and laterally down the thigh to eventually insert at the anterior surface of the tibia, just inferomedial to the tibial

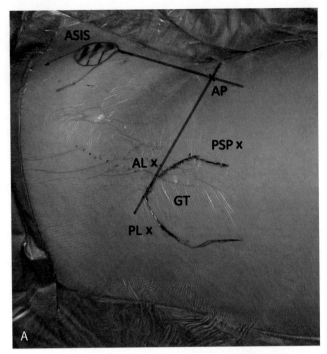

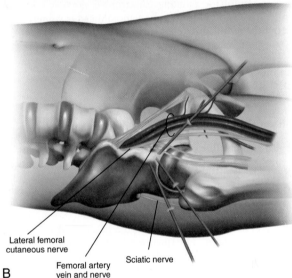

**Figure 2–1** Surface anatomy of the anterior, anterolateral, and posterolateral portals. **A,** Preoperative planning. The superficial location of the anterior portal *(AP)* lies at the intersection of a vertical line drawn from the anterosuperior iliac spine *(ASIS)* and a horizontal line drawn from the superior aspect of the greater trochanter *(GT)*. The anterolateral portal *(AL)* and the posterolateral portal *(PL)* are made anterior and posterior to the superolateral aspect of the greater trochanter. Peritrochanteric Space Portal *(PSP)*. **B,** Neurovascular structures that are in close proximity to the three arthroscopic hip portals.

tuberosity, as part of the pes anserinus. In addition to flexing the hip and knee, the sartorius aids in the abduction of the hip. It is innervated by the femoral nerve (i.e., the posterior division of L2 and L3).

Other muscles that can be recruited to assist with hip flexion include the tensor fascia latae (TFL), the pectineus, the adductors, the gracilis, and the anterior aspects of the gluteus medius and the gluteus minimus. The contribution of these secondary hip flexors largely depends on the position of the hip at the time at which movement is initiated.

## Hip Extensors

The major contributors to hip extension are the gluteus maximus, the ischiocondylar part of the adductor magnus, the semimembranosus, the semitendinosus, and the biceps femoris (i.e., the long and the short heads). The most powerful muscle of this group is the gluteus maximus, which is responsible for more than 75% of the total power output of the extensor group. The gluteus maximus originates at the posteromedial outer rim of the iliac wing (i.e., behind the posterior gluteal line), the sacrococcygeal junction, the sacrotuberous ligaments, and the aponeurosis of the gluteus medius origin. Distally, the majority of the muscle inserts at the posterior aspect of the iliotibial tract of fascia lata, whereas the remainder inserts at the gluteal tuberosity of the proximal femur. In addition to extending the flexed femur, the gluteus maximus assists with lateral rotation and abduction of the thigh, and it stabilizes both the hip and knee joints through its influence on the iliotibial tract. It is innervated by the inferior gluteal nerve (i.e., the posterior divisions of L5 to S2).

The hamstring muscles also collaboratively assist with the extension of the hip. The long head of the biceps femoris, the semitendinosus, and the semimembranosus originate at the ischial tuberosity and insert below the knee. The combined hip extensor strength of these three hamstring muscles is still significantly lower than that of the gluteus maximus. However, in maximal hip flexion, the gluteus maximus loses its mechanical advantage, and the hamstrings become the dominant hip extensors. Because the hamstrings cross the knee joint, they are also able to flex and rotate the leg at the knee. They are innervated by the sciatic nerve (i.e., the posterior divisions of L5 to S2).

## Adductors

The adductors of the hip are the adductor brevis, the adductor longus, the anterior part of the adductor magnus, the pectineus, and the gracilis. The adductors originate at the inferior pubic ramus and the ischial tuberosity, whereas distally their attachments are along the linea aspera of the femur. The adductors are innervated by the obturator nerve (i.e., the anterior division of L2 to L4). The adductor longus is the most commonly damaged muscle of this group. Unlike most tendinous attachments to bone, the adductor longus attachment at the external surface of the pubic ramus is comprised of 62% muscle and only 38% tendon. It is postulated that this abnormal muscle-to-tendon ratio at the bony attachment creates a vulnerability to injury. However, given its medial location, the adductor musculature is rarely at risk during standard open or arthroscopic approaches to the hip, except in the pediatric population.

## Abductors

The abductors consist of the gluteus medius and gluteus minimus muscles. Both of these muscles are innervated by the superior gluteal nerve (i.e., the posterior division of L5 to S2). The TFL and the iliotibial band also contribute to hip abduction. This action is only apparent with the hip in a flexed position, and the TFL and the iliotibial band are therefore considered secondary abductors. The gluteus medius, which is the primary hip abductor, originates at the posterior external table of the iliac wing. It is completely covered by the overlying gluteus maximus as it travels distally toward its insertion at the lateral and superoposterior facet of the greater trochanter (Figure 2-3, *A*). The gluteus minimus fibers run in close approximation to the

**Table 2–1** MUSCULATURE OF THE PELVIS AND THE LOWER LIMB: FUNCTION AND INNERVATION

| Action | Muscle | Origin | Insertion | Nerve | Segment |
|---|---|---|---|---|---|
| Flexors | Iliacus | Iliac fossa | Lesser trochanter | Femoral | L2 to L4 (P) |
| | Psoas | Transverse processes of L1 to L5 | Lesser trochanter | Femoral | L2 to L4 (P) |
| | Pectineus | Pectineal line of pubis | Pectineal line of femur | Femoral | L2 to L4 (P) |
| | Rectus femoris | Anteroinferior iliac spine and acetabular rim | Patella and tibial tubercle | Femoral | L2 to L4 (P) |
| Adductors | Adductor magnus | Inferior pubic ramus and ischial tuberosity | Linea aspera and adductor tubercle | Obturator (P) and sciatic (Tib) | L2 to L4 (A) |
| | Adductor brevis | Inferior pubic ramus | Linea aspera and pectineal line | Obturator (P) | L2 to L4 (A) |
| | Adductor longus | Anterior pubic ramus | Linea aspera | Obturator (A) | L2 to L4 (A) |
| | Gracilis | Inferior pubic symphysis | Proximal medial tibia | Obturator (A) | L2 to L4 (A) |
| External rotators | Gluteus maximus | Ilium to postgluteal line | Iliotibial band | Inferior gluteal | L5 to S2 (P) |
| | Piriformis | Anterior sacrum and sciatic notch | Proximal greater trochanter | Piriformis | S1 to S2 (P) |
| | Obturator externus | Ischiopubic rami and obturator membrane | Trochlear fossa | Obturator (P) | L2 to L4 (A) |
| | Obturator internus | Ischiopubic rami and obturator membrane | Medial greater trochanter | Obturator internus | L5 to S2 (A) |
| | Superior gemellus | Outer ischial spine | Medial greater trochanter | Obturator internus | L5 to S2 (A) |
| | Inferior gemellus | Ischial tuberosity | Medial greater trochanter | Obturator femoris | L4 to S1 (A) |
| | Quadratus femoris | Ischial tuberosity | Quadrate line of femur | Obturator femoris | L4 to S1 (A) |
| Abductors | Gluteus medius | Ilium between posterior and anterior gluteal lines | Greater trochanter | Superior gluteal | L4 to S1 (P) |
| | Gluteus minimus | Ilium between anterior and inferior gluteal lines | Anterior border of greater trochanter | Superior gluteal | L4 to S1 (P) |
| | Tensor fascia latae | Anterior iliac crest | Iliotibial band | Superior gluteal | L4 to S1 (P) |

A, Anterior; P, Posterior; Tib, Tibial.

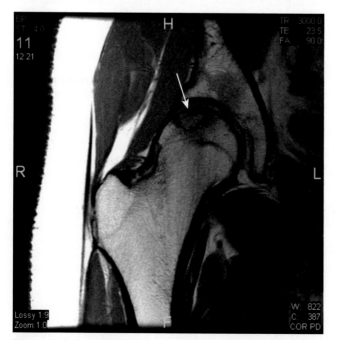

**Figure 2–2** Coronal T1-weighted magnetic resonance image of avascular necrosis of the anterolateral aspect of the femoral head (*arrow*).

lateral hip capsule, onto which some of the muscle may also insert. These fibers are often the first to be encountered during hip arthroscopy procedures when establishing the anterolateral portal. The gluteus minimus, which is responsible for 25% of abduction power, runs in the same plane deep to the gluteus medius. It inserts more anteriorly on the greater trochanter, and it has a separate long head component. Recent evidence suggests that a common cause of lateral hip pain may be tears of the hip abductor insertion and not simply trochanteric bursitis. These tears are referred to as *rotator cuff tears of the hip.* Anatomic restoration of the insertion of the torn gluteus medius can be achieved with standard arthroscopic technique in the recently described peritrochanteric compartment. When trochanteric bursitis does exist in isolation, it is most likely located at the posterior facet or the bald spot of the trochanter (see Figure 2-3, *B*).

Functionally, the gluteus medius and gluteus minimus are critical to the gait cycle, and they assert the major stabilizing force during the end of the terminal swing phase. This force provides tension among the pelvis, the iliotibial band, and the greater trochanter; it peaks during the initial part of the stance phase, and it persists through the middle of the stance. Injury to the gluteus medius or indeed to the superior gluteal nerve can be clinically recognized by the presence of a Trendelenburg sign, which is classically described as the dropping of the pelvis on the opposite side of the pathology.

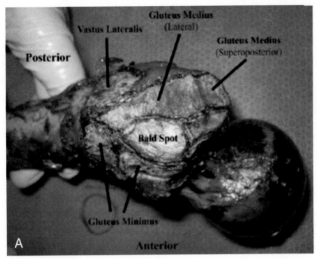
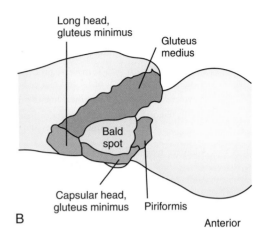

**Figure 2–3 A,** Superolateral view of a cadaveric right proximal femur that shows the attachment footprints of muscles on the greater trochanter. **B,** Computer-generated model of the proximal femur that shows muscular insertional sites on the greater trochanter.

## External and Internal Rotators

The external rotators include the obturator internus, the obturator externus, the superior and inferior gemelli, the quadratus femoris, and the piriformis muscles (see Figure 2-3). These small but powerful musculotendinous units act synergistically to provide the external moments that are necessary to generate lateral and rotational activities. The piriformis is the common denominator of the external rotators, and it serves as an important anatomic landmark during both the posterior approach and the surgical dislocation of the hip.

The internal rotation of the hip occurs primarily through the combined efforts of the TFL, the anterior gluteus medius, and the gluteus minimus. There are no primary internal hip rotators, and, consequently, the internal rotational moments of the hip are the weakest of all functional movements. Other secondary hip internal rotators include the hamstring muscles and the pectineus.

## NEUROVASCULAR SUPPLY OF THE HIP

### Vasculature of the Hip

The common iliac arteries provide the primary blood supply to the lower limbs. Each artery divides into the external and internal iliac arteries. These vessels run parallel with their venous counterparts, the internal and external iliac veins, which join to form the inferior vena cava. The external iliac artery, which travels obliquely over the psoas muscle, is particularly vulnerable to injury. Damage can occur during hip arthroplasty when accessing the acetabulum, during the placement of screws in the anterior quadrant, or, more commonly, from the aberrant placement of anterior acetabular retractors. Excessive medial reaming can also put the external iliac vessels at risk, especially during revision acetabular surgery. If iatrogenic injury does occur, the external iliac artery and vein can be accessed most easily through the ilioinguinal approach.

The obturator vessels arise from the internal iliac vessels. They pass over the quadrilateral surface of the pelvis to the upper part of the obturator foramen to emerge from the obturator canal. The obturator artery divides into anterior branch, which supplies the obturator externus and the adjacent bone, and the posterior branch, which supplies the soft tissue of the acetabular fossa. The obturator nerve mimics the course and divisions of the obturator vessels. It is responsible for the sensory cutaneous innervation of the medial thigh and the motor innervation of the adductor muscles. Overlying these neurovascular structures is a reflected portion of the parietal peritoneum and the obturator internus muscle. These structures are fairly consistent, and they are anchored firmly by the obturator membrane as they pass through the obturator foramen. Occasionally, an aberrant vessel may traverse the pelvic brim that connects the external iliac vessels and the obturator vessels. Although the obturator vessels are usually safe during arthroscopic approaches to the hip, errant passes of an inferomedially directed arthroscopic cannula can be potentially injurious. Similarly, there is little risk to the obturator vessels and nerve during open approaches for primary hip arthroplasty, but one still has to be cautious around the transverse acetabular ligament, because distal branches of the obturator vessels can be injured here. In addition, anteroinferior screw placement or excess traction on the proximal femur during an anterior approach to the hip can also be potentially harmful.

The common femoral artery is the first branch of the external iliac artery, and it traverses just anteromedial to the hip capsule as it travels distally. It is at high risk for damage during both arthroscopic and open anterior approaches to the hip. In fact, the traditional anterior arthroscopic portal is approximately 3.5 cm from the femoral neurovascular bundle (Table 2-2). During total hip arthroplasty (THA), femoral vessel injury and femoral nerve palsy have been described as arising from the incorrect placement of retractors, which can occur with all approaches to the hip. However, because the artery is a large, fairly superficial, and therefore readily palpable vascular structure, its exact location should be routinely identified and thus easily avoided.

The profundus femoris artery, which is also known as the *deep femoral artery*, is the first branch of the common femoral artery. It penetrates posteriorly between the pectineus, the adductor longus, and the adductor brevis, lying behind the femoral artery and vein on the medial side of the femur. The profundus femoris artery gives rise to the lateral circumflex femoral artery 90% of the time and the medial circumflex femoral artery only 30% of the time. Injuries to the profundus femoris and its branches have been described during arthroplasty approaches to the hip, but they are fairly unusual. When they do occur, it is usually as a result of anteriorly placed deep retractors or during cement extrusion in this region.

The superior gluteal vessels are branches of the internal iliac artery (i.e., the posterior branches). The vessels, along with the gluteal nerve, traverse the posterior column of the acetabulum as they exit through the sciatic notch. They emerge superior to the piriformis and then terminate in the gluteus medius and

**Table 2-2** PROXIMITY OF ARTHROSCOPIC PORTALS TO NEUROVASCULAR STRUCTURES

| Compartment | Portal | Anatomic Structure | Mean Distance |
|---|---|---|---|
| Central | Anterior | Lateral femoral cutaneous nerve | 15 mm |
| | | Femoral nerve at sartorius | 54 mm |
| | | Femoral nerve at rectus femoris | 45 mm |
| | | Femoral nerve at capsule | 35 mm |
| | | Ascending lateral femoral cutaneous artery | 31 mm |
| | | Terminal branch of ascending lateral femoral cutaneous artery | 15 mm |
| | Anterolateral | Superior gluteal nerve | 64 mm |
| | | Sciatic nerve | 40 mm |
| | Mid-anterior | Lateral femoral cutaneous nerve | 25 mm |
| | | Femoral nerve at sartorius | 64 mm |
| | | Femoral nerve at rectus femoris | 53 mm |
| | | Femoral nerve at capsule | 40 mm |
| | | Ascending lateral femoral cutaneous artery | 19 mm |
| | | Terminal branch of ascending lateral femoral cutaneous artery | 10 mm |
| | Posterolateral | Sciatic nerve | 22 mm |
| Peripheral | Anterolateral | Superior gluteal nerve | 69 mm |
| | | Sciatic nerve | 58 mm |
| | Mid-anterior | Lateral femoral cutaneous nerve | 30 mm |
| | | Femoral nerve at sartorius | 70 mm |
| | | Femoral nerve at rectus femoris | 57 mm |
| | | Femoral nerve at capsule | 39 mm |
| | | Ascending lateral femoral cutaneous artery | 21 mm |
| | | Terminal branch of ascending lateral femoral cutaneous artery | 15 mm |
| | | Sciatic nerve | 58 mm |
| | Posterolateral | Sciatic nerve | 34 mm |

Adapted from Robertson WJ, Kelly BT. The safe zone for hip arthroscopy: a cadaveric assessment of central, peripheral, and lateral compartment portal placement. *Arthroscopy.* 2008;24(9):1019-1026.

gluteus minimus muscles. The inferior gluteal and internal pudendal vessels are also branches of the internal iliac artery (i.e., the anterior branches). They exit inferior and medial to the piriformis. The inferior gluteal vessels pass through the lower part of the greater sciatic foramen. The internal pudendal vessels exit the greater sciatic notch and then reenter the pelvis via the lesser sciatic notch. Erroneous posterior screw placement can cause the disruption of these structures. Palpation of the sciatic notch and the posterior column can help to prevent the placement of proud screws and further decrease the risk of injury. However, arthroscopic approaches in the safe zones as described by Byrd and colleagues pose very little risk to these neurovascular structures.

Four sets of arteries are responsible for the arterial blood supply to the femoral head: 1) the medial circumflex artery; 2) the lateral circumflex artery; 3) the medullary artery from the shaft of the femur; and 4) the artery of the ligamentum teres. The last one provides minimal if any contribution to the vascular integrity to the femoral head, although the vessel remains patent in approximately 20% of the adult population. The exact contribution of the medullary artery to the femoral head is unknown, but it is believed that this also plays a relatively minor role in vascularization.

Therefore, the vessel that supplies the majority of the arterial supply to the head is the medial circumflex femoral artery, with varying contributions from the lateral circumflex femoral artery. These vessels branch off at the base of the femoral neck and then ascend toward the femoral head via the posterolateral and posteroinferior synovial retinacular folds (Figure 2-4, *A* and *B*). It is believed that disruption at this level (e.g., by a femoral neck fracture) poses the greatest risk for avascular necrosis. The lateral synovial folds, which contain the terminal branches of the medial circumflex femoral artery, can also be injured as a result of aggressive arthroscopic dissection (Figure 2-5) or open approaches. Therefore, they should be routinely identified and protected during peripheral compartment arthroscopy and during open joint-preserving hip surgery.

## Neural Supply of the Hip

The sciatic nerve is the largest nerve in the body, and it is the main branch of the sacral plexus. It contains nerve branches primarily from L4 to S3. It consists of two main peripheral nerves contained within a single sheath: the tibial nerve (anterior division) and the common fibular or peroneal nerve (posterior division). These branches enter the gluteal region just inferior to the piriformis via the greater sciatic foramen. The sciatic nerve then descends in the plane between the superficial and deep group of gluteal region muscles, crossing the posterior surfaces first of the obturator internus and associated gemellus muscles and then of the quadratus femoris muscle. It lies just deep to the gluteus maximus at the midpoint between the ischial tuberosity and the greater trochanter. At the lower margin of the quadratus femoris muscle, the sciatic nerve enters the posterior thigh. The hip surgeon should be aware that, in a small subset of the population (i.e., 10% to 12%), the sciatic nerve can bifurcate proximal to the piriformis and pass through the piriformis.

The sciatic nerve is one of the most commonly injured structures during THA. The incidence ranges from 0.4% to 2.0%.

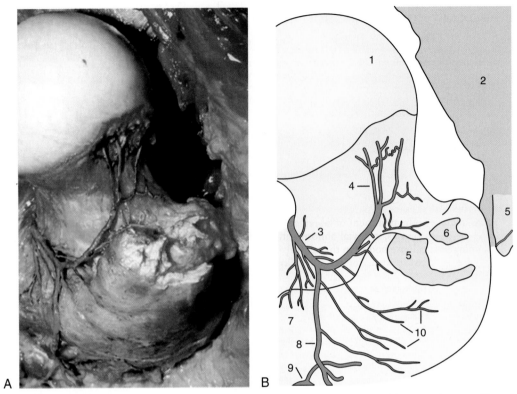

**Figure 2–4** Blood supply to the femoral head. **A,** Photograph that shows the posterosuperior proximal femur, with terminal branches of medial femoral circumflex artery (MFCA) perforating the femur. *With permission from Gautier E, Ganz K, Krugel N, Gill T, Ganz R. Anatomy of the medial femoral circumflex artery and its surgical implications. J Bone Joint Surg Br. 2000;82(5):679-683.* **B,** Illustration of posterosuperior proximal femur that shows the following: 1) the head of the femur; 2) the gluteus medius; 3) the deep branch of the MFCA; 4) the terminal branches of the MFCA; 5) the insertion of the tendon of the gluteus medius; 6) the insertion of the tendon of the piriformis; 7) the lesser trochanter with its nutrient vessels; 8) the trochanteric branch of the MFCA; 9) the branch of the first perforating artery; and 10) the trochanteric branches.

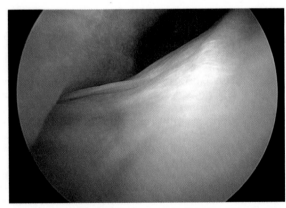

**Figure 2–5** An arthroscopic photograph of the lateral retinacular fold, which contains the ascending vessels of medial circumflex femoral artery en route to the femoral head.

The inadvertent lengthening of the operative limb is the most common cause for sciatic and peroneal palsies. Other risk factors include revision THA, increased intraoperative blood loss, the aberrant placement of retractors, and congenital hip deformities. As with THA, prolonged distraction time of the operative limb during arthroscopy is associated with sciatic nerve injury. Some studies have suggested that sciatic and femoral nerve distress is seen on intraoperative monitoring during hip arthroscopy. Fortunately, the clinical manifestation of sciatic nerve stretch palsy is very rare during hip arthroscopy. Despite this, it is still recommended that traction on the operative limb

be let down within 2 hours in an effort to further reduce the risk of neurovascular distress.

The pudendal nerve, which supplies structures within the perineum, and the nerve to the obturator internus, which supplies the obturator internus muscle on its pelvic surface, are branches of the sacral plexus. They leave the pelvis via the greater sciatic foramen and below the piriformis before crossing the ischial spine and entering the pelvis via the lesser sciatic foramen. Neuropraxia of the pudendal nerve and its branches (including the perineal nerve) is a more common complication of hip arthroscopy. This is usually a compression phenomenon seen during limb traction and caused by the direct abutment of the perineal post on the groin. The genitofemoral nerve is also at risk here. These traction injuries manifest as a loss of cutaneous sensation around the labia or scrotum and the inner thigh; they are minimized intraoperatively by abundantly padding the perineal post.

The femoral nerve (L2 to L4) arises from the lumbar plexus and descends between the psoas and the iliacus. It enters the thigh posterior to the inguinal ligament, lateral to the femoral artery, and outside of the femoral sheath. The femoral nerve supplies muscles in the anterior thigh compartment, including the iliacus, psoas major, pectineus, and quadriceps muscles. In addition, it has several cutaneous branches that supply the skin over the medial and anterior thigh. The distal branches supply sections of skin that overlie the knee, leg, and foot. The lateral femoral cutaneous nerve (LFCN), however, provides the lateral cutaneous innervation of the thigh and knee. Finally, the superior gluteal nerve is also of particular importance to the hip arthroscopist. It leaves the pelvis through the greater sciatic foramen and above the piriformis to supply the gluteus medius, the gluteus minimus, and the TFL.

## ARTHROSCOPIC ANATOMY OF THE HIP

Hip arthroscopists divide the femoroacetabular joint and its surrounding areas into three compartments. The central compartment refers to the confines of the hip joint proper; the peripheral compartment provides access to the femoral neck and the outer acetabular rim. More recently, Kelly and colleagues described the peritrochanteric compartment, which lies between the iliotibial band and the proximal femur. Each compartment can be accessed by a number of arthroscopic portals and has pathologies that are individual to the specific area.

Hip arthroscopy has evolved with improvements in surgical equipment and technical skill. In addition, advances in magnetic resonance imaging have heralded the diagnosis of previously unrecognized intra-articular pathology. Arthroscopy now has numerous indications, including the treatment of labral lesions, degenerative disease, articular injuries, synovial abnormalities, femoroacetabular impingement, loose bodies in the central and peripheral compartments, gluteus medius tendon tears, iliotibial band problems, and trochanteric bursitis.

The biggest challenge in hip arthroscopy is gaining safe access to the various compartments of the hip. A detailed understanding of local anatomy is therefore intrinsic to establishing a safe and effective portal to the hip. In addition to negotiating neurovascular structures, the arthroscopist is confronted by the large soft-tissue envelope that encases the femoroacetabular joint. In obese patients, this envelope may make an arthroscopic approach to the hip an impossible endeavor, even with specialized long instrumentation. Even in the thinner patient, the tough, fibrous hip capsule can still make access problematic. Precise arthroscopic technique and adherence to established principles for the management of the soft-tissue envelope can make hip arthroscopy a reliable and successful procedure for the relief of hip symptoms.

### Surface Anatomy

An accurate understanding of the surface anatomy is crucial for anatomic orientation and initial trocar insertion. Typically, the outlines of the greater trochanter and the ASIS are drawn, followed by the intersecting horizontal and vertical lines from each point, respectively. With the use of these basic landmarks, the three most commonly used portals as described by Thomas Byrd—the anterior, anterolateral, and posterolateral portals—can be accurately placed (see Figure 2-1, *B*).

Anterolaterally, the arthroscopist should understand the course of the LFCN, which travels approximately 1 cm medial to the ASIS just below the epidermal layer and subsequently branches out in a fan-like distribution (Figure 2-6). Although the incidence of complications during hip arthroscopy is low, the LFCN branches are in close proximity to the anterior portals, and localized paresthesias of the thigh as a result of damage of this nerve are not uncommon. Although blunt trauma during portal placement can cause damage to the LFCN branches, the more likely culprit is inadvertent scalpel injury, which reiterates the importance of a careful skin incision.

It is also important to palpate and mark the main neurovascular bundle that traverses just anteromedial to the hip joint, which contains the femoral nerve, artery, and vein and the associated lymphatics. These structures are only a few centimeters medial to the anterior portal, so the arthroscopist should be keenly aware of their location when establishing anterior or medial portals. One should rarely if ever be medial to the imaginary line that extends distally from the ASIS. In addition, in the peripheral compartment, the distal part of the iliopsoas is within 3 cm of the femoral vessels, and care must be taken when performing an iliopsoas release at this level. Fortunately,

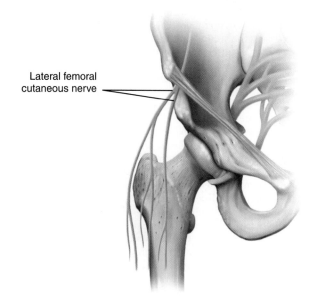

Lateral femoral cutaneous nerve

**Figure 2–6** A diagram that illustrates the fan-like distribution of the branches of lateral femoral cutaneous nerve and its proximity to the anterolateral and posterolateral portals.

these complications are extremely rare during arthroscopy of the hip. Finally, the arthroscopist should be familiar with the sciatic nerve and the gluteal vessels posteriorly and proximally. Localization of the portal pathway is then typically achieved with the use of a long 18-gauge spinal needle and image intensification. One measure that helps to avoid injury is to make skin incisions only after proper intra-articular placement has been achieved.

### The Arthroscopic Portals

A keen appreciation of hip anatomy in combination with proper positioning and distraction is fundamental to safe and successful portal placement. Portals should be established in zones that minimize the risk of soft-tissue damage and that maximize arthroscope maneuverability and the visualization of anatomic structures. This is of particular importance in the hip joint, because it is deeply recessed and enveloped by the thick, fibrous capsule.

The anterolateral portal is the workhorse of all of the arthroscopic portals around the hip. It is considered to be the safest portal, and it is therefore established first and "blindly" (i.e., with the assistance of fluoroscopy alone). It is useful for the visualization of the central, peripheral, and peritrochanteric compartments. To create an anterolateral portal, an initial superficial incision no deeper than the subcutaneous adipose tissue is made over the anterosuperior tip of the greater trochanter. A fascial band just posterior to the skin incision is commonly encountered, and it can be used as a reference mark. A sheathed blunt trocar or snap is used to pass through the adipose tissue, fascia, and muscle tissue to the hip capsule. The superior gluteal nerve lays approximately 4.5 cm superiorly to this portal (see Table 2-2). A spinal needle is then used to enter the hip joint, and this is followed by a guidewire and a trocar. After the surgeon has entered the joint space, the superolateral labrum, the acetabular articular cartilage, and the femoral head are vulnerable to iatrogenic damage. Therefore, blunt trocars are preferred. Finally, image intensification and the injection of saline can confirm the proper positioning of the intra-articular spinal needle. Subsequent portals are established with intra-articular arthroscopic guidance.

After the anterolateral portal is established, the anterior portal is typically the second and most difficult portal to establish. It allows for the observation of the anterior femoral neck, the superior retinacular fold, the lateral acetabular labrum, portions of the transverse acetabular ligament, and the ligamentum teres. Traditionally, this portal is placed directly at the intersection of the lines drawn vertically from the ASIS and horizontally from the greater trochanter. However, this approach involves the direct penetration of the origin of the rectus femoris tendon. It has been suggested that a resultant tendinopathy causes increased soreness in the anterior groin region. Therefore, a recent a trend has emerged with the anterior portal placed just distal and lateral to the traditional portal site: the mid-anterior portal (Figure 2-7). To establish any anterior portal, one must be careful to superficially avoid the LFCN and its branches. On deeper exploration, the surgeon should be familiar with the ascending branch of the lateral circumflex femoral artery, which can be only 1.9 cm away; a small terminal branch of this artery can be as close as 1 cm away. As stated previously, one must also be aware of the femoral neurovascular bundle, which is located approximately 3.5 cm to 4 cm medially (see Table 2-2).

When creating an anterior or mid-anterior portal, it is important to penetrate the hip capsule with firm and controlled pressure so that the joint space is accessed without damage to the intra-articular anterior femoral head and the anterior labrum. Indeed, inadvertent plunging and sudden penetration of the obturator and cannula can have devastating results.

The final central compartment portal is the posterolateral portal. It is placed under direct arthroscopic visualization, and it is considered the easiest to establish because of a relative "soft spot" in the posterior soft-tissue envelope. The hip capsule is thinnest in this zone. The portal is placed on the same transverse line as the anterolateral portal but just posterior to the greater trochanter. It traverses the gluteus medius and the gluteus minimus before entering the posterior capsule. The most obvious

extra-articular structure at risk is the sciatic nerve, which is approximately 2.9 cm away (see Table 2-2). Fortunately, sciatic nerve injury is extremely rare. Most surgeons do not routinely make use of the posterolateral portal, because the majority of intra-articular pathology is localized to the anterolateral zones. Instead, the main purpose of this portal is to provide access for observation of the posterior aspect of the hip.

In addition to these three traditional portals, cadaveric studies have provided an understanding of the relationship between anatomic structures and portal placement. More recently, Kelly and colleagues have demonstrated that, including the three standard portals (i.e., anterolateral, anterior, and posterolateral), eleven arthroscopic portals may be placed for correcting pathology in the central, peripheral, and peritrochanteric compartments. Caution should be employed when attempting portal placement out of the relative "safe zone," which is considered to lie within approximately 4 cm superior and 6 cm to 8 cm inferior to the anterior and anterolateral portals. This is especially important when attempting to establish access posterior to the posterolateral portal or medial to the anterior portal.

## EXAMINATION OF THE HIP THROUGH ARTHROSCOPIC COMPARTMENTS

During the early days of hip arthroscopy, the most common indications were infection, loose body removal, and labral tears. Hip arthroscopy was confined to the central compartment, which included only the intra-articular region of the femoroacetabular joint. As the indications for hip arthroscopy have grown, the orthopedic surgeon must now routinely explore the areas of the joint outside of the central compartment. If surgery is confined to the central compartment, then overall mean accessible surface area is limited to 68% to 75% of the joint (Figure 2-8, *A* through *D*). However, by expanding arthroscopy to include the peripheral and peritrochanteric compartments, the surgeon can access more than 90% of the hip. Therefore, only the most posteromedial zones of the hip have limited accessibility. In addition, the indications for extra-articular procedures have recently expanded. Surgeons are now successfully navigating areas such as the iliopsoas bursa and the peritrochanteric space. Therefore, it is essential to appreciate the anatomic contents of the three hip compartments (Figure 2-9) and to familiarize oneself with the indications that are characteristic of each.

### Central Compartment

#### The Capsule

The hip capsule consists of three discrete ligaments: 1) the ischiofemoral (posterior) ligament; the iliofemoral (anterior) ligament; and the pubofemoral (anterior) ligament. These form a thick and fibrous wrap around the femoroacetabular joint, and they result in more than 95% of the femoral neck being intracapsular. The ischiofemoral ligament is located posteriorly. It is thin and pliable, and it generally poses few problems for the hip arthroscopist, because the majority of the work in hip arthroscopy is located anteriorly. The iliofemoral and pubofemoral ligaments are located anteriorly, and together they combine to make one of the thickest and toughest capsules of the entire body. A traditional open anterior capsulotomy directly involves the release of these two adherent structures. The pubofemoral ligament is located anteromedially; it spans from the pubic ramus and the anteroinferior acetabular wall to the anteromedial femoral neck. Distally, it becomes confluent with the fibers of the iliofemoral ligament. Its functions are primarily to resist hip extension and to prevent excessive abduction. In patients with a soft-tissue contracture of the hip, the release of the pubofemoral ligament will effectively increase abduction.

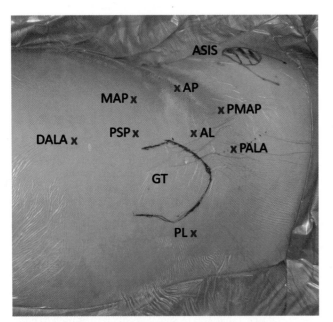

**Figure 2–7** Commonly employed accessory portals for hip arthroscopy with associated palpable landmarks. *AL,* Anterolateral portal; *AP,* anterior portal; *ASIS,* anterosuperior iliac spine; *DALA,* distal anterolateral accessory portal; *GT,* greater trochanter; *MAP,* mid-anterior portal; *PALA,* proximal anterolateral accessory portal; *PL,* posterolateral portal; *PMAP,* proximal mid-anterior portal; *PSP,* peritrochanteric space portal.

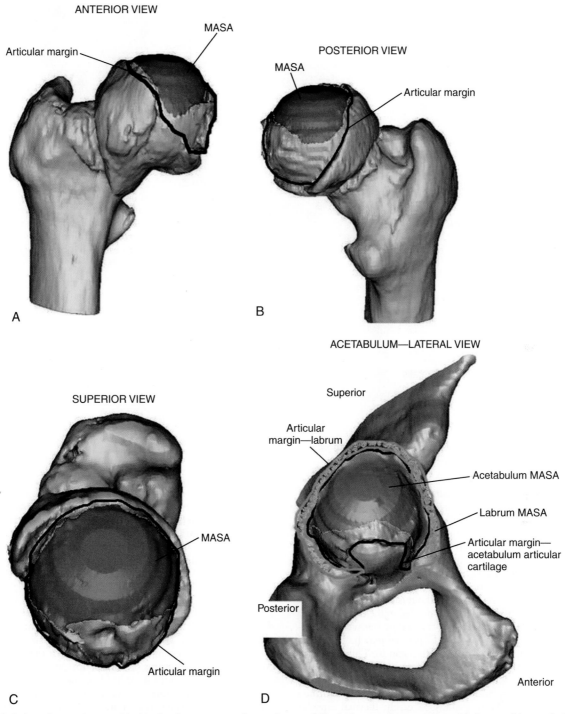

**Figure 2–8** An arthroscopic map of the hip that demonstrates arthroscopic accessibility in the central compartment with the use of the standard three-portal technique. **A,** AP view of CT scan of right femur showing the mean accessible surface area (MASA), i.e. accessible part of the femur during standard hip arthroscopy. **B,** PA view of CT scan of right femur showing the MASA during standard hip arthroscopy. **C,** Superior view of CT scan of right femur showing the MASA during standard hip arthroscopy. **D,** CT scan lateral view of a right acetabulum showing the MASA during standard hip arthroscopy.

The iliofemoral ligament, which is located anterolaterally, is of particular clinical importance when establishing the anterior portal. It is perhaps the single biggest impediment to the hip arthroscopist. The iliofemoral ligament (i.e., the Y ligament of Bigelow) arises from the AIIS and spreads obliquely and inferolaterally to insert into the intertrochanteric line on the anterior femoral head. This is the strongest ligament in the human body, and it prevents anterior translation of the hip in positions of extension and external rotation, especially when the pelvis is posteriorly tilted. The intra-articular medial and lateral limbs of the iliofemoral ligament form an anterior triangle. The terminal fibers of the ligament form the zona orbicularis; this is a circular leash around the femoral neck that tightens during extension and loosens during flexion.

The thickest part of this ligament lies anteriorly and coincides with the location of the majority of hip pathology that is amenable to arthroscopic intervention. Even after the portals are established, the capsule limits the maneuverability of the

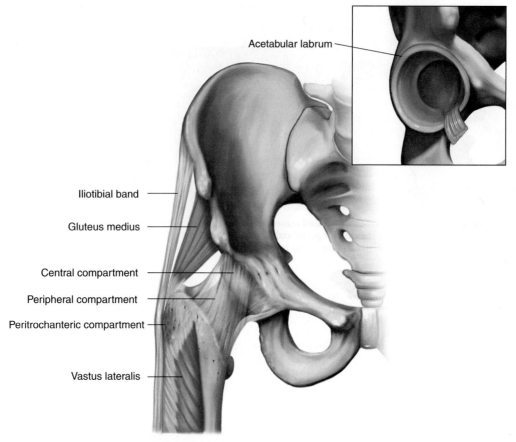

Acetabular labrum

Iliotibial band

Gluteus medius

Central compartment

Peripheral compartment

Peritrochanteric compartment

Vastus lateralis

**Figure 2–9** The three arthroscopic compartments of the hip joint.

instrumentation and the arthroscope within the central compartment. Therefore, a limited capsulotomy is recommended to enhance mobility. This is usually accomplished with the assistance of a beaver blade or a radiofrequency device. If work is confined to the central compartment, it is sufficient to make mini-capsulotomy incisions in the areas in which the portals are penetrating the capsule. This allows the surgeon to access the femoroacetabular articular cartilage, the labrum, and the contents of the cotyloid fossa without significant challenge. However, if any substantial work is needed in the extra-articular areas (e.g., osteoplasty), then a horizontal or transverse capsular release in a "fish-mouth" or "T" pattern may be necessary, anteriorly or posteriorly (Figure 2-10, *A* and *B*). This allows for increased visualization and the ability to work in the peripheral compartment. Currently, the incision of the capsule, the extent of this incision, and the subsequent repair are performed at the discretion of the surgeon. Conversely, thermal capsular shrinkage can also be achieved by hip arthroscopy to stabilize the joint. Capsular plication in combination with shrinkage has also been shown to have good short-term results among patients with recurrent instability in the presence of an intact ligamentum teres.

*The Labrum*

The acetabular labrum is made predominantly of fibrocartilage supported by a collagen scaffold. It runs circumferentially around the acetabular rim and the fovea. This scaffold is oriented in both a longitudinal and radial direction, which confers stability to the femoroacetabular articulation. The sensory innervation of this scaffold provides the hip with both proprioception and nociceptive function, and it participates in hip

stability and pressure distribution in the joint. The labrum attaches to the transverse acetabular ligament anteriorly and posteriorly; it has a vascular peripheral capsular surface with a less-vascular central articular margin.

The labrum and the capsule help to contain the femoral head in extreme ranges of motion, and they act as load-bearing structures during flexion. Therefore, patients who have undergone extensive labrectomy may complain of significant rotational instability or hypermobility. The capsulolabral disruption may result in transient micro motion, abnormal load distribution, and redundant capsular tissue. This allows for redundancy of the anterior capsule, which can then lead to microinstability. Recent studies have shown that the labrum contains neural structures of both proprioceptive and nociceptive function. In addition, it has been shown that the majority of these mechanoreceptors and sensory nerve endings are most highly concentrated anteriorly, which is where the majority of symptomatic hip pathology is seen. Excessive debridement of the labral tissue not only involves the mechanical implications discussed previously, but it may also result in altered joint proprioception, which may further lead to joint derangement.

It has been suggested that the labrum enhances stability by maintaining negative intra-articular pressure in the hip joint and that it acts as a tension band for preventing joint expansion as part of a normal gait. In addition, the negative pressure creates a suction-seal effect at the innermost aspect of the joint by forming a seal between the femoral head and the acetabular rim and thus enhancing hip stability. Fluid mechanics models have provided evidence that, in a hip with a discontinuous labrum, the joint contact pressure distribution is greatly diminished and can lead to decreased cartilage surface consolidation.

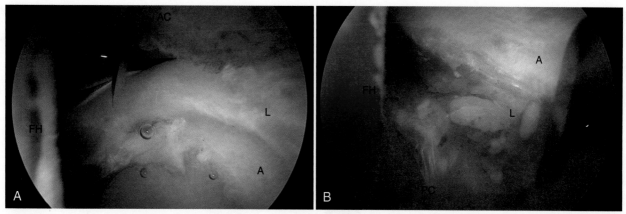

**Figure 2–10** Arthroscopic capsule release provides increased maneuverability within the central and peripheral compartment. **A,** Central compartment view of the connection between the anterior portal and the anterolateral portal during anterior capsule release of the left hip. **B,** Central compartment view from the anterolateral portal of the left hip during posterior capsule release. *A,* Acetabulum; *AC,* anterior capsule; *FH,* femoral head; *L,* labrum; *PC,* posterior capsule.

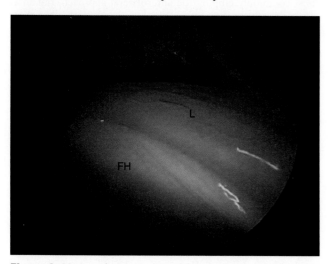

**Figure 2–11** An arthroscopic view of the capsulolabral junction and the vascularization of the labrum. *FH,* Femoral head; *L,* labrum.

The obturator artery, with contributions from the inferior and superior gluteal vessels, provides the blood supply to the labrum (Figure 2-11). Histologic studies have shown that the blood supply to the labrum is analogous to that of the knee menisci. The majority of the microvascular supply proliferates the capsulolabral junction with a relative paucity of vascularization to the innermost aspect of the labrum. Therefore, like the meniscus, the labrum may have the greatest healing potential at the peripheral capsulolabral junction.

Magnetic resonance imaging is becoming more effective for detecting labral lesions. Most are encountered in the relatively avascular zone and thus warrant debridement. If the tear is located adjacent to the more vascular capsulolabral junction in a longitudinal peripheral orientation, then primary labral repair may be possible. However, many "labral repairs" that are currently performed are in fact labral refixation procedures after acetabular rim trimming in patients with pincer-type femoroacetabular impingement. Normal variants (e.g., a labral cleft) should not be interpreted as traumatic detachment.

### The Cotyloid Fossa

The cotyloid fossa is roughly hemispheric. It has a wave-like profile of three peaks and three troughs, including the acetabular notch. The most clinically relevant anatomic structure within the cotyloid fossa is the ligamentum teres. The ligamentum teres is a highly variable structure, but it is generally described as a thin, flat ligament with a triangular cross section that originates from the fovea capitus on the femoral head. It is shrouded by synovium throughout its entirety, and it is often obscured by the prolific fat pad of the cotyloid fossa. The ligament is between 30 mm and 35 mm in length, and it consists structurally of two main bundles (i.e., anterior and posterior) that insert medially into the base of the cotyloid fossa adjacent to the transverse acetabular ligament. The function of the ligamentum teres in the adult is controversial. In the immature hip, it is clear that the ligamentum teres serves as a conduit for the arterial supply to the femoral head via the artery of the ligamentum teres, which is a branch of the obturator artery. However, as the human hip matures, the main blood supply to the femoral head is via the medial circumflex artery and the intracapsular perforating arteries, and the joint does not rely on direct vascularization from the ligamentum teres.

It has been suggested that the ligamentum teres contributes to the stability of the joint, especially in the presence of dysplasia. In addition, the bundles tighten in hip flexion, external rotation, and abduction, which is the common hip position during a dashboard injury; it may therefore play a role as a secondary restraint to a posterior hip dislocation. Others have postulated that the ligamentum teres has a proprioceptive function. However, recent studies have shown a paucity of mechanoreceptors in the bundles. In addition, the surgical debridement of the ligament after rupture shows excellent results, even in high-level athletes, thus further undermining its possible role in proprioception.

### Peripheral Compartment

The peripheral compartment is an area of the hip that is considered to be extra-articular yet intra-capsular; it lies along the anterior femoral neck. Loose bodies commonly collect here, and cam-type bony lesions are largely localized to this compartment. Labral surgery can also be performed here in an "outside-in" fashion. Therefore, a systematic examination of the compartment is routine. After the inspection of the central compartment is complete, the peripheral compartment is most easily viewed from the anterior portal and accessed by flexing and externally rotating the hip without traction, thus atraumatically avoiding the femoral head. Other techniques have described a "peripheral-first" method.

After entry into the peripheral compartment, the first anatomic landmark that can be readily identified is the medial synovial fold (Figure 2-12). The synovial folds are sheet-like

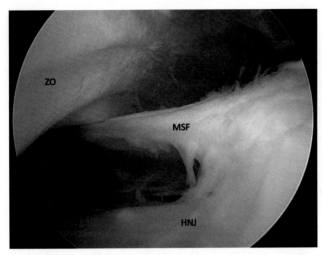

**Figure 2–12** An arthroscopic view of the femoral head through the anterolateral portal. *HNJ*, Head–neck junction; *MSF*, medial synovial fold; *ZO*, zona orbicularis.

collections of synovial tissue that run longitudinally in various parts of the peripheral compartment. The medial synovial fold is located at the anteromedial aspect of the femoral neck. The lateral synovial fold is located at the junction between the lateral and posterior femoral neck. It is important to closely inspect both of these structures, because their redundant tissue can easily obscure loose bodies. In addition, when significant synovitis is present, these synovial folds become inflamed and need to be thoroughly debrided as part of a synovectomy procedure.

The synovial folds can serve as important landmarks in the peripheral compartment. It is unusual for a cam-type lesion of the femoral head–neck junction to extend more medial than the medial synovial fold, so this can be used as a rough guide to the 6-o'clock position. The lateral synovial fold contains the lateral retinaculum and the intracapsular penetrating arteries from the lateral epiphyseal vessels. It is essential to employ great caution when working near and posterior to the lateral synovial fold to avoid iatrogenic injury to these vessels. The lateral synovial fold can also be used a rough landmark for the 12-o'clock position.

Another important landmark in the peripheral compartment is the zona orbicularis, which refers to the thickening of the hip capsule as it forms a ring around the circumference of the femoral neck. Although the exact function of the zona orbicularis is not entirely known, it has particular use as an arthroscopic anatomic landmark of the peripheral compartment. Just cranial to the zona orbicularis, by the anterior capsular recess, and in line with the medial synovial fold lies the psoas tendon. Anteromedially, the tendon may be covered by a thin, transparent capsule that leads directly to the iliopsoas bursa. In fact, in approximately 20% of the population, the iliopsoas bursa may be in direct communication with the peripheral compartment. This is of particular clinical relevance: coxa saltans interna (i.e., internal snapping hip) can be related to iliopsoas bursitis or iliopsoas tendonitis. This condition can be surgically treated by partially releasing or lengthening the iliopsoas tendon from the lesser trochanter. Arthroscopically, the tendon is visualized and released in the peripheral compartment just proximal to the zona orbicularis and deep to the thin anteromedial capsule in this region.

### Peritrochanteric Compartment

The peritrochanteric compartment of the hip joint, which is also known as the *lateral compartment*, lies between the iliotibial band and the proximal femur. This space may typically be accessed after the routine evaluation and treatment of central and peripheral compartment pathology. Anatomically, arthroscopists can examine the insertion of the gluteus maximus into the posterior border of the iliotibial band. Proximally, the longitudinal lines of the vastus lateralis can be identified; anterosuperiorly, the gluteus medius and gluteus minimus tendon insertions on the greater trochanter can be visualized. Although the arthroscopic anatomy in this compartment has been well defined, the treatment of greater trochanteric pain syndrome and the arthroscopic repair of abductor tendon tears are only beginning to be reported. Improved techniques and longer-term outcome studies will further define the optimal role of hip arthroscopy in this compartment.

## OPEN APPROACHES TO THE HIP JOINT

There are a number of open approaches to the hip that have been advocated for ideal anatomic exposure with minimal dissection and low patient morbidity. Surgeons who perform THA most commonly employ the anterolateral approach, the anterior approach, or the posterolateral approach, with all of these approaches now having new modifications. For acetabular access and reconstruction, the ilioinguinal and iliofemoral approaches are often recommended, whereas a surgical hip dislocation is now commonly performed for femoroacetabular impingement, arthroplasty, or fracture treatment.

### The Watson-Jones Anterolateral Approach

The anterolateral approach is now most commonly used for THA. The hip is exposed through a lateral skin incision that is centered over the trochanter. After the initial superficial incision and dissection, splitting and retraction of the TFL exposes the vastus lateralis and the gluteus medius. The hip joint can be entered by partial detachment of the abductor mechanism or a trochanteric osteotomy. After the capsule is identified, the reflected head of the rectus and the capsule can be incised. The surgeon should be aware of potential femoral nerve damage as a result of excessive medial retraction and unnecessary splitting of the gluteus medius, which can injure the superior gluteal nerve. The anterolateral approach demands a meticulous dissection; it has been associated with weakness and limping from abductor attachment site disruption. However, it has been suggested that it is the least traumatic and most direct approach to the hip.

### The Kocher-Langenbeck Posterolateral Approach

The posterolateral approach or Southern approach was first developed by Langenbeck and Kocher, and it was more recently modified by Marcy and Fletcher. It is indicated for THA, internal fixation, and revision surgery. The hip joint is accessed via a gluteus maximus splitting incision. A curvilinear incision is made proximal to the greater trochanter and then straight down the posterior border of the trochanter distally down the femur. The short external rotators are exposed close to their insertion points into the greater trochanter, and the hip is dislocated by internally rotating the femur. The sciatic nerve runs just deep to the gluteus maximus at the midpoint between the ischial tuberosity and the greater trochanter. The short external rotators should be reflected onto the sciatic nerve to protect it from sciatic neuropraxia. In addition, the splitting of the gluteus maximus may damage the inferior gluteal nerve. The posterolateral approach (as compared with the anterolateral approach) requires little soft-tissue dissection, and it has historically been associated with a significantly shorter operation time but an increased risk of dislocation.

## The Smith-Peterson Anterior Approach

The anterior approach to the hip joint is used for hemiarthroplasty, THA, resurfacing, fracture surgery, and anterior femoroacetabular impingement surgery. An incision is made just distal to the ASIS down the anterior aspect of the proximal thigh. The anterior hip is exposed via the internervous plane between the femoral nerve (i.e., the sartorius muscle and the rectus femoris) and the superior gluteal nerve (i.e., the TFL and the gluteus medius). The LFCN is encountered as it passes distal to the AIIS and should be protected, whereas the ascending branch of the lateral femoral cutaneous artery will commonly be encountered at the inferior aspect of the wound. A modification of this technique is the anterior Hueter approach, which diminishes the risk of injury to the LFCN by having the surgeon incise the fascia of the TFL longitudinally and then use the fascia to retract the nerve medially. Thus, the interval is slightly lateral to the classic Smith-Peterson approach. However, the downside of this approach is that the TFL does sustain muscle injury.

## Open Surgical Dislocation of the Hip

A safe surgical dislocation of the hip has been described and championed by Ganz. The surgeon must take care to not compromise the blood supply of the femoral head, which arises from the deep branch of the medial femoral circumflex artery. This is done by a careful trochanteric osteotomy to a level no deeper than that of the piriformis insertion, followed by an anterior dislocation. The role of this procedure for femoroacetabular impingement, fracture surgery, and arthroplasty is constantly growing.

## CONCLUSION

The human hip is a challenging joint as a result of its complex anatomy, orientation, and biomechanics. It is no longer adequate to understand and employ only the classic open surgical approaches to this joint. With the gaining popularity of new open techniques and arthroscopic interventions, the surgeon must have a sound understanding of hip anatomy to gain safe access to the hip. With the advent of new instruments and techniques, the indications for hip arthroscopy have expanded tremendously during recent years. Although the procedure carries a low risk of significant complications, it is critical for hip arthroscopists to avoid iatrogenic injury. However, this feat is only achieved with a comprehensive anatomic knowledge base.

## ANNOTATED REFERENCES

**Bardakos NV, Villar RN. The ligamentum teres of the adult hip.** *J Bone Joint Surg Br.* 2009;91(1):8–15.

Although once thought to be a developmental vestige, the ligamentum teres is now considered an important source of pain and mechanical symptoms. The authors, orthopaedic surgeons from The Richard Villar Practice, London, provide an update on the development, structure and function of the ligamentum teres, and its critical relevance to both arthroscopic and open hip procedures.

**Barrack RL, Butler RA. Avoidance and management of neurovascular injuries in total hip arthroplasty.** *Instr Course Lect.* 2003;52:267–274.

This instructional review outlines operative techniques to avoid common neurovascular pitfalls during THA. In addition it discusses the mechanisms by which both the central and peripheral nervous system and vasculature may be damaged

**Byrd JW. Avoiding the labrum in hip arthroscopy.** *Arthroscopy.* 2000;16(7):770–773.

The labrum is easily perforated during hip arthroscopy. The author of this short technical piece, an accomplished orthopaedic surgeon and founder of the Nashville Sports Medicine Centre, acknowledges that occasional damage is unavoidable. He highlights the importance of careful technique when establishing initial access into the capsule and provides surgeons with procedural guidance to avoid iatrogenic trauma of the labrum.

**Byrd JW. Labral lesions: an elusive source of hip pain case reports and literature review.** *Arthroscopy.* 1996;12(5):603–612.

This review, from the Nashville Orthopaedic Centre uses case reports and a literature review to discuss the relative contributions of clinical history, non-invasive imaging, and arthrography to the diagnosis of labral pathology.

**Byrd JW, Pappas JN, Pedley MJ. Hip arthroscopy: an anatomic study of portal placement and relationship to the extra-articular structures.** *Arthroscopy.* 1995;11(4):418–423.

This cadaveric anatomic study describes the proximity of the anterior, anterolateral and posterolateral arthroscopic hip portals to neurovascular structures. Although all measurements were made without distraction of the hip joint, the authors bring attention to the importance of negotiating anatomical structures, particularly the LFCN and sciatic nerve, when accessing the joint.

**Clarke MT, Arora A, Villar RN. Hip arthroscopy: complications in 1054 cases.** *Clin Orthop Relat Res.* 2003;(406)84–88.

This prospective study of a large sample of consecutive hip arthroscopies performed at one centre reports an overall complication rate of 1.4%. The authors are orthopaedic arthroscopy specialists, and the results are therefore perhaps not reflective of general practice. However, it is clear that with careful technique and via low-risk portals, arthroscopy of the hip has a low safety profile that is comparable to other orthopaedic procedures.

**Dandachli W, Kannan V, Richards R, Shah Z, Hall-Craggs M, Witt J. Analysis of cover of the femoral head in normal and dysplastic hips: new CT-based technique.** *J Bone Joint Surg Br.* 2008;90(11):1428–1434.

The femoroacetabular joint is a complex three-dimensional construct. This non-interventional case-control study uses novel 3D-CT methodology to describe femoral head coverage. The authors, from London, UK, are able to distinguish dysplastic and normal femoral head coverage - mean cover was 73% and 51% respectively. This is useful for anatomical understanding and has application in post-operative assessment of corrected hips.

**Ferguson SJ, Bryant JT, Ganz R, Ito K. An in vitro investigation of the acetabular labral seal in hip joint mechanics.** *J Biomech.* 2003;36(2):171–178.

The authors harvest four human cadaveric pelvises and investigate the load- and stress-limiting role of the acetabular labrum in preventing cartilage layer consolidation and early joint degeneration. They demonstrate that the sealing mechanism of an intact labrum creates a hydrostatic fluid pressure in the intra-articular space, which may enhance joint lubrication. The labrum may be partially debrided prior to acetabular rim resection, or torn during acetabular trauma. This study emphasizes the importance of labral restoration in preventing functional deterioration of the hip joint .

**Ganz R, Gill TJ, Gautier E, Ganz K, Krugel N, Berlemann U. Surgical dislocation of the adult hip a technique with full access to the femoral head and acetabulum without the risk of avascular necrosis.** *J Bone Joint Surg Br.* 2001;83:1119–1124.

The authors describe their experience of surgical dislocation of the hip in 213 hips over seven years. Their technique is an anterior dislocation through a posterior approach with a 'trochanteric flip' osteotomy. The external rotator muscles are not divided and the medial femoral circumflex artery is protected by the intact obturator externus. Their results suggest adequate preservation of the vascularity of the femoral head can be achieved with little morbidity.

**Gautier E, Ganz K, Krugel N, Gill T, Ganz R. Anatomy of the medial femoral circumflex artery and its surgical implications.** *J Bone Joint Surg Br.* 2000;82(5):679–683.

The classic description of the approach and technique commenting on the advantages of a posterior exposure of the hip joint.

**Glick JM. Hip arthroscopy. The lateral approach.** *Clin Sports Med.* 2001;20(4):733–747.

It is of the author's opinion that the lateral approach is the safest, simplest and most versatile of arthroscopic hip approaches. This review presents technical operative direction for the arthroscopist, particularly highlighting techniques to prevent sciatic neuropraxia during traction.

**Kagan A 2nd. Rotator cuff tears of the hip.** *Clin Orthop Relat Res.* 1999;(368)135–140.

Partial tears of the gluteus medius, near its attachment to the greater trochanter, are often misdiagnosed as greater trochanteric pain syndrome (GTPS). This seminal paper describes the diagnostic process and operative treatment of 7 patients with 'rotator cuff tears of the hip', and provides informative guidance for distinguishing this hip pathology. It is particularly illuminating given the recent advances in the peritrochanteric arthoscopic compartment.

**Kelly BT, Shapiro GS, Digiovanni CW, Buly RL, Potter HG, Hannafin JA. Vascularity of the hip labrum: a cadaveric investigation.** *Arthroscopy.* 2005;21(1):3–11.

The function of the damaged hip labrum is notoriously difficult to restore. This study uses MRI-based ink-injection analysis to measure its vascularity. The authors found that although the labrum is a largely avascular structure, its capsular contribution is significantly more vascular. The authors propose that tears of the vascular portion may be more amenable to surgical repair and subsequent physiological healing, while tears in the articular, avascular portion are better debrided.

**Mason JB, McCarthy JC, O'Donnell J, et al. Hip arthroscopy: surgical approach, positioning, and distraction.** *Clin Orthop Relat Res.* 2003;(406)29–37.

This is a comprehensive technical overview of operative techniques in hip arthroscopy. In addition to discussing the lateral approach, portals, patient positioning and portal placement, the paper provides a balanced review of the use of distraction in arthroscopy.

**Murtha PE, Hafez MA, Jaramaz B, DiGioia AM 3rd. Variations in acetabular anatomy with reference to total hip replacement.** *J Bone Joint Surg Br.* 2008;90(3):308–313.

This descriptive study of 42 pelvises using three-dimensional CT imaging analyses the orientation of the human acetabulum. It rejects the gold standard of the Lewinnek's 'safe zone' for the ideal position of the acetabular component in hip arthroplasty. It also shows that female acetabulae are more anteverted than their male counterparts. The paper raises questions about following the orientation of the native acetabulum for component placement, and whether gender-specific components better mimic normal anatomy.

**Philippon MJ. The role of arthroscopic thermal capsulorrhaphy in the hip.** *Clin Sports Med.* 2001;20(4):817–829.

Hip instability is associated with capsular laxity. The author discusses the role of arthroscopic thermal shrinkage of type 1 collagen in the hip tissue to reduce capsular redundancy, restore stability and decrease the development of arthrosis. Although this practice is well established in the treatment of posterior shoulder instability, the author reviews its early results in the hip.

**Rachbauer F, Kain MS, Leuing M. The history of the anterior approach to the hip.** *Orthop Clin North Am* 2009;40(3):311–320.

The anterior approach to the hip has evolved since its description in 1881. This historical review details the changes and adaptations since its inception, and describes both the open and arthroscopic potential of this internervous and muscle sparing approach.

**Robertson WJ, Kelly BT. The safe zone for hip arthroscopy: a cadaveric assessment of central, peripheral, and lateral compartment portal placement.** *Arthroscopy.* 2008;24(9):1019–1026.

In addition to the three traditional arthroscopic portals to the hip, this cadaveric study measures the proximity of accessory portals to the central, peripheral and trochanteric compartments. A total of 11 portals were determined to provide viable access to the joint. The article provides a valuable anatomical insight into accurate and safe access for the arthroscopic hip surgeon.

**Schmalzried TP, Amstutz HC, Dorey FJ.. Nerve palsy associated with total hip replacement. Risk factors and prognosis.** *J Bone Joint Surg Am.* 1991;73(7):1074–1080.

In this retrospective analysis of 3126 consecutive operations performed over 17 years, the authors discuss the prevalence and aetiology of nerve palsy as a complication of total hip arthroplasty via an open lateral transtrochanteric approach. The study documents that while nerve palsy was the most debilitating of post-operative complications, there is a low prevalence rate of 1.7% and the sciatic nerve is involved in the majority of cases. The positioning of the limb and placement of the retractors play an important role in these injuries.

**Strauss EJ, Campbell K, Bosco JA. Analysis of the cross-sectional area of the adductor longus tendon: a descriptive anatomic study.** *Am J Sports Med.* 2007;35(6):996–999.

This descriptive anatomical cadaveric study demonstrates that the origin of the adductor magnus muscle has minimal tendinous content. The authors propose that this feature both contributes to the adductor longus' propensity for damage during eccentric contraction and the relative difficulty experienced by surgeons when repairing it.

**Vail TP, Mariani EM, Bourne MH, Berger RA, Meneghini RM. Approaches in primary total hip arthroplasty.** *J Bone Joint Surg Am.* 2009;91(Suppl 5):10–12.

Following on from the review of the anterior approach to the hip, above, this three part multicentre paper compares the anterolateral and posterolateral approaches to THA. It presents novel data supporting the anterolateral approach, suggests a novel minimally invasive rethink of the classic posterolateral approach, and discusses the ongoing disagreement regarding the merits of different/minimally invasive approaches. The choice of approach in THA remains contentious, and the article's moderator ultimately states that there is insufficient long-term data to support any particular preference.

**Voos JE, Ranawat AS, Kelly BT. The peritrochanteric space of the hip.** *Instr Course Lect.* 2009;58:193–201.

This instructional article discusses a recent addition to the hip arthroscopist's armamentarium - the peritrochanteric space. It details the disorders, including tears of the gluteus maximus and recalcitrant trochanteric bursitis, which are amenable to endoscopic access and treatment. The authors discuss patient orientation and portal placement necessary for successful intervention, as well as outlining the relevant local anatomy.

# CHAPTER 3

# Imaging: Plain Radiographs

*Moritz Tannast and Klaus A. Siebenrock*

## INTRODUCTION

Despite modern radiographic technologies such as computed tomography scanning and magnetic resonance imaging, conventional radiographic evaluation of the hip and the bony pelvis remains the fastest and most inexpensive imaging modality in daily clinical practice. Every orthopedic surgeon should be familiar with basic imaging principles, including patient positioning and radiographic projections. This chapter does not provide a complete overview of all previously described projections around the hip and pelvis. Rather, it focuses on recently described observations and the technical pitfalls of conventional radiographs in the context of the pathomorphologies associated with early osteoarthritis of the hip, particularly femoroacetabular impingement (FAI) and developmental dysplasia of the hip (DDH).

During the initial stage of early hip osteoarthritis, conventional pelvic radiographs typically do not display features of reactive degenerative changes, such as subchondral sclerosis, cysts, joint space narrowing, or osteophytes. Therefore, it is important to recognize typical prearthritic hip pathomorphologies on conventional radiographs before radiographically evident joint degeneration develops.

## BASIC SCIENCE

To understand the projected anatomy of the hip and the potential technical pitfalls related to it, it is essential to know the basic geometric radiographic principles. Conventional radiography is based on a point-shaped radiation source. In contrast with computed tomography scanning and magnetic resonance imaging, the image shows a distorted projection of the real anatomy. This conical projection implies that objects lying closer to the x-ray source necessarily will be projected more laterally (Figure 3-1).

To obtain reproducible x-ray projections, it is mandatory that the film-focus distance is standardized. A radiograph with a very small film-focus distance can lead to a magnification of anatomic structures that are lying closer to the x-ray beam and vice versa (Figure 3-2).

In addition, the proper centering of the x-ray beam is crucial. Two radiographs of the same patient taken with different beam centers can reveal a substantially different radiographic joint anatomy of the hip; this can typically be seen when radiographs of the entire pelvis are compared with radiographs of an individual hip (Figure 3-3).

## INDICATIONS

Imaging is fundamental for the screening, diagnosis, treatment, and follow up of patients with hip disorders. Basically, standard, routine, conventional radiographs should be obtained initially for evaluation before additional imaging modalities are considered.

Young patients with painful hip disorders often present with groin pain of slow onset, which may optionally first be noticed after a minor trauma incident. The pain is typically intermittent, and it may be exacerbated by excessive demand on the hip

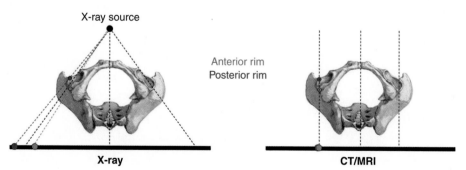

**Figure 3–1** The effect of the conical projection in conventional radiographs as a result of the point-shaped radiation source is shown. **Left,** X-ray beams lead to a distortion of the image; points that lie closer to the x-ray source (the blue point on the anterior acetabular rim) are projected more laterally than points that are closer to the x-ray plate (the red point on the posterior acetabular rim). **Right,** With computed tomography (CT) scanning and magnetic resonance imaging (MRI), no distortion is present.

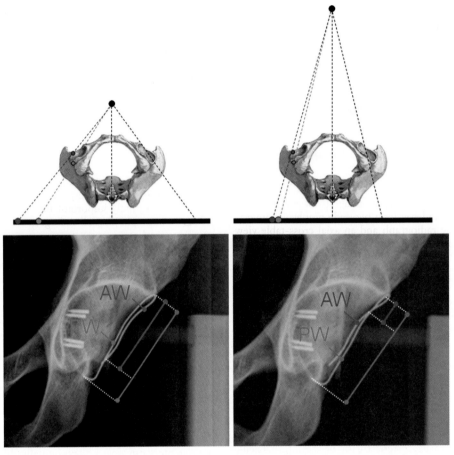

**Figure 3–2** Demonstration of how the projected acetabular morphology depends on the film-focus distance. **Left,** A decreased distance (here, 80 cm) leads to magnification of the anterior rim (blue), with the appearance of a more pronounced retroversion sign. **Right,** An increased distance (here, 140 cm) leads to a less-pronounced retroversion sign. *AW,* anterior wall; *PW,* posterior wall.

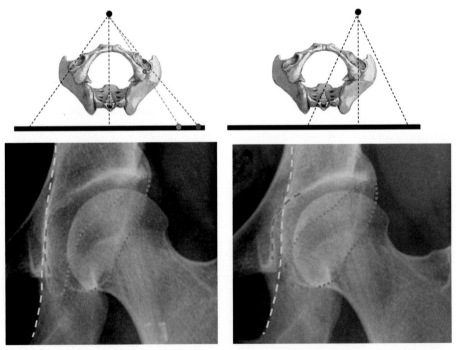

**Figure 3–3** The influence of the position of the x-ray beam on the projected acetabular morphology is shown. **Left,** A normal acetabular morphology is seen, with the x-ray beam centered on the entire pelvis. **Right,** A coxa profunda with an increased acetabular anteversion can be created if the x-ray beam is centered over the hip. *Yellow,* Ilioischial line; *green,* acetabular fossa; *blue,* anterior acetabular rim; *red,* posterior acetabular rim.

(e.g., athletic activities) or by normal activities of daily living (e.g., walking). The pain may also present after sitting for a prolonged period. Depending on the underlying pathology, physical examination can reveal an increased (DDH) or decreased (FAI) range of motion. A positive anterior impingement sign can be present with either DDH or FAI. This condition is characterized by painful internal rotation in 90 degrees of flexion, and it represents a clinically reproducible sign for the detection of labral pathologies.

## RADIOGRAPHIC TECHNIQUE FOR SPECIFIC PROJECTIONS

Standard conventional radiographic imaging for the detection of hip pathologies includes at least two radiographs: an anteroposterior (AP) pelvic radiograph and an axial cross-table view of the proximal femur. Optionally, depending on the indication and the findings of these two x-rays, a false profile and an abduction view can also be obtained. In general, gonadal shielding is not recommended, at least for the initial diagnostic analysis, because it can potentially hide important anatomic landmarks for quantifying pelvic tilt and rotation; these landmarks will be described later in this chapter.

### Anteroposterior Pelvic Radiograph

To correctly analyze hip joint morphology, an entire pelvic view—not only imaging of the affected hip—is mandatory. The AP pelvic radiograph is taken as a standard in our department, with the patient lying supine (Figure 3-4, *A*). This can be directly compared with intraoperative AP pelvic radiographs while the patient is under general anesthesia or with follow up radiographs during the early rehabilitation period. The legs have to be internally rotated to adjust for femoral antetorsion, and the film-focus distance should be 1.2 m. The central beam should be directed to the midpoint between the superior border of the symphysis and a line that connects both of the anterior superior iliac spines; these landmarks can easily and reproducibly be palpated by the radiology technician. It is extremely important for the correct interpretation of the radiographs that all radiographs are obtained with the same protocol.

### Axial Cross-Table View of the Proximal Femur

The axial cross-table view of the proximal femur visualizes the anterior and posterior contour of the femoral head–neck junction, which cannot be seen on the AP pelvic radiograph.

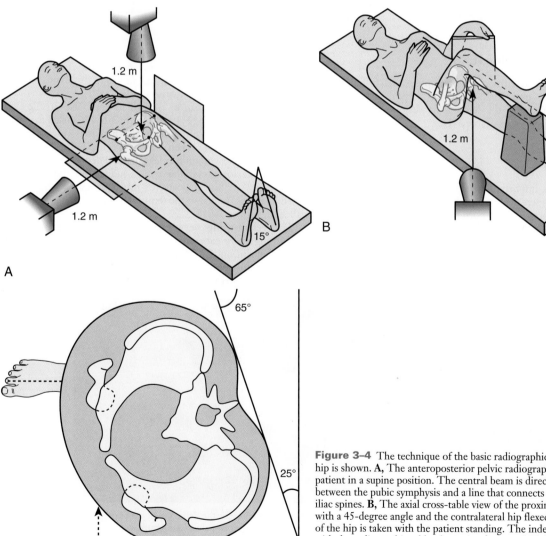

**Figure 3–4**  The technique of the basic radiographic projections of the hip is shown. **A,** The anteroposterior pelvic radiograph is taken with the patient in a supine position. The central beam is directed to the midpoint between the pubic symphysis and a line that connects the anterior superior iliac spines. **B,** The axial cross-table view of the proximal femur is taken with a 45-degree angle and the contralateral hip flexed. **C,** The false profile of the hip is taken with the patient standing. The index hip is in contact with the radiographic table, the patient is rotated 25 degrees backward, and the long axis of the foot remains parallel with the x-ray table.

This image is taken with the patient in the supine position with the contralateral hip flexed and the ipsilateral leg internally rotated (Figure 3-4, *B*). Again, the film-focus distance is 1.2 m, and the central beam is directed to the inguinal fold with an angle of 45 degrees. As an alternative to this view, a Dunn-Rippstein view or a frog-leg lateral radiograph may be obtained.

### False Profile

The false profile of the hip is taken with the patient standing (Figure 3-4, *C*). The index hip is in contact with the radiographic table, and the patient is rotated 25 degrees backward while the long axis of the foot remains parallel with the x-ray table. This view is used to quantify anterior acetabular coverage, the narrowing of the joint space posteroinferiorly or anterosuperiorly, and the decentration of the femoral head into the defect.

### Abduction View

The abduction view is an analogous view to the AP pelvic radiograph, with the patient's legs positioned in approximately 20 degrees of abduction and with the internal rotation of both legs. This view is used to simulate the appearance—particularly the congruency—of the hip after a planned hip reorientation osteotomy (Figure 3-5).

## RADIOGRAPHIC PARAMETERS

When evaluating conventional radiographs, the following features have to be evaluated: acetabular depth; acetabular coverage; the sphericity of the femoral head; joint incongruency; and additional findings (Table 3-1).

### Acetabular Depth

Acetabular depth is important to evaluate, because it is often correlated with an increased acetabular coverage that can lead to symptomatic pincer FAI. A normal depth is defined as the acetabular fossa being lateral to the ilioischial line (Figures 3-6, *A*, and 3-7, *left*; see Table 3-1). A coxa profunda is characterized as the acetabular fossa touching or crossing the ilioischial line (Figures 3-6, *B*, and 3-7, *middle*). In a protrusio acetabuli, which represents the deepest form of acetabular depth, the even

femoral head crosses the ilioischial line (Figures 3-6, *C*, and 3-7, *right*). These joint configurations are primary pathologies and should not be mixed up with secondary acetabular protrusion in patients with end-stage osteoarthritis.

Care must be taken if an AP view of the hip (rather than the entire pelvis) is evaluated. Here, because of the particular x-ray beam centering, a false-positive coxa profunda can be created with a normal-appearing AP radiograph that is centered over the entire pelvis (see Figure 3-3). The only quantitative parameter that describes acetabular depth is the ACM angle (Figure 3-6, *D*; values given in Table 3-1). This view is rarely used in daily clinical practice.

### Acetabular Coverage

Acetabular coverage has to be judged laterally, anteriorly, posteriorly, and in relation to each other.

Lateral coverage can be characterized by the lateral center edge (LCE) angle, the acetabular index, and the extrusion index (values given in Table 3-1). Normally, the LCE angle varies between 25 degrees, which defines a deficient acetabular coverage, and 39 degrees, which defines excessive coverage (Figure 3-6, *E*).

The acetabular index, which is also called the *acetabular roof angle*, is formed by a horizontal line and a line through the medial edge of the sclerotic zone and the lateral edge of the acetabulum (Figure 3-6, *F*). In patients with hips with coxa profunda or protrusio acetabuli, this index is typically 0 degrees, or it may even be negative (see Figures 3-6, *C*, and 3-7, *B*). The femoral head extrusion index is defined as the horizontal portion of the femoral head in a horizontal direction that is uncovered by the acetabulum (Figure 3-6, *G*). Although there is a maximum extrusion of 25%, which indicates dysplasia, no study has defined a minimum extrusion index.

Anterior coverage can be quantified on a false-profile view. The anterior center edge angle (Figure 3-6, *H*) is used for quantification. It is regarded as normal when it is more than 25 degrees, as borderline when it is between 20 and 25 degrees, and as pathological when it is less than 20 degrees.

The posterior acetabular rim is judged on the AP pelvic radiograph. A deficient posterior rim is present when its projected line runs medial to the femoral head center (i.e., posterior wall sign; Figure 3-6, *J*).

The relationship between anterior and posterior coverage is judged by carefully tracing the anterior and posterior acetabular rim on the AP pelvic radiograph. In a patient with normal hip morphology, the posterior rim typically lies laterally to the anterior rim. In addition, the posterior rim runs

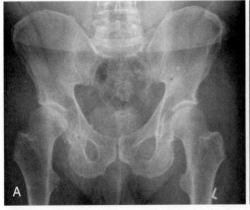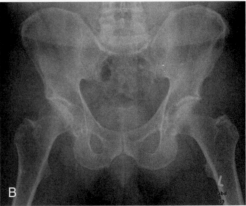

**Figure 3–5** The abduction view is used for patients with developmental dysplasia of the hip for the detection of joint congruency after acetabular reorientation procedures and to simulate postoperative coverage. **A,** Preoperative anteroposterior pelvic radiograph with an incongruent hip joint on the right and a congruent hip joint on the left side. **B,** Abduction/internal rotation view. A persistent joint incongruency is visible on the right side, which represents a relative contraindication for joint-preserving surgery.

## Table 3-1 DEFINITIONS OF RELEVANT HIP PARAMETERS

| Category | Parameter | Radiograph | Definition |
|---|---|---|---|
| Depth | Coxa profunda | Anteroposterior pelvic | The floor of the fossa acetabuli touches the ilioischial line |
| | Protrusio acetabuli | Anteroposterior pelvic | The femoral head overlaps the ilioischial line medially |
| | ACM angle | Anteroposterior pelvic | The angle formed by a line through the middle between the lateral (E) and inferior acetabular edge and the deepest acetabular point (P) and a line through (P) and (E) |
| Coverage | Extrusion index | Anteroposterior pelvic | The ratio of the uncovered femoral head part to the total femoral head width |
| | Lateral center edge angle | Anteroposterior pelvic | The angle formed by a vertical line and a line through the center of the head and the lateral acetabular edge on an anteroposterior pelvic radiograph; a lateral center edge angle of less than 20 degrees indicates dysplasia |
| | Acetabular index | Anteroposterior pelvic | The angle formed by a horizontal line and a line through the medial and lateral acetabular edge |
| | Acetabular retroversion | Anteroposterior pelvic | The anterior wall crosses the posterior wall |
| | Anterior center edge angle | False profile | The angle formed by a vertical line and a line that connects the center of the femoral head with the anterior portion of the acetabular roof |
| | Posterior wall sign | Anteroposterior pelvic | The posterior wall sign is negative if the posterior wall runs laterally to the femoral head center |
| | Sharp angle | Anteroposterior pelvic | The angle between a horizontal line and a line that connects the acetabular teardrop with the lateral edge of the acetabular roof |
| | Ischial spine sign | Anteroposterior pelvic | The ischial spine protrudes into the true pelvis; this is an indicator of acetabular retroversion |
| Sphericity | Alpha angle | Cross-table lateral view | The angle formed by the femoral neck axis and a line that connects the center of the femoral head with the point of beginning asphericity |
| | Offset | Cross-table lateral view | The difference in radius between the anterior femoral head and the anterior femoral neck |
| | Offset ratio | Cross-table lateral view | The ratio between the anterior offset and the diameter of the head |
| | Triangular index | Anteroposterior pelvic | The triangular index is positive if $R > r + 2$ mm |
| Joint Congruency | Integrity of the Shenton line | Anteroposterior pelvic | The radiographic line formed by the top of the obturator foramen and the inner side of the neck of the femur; this is an indicator of subluxation of the joint |
| | Lateralization of the femoral head | Anteroposterior pelvic | The shortest distance between the medial aspect of the femoral head and the ilioischial line |
| Additional Findings | Centrum collum diaphyseal angle | Anteroposterior pelvic | The angle formed by the femoral head–neck axis and the femoral shaft axis |
| | Fovea alta | Anteroposterior pelvic | The cranial edge of the fovea is in contact with the weight-bearing zone |

A scheme that describes each parameter is given in Figure 3–6.

more vertically (see Figure 3-6, *J*). Sometimes, distinguishing between the two portions of the acetabular rim can be difficult. The posterior rim line can always be readily identified when starting from the inferior edge of the acetabulum. A too-prominent anterior acetabular rim is present when its projected line runs laterally to the posterior line in the cranial portion of the acetabulum, thus causing a "figure-of-8" sign (Figures 3-6, *J*, and 3-8, *A*). This relative anterior overcoverage can cause the pincer type of FAI, and it is occasionally seen in hips with DDH. Because it is assumed that the entire affected inferior hemipelvis is rotated, these "retroverted" hips usually show an ischial spine that protrudes into the true pelvis (i.e., ischial spine sign; Figure 3-6, *K*).

Care has to be taken with regard to the interpretation of the projected acetabular rim, because it strongly depends on the position of the pelvis on the x-ray table. An acetabular retroversion can be created by an increased pelvic tilt or rotation to the ipsilateral side of the patient (Figure 3-9). Similarly, other radiographic parameters (e.g., the LCE angle) can substantially change with different pelvic orientations (Figure 3-10). Neutral pelvic rotation around the longitudinal axis is a given when the tip of the coccyx points toward the middle of the symphysis. As an indicator of neutral pelvic tilt, the distance between the upper border of the symphysis and the middle of the sacrococcygeal joint should be 3.2 cm ± 1 cm for men and 4.7 cm ± 1 cm for women. To accurately determine the individual pelvic tilt of the patient, a strong

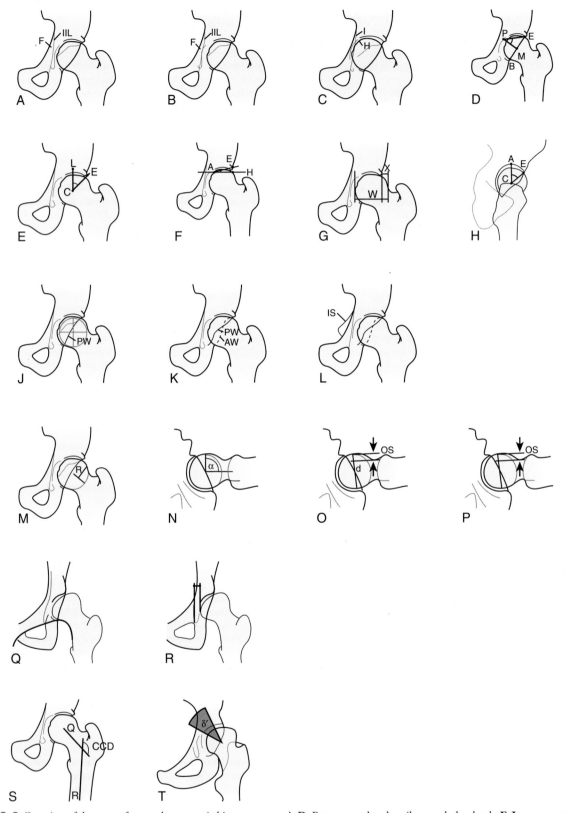

**Figure 3–6** Overview of the most often used coxometric hip parameters. **A-D,** Parameters that describe acetabular depth; **E-L,** parameters that describe acetabular coverage; **M-P,** parameters that describe femoral asphericity; **Q,R,** parameters that describe joint congruency; **S,T,** additional findings.

lateral pelvic radiograph is very useful (Figure 3-11). A neutral pelvic tilt is defined by 60 degrees of pelvic inclination, which is determined by a horizontal line and a line that connects the symphysis with the sacral promontory (see Figure 3-11). Specific software called *Hip²Norm* is available to correct the individual acetabular morphology to a standardized neutral orientation (see Figure 3-11); this will allow for differences between anatomic and functional differences in acetabular pathomorphology. The further use of this software in clinical practice is currently being evaluated.

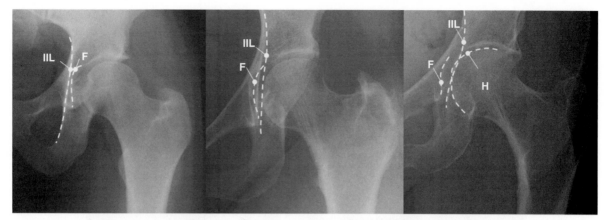

**Figure 3–7** Evaluation of acetabular depth. **Left,** Normal acetabular depth with the acetabular fossa *(F)* lying lateral to the ilioischial line *(IIL)*. **Middle,** With a coxa profunda, the acetabular fossa is touching or overlying the ilioischial line. **Right,** With a protrusio acetabuli, even the femoral head is touching the ilioischial line.

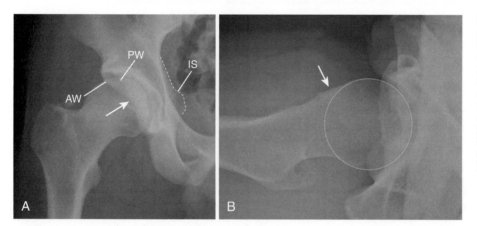

**Figure 3–8** A 27-year-old male patient with mixed femoroacetabular impingement. The figures show images of the hip taken from an anteroposterior pelvic radiograph. **A,** An acetabular retroversion is seen with the projected anterior acetabular wall *(AW)* crossing *(arrow)* the posterior wall *(PW)*. As an indirect sign, the ischial spine *(IS)* protrudes into the true pelvis. **B,** The axial cross-table view shows a typical aspherical anterior femoral head–neck junction.

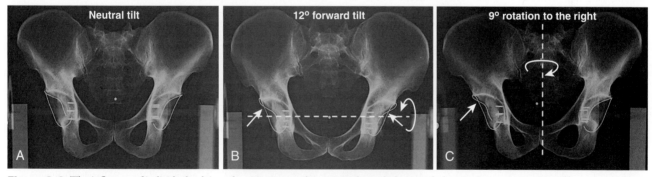

**Figure 3–9** The influence of individual pelvic malpositioning on the projected acetabular morphology is shown. **A,** In a hip with a normal tilt, no retroversion is visible. **B,** In a hip with increased pelvic tilt, a crossover can be created. **C,** The same effect can be obtained with an ipsilateral rotation around the longitudinal axis.

## Sphericity of the Femoral Head

The assessment of sphericity of the femoral head is important because it can lead to the symptomatic cam type of FAI. A nonspherical, oval-shaped femoral head is often seen in the hips of patients with DDH, and this is routinely treated with an intraoperative capsulotomy and osteochondroplasty during acetabular reorientation procedures. Head asphericity may become especially clinically relevant when it is located in the lateral or anterior aspect of the femoral head–neck junction.

Lateral asphericity is also called the *pistol grip deformity*, and it can be quantified with the triangular index (see Figure 3-6, *L*;

see Table 3-1). Therefore, on the femoral neck axis, half of the radius $r$ of the femoral head is measured, and a perpendicular line is drawn. A new radius $R$ is defined as the distance between the femoral head center and the intersection point of the perpendicular line with the superior femoral head–neck contour. It is considered to be pathological if $R \geq r + 2$ mm (with an estimated magnification of 1.2).

Anterior asphericity is clinically relevant in end-range flexion and internal rotation because it can cause the cam type of FAI. It is invisible on an AP pelvic radiograph, and it can be better visualized on a lateral cross-table projection. Three parameters are measured for assessment: the alpha angle, the

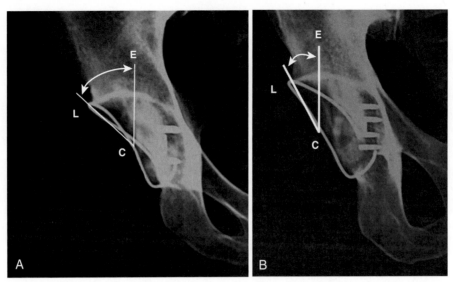

**Figure 3–10** The influence of pelvic tilting on the lateral center edge *(LCE)* angle is shown. **A,** X-ray of a cadaver pelvis with a wire-marked acetabular rim in a neutral pelvic orientation. The LCE angle is 28 degrees. **B,** With excessive pelvic tilt, the same pelvis shows an LCE angle of 48 degrees. A retroversion with a positive ischial spine sign is created.

femoral offset, and the femoral offset ratio. The alpha angle is formed by the femoral neck axis and a line that connects the femoral head center with the point of beginning asphericity of the anterosuperior femoral head contour (Figure 3-6, *M*). An alpha angle that exceeds 50 degrees is an indicator of an abnormally shaped femoral head–neck contour. The anterior offset is defined as the difference in radius between the anterior femoral head and the anterior femoral neck (Figure 3-6, *N*). In asymptomatic hips, the anterior offset is 11.6 mm ± 0.7 mm; hips with cam impingement have a decreased anterior offset of 7.2 mm ± 0.7 mm. The offset ratio is defined as the ratio between the anterior offset and the diameter of the head (Figure 3-6, *O*). It is 0.21 ± 0.03 in asymptomatic patients and 0.13 ± 0.05 in patients with hips with relevant asphericity that causes the cam type of FAI.

The triangular index has a better reproducibility than the alpha angle because it is defined by clearer geometric landmarks, whereas the alpha angle can sometimes be difficult to pinpoint. In addition, the triangular index is more independent of femoral rotation.

### Joint Incongruency

Joint congruency is difficult to assess, and it is more relevant in patients with DDH than in those with FAI. Because there are no parameters that describe the three-dimensional incongruency of the joint rotation centers, joint congruency can only be assessed indirectly by the degree of joint subluxation. Subluxation in the vertical direction can be objectified with the intactness of the Shenton line, which consists of the medial border of the femoral head and the superior border of the obturator foramen (see Figures 3-6, *P*, and 3-12, *C*). Subluxation of the femoral head in the horizontal direction can be measured as the shortest distance between the medial aspect of the femoral head and the ilioischial line (see Figure 3-6, *Q*).

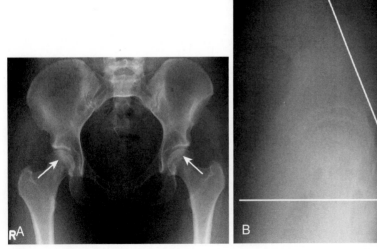

**Figure 3–11 A,** An anteroposterior pelvic radiograph of a 26-year-old patient that shows a bilateral acetabular retroversion. **B,** The strong pelvic lateral radiograph shows an increased pelvic inclination of 69 degrees. **C,** After computerized correction to the neutral pelvic orientation of 60 degrees of pelvic inclination with Hip²Norm software (University of Bern, Switzerland), a more or less normal acetabular configuration without a crossover sign is present.

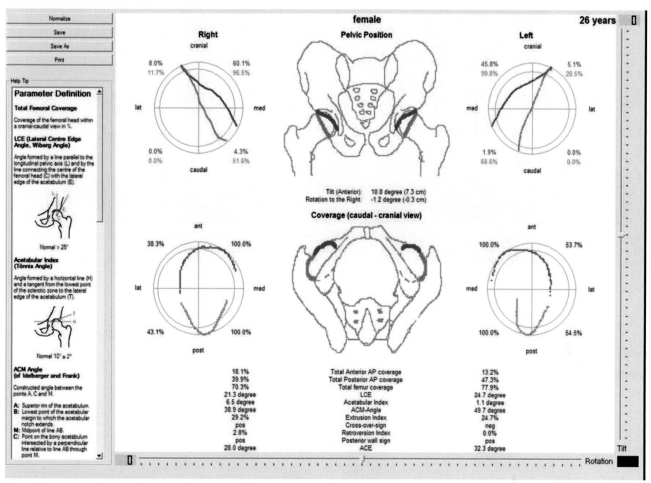

**Figure 3–11 —cont'd**

## Additional Findings

The centrum collum diaphyseal angle is different in patients with hips with dysplasia as compared with those with impingement (see Figure 3-6, *R*). Hips with the global pincer type of FAI (i.e., coxa profunda, protrusion acetabuli) often have a varus type of morphology (Figure 3-12, *A*). In these hips, the horizontal line through to the tip of the greater trochanter runs cranial to the center of the femoral head. In a normal hip, the horizontal line runs approximately through the joint center (Figure 3-12, *B*). Patients with DDH frequently present with a valgus configuration of the proximal femur (Figure 3-12, *C*), which is defined as when the horizontal trochanteric line lies inferior to the head center. Subsequently, the fovea capitis femoris lies more cranial than it does in the normal hip morphology (see Figure 3-12, *C*). This so-called fovea alta can further reduce the weight-bearing zone between cartilaginous joint surfaces, thus causing the condition to worsen and leading to the early degeneration of the joint.

## OVERVIEW OF RADIOGRAPHIC PARAMETERS

Table 3-2 gives an overview of the described characteristic individual radiographic parameters for hips with a normal configuration, DDH, and the two types of FAIs (i.e., cam and pincer). Each hip is unique, and allocation to one of the pathologies will be difficult, because there is often a mixture of pathomorphologies that may even lead to segmental undercoverage and overcoverage in the same hip. For example, a hip with a lateral undercoverage can present with an acetabular retroversion that indicates a relative anterior overcoverage (Figure 3-13).

Care has to be taken when interpreting radiographs when a patient's pelvis is in extreme pelvic tilt or rotation to either side. In this case, the correct diagnosis is only possible if a positive correlation among symptoms, physical findings on examination, and additional imaging means are present.

## SECONDARY CHANGES OF EARLY HIP OSTEOARTHRITIS

Repetitive irritation in unrecognized FAI leads to reactive ossification of the labral basis (Figure 3-14, *A*); this can be seen as a double contour of one of the projected acetabular rims. Typically, it is well visible on the superolateral edge of the acetabulum, because the x-ray beams hit the labrum tangentially. Although significant and irreversible damage of the cartilage may already be present, there is no joint space narrowing, because only the quality of the cartilage—not its diameter—is impaired during the early stage of the disease. Classic radiographic signs of osteoarthritis only occur late; these indicate an already advanced joint degeneration, which is a relative contraindication for joint-preserving surgery.

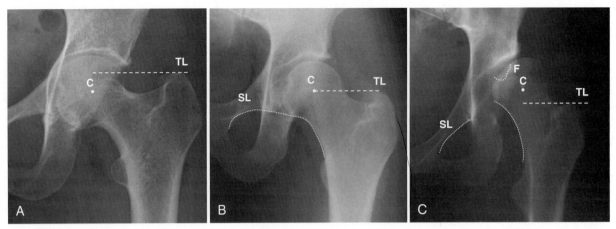

**Figure 3–12** The trochanteric line *(TL)* runs inferior to the femoral head center *(C)*. This leads to a fovea alta *(F)*, which is in contact with the weight-bearing zone of the acetabulum. If a subluxation is present, the Shenton line *(SL)* is interrupted. **A,** In a hip with the pincer type of femoroacetabular impingement, more varus configurations are seen. As a result, the trochanteric line runs cranial to the femoral head center. **B,** In a normal hip, the Shenton line is intact, and the trochanteric line runs approximately through the femoral head center. **C,** Dysplastic hips typically have a coxa valga.

## Table 3–2 NORMAL AND PATHOLOGIC VALUES OF ALL DESCRIBED RADIOGRAPHIC PARAMETERS

| Criteria | Normal | Hip Dysplasia | Pincer Impingement | Cam Impingement |
|---|---|---|---|---|
| Main cause | — | Undercoverage | Focal or general overcoverage | Aspherical head |
| Mechanism | Unrestricted range of motion | Overload stress | Linear contact between overcovering rim and head–neck junction | Jamming of the aspherical head portion into the acetabulum |
| **Depth** | | | | |
| Acetabular fossa | Normal | Normal | Coxa profunda or protrusio acetabuli | Normal depth |
| ACM angle | 39 to 51 degrees | <39 degrees | >51 degrees | >51 degrees |
| **Acetabular Coverage** | | | | |
| Extrusion index | 10% to 20% | >20% | <10% | <10% |
| Lateral center edge angle | 20 to 39 degrees | <20 degrees | >39 degrees | Normal |
| Acetabular index | 0 to 14 degrees | >14 degrees | <0 degrees | 0 to 14 degrees |
| Acetabular retroversion | No | Often | Often | No |
| Anterior center edge angle | >25 degrees | <20 degrees | Not described | Not described |
| Posterior wall sign | Not described | Not described | Positive with retroversion; negative with protrusio acetabuli | Normal |
| Sharp angle | 33 to 38 degrees | >47 degrees | Not described | Not described |
| Ischial spine sign | Negative | Not described | Positive with retroversion | Negative |
| **Sphericity** | | | | |
| Alpha angle | >50 degrees | Often >50 degrees | <50 degrees | >50 degrees |
| Offset | >10 mm | Not described | >10 mm | <8 mm |
| Offset ratio | <0.18 | Not described | >0.20 | <0.18 |
| Triangular index | Negative | Not described | Negative | Positive |
| **Joint Congruency** | | | | |
| Integrity of the Shenton line | Intact | Often interrupted | Intact | Intact |
| Lateralization of the femoral head | Not described | ~16 mm | Not described | Not described |
| **Additional Findings** | | | | |
| Centrum collum diaphyseal angle | 125 to 130 degrees | >135 degrees | <130 degrees | Not described; often seen in hips with coxa vara |
| Fovea alta | Not present | Present | Not described | Not described |

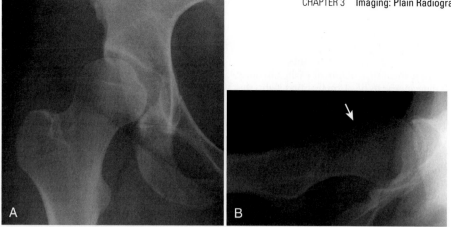

**Figure 3–13**  This section of an anteroposterior pelvic radiograph shows a mixed form of developmental dysplasia and femoroacetabular impingement. **A,** This 34-year-old male patient with a lateral undercoverage presents with relative anterior overcoverage (i.e., positive crossover sign, positive ischial spine sign). When an acetabular reorientation procedure is planned, the correction has to include an improvement of lateral coverage by abduction of the acetabular fragment in combination with an anteversion (i.e., internal rotation of the fragment). **B,** With the axial cross-table view, an aspherical portion is visible that can potentially cause the cam type of impingement after an acetabular reorientation procedure.

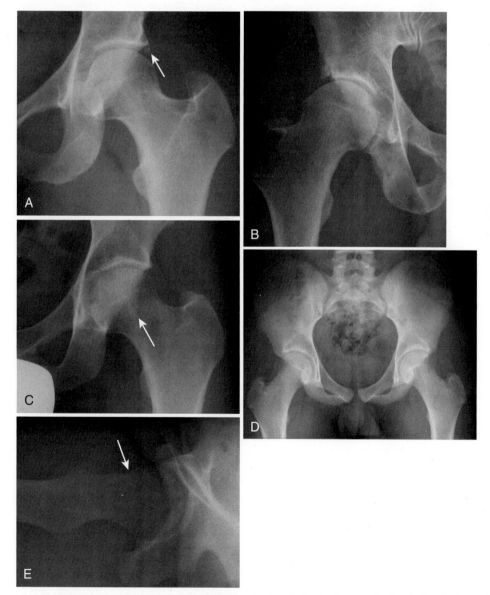

**Figure 3–14**  Secondary changes in hips with FAI. **A,** Labral ossification. **B,** Acetabular rim fracture. **C,** Herniation pit *(arrow)*. **D,** A 35-year-old patient with the pincer type of femoroacetabular impingement. **E,** As a result of the recurrent linear contact between the femoral head–neck junction and the excessive acetabular rim, an indentation sign is visible *(arrow)*.

The recurrent abutment against the acetabular rim by the aspherical portion of the femoral head can cause stress fractures of the acetabulum (Figure 3-14, *B*), especially in substantial retroverted acetabula. Because the initial judgment of the hip on an AP pelvic radiograph may appear to be normal at first sight, this damage pattern can eventually be misinterpreted as incidental os acetabuli. However, the presence of a radiodense structure at the edge of the acetabular roof must raise the suspicion of FAI.

Hips with FAI have a higher prevalence of herniation pits (Figure 3-14, *C*), which are initially thought to be benign. These present as radiolucencies that are surrounded by sclerotic margins and typically located in the anterosuperior quadrant of the femoral neck. They are thought to be intraosseous ganglia at the femoral zone of FAI. Therefore, hips with these juxta-articular cysts should be considered to be at risk for FAI. However, herniation pits are not always associated with symptomatic impingement.

Hips with the pincer type of FAI can present with an indentation on the lateral cross-table radiograph (Figure 3-14, *D* and *E*). This is the result of the recurrent linear contact between the excessive acetabular rim and the femoral head–neck junction.

## ANNOTATED REFERENCES

**Davies AM, Johnson K, Whitehouse RW:** *Imaging of the hip and the bony pelvis.* **New York: Springer, 2006.**

This book serves as a usefool reference for the acquisition and interpretation of different radiographic projections of the pelvis.

**Ganz R, Parvizi J, Beck M, Leunig M, Nötzli H, Siebenrock KA: Femoroacetabular impingement: a cause for osteoarthritis of the hip.** *Clin Orthop Relat Res.* **2003 Dec;(417):112–120.**

The first and the best overview on the pathomechanical and radiographical findings of femoroacetabular impingement.

**Murphy SB, Ganz R, Müller ME: The prognosis of untreated dysplasia of the hip. A study of radiographic factors that predict the outcome.** *J Bone Joint Surg.* **1995 July;77A(7):985–989.**

This classic article analyzes specific radiographic parameters in hip dysplasia and correlates them with their natural course.

**Tannast M, Siebenrock KA, Anderson SE: Femoroacetabular impingement: radiographic diagnosis—what the radiologist should know.** *AJR Am J Roentgenol.* **2007 Jun;188(6):1540–1552.**

This article gives an easy-to-understand but comprehensive overview of different aspects of femoroacetabular impingement.

# CHAPTER 4

# Magnetic Resonance Imaging of the Hip Joint

*Stefan Werlen, Tallal Charles Mamisch, Reinhold Ganz, and Michael Leunig*

## INTRODUCTION

For years, classic magnetic resonance imaging (MRI) has been performed in three planes to identify hip pathologies such as avascular necrosis, loose bodies, and labral pathologies. Recently, there has been a need for more information to help diagnose the early stages of osteoarthritis, which are not well visible on standard radiographs or with MRI. Magnetic resonance arthrography (MRA) of the hip has been used with increasing frequency to identify pathomorphologies of the hip such as femoroacetabular impingement (FAI) or developmental dysplasia of the hip (DDH). For these conditions, plain radiographs give insufficient information about cartilage, labral, and even osseous abnormalities. MRA has been used since 1992 at our institution for the visualization of the acetabular labrum and the articular cartilage, especially for patients with FAI and DDH. During the past decade, various modifications of our MRA technique have been implemented, and these have led to considerable improvements in our ability to visualize pathologic changes of the hip.

MRA is a minimally invasive method of assessing the extent of cartilage damage, which has numerous implications for both the surgeon and the patient. Knowing the extent of damage—particularly of the cartilage—is essential in helping the surgeon to determine the correct surgical strategy (i.e., to preserve or replace the joint). Moreover, it provides detailed preoperative information so that the surgeon can inform the patient about potential long-term outcomes of a surgical procedure. In this chapter, we explain our current technique of 1.5-T MRA of the hip, and we demonstrate some of the findings and their interpretations with regard to bone, cartilage, labral, and capsular tissue in patients with FAI. Given the fact that the current protocols of 1.5-T scanners have limitations, we will also present more recent technologic advances in MRI: 3 T[16] and dGEMRIC biochemical imaging of the hip.

## 1.5-T MORPHOLOGIC IMAGING

During the past 15 years, we examined approximately 3500 hips with the use of MRA. The MRA technique was constantly refined during this time. Our 1.5-T protocol is the result of a close collaboration between radiologists (SW) and surgeons (RG and ML).

### Examination Protocol

All patients are examined with the use of a Siemens Vision and Avanto 1.5-T, or Trio 3T high-field scanner (Erlangen, Germany). A flexible surface coil is used exclusively for high spatial resolution and signal-to-noise ratio. Before the MRA examination, all patients receive an intra-articular injection of 10 mL to 20 mL of saline-diluted Gd-DOTA 0.0025 mmolGd/mL (Artirem^R, Guerbert AG, Paris) into the hip joint with the use of fluoroscopic guidance. Patients are positioned supine under a C-arm, and the hip is placed slightly in external rotation to relax the anterior capsule. After the disinfection and sterile draping of the injection site, the injection is performed with a 22-gauge, spinal, obtuse-cut–angle needle, which helps to prevent injection into the capsular tissue or any extravasation. Between the injection and MR examination, a maximum time allowance of 10 minutes is preferred. The patients are then positioned supine, and the lower extremities are fixed with 20 degrees of internal rotation to prevent motion during scanning, to generate a standard version of the femoral neck, and to control the position of the pelvis.

After a short localizer in three planes, the examination continues with an axial T1-weighted sequence (repetition time [TR] 650, echo time [TE] 20, 200 mm × 200 mm field of view, 224 × 512 matrix, 4-mm section thickness with a 0.2-mm section gap, 17 slices, 3 minutes and 44 seconds). The sequence is centered on the femoral head, and it covers the whole joint (Figure 4-1).

The second sequence is an axial FLASH sequence with a few thin slices that is centered on the upper joint space. This sequence is used to evaluate the version of the acetabulum, and it also helps with the assessment for subcortical hypersclerosis of the rim as well as for the presence of synovial cysts (TR 550, TE 10, flip angle of 90 degrees, 120 mm × 120 mm field of view, 256 × 256 matrix, 2-mm section thickness with a 0.1-mm section gap, 11 slices, 3 minutes and 6 seconds; Figure 4-2).

Next is a coronal–oblique proton-density l–weighted (PDW) thin-slice sequence (TR 3200, TE 15, 120 mm × 120 mm field of view, 256 × 256 matrix, 2-mm section thickness with a 0.1-mm section gap, 23 slices, 5 minutes). This sequence is aligned perpendicular to the femoral neck, and it is marked on the axial T1W sequence (Figure 4-3).

A second PDW sequence in the sagittal direction (TR 3200, TE 15, 120 mm × 120 mm field of view, 256 × 256 matrix, 2-mm section thickness with a 0.2-mm section gap, 23 slices, 5 minutes and 37 seconds) is applied as the next step (Figure 4-4).

Finally, a radial PDW sequence (Figure 4-5) is used in which all slices are oriented basically orthogonal to the acetabular rim and labrum. This sequence is based on a sagittal oblique localizer, which is marked on the PDW coronal sequence, and it runs parallel with the sagittal oblique course of the acetabulum. The MRA imaging parameters are as follows: TR 2000, TE 15, 260 mm × 260 mm field of view, 266 × 512 matrix,

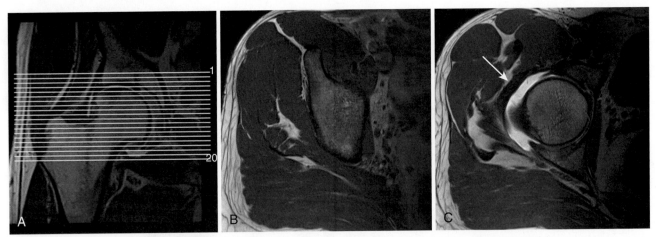

**Figure 4–1 A,** Coronal scout view showing the right hip joint. The white lines overlying the joint represent the slices of the transverse T1-weighted sequence. **B,** Transverse slice through the acetabulum just above the joint space. **C,** Transverse slice through the midsection of the joint. The white arrow shows the normal anterior joint capsule.

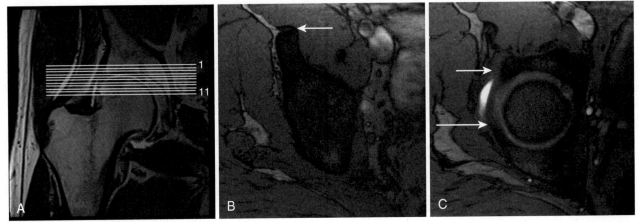

**Figure 4–2 A,** Coronal scout view showing the right hip joint. The white lines overlying the joint represent the slices of the transverse FLASH sequence. **B,** Transverse slice through the acetabulum just above the joint space. The white arrow points to the attachment of the rectus femoris tendon (pars recta) at the spina iliaca anterior inferior. **C,** Transverse slice through the uppermost part of the joint. The short white arrow points to the anterior acetabular rim; the long white arrow points to the posterior acetabular rim.

4-mm section thickness, 16 slices, 4 minutes and 43 seconds. In the center of the radial sequence, where the slices cross over, the signal wipes out. This produces a broad line without signal on the image, which affects the quality of the image. The more slices in a sequence, the broader the no-signal line gets. To reduce this artifact, this sequence is split into two sequences of eight slices each. The whole examination, including the hip injection, lasts about 50 to 60 minutes.

### Interpretation and Findings

There are numerous methods that address how best to interpret MR images of the hip. We prefer to look first at the bony structures, beginning with the acetabulum, and we then proceed to the soft-tissue structures.

#### Osseous structures

Normally, the acetabulum has an anteversion of between 14 and 26.5 degrees (men: 18.5 ± 4.5 degrees; women: 21.5 ± 5 degrees). To determine the version, we use the axial FLASH sequence with few but very thin (2-mm) slices. Because acetabular version in the cranial third of the acetabulum contributes

to the development of osteoarthritis of the hip, we measure the version at the superior portion of the acetabulum and use the first slice, where the anterior rim can be differentiated from the posterior. When a retroversion is present (e.g., in a conventional radiograph of the pelvis), the posterior acetabular rim lies laterally to the anterior rim at the uppermost part of the hip.

Further caudally, all acetabuli have an anteversion. The angle of version is measured and mentioned in the report. We then look for signs of hypersclerosis of the subchondral bone in the FLASH sequence but also in all other sequences as a very hypointense subcortical signal. If this is present, it is a sign of overload. We also note whether ganglia are present at the subchondral bone; this is also a sign of overload. These cyst formations are of various diameters, from a few millimeters to several centimeters. Because they contain fluid or synovia, they have a bright signal intensity in the FLASH and PDW sequences, and they are hypointense in the T1W sequence. They are mostly located at the superomedial area and next to the rim of the acetabulum. Occasionally, one can see a tiny channel of connection with the joint.

For patients with a local or global overcoverage, one can observe a bone apposition at the rim, often anterolaterally but also posteriorly, where impingement takes place. We believe

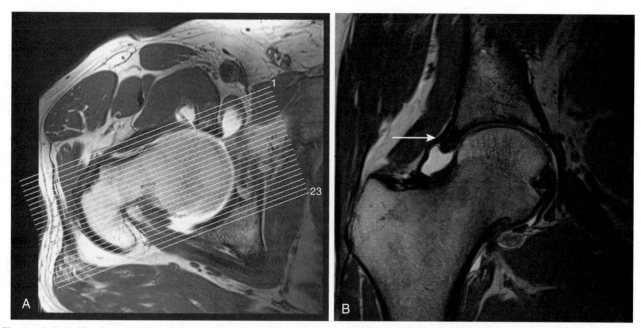

**Figure 4–3  A,** Slice from the T1-weighted transverse sequence as a localizer for the coronal-oblique PDW sequence. The white lines overlying the joint represent the coronal-oblique PDW sequence. **B,** Coronal-oblique slice through the midsection of the joint. The white arrow points at a slightly enlarged, hypointense lateral labrum.

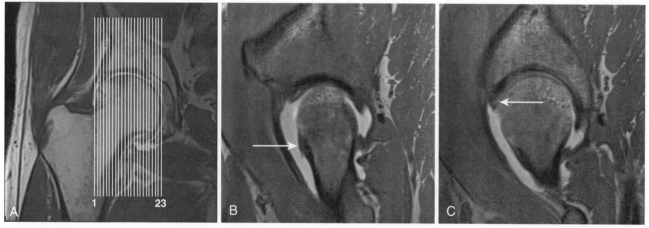

**Figure 4–4  A,** Coronal scout view showing the right hip joint. The white lines overlying the joint represent the slices of the sagittal PDW sequence. Sagittal slices through the hip joint showing **B,** a bony apposition at the femoral neck *(white arrow)*, and **C,** a torn labrum *(white arrow)*.

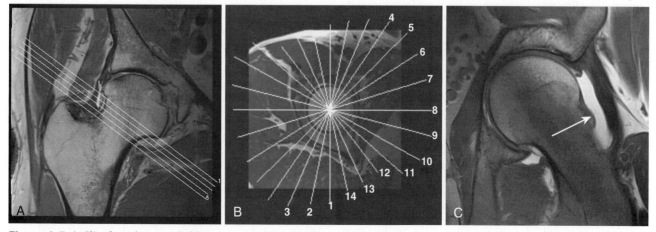

**Figure 4–5  A,** Slice from the coronal-oblique sequence. The white lines overlying the femoral neck represent the slices of the radial scout view plane. **B,** Radial scout view with overlying slices of the radial PDW sequence. **C,** Slice from the radial PDW sequence showing a secondary metaphyseal bump at the femoral neck, characteristic for pincer impingement *(white arrow)*.

that this is a bony reaction to repetitive microtrauma, and it can be seen on a standard radiograph as a double line. This "osteophyte" is obtuse or sharp at the edge, and it is broad based. The labrum becomes thinned in this area, and, in some cases, it fully disappears. The latter observation gives the false interpretation of an ossification of the labrum.

At the femoral head and neck, we first look at the shape of the neck and femoral head and also at the transition zone between head and neck. A normal femoral head is spherical in shape, and the neck is waisted or concave. In hips with cam FAI, several differently shaped femoral necks can be encountered. In some cases, there is an isolated bump that is localized to the anterolateral face of femoral neck, whereas other necks are circumferentially thicker throughout; in some cases, there is the pistol grip deformity as a result of a more laterally located lesion. In hips with pincer FAI, there is often concavity in the contour of the femoral neck, followed by a distal osseous bump. This is a reaction that is mostly located on the anterolateral cortex of the femoral neck.

Impingement cysts of the head–neck junction are closely related to site of maximal impingement. They are usually located anterior on the femoral neck, and they vary in size from 3 mm to more than 12 mm in length. Mostly they are seen as bright, fluid-filled, spheric lesions, but sometimes they are composed of fibrous tissue. In this case, they are hypointense in all sequences. In most cases, there is a hypersclerotic rim around the cyst.

### Cartilage

The zone of maximum acetabular articular damage is located at the anterosuperior rim near the labral attachment to the acetabular rim. In most cases of cam FAI, there is a small cartilage flap along the outer rim of the acetabulum. When these flap tears progress, the damage can be illustrated when contrast material gets between the acetabular cartilage and the subchondral bone. In advanced cases, the cartilage thins to the point of full-thickness ulceration, and this can extend toward the center of the acetabulum. With pincer FAI, there is also a cartilage abrasion posteroinferiorly; this is explained as a contrecoup lesion related to the leverage of the femoral head in that direction.

As the disease progresses, the cartilage of the femoral head becomes thin at the analogous site of impingement. The head then migrates into the acetabular defect. Later, the femoral disease progresses to the center of the head, near the fovea, with further flap tears of the femoral cartilage. These flap tears extend into sheets of cartilage that are separated from the bone and that can fill with contrast medium between the bone and the flap tear. Cartilage, which is separated from its bony base, will undergo malacic change and therefore change intensity to a brighter signal, whereas fresh flaps are hardly visible when the flap is reduced and pressed against the subchondral bone.

### Labrum

A normal labrum appears as a triangular structure with a low signal intensity. It attaches with a broad base to the acetabular rim and cartilage, and the border is distinct on all sides. At the incisura acetabuli, the ligamentum transversum replaces the rim. In patients with FAI, there are signal-intensity changes, with the labrum having higher intensity as a result of excessive edema. In a patients with cam impingement, an undersurface separation of the base of the labrum is commonly seen as a bright linear structure between the acetabular cartilage and the base. This is not really a labral tear but rather a rupture of the cartilage from the labrum. This tear pattern is partial thickness at this stage. Later, as the disease progresses, the tear may propagate to the bony rim, thus creating a full-thickness tear. This is typically seen in hips with DDH and FAI, although in cases of DDH the labrum is bigger than normal. The tear can also extend toward the tip of the labrum as a longitudinal tear, which is seen as a bright linear lesion from the base to the tip. Alternatively, with long-standing pincer FAI, the labrum is thinned from the base to the tip by bony apposition of the acetabular rim; this is seen as the signal intensity changes into bone marrow intensity, and it can be localized (anterior overcoverage) or generalized (coxa profunda).

Because of the high pressure in the joint as compared with the periarticular soft tissues, synovial fluid can be forced out through these tears, thus creating soft-tissue ganglia. In cases that involve longitudinal intralabral tears, intralabral ganglia can also occur.

### Joint capsule

In FAI cases that involve advanced involvement of the joint capsule, the capsule can be thickened with higher signal intensity. This process is felt to be the result of direct trauma from impingement between the acetabular rim and the femoral neck. Another cause may be an arthritic microenvironment in which tissue factors are released and contribute to capsular alterations. After the surgical treatment of FAI, scarring of the capsule to the anterolateral femoral neck has been observed; these adhesions may be a cause of continued symptoms. The adhesions are seen as string-like hypodense structures that are located between the capsule and the anterior femoral neck. These adhesions can best be seen after the administration of intra-articular contrast.

### Periarticular soft tissues

A bursa is commonly encountered around the iliopsoas tendon. In such cases, a connection between the joint and the iliopectineal bursa must be postulated. The bursal tissue is smooth and thin walled, and the cavity may fill with medium. In some cases, the thin bursal tissue bursts during the intra-articular injection of contrast medium. When this happens, most of the gadolinium flows out in the surrounding tissues. The bursae vary in extent from very small to very large; they can reach the extraperitoneal space in the pelvis.

## 3-T MORPHOLOGIC IMAGING

In addition to novel MR sequences, imaging quality can also be improved with the use of higher field strengths, because they provide a higher intrinsic signal-to-noise ratio, which is critical for high-resolution imaging. Two preliminary studies have been published about the use of 3-T imaging of the hip, which may help to improve the MR diagnostic accuracy of diagnosis with the use of high-resolution imaging. In addition, 3-T imaging may obviate the need for a contrast medium (Figure 4-6). The visualization of acetabular and femoral cartilage separation and the assessment of the acetabular labrum and adjacent cartilage—both of which are essential for an accurate diagnosis of FAI—can be improved with the use of high-resolution techniques. These advantages can also improve the usefulness of postoperative MR by monitoring cartilage integrity, which is a useful measure for evaluating surgical outcomes (Figure 4-7).

## 3-T ISOTROPIC IMAGING

Isotropic three-dimensional sequences may provide for the diagnosis and characterization of acetabular and femoral cartilage on the basis of their anatomic correlation with the acetabular version or the femoral head–neck offset. A more precise overview of the different 3-T techniques is described in the

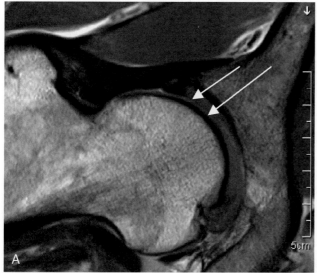

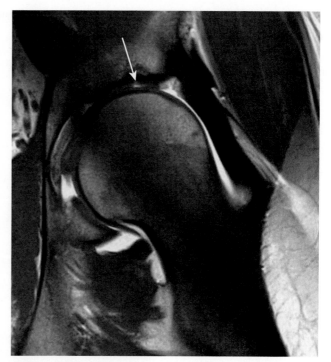

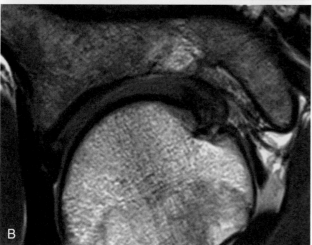

**Figure 4–7** Proton-density turbo spin-echo radial view of a patient with persisting hip pain 6 months after an arthroscopic labrum resection. Note the signal alteration within the acetabular cartilage (*white arrow*) showing a cartilage defect as a result of the insufficient correction of the femoroacetabular impingement.

**Figure 4–6 A,** Proton-density turbo spin-echo oblique coronal view. Note the separation of the femoral and acetabular cartilage (noncontrast) and the clear assessment of the acetabular labrum and the adjacent cartilage, represented by the thin black line between the two cartilage (gray) layers (*white arrows*). **B,** magnification of A rotated 90 degrees counterclockwise.

review article by Philipp Lang, Farimah Noorbakhsh, Hiroshi Yoshioka. Figure 4-8 is an image from a patient with a cam-type impingement and cartilage degeneration with multiplanar reconstruction around the femoral neck that was obtained with the use of a three-dimensional true fast imaging with steady precession (FISP) sequence.

## 3-T BIOCHEMICAL IMAGING

Another promising new technique is contrast-enhanced MRI, which is referred to as *dGEMRIC* or *delayed gadolinium-enhanced MRI of cartilage*. This technique is based on findings that glycosaminoglycans (GAGs) contribute a strong negative charge to the cartilage matrix. Therefore, if a negatively charged contrast agent (e.g., gadolinium–diethylenetriamine penta-acetic acid 2) is given time to distribute in the cartilage, it will distribute in inverse proportion to the GAG content. By means of gadolinium enhancement within the cartilage and subsequent T1 quantification, the T1 value can be used as an index for GAG concentration within the cartilage. Because

GAG seems to be lost early during cartilage degeneration, this technique may improve osteoarthritis diagnosis during the early stages. Despite promising results in patients with hip dysplasia, the described method is limited in the hip in terms of reproducibility and imaging planes, and it is additionally hindered by the requirement of additional sequences for the assessment of the acetabular labrum and the femoral head–neck junction morphology.

T2 mapping for biochemical imaging may be an alternative to the use of a contrast agent. T2 techniques make use of the T2 relaxation constant, which is affected by water–collagen interactions and, therefore, by water concentration, collagen concentration, and collagen alignment. In normal hyaline cartilage, there is a spatial variation of T2 with increasing values from the deep aspect to the superficial layer that are based on cartilage composition and structure within each layer. The influence of cartilage degeneration or alteration (e.g., cartilage repair tissue on the spatial T2 variation) has been investigated. The advantage of T2 mapping is that it does not require the use of a contrast agent. The drawbacks, however, are the nonspecificity of T2, as described previously, and the relatively long acquisition times required for the long echo trains needed for accurate T2 decay assessment (Figure 4-9).

## CONCLUSION

It has been shown that plain films are not as accurate as MR to assess the extent of intra-articular damage in patients with FAI. MRI can provide views of osseous and soft-tissue anatomy. Presently, MRI is the best available imaging tool for hip evaluation; however, it still has limitations for the diagnosis of cartilage and labrum lesions during the early stages of disease. In these cases, the relative thin cartilage, the spherical

**Figure 4–8** Isotropic three-dimensional true-fast imaging with steady-state precession (0.53 mm × 0.53 mm × 0.53 mm voxel size; TA (acquisition time), 7:32 minutes) of a patient with **A**, localizer slice perpendicular to the long femoral neck axis, showing the radial slice plan. **B**, **C**, and **D** are radial slices in different positions. Radial reconstruction was performed around the femoral neck to assess the femoral metaphysis morphology and the cartilage and labrum degeneration.

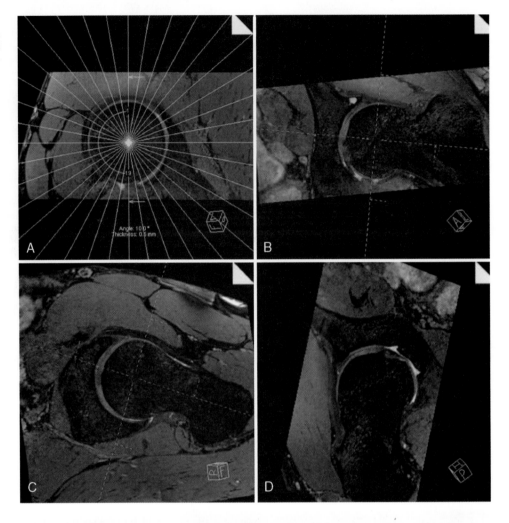

**Figure 4–9** Color-coded T2 relaxation times in the acetabular cartilage based on a three-dimensional gradient-recalled echo sequence with different echoes. Note the altered T2 values in the anterosuperior (**A**) and the anterior acetabulum (**B**, *cartilage damage more extensive*) in the expected area of femoroacetabular impingement.

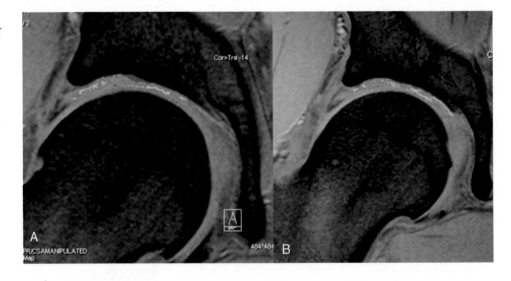

joint shape, and the narrowness of tissue structures pose logistical difficulties and demand high MR technology standards. So far, MR arthrography in combination with radially reconstructed planes is the method of choice for the assessment of FAI as a result of the improved detection of labral lesions. As compared with MR arthrography, the results of noncontrast techniques are less promising. In terms of cartilage evaluation, study results are still moderate, and the detection of cartilage delamination remains difficult. Recent developments in high-resolution isotropic imaging, cartilage-specific MR sequences, local gradient and radiofrequency coils, and high-field MR systems will improve diagnostic capabilities in terms of signal-to-noise ratio, contrast-to-noise ratio (CNR), shorter acquisition times, three-dimensional imaging, and the reduction of the need for a contrast agent. In addition to morphologic MRI, biochemical MR (i.e., dGEMRIC and T2 mapping) approaches that characterize cartilage microstructure and biochemical content will contribute to a better understanding of cartilage degeneration.

## ANNOTATED REFERENCES AND SUGGESTED READINGS

**Ganz R, Beck M, Leunig M, Nötzli H, Siebenrock H. Femoroacetabuläres impingement. In: Wirth CJ, Zichner L, eds. *Handbuch der Orthopädie*. Stuttgart, New York: Thieme; 2003.**

This is a complete review of the work on FAI from the Bern group, which summarized different articles. This article very well summarizes the image findings that occur with FAI on x-ray and MRI.

**Ganz R, Parvizi J, Beck M, Leunig M, Nötzli H, Siebenrock KA. Femoroacetabular impingement: a cause for osteoarthritis of the hip. *Clin Orthop Relat Res*. 2003;(417):112–120.**

This is the first overview manuscript by Ganz and colleagues about femoroacetabular impingement as a disease, and the significant image findings are described. This is a basic article to read to understand FAI in the context of our chapter.

**Ito K, Minka MA 2nd, Leunig M, Werlen S, Ganz R. Femoroacetabular impingement and the cam-effect. A MRI-based quantitative anatomical study of the femoral head-neck offset. *J Bone Joint Surg Br*. 2001;83(2):171–176.**

Ito and colleagues assessed morphologic changes seen on MRI from patients with CAM impingement. They described the measurement of the head–neck offset at different positions on the MRI and compared these measurements with those of volunteers. This is one method that was used with MRI for the diagnosis of FAI as described in our chapter.

**Jager M, Wild A, Westhoff B, Krauspe R. Femoroacetabular impingement caused by a femoral osseous head-neck bump deformity: clinical, radiological, and experimental results. *J Orthop Sci*. 2004;9(0):256–263.**

Jager and colleagues compared radiographic image findings before and after therapy with patient outcomes. This is one clinical study that addressed the value of image findings for patients with FAI.

**Kim YJ, Jaramillo D, Millis MB, Gray ML, Burstein D. Assessment of early osteoarthritis in hip dysplasia with delayed gadolinium-enhanced magnetic resonance imaging of cartilage. *J Bone Joint Surg Am*. 2003;85-A(10):1987–1992.**

This article was the first to describe the use of dGEMRIC for the assessment of early cartilage lesions of the hip joint. On the basis of these findings, the technique was found to be transferrable for clinical use for patients with FAI.

**Leunig M, Beck M, Kalhor M, Kim J, Werlen S, Ganz R. Fibrocystic changes at the anterosuperior femoral neck: prevalence in hips with femoroacetabular impingement. *Radiology*. 2005;236(1):237–246.**

Leunig and colleagues described the diagnosis of cystic formation in the femoral neck in patients with FAI. This added an additional factor to the MRI assessment of FAI, and it is therefore described in our chapter.

**Leunig M, Podeszwa D, Beck M, Werlen S, Ganz R. Magnetic resonance arthrography of labral disorders in hips with dysplasia and impingement. *Clin Orthop Relat Res*. 2004;(418):74–80.**

This is the first clinical article about the value of MRA as a standard technique for the assessment of labrum morphology in patients with hip impingement. This is basic information for understanding the techniques that we describe in this chapter.

**Leunig M, Werlen S, Ungersbock A, Ito K, Ganz R. Evaluation of the acetabular labrum by MR arthrography. *J Bone Joint Surg Br*. 1997;79(2):230–234.**

This article is important for understanding the value of MRA for imaging of the hip. It also provides a detailed description of the technique of MRA.

**Locher S, Werlen S, Leunig M, Ganz R. [Inadequate detectability of early stages of coxarthrosis with conventional roentgen images]. *Z Orthop Ihre Grenzgeb*. 2001;139(1):70–74.**

**Locher S, Werlen S, Leunig M, Ganz R. [MR-Arthrography with radial sequences for visualization of early hip pathology not visible on plain radiographs]. *Z Orthop Ihre Grenzgeb*. 2002;140(1):52–57.**

These two articles by Locher and colleagues describe in two consecutive steps the limitations of plain radiography for assessing hip-joint degeneration and the value of radial imaging of the hip joint with the use of MRI. Radial MRI is one of the most important parts of the Bern hip protocol described in this chapter.

**Murphy S, Tannast M, Kim YJ, Buly R, Millis MB. Debridement of the adult hip for femoroacetabular impingement: indications and preliminary clinical results. *Clin Orthop Relat Res*. 2004;(429):178–181.**

This articles describes FAI and summarizes the results of therapy. It demonstrates the value of the imaging methods described within this chapter.

**Philipp Lang, Farimah Noorbakhsh, Hiroshi Yoshioka. MR Imaging of Articular Cartilage: Current State and Recent Developments. *Radiol Clin N Am*. 2005;(43):629–639.**

**Recht MP, Goodwin DW, Winalski CS, White LM. MRI of articular cartilage: revisiting current status and future directions. *AJR Am J Roentgenol*. 2005;185(4):899–914.**

This is an overview of all of the current techniques that are used for cartilage imaging. This gives the reader a better understanding of the different techniques described in the chapter, and it also discusses possible future techniques.

**Reynolds D, Lucas J, Klaue K. Retroversion of the acetabulum. A cause of hip pain. *J Bone Joint Surg Br*. 1999;81(2):281–288.**

This article describes the role of retroversion. The MR assessment of retroversion is described within our chapter, and this article provides a good overview of the subject.

**Schmid MR, Notzli HP, Zanetti M, Wyss TF, Hodler J. Cartilage lesions in the hip: diagnostic effectiveness of MR arthrography. *Radiology*. 2003;226(2):382–386.**

This article describes the limited value of standard MRA for assessing early lesions of the cartilage in the hip. These findings led to the need for advanced imaging techniques, as described in this chapter.

**Siebenrock KA, Wahab KH, Werlen S, Kalhor M, Leunig M, Ganz R. Abnormal extension of the femoral head epiphysis as a cause of cam impingement. *Clin Orthop Relat Res*. 2004;(418):54–60.**

This article shows the value of measurements of the femoral epiphysis in patients with FAI. As the development of FAI becomes increasingly important, these measurements are needed to demonstrate the impact of epiphyseal development for patients with FAI.

**Smith HE, Mosher TJ, Dardzinski BJ, et al. Spatial variation in cartilage T2 of the knee. *J Magn Reson Imaging*. 2001;14(1):50–55.**

This is an article about the use of T2 for the assessment of cartilage. T2 mapping is a commonly used method for diagnosing cartilage issues of the knee, and it is currently being looked at for the diagnosis of hip cartilage problems. This article provides a background and better understanding of T2.

Sundberg TP, Toomayan GA, Major NM. Evaluation of the acetabular labrum at 3.0-T MR imaging compared with 1.5-T MR arthrography: preliminary experience. *Radiology.* 2006;238(2):706–711.

This article provides initial results of a comparison of high-field imaging with standard MRA. This is a future direction for the imaging of FAI, and 3-T imaging is discussed in this chapter. This article gives the reader some background information about high-field imaging.

Tanzer M, Noiseux N. Osseous abnormalities and early osteoarthritis: the role of hip impingement. *Clin Orthop Relat Res.* 2004;(429):170–177.

This article describes the osseous abnormalities and image findings in clients with FAI with hip pain and labral damages in three different patient groups. It gives the reader an overview of the clinical findings of hip arthroscopy as compared with the image findings described in this chapter.

Trattnig S, Marlovits S, Gebetsroither S, et al. Three dimensional delayed gadolinium-enhanced MRI of cartilage (dGEMRIC) for in vivo evaluation of reparative cartilage after matrix-associated autologous chondrocyte transplantation at 3.0T: preliminary results. *J Magn Reson Imaging.* 2007;26(4):974–982.

This article describes the three-dimensional dGEMRIC technique for the assessment of cartilage. This new technique enables the radial use of dGEMRIC in the hip joint to assess the cartilage damage pattern found in patients with FAI.

Wagner S, Hofstetter W, Chiquet M, et al. Early osteoarthritic changes of human femoral head cartilage subsequent to femoro-acetabular impingement. *Osteoarthritis Cartilage.* 2003;11(7):508–518.

This work correlates the imaging findings of the femoral head–neck offset with histologic findings. It also helps to identify the background of the femoral–head–neck abnormalities and therefore their signal presence on MRI.

Welsch, TC, Mamisch GH, Domayer SE, et al. Cartilage T2 assessment at 3-T MR imaging: in vivo differentiation of normal hyaline cartilage from reparative tissue after two cartilage repair procedures—initial experience. *Radiology.* 2008;247(1):154–161.

This article describes the initial results of the use of biochemical imaging techniques and T2 mapping for the comparison of different surgical therapy concepts of cartilage repair. These techniques could potentially also be used for therapy assessment among patients with FAI, and early image examples are shown.

Xia Y. Magic-angle effect in magnetic resonance imaging of articular cartilage: a review. *Invest Radiol.* 2000;35(10):602–621.

This article describes the limitations of the use of T2 mapping in the hip joint as a result of the magic-angle effect.

# CHAPTER 5

# Computed Tomography, Ultrasound, and Imaging-Guided Injections of the Hip

*Jon A. Jacobson*

## COMPUTED TOMOGRAPHY

There are many applications for imaging the hip with computed tomography (CT). Because CT is ideal for evaluating cortical bone, one common indication is the characterization of acetabular fractures. Another indication is the evaluation of the proximal femur and hip for causes of osseous impingement. In combination with intra-articular contrast, CT arthrography can also be used to diagnose labral and hyaline cartilage abnormalities. Other indications for CT of the hip include the evaluation of osteolysis after hip arthroplasty in the setting of particle disease, evaluation for osteoid osteoma, and evaluation for intra-articular bodies. Many of these applications are successful because of advances in CT technology. One of the key aspects of newer CT techniques is the ability to reformat axial images in any plane and to perform surface rendering, which is directly linked to improvements in CT technology.

### Computed Tomography Scanner Technology

The original CT scanners were introduced for clinical medical imaging in 1972. These first-generation CT scanners consisted of a gantry in which x-rays produced at one end traveled through the patient and then to a detector 180 degrees away, which would measure the amount of attenuation of the x-ray beam. The x-ray source and the detector would translate around the patient, and the information from this slice would be converted to a gray-scale, cross-sectional image with the use of a computerized filtered back projection. In this image, each pixel represented a measurement of the mean x-ray attenuation. Structures that attenuate x-rays more than water (i.e., cortical bone and muscle) will have positive CT numbers or Hounsfield units, whereas structures that attenuate x-rays less than water (i.e., air and fat) have negative CT Hounsfield units. High-attenuation structures would appear white whereas at the opposite end of the scale would appear black. The imaging of the patient would take up to 30 minutes as the patient moved through the gantry in a stepwise manner, 1 cm at a time, until the region of interest was imaged. The next-generation CT scanners increased the number of detectors in one row so that the x-ray beam fanned out from its source and hit multiple detectors at one time; this reduced imaging time. Additional improvements in 1989 included the spiral or helical scanning of the patient so that the patient would move continuously through the gantry; this again reduced imaging time. With this technique, a series of images could be obtained during the holding of a single breath.

The next generation of CT scanners then added rows of detectors; this technology is referred to as *multislice CT, multichannel CT,* or *multidetector CT* (MDCT). The initial MDCT scanners introduced in 1992 could image only two slices at the same time, but this number has since increased; currently available commercial scanners can image 64, 128, or even 256 rows or slices. There are several benefits of such MDCT scanners. One significant benefit is the markedly reduced time that it takes to acquire images; an entire extremity can be imaged with this type of CT with less than 1 minute of imaging time. Another benefit is that high x-ray tube current, which is measured as milliampere-seconds, can be achieved to allow imaging through metal hardware; however, this advantage is offset by the increased radiation dose required. Another significant benefit is that slice thicknesses of less than 1 mm are now attainable, which allows for high-resolution imaging and, more important, for high-resolution reformatted images in any plane.

### Two- and Three-Dimensional Reformatted Computed Tomography Images

Before the invention of MDCT scanners, the ability to reformat the original axial data set into other imaging planes was markedly limited. The resulting images were often distorted with a venetian-blind effect with steplike contours, and thus they were of limited diagnostic quality. With the advent of MDCT scanners, however, this has dramatically improved. The reason behind this is the concept of isotropic imaging. If a volume of tissue (i.e., a voxel) is imaged at a very small quantity such that the length, width, and height of the volume are equal, then a reformatted image retains high resolution as compared with the axial images (Figure 5-1, *A* and *B*). It is possible to obtain these images with the use of MDCT scanners with 16 or more detector rows that allow for a slice thickness of less than 1 mm. A standard protocol for the imaging of any extremity with CT is to reconstruct the original data at a slice thickness of less than 1 mm with 50% overlap of each slice and to then produce two-dimensional reformatted images 1- to 2-mm thick in the axial, sagittal, and coronal planes. MDCT scanners now have several options or tools that allow for three-dimensional reformatted imaging and surface rendering. At an independent workstation, these data can be manipulated to remove overlying soft tissues, osseous structures, or hardware and to produce a rotating volumetric data set (Figure 5-1, *C* and *D*).

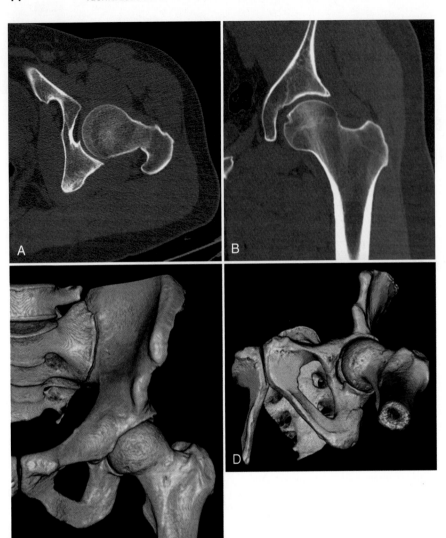

**Figure 5–1** Normal CT of the hip. **A,** Axial CT image. **B,** Coronal multiplanar reformatted CT image. **C** and **D,** Surface rendering three-dimensional CT images show a normal left hip.

## Radiation Exposure

Although imaging quality and resolution improve with the use of MDCT, one must understand that this is at the expense of radiation dose. The effective radiation dose takes into account the tissue being irradiated and the type of radiation, and it is measured in units of rem or sievert (Sv), with 100 rem being equal to 1 Sv. The effective patient dose for CT of the pelvis is approximately 3 mSv to 4 mSv. To put this into perspective, a single posteroanterior chest radiograph is approximately 0.02 mSv, and the average annual background radiation dose in the United States is 3.6 mSv. A statistically significant increase in cancer is seen among individuals who have been exposed to 50 mSv or more; this was determined on the basis of a study of atomic bomb survivors in Japan. The radiation dose from CT is not insignificant, and this becomes even more problematic in the patient who is young or potentially wants to bear children. As with any imaging study, the medical necessity of the test should be weighed against the risks of the examination.

## Femoroacetabular Impingement and Computed Tomography Arthrography

Impingement between the proximal femur and the acetabulum may be classified as cam type, pincer type, or mixed type. With the cam type of femoroacetabular impingement (FAI), a nonspheric femoral head with an abnormal contour of the femoral head–neck junction directly impinges on the acetabulum and labrum with flexion, adduction, and internal rotation of the hip. Proposed causes for this type of impingement include prior slipped capital femoral epiphysis, prior trauma, and growth disturbance with distortion of the physis. With the pincer type of FAI, there is abnormal contact between the acetabulum and the proximal femur from acetabular causes (e.g., retroversion, protrusio, acetabular rim prominence) or femoral causes (e.g., coxa magna, coxa profunda).

Many of the imaging features of FAI include bony abnormalities. Although magnetic resonance imaging (MRI) has also been used to demonstrate these findings, CT is well suited for characterizing bone abnormalities (Figure 5-2, *A*). With the

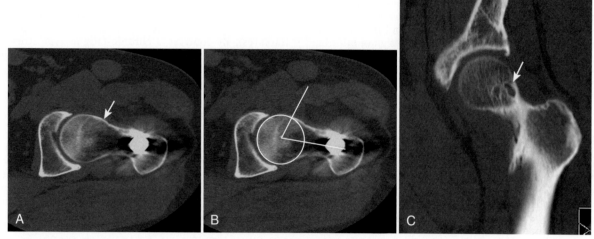

**Figure 5–2** Femoroacetabular impingement, cam type. **A,** Axial CT image shows abnormal contour *(arrow)* at the femoral head–neck junction. **B,** Abnormal alpha angle, which measures more than 55 degrees, and incidental proximal femur intramedullary nail. **C,** Coronal multiplanar reformatted CT image from a different patient shows cortical defects with sclerotic margins *(arrow).*

cam type of FAI, the abnormal contour at the femoral head–neck junction is measured as the alpha angle, which indicates where the bone contour of the femoral head extends beyond the confines of the femoral head. An angle of more than 55 degrees measured on a sagittal–oblique image parallel to the femoral neck is considered abnormal and correlates with the cam type of FAI (Figure 5-2, *B*). Other bony changes associated with the cam type of FAI are well demonstrated with CT, including fibrocystic changes at the anterosuperior femoral neck (Figure 5-2, *C*). Such fibrocystic changes are more common among patients with FAI, and they may be directly caused by impingement. CT has an advantage over radiography for showing such cortical changes. Other radiographic signs of the cam type of FAI, such as the abnormal contour of the femoral head–neck junction (pistol grip deformity), are also well delineated on CT, because patient positioning may not optimally profile the bone contour deformity.

With regard to CT of the pincer type of FAI, bony abnormalities such as acetabular protrusion (Figure 5-3) and acetabular retroversion may be demonstrated. When assessing for acetabular retroversion on radiography, the crossover sign (i.e., the anterior acetabular wall projects lateral to the posterior acetabular wall) may be affected by patient positioning. CT avoids this pitfall by directly measuring the acetabular version, which is described as 23 degrees in females (range, 10 to 37 degrees) and 17 degrees in males (range, 4 to 30 degrees). A retroverted acetabulum is associated with the pincer type of FAI and with hip osteoarthrosis. CT is also effective for measuring anterior and posterior acetabular sector angles in the setting of hip dysplasia.

One of the benefits of MRI and, more important, of MR arthrography for the assessment of FAI is that cartilage abnormalities may also be diagnosed in addition to the previously described bony abnormalities. Although the evaluation of the cartilaginous structures is limited with routine CT, the use of intra-articular iodinated contrast in conjunction with CT (or CT arthrography) can effectively diagnose labral and hyaline cartilage abnormalities, which are seen with FAI. With the use of isotropic imaging that can produce a submillimeter slice thickness, CT arthrography can diagnose a labral tear with 97% sensitivity, 87% specificity, and 92% accuracy. Similarly, CT arthrography can diagnose articular cartilage disorders with 88% sensitivity, 82% specificity, and 85% accuracy. In the setting of hip dysplasia, labral and hyaline cartilage abnormalities commonly coexist. The use of radial reformatted CT is also possible with submillimeter slice thicknesses and isotropic imaging.

## Hip Trauma

CT is often used to evaluate the hip and acetabulum after hip dislocation and other pelvic trauma (Figures 5-3 and 5-4). When an acetabular fracture is identified by radiography, CT can further characterize the fracture pattern with the use of multiplanar reformatted images and three-dimensional

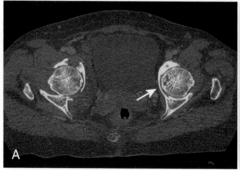

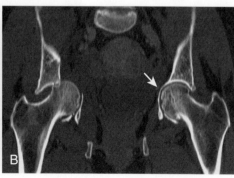

**Figure 5–3** Femoroacetabular impingement, pincer type. **A,** Axial and **B,** coronal multiplanar reformatted CT images show *(arrow)* left acetabular protrusio. Note the right acetabular fracture.

surface rendering (see Figure 5-3). Associated abnormalities such as intra-articular bodies and pelvic hematoma are also well demonstrated with CT. After hip dislocation, CT demonstrates the position of the femoral head and the coexisting femoral head fracture (see Figure 5-4, *A*). A sign of prior hip dislocation on CT is the presence of a bubble of gas, which is most commonly seen at the anterior aspect of the hip joint (see Figure 5-4, *B*).

It is important to understand the advantages and disadvantages of CT for the evaluation of fracture. CT is most accurate for demonstrating fractures of cortical bone (Figure 5-5, *A*). In an osteopenic patient in whom the cortex is thin, accuracy will decrease, especially when the fracture is not displaced. This becomes even more problematic for the diagnosis of an intramedullary fracture. In an osteopenic patient in whom the trabeculae are thin or resorbed, a fracture may not be apparent on CT. MRI has been shown to be more accurate than CT for the evaluation of proximal femur fractures in patients more than 50 years old where CT led to a misdiagnosis in 66% of patients. In addition, CT may not show the entire intramedullary extent of a presumed isolated greater trochanteric fracture.

As a general rule, CT is most effective for diagnosing fractures of cortical bone in younger patients, and it is relatively limited with regard to intramedullary fractures among the elderly (e.g., insufficiency-type stress fractures). By contrast, a chronic-fatigue–type stress fracture is well demonstrated with CT given the associated sclerosis (Figure 5-5, *B*).

## Hip Arthroplasty

Although radiography is the imaging method of choice for the routine evaluation of the hip after arthroplasty, CT does have a role in specific scenarios, such as the evaluation of infection, osteolysis, and component position. The technical advance that permits for the CT evaluation of metal with reduced artifact is MDCT, which allows increased x-ray tube current to image through metal. The individual components of an arthroplasty as well as the adjacent soft tissues and bone can be visualized with CT (Figure 5-6). This is helpful for displaying fracture (Figure 5-7) and for the diagnosis of soft-tissue infection adjacent to a prosthesis (Figure 5-8). In the presence of component wear

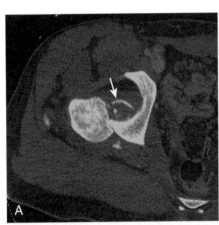
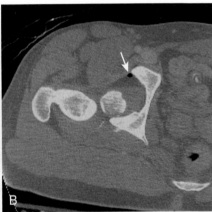

**Figure 5–4** Femoral head fracture and dislocation. **A,** Axial CT image shows a posterior dislocation of the right hip with a comminuted femoral head fracture *(arrow)*. **B,** Axial CT image with soft-tissue windows shows an air bubble *(arrow)* anterior to the hip joint.

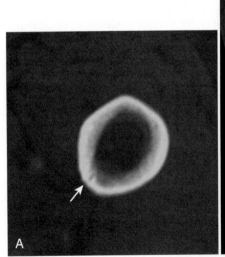
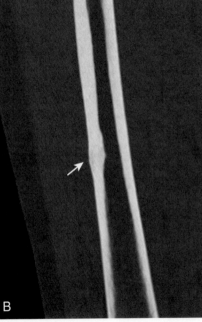

**Figure 5–5** Stress fracture, fatigue type. **A,** Axial CT image shows an acute cortical fracture as linear low attenuation *(arrow)*. **B,** Coronal multiplanar reformatted CT image from a different patient shows a chronic cortical fracture *(arrow)* as a linear low-attenuation fracture line and a thickened high-attenuation cortex.

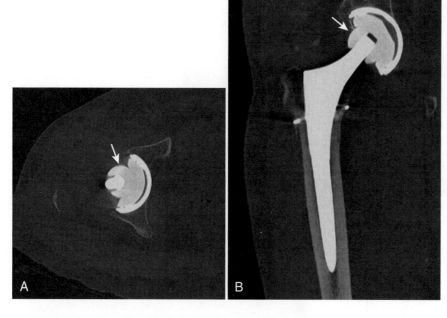

**Figure 5–6** Total hip arthroplasty, normal. **A,** Axial and **B,** coronal multiplanar reformatted CT images show a cementless total hip arthroplasty. Note the ceramic acetabular and femoral head *(arrow)* surfaces, which are lower in attenuation as compared with metal.

and particle disease, CT can directly show the polyethylene component wear as well as the adjacent osteolysis (Figure 5-9). Although radiography adequately screens for osteolysis, CT more accurately measures the volume of osteolysis. CT can also be used to measure component version after hip arthroplasty.

## Miscellaneous Hip Abnormalities

Other hip disorders that involve the bone or that produce calcification or ossification can be evaluated with CT. Primary synovial osteochondromatosis is a benign neoplastic condition in which hyaline cartilage nodules form in the subsynovial tissue of a single large joint. If these nodules ossify, they are readily demonstrated on CT as multiple uniform ossific bodies in the joint (Figure 5-10). Secondary osteoarthrosis and associated erosions may also be present. The hip is the second most common joint affected by this condition, after the knee.

Osteoid osteoma is a benign bone lesion of uncertain origin that involves a vascularized nidus being present within the bone, typically the cortex. When this occurs in an extra-articular location, the nidus is associated with significant sclerosis and periostitis (Figure 5-11). When it is intra-articular, there is associated effusion and synovitis. CT shows the nidus as a round area of low attenuation with surrounding sclerosis that may calcify. CT can be used to effectively guide the percutaneous thermoablation of osteoid osteomas.

CT may also be used to characterize other bone abnormalities. When a sclerotic focus is present within the bone, CT can show the uniform sclerotic density and spiculated margins that are typical of a bone island or enostosis (Figure 5-12). The calcified matrix of a chondroid tumor such as chondroblastoma or chondrosarcoma (Figure 5-13) or the ossified matrix of an osteosarcoma can be demonstrated with CT, which assists with the characterization of a primary bone tumor. CT is the typical imaging method used for the percutaneous imaging-guided biopsy of a bone tumor that involves the pelvis or the proximal femur.

## ULTRASOUND

The primary use of ultrasound in areas around the hip is for the evaluation of soft tissues (e.g., joint effusion, bursa, tendon). Ultrasound is most effective when an abnormality is superficial or when the patient does not have a large body habitus, because image resolution decreases with increased depth. In the hip region, ultrasound is therefore more accurate for children than for adults, especially when evaluating for abnormalities in the deep soft tissues. Advantages of ultrasound include dynamic imaging, evaluation around hardware, lack of radiation, the ability to compare the affected side with the contralateral side, and decreased cost as compared with MRI.

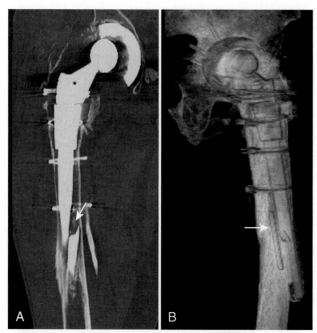

**Figure 5–7** Component failure, total hip arthroplasty revision. **A,** Coronal multiplanar reformatted CT image, and **B,** three-dimensional rendering with partially transparent bone and red-colored metal shows femoral component failure *(arrow)*.

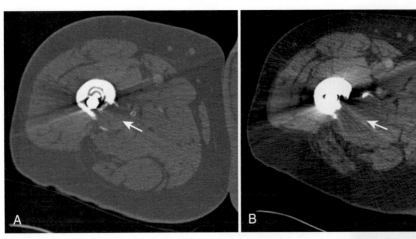

**Figure 5–8** Infection, total hip arthroplasty. Axial CT images after intravenous contrast in **A,** bone, and **B,** soft-tissue windows, show cortical destruction and adjacent soft-tissue fluid collection *(arrow)*.

## Ultrasound Technology

Ultrasound is a unique imaging method in that it does not involve ionizing radiation but rather makes use of sound waves to produce images. A sound wave is transmitted from the ultrasound transducer, which is placed on the skin surface with acoustic coupling

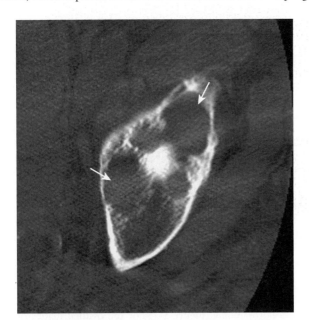

**Figure 5–9** Particle disease, total hip arthroplasty. Axial CT image in soft-tissue windows shows focal areas of bone lysis *(arrows)* of the acetabulum replaced with soft-tissue attenuation.

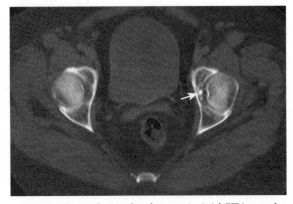

**Figure 5–10** Synovial osteochondromatosis. Axial CT image shows several ossified cartilaginous bodies *(arrow)*.

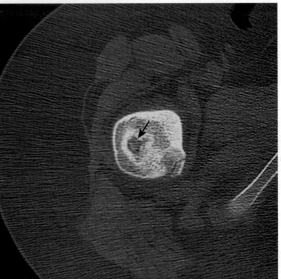

**Figure 5–11** Osteoid osteoma. Axial CT image shows a low-attenuation nidus *(arrow)* with partial calcification. Note the surrounding high-attenuation sclerosis.

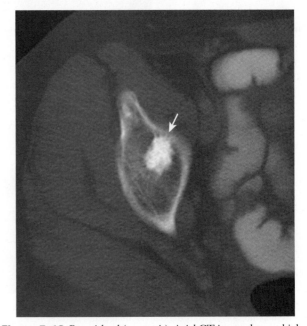

**Figure 5–12** Bone island (enostosis). Axial CT image shows a high-attenuation sclerotic focus with speculated margins *(arrow)*.

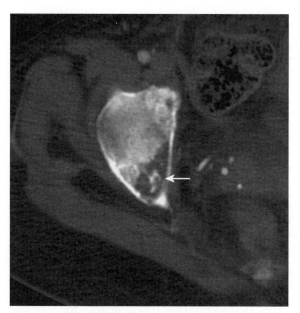

**Figure 5–13** Chondrosarcoma. Axial CT image shows low-attenuation bone destruction with a calcified matrix *(arrow)*.

gel. The sound wave propagates through the soft tissues, interacts at soft-tissue interfaces, and then returns to the transducer, where the sound waves are converted into an image. At interfaces where there is a significant difference in impedance, nearly all of the sound waves are reflected back to the transducer, which produces a bright echo that is displayed on the image. The echoes on the ultrasound image are described as hyperechoic (bright echo), isoechoic (equal echo), hypoechoic (low echo), or anechoic (no echo) as compared with the surrounding tissues. Cortical bone is hyperechoic with shadowing, tendon is hyperechoic and fibrillar, muscle is hypoechoic with interspersed hyperechoic fibroadipose septae, and simple fluid is anechoic. An important technical option on most ultrasound machines is color or power Doppler imaging, which shows blood flow as color on the ultrasound image.

## Joint Abnormalities

Ultrasound can be used to identify a hip effusion, which characteristically distends the anterior recess over the femoral neck (Figure 5-14). Joint effusion is diagnosed when there is 2 mm or more of fluid between the anterior capsule and posterior capsular reflection, when the hip capsule over the femoral neck measures 7 mm or more, or when there is a difference in distention of more than 1 mm as compared with the normal contralateral side. The collapsed joint recess with its capsular

reflection may measure up to 7 mm and appear to be hyperechoic, but this can appear hypoechoic if it is not imaged perpendicular to the ultrasound beam or if the patient is large. A simple effusion is anechoic, whereas complex fluid will appear to be hypoechoic with possible internal echoes. Synovitis is characterized by hypoechoic to variable echogenicity distention of the joint recess with possible increased flow on color or power Doppler imaging (Figure 5-15). Ultrasound cannot differentiate septic from aseptic effusion; therefore, aspiration should be considered when there is concern about infection. The accuracy of ultrasound for the diagnosis of hip effusion depends on the quantity of fluid and the size of the patient; ultrasound is very accurate in children and thin adults, whereas the diagnosis may be difficult in adults with a large body habitus. When screening for joint effusion, a negative ultrasound should be followed with a fluoroscopy-guided aspiration in a large patient when there is high clinical concern regarding infection. Although the anterior labrum can be visualized with ultrasound as a hyperechoic triangle-shaped structure, the diagnosis of labral tear is limited as a result of the thickness of the soft tissues over the labrum and the inability to visualize the entire labrum.

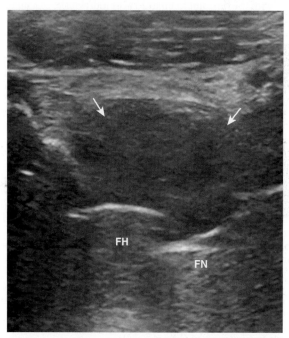

**Figure 5–15** Synovitis. Sagittal–oblique ultrasound image shows hypoechoic synovitis *(arrows)*. Note the reflective surface and artifact deep to the femoral head and neck of the total hip arthroplasty. The left side of the image is superior, and the right side is inferior. *FH,* Femoral head; *FN,* femoral neck.

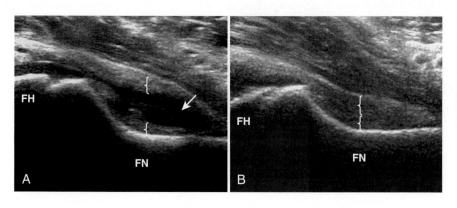

**Figure 5–14** Hip joint effusion. **A,** Sagittal–oblique ultrasound image parallel to the femoral neck shows anechoic joint fluid *(arrow)* in between the anterior capsule and the posterior capsular reflection *(braces)*. **B,** Normal contralateral hip joint with opposed capsule layers *(braces)*. In both images, the left side of the image is superior, and the right side is inferior. *FH,* femoral head; *FN,* femoral neck.

Ultrasound for the diagnosis of hip joint effusion after hip arthroplasty is more limited as compared with a native adult hip, likely as a result of postsurgical changes in the soft tissue and possible patient body habitus size. Although ultrasound may show a large effusion, a small effusion may be overlooked. A negative ultrasound should be followed with a fluoroscopic-guided hip joint aspiration if there is a high concern about infection. Ultrasound does have a significant role in the evaluation of infection after arthroplasty for evaluating the overlying soft tissues for abscess before fluoroscopic aspiration, thereby avoiding the passage of a needle through an occult abscess with resulting contamination of the joint. Ultrasound may also show bursae or other fluid collections that will not be visible during fluoroscopy (Figure 5-16). The region deep to a skin incision should be evaluated for postoperative fluid collection or abscess. The identification of soft-tissue fluid that extends from the hip joint suggests infection.

### Bursal Abnormalities

The iliopsoas bursa is located anterior to the hip and communicates with the hip joint in up to 15% of individuals; this number is increased in the presence of hip pathology. Distention of the iliopsoas bursa produces a characteristic shape that is concave lateral as it wraps around the iliopsoas tendon (Figure 5-17). Communication between the iliopsoas bursa and the hip joint can be demonstrated with imaging. Similar to the hip joint, the distention of the bursa may appear as anechoic simple fluid, mixed echogenicity complex fluid, and hypoechoic to variable echogenicity synovitis with possible flow on color or power Doppler imaging. A chronically distended iliopsoas bursa may enlarge significantly and extend cephalad into the abdomen. It is important in this situation to not mistake a large iliopsoas bursa for a psoas abscess.

There are three bursa that are located near the greater trochanter of the femur: the subgluteus minimus bursa (anterolaterally between the gluteus minimus and greater trochanter), the subgluteus medius bursa (laterally between the gluteus medius and the greater trochanter), and the trochanteric bursa (posterolaterally between the gluteus maximus and the greater trochanter with some extension over the gluteus medius). It is important to evaluate the circumference of the greater trochanter and to evaluate for the distention of these bursae between their respective tendons and the greater trochanter. As with the iliopsoas bursa, distention can range from anechoic to mixed echogenicity, depending on whether there is simple fluid, complex fluid, or synovitis distention (Figure 5-18).

### Muscle and Tendon Abnormalities

Muscle or tendon tear is characterized as the disruption of tendon fibers with anechoic or hypoechoic fluid or hemorrhage. The presence of tendon retraction suggests a full-thickness tear. By contrast, the hypoechoic thickening of a tendon without tendon fiber disruption is characteristic of tendinosis. If a tendon has a tendon sheath, the distention of the tendon sheath indicates tenosynovitis; similar to joint recess distention, this can range from anechoic to mixed echogenicity distention. Ultrasound is useful for the diagnosis of iliopsoas impingement from an adjacent hip arthroplasty, because prosthesis artifact occurs deep and away from the overlying soft tissues (Figure 5-19).

Ultrasound is well suited for evaluating for snapping tendon abnormalities around the hip given its dynamic capabilities, which allow for examination during hip or leg motion. Snapping hip syndrome represents a number of pathologies that cause painful snapping of the hip during motion. These conditions can be divided into internal (hip joint) and external (iliopsoas, iliotibial tract, or gluteus maximus) causes. With regard to the external causes, these relate to the abnormal snapping of a tendon or muscle during motion. Iliopsoas tendon snapping occurs when the leg is straightened from a frog-leg position, which causes the abrupt movement of the iliopsoas tendon in the region of the iliopectineal eminence of the ilium (Figure 5-20). Iliotibial tract or gluteus maximus snapping may occur over the greater trochanter with hip flexion and extension, and there will be abrupt snapping of the representative structure. In each situation, a palpable snap may be felt through the transducer, which corresponds with the abrupt motion of the structure during ultrasound and when the patient is experiencing symptoms. Ultrasound-guided injection may be used for treatment.

### Other Hip Abnormalities

Ultrasound has been used effectively for the evaluation for hip dysplasia, and it is accepted as a screening tool for this diagnosis. The ultrasound examination includes static images with measurements and various dynamic stress maneuvers similar to Barlow or Ortolani tests to demonstrate subluxation and dislocation. A newborn with abnormal clinical findings and an unstable hip has an ultrasound examination at 2 weeks of age, whereas one with abnormal clinical findings and a stable click will have ultrasound at 4 to 6 weeks of age. A newborn with normal clinical findings and the presence of risk factors will also

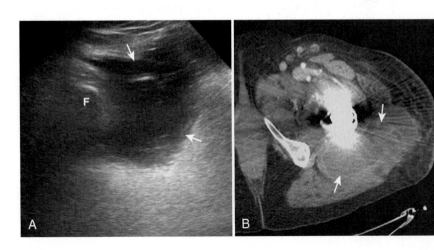

**Figure 5–16** Infection, total hip arthroplasty. **A,** Axial ultrasound image shows hypoechoic and heterogeneous fluid collection *(arrows)* adjacent to the femur. Note the bright artifact deep to the fluid collection. **B,** Corresponding CT image after intravenous contrast administration. *F,* Femur.

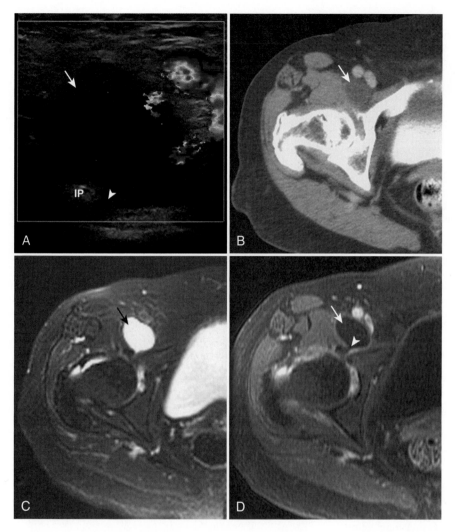

**Figure 5–17** Iliopsoas bursa. **A,** Axial color Doppler ultrasound image of right hip shows hypoechoic distention of the iliopsoas bursa *(arrow)*. Note the communication with the hip joint *(arrowhead)* medial to the iliopsoas tendon and the color flow in the adjacent femoral artery and vein. The iliopsoas bursa *(arrow)* is also shown on the following: **B,** corresponding axial CT image as low attenuation; **C,** T2-weighted axial MRI as high signal; and **D,** T1-weighted fat-saturation axial MRI after intravenous gadolinium administration as ring enhancement. Note the communication between the iliopsoas bursa and the hip joint *(arrowhead)*. *IP,* Iliopsoas tendon.

have an ultrasound at 4 to 6 weeks of age. The benefit of ultrasound is its ability to visualize the unossified epiphysis and to incorporate stress maneuvers. As the epiphysis ossifies, ultrasound becomes more limited for the evaluation for dysplasia as radiographs become more important.

Soft-tissue abscess and other fluid collections can be demonstrated with ultrasound in a way that is similar to what was described previously with regard to hip joint effusion and bursal

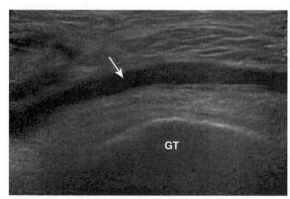

**Figure 5–18** Trochanteric bursitis. Axial ultrasound image shows anechoic distention of the trochanteric bursa *(arrow)* adjacent to the greater trochanter. *GT,* Greater trochanter.

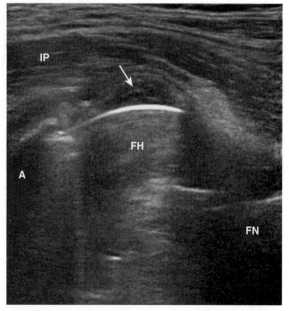

**Figure 5–19** Iliopsoas impingement after arthroplasty. Sagittal–oblique ultrasound image shows abnormal hypoechoic soft tissue *(arrow)* between the metal femoral head and the overlying iliopsoas. *A,* Acetabulum; *FH,* femoral head; *FN,* femoral neck; *IP,* iliopsoas.

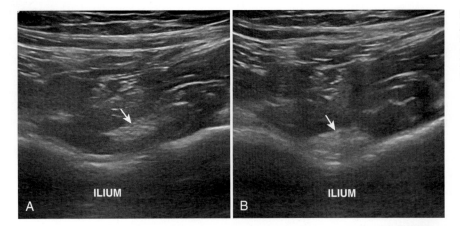

**Figure 5–20** Snapping iliopsoas tendon. Axial–oblique ultrasound images of left hip show abrupt movement of the iliopsoas tendon (*arrow*) when comparing **A** with **B.** The left side of each image is medial, and the right side is lateral.

fluid. The patient typically can indicate the area of concern, or signs and symptoms may help to localize the area to be imaged. The limitation of ultrasound is difficulty with screening large areas of soft tissue, especially when the pathology is located deep, where resolution will be lower. In addition, the involvement of adjacent bone may be overlooked. In the setting of a negative ultrasound examination, MRI is usually considered if there is high clinical concern for occult infection or other pathology.

## IMAGING-GUIDED INJECTIONS

Percutaneous imaging-guided injections may be diagnostic or therapeutic in nature, and they may be guided with fluoroscopy, CT, or ultrasound. Possible anatomic targets include the hip joint, a bursa, or the region around a tendon. Typically, any fluid present at the time of an injection is aspirated and sent for appropriate laboratory tests (i.e., Gram staining, culture and sensitivity, cell count and differential, and possible crystal analysis). An injection may consist of short- and long-acting anesthetic agents as well as corticosteroids or hyaluronate. The quantity of the injection depends on the capacity of the space being injected. The goal of a therapeutic injection is to relieve symptoms by reducing pain and inflammation. A diagnostic injection plays a role in determining the source of symptoms and in predicting whether the patient's symptoms will improve with surgical treatment. To that end, it is critical that the therapeutic injection is accurate. In addition, if fluoroscopy or CT guidance is used, it is important to combine the diagnostic or therapeutic agents with iodinated contrast so that any extension of the agents beyond the intended target is visualized and subsequently reported.

### Joint Injection

Percutaneous injection of the hip joint may be guided with fluoroscopy, CT, or ultrasound. The use of fluoroscopy is most common, and it can be completed in minutes with few complications. With the patient supine and oblique toward the opposite hip, the femoral artery is identified, and the skin directly over the femoral neck (lateral to the artery) is marked and prepared in typical sterile fashion. A 20-gauge spinal needle with a stylet is inserted into the femoral neck from an anterior or anterolateral approach. Needle-tip placement laterally near the femoral head–neck junction is usually successful, although any location along the femoral neck to the level of the intertrochanteric line is intra-articular (Figure 5-21). Because the needle tip may be located within the capsular reflection immediately

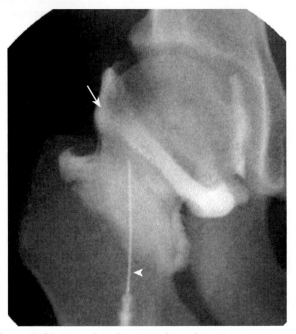

**Figure 5–21** Normal single-contrast hip arthrogram. Anteroposterior fluoroscopic image of the right hip shows high-attenuation iodinated contrast (*arrow*) distending the hip joint. Note the 20-gauge spinal needle (*arrowhead*).

adjacent to the bone, thus inhibiting low-resistance injection, minimal rotation of the needle or backing the needle out 1 mm during a test injection will assist with the finding of the joint recess. Before injecting the diagnostic or therapeutic agents, a test injection with iodinated contrast is used to confirm correct needle placement; the needle can then be repositioned as necessary with a repeat test injection of iodinated contrast. It is important to combine the diagnostic or therapeutic agents with iodinated contrast to visualize the structures that are being injected. The extension of diagnostic or therapeutic agents beyond the intended target (e.g., the filling of the iliopsoas bursa) must be reported. A diagnostic or therapeutic injection may be combined with dilute gadolinium for subsequent MR arthrography. The technique of hip injection with the use of CT is the same as described previously with the use fluoroscopy, in which a test injection of iodinated contrast is used before the injection of contrast with the diagnostic and therapeutic agents. CT is not typically used for hip injections, except for cases in which extensive heterotopic ossification may make fluoroscopic-guided injection difficult.

Ultrasound may also be used when injecting the hip joint. The benefit of ultrasound is the lack of ionizing radiation and the real-time visualization of the needle entering the hip joint with capsular distention during injection. Ultrasound guidance is most successful for smaller patients (i.e., resolution improves when imaging near the transducer) and when there is a sonographic target (e.g., a distention of the hip joint recess). The technique is similar to that described with fluoroscopy because of where the femoral artery is located and because the 20-gauge spinal needle is inserted into the femoral neck. The imaging and needle plane when ultrasound is used is typically parallel to the femoral neck, with the needle angled cephalad. Ultrasound may be difficult in larger patients, because the needle may be difficult to visualize. In addition, one significant disadvantage of ultrasound as compared with fluoroscopy or CT is that the extension of diagnostic and therapeutic agents beyond the hip joint may not be easily identified. One solution to this limitation is mixing iodinated contrast with the diagnostic and therapeutic agents and then immediately obtaining a radiograph to show the extent of the injection.

## Bursa Injection

Both CT and ultrasound can be used to inject the bursae near the hip. Each imaging test is most accurate when there is distention of the bursa before the procedure, because the bursa is then visible and can be used as a target. With the use of sterile technique, a spinal needle is guided to the bursa for the injection, which will demonstrate low resistance to injection as compared with the surrounding soft tissues (Figure 5-22). A collapsed hip bursa is usually not identified during CT or ultrasound, which makes the injection of a collapsed bursa near the hip very difficult and most times unsuccessful. In this scenario, the needle is guided to where the bursa should be located, and test injections of an anesthetic agent are used while the needle is repositioned until the low resistance and distention of a bursa are found. If a bursa is not located, many times the area around the bursa is infiltrated with the agent, and this is noted in the procedural report. Fluoroscopy has also been described for the injection of the iliopsoas bursa, although ultrasound has the advantage of direct visualization of the bursa.

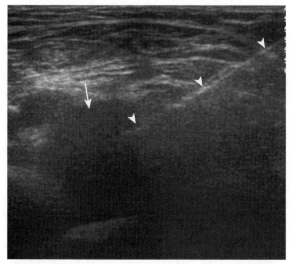

**Figure 5–22** Iliopsoas bursal injection. Axial ultrasound image shows a hyperechoic needle (*arrowheads*) entering into the hypoechoic iliopsoas bursa (*arrow*) from lateral to medial.

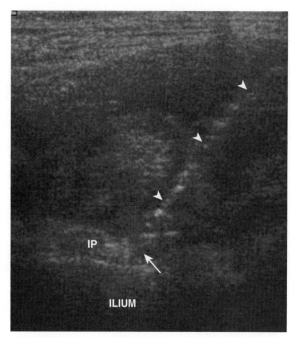

**Figure 5–23** Iliopsoas peritendinous injection. Axial ultrasound image shows a hyperechoic needle (*arrowheads*) with the needle tip (*arrow*) located where the iliopsoas tendon is adjacent to the ilium. *IP*, Iliopsoas.

## Peritendinous Injection

In the setting of snapping hip syndrome, the soft tissues between the snapping tendon or muscle and the adjacent bone may be injected. Ultrasound is ideal for this procedure, because, unlike CT, it allows for real-time imaging during needle positioning and for the targeting of soft tissues between the snapping structure and the bone, which is difficult with fluoroscopy. During ultrasound, if a bursa is identified, this can be the target of the injection. If a bursa is not visualized and not found during test injections, the tissues between the snapping structure and the bone are targeted. Injection for a snapping iliopsoas tendon under ultrasound guidance is completed in the axial plane, with the spinal needle entering from lateral to medial. The needle tip is placed between the iliopsoas tendon and the adjacent iliopectineal eminence, and the diagnostic and therapeutic agents are injected (Figure 5-23). During injection, fluid will be demonstrated to be pooling between the iliopsoas tendon and the ilium. It is important to inject around a tendon and to not place corticosteroids within the tendon because of the theoretic risk of tendon rupture. It is also important to avoid the injection of other structures (e.g., the hip joint), because this would create confusion with regard to the anatomic origin of symptoms and limit the effectiveness of diagnostic injection. Therapeutic injection around the iliopsoas tendon has been described for the treatment of impingement after total hip arthroplasty. With regard to a snapping iliotibial tract or gluteus maximus over the greater trochanter, ultrasound guidance is similarly used to inject the soft tissues between the snapping structure and the adjacent bone, including a bursa, if present.

## SUMMARY

CT is effective for the evaluation of abnormalities around the hip, such as fractures and complications after hip arthroplasty. The use of intra-articular contrast with CT allows for the visualization of cartilage abnormalities. The use of multislice CT has dramatically improved resolution and allows for the reconstruction of images in any plane. Ultrasound is effective for the evaluation of soft tissues near the hip, such as joint recess, bursa, and tendon. The benefit of ultrasound is the lack of ionizing radiation and the ability to dynamically assess the joint, which is useful for the diagnosis of snapping hip syndrome. Although imaging-guided percutaneous injections may be completed with the use of fluoroscopy, CT, or ultrasound, the hip joint is most commonly injected with the use of fluoroscopy or ultrasound guidance, whereas other soft-tissue structures such as the bursae are ideally injected with the use of ultrasound guidance. The accurate injection of a diagnostic agent is critical to identify the source of symptoms and to predict the potential success of surgical treatment.

## ANNOTATED REFERENCES

Adler RS, Buly R, Ambrose R, et al. Diagnostic and therapeutic use of sonography-guided iliopsoas peritendinous injections. *AJR Am J Roentgenol.* 2005;185:940–943.

The authors describe ultrasound-guided iliopsoas injection, which may identify the cause of hip pain, determine who may benefit from tendon release, and also treat iliopsoas-related symptoms after hip replacement.

Amis Jr ES, Butler PF, Applegate KE, et al. American College of Radiology white paper on radiation dose in medicine. *J Am Coll Radiol.* 2007;4:272–284.

The authors conclude that expanding use of imaging methods using ionizing radiation may result in an increased incidence of cancer, although this can be minimized with appropriate use of imaging at the lowest possible radiation dose while preserving image quality.

Anda S, Terjesen T, Kvistad KA. Computed tomography measurements of the acetabulum in adult dysplastic hips: which level is appropriate? *Skeletal Radiol.* 1991;20:267–271.

The authors conclude that a single axial CT image through the center of the femoral heads is most appropriate for acetabular measurements in hip dysplasia.

Assoun J, Richardi G, Railhac JJ, et al. Osteoid osteoma: MR imaging versus CT. *Radiology.* 1994;191:217–223.

The authors conclude that CT is more accurate than MRI in visualization of an osteoid osteoma nidus, while MRI shows more marrow and soft-tissue changes.

Beall DP, Sweet CF, Martin HD, et al. Imaging findings of femoroacetabular impingement syndrome. *Skeletal Radiol.* 2005;34:691–701.

The authors review the clinical presentation, mechanism, anatomy, and imaging findings of cam-type and pincer-type femoroacetabular impingement.

Bianchi S, Martinoli C, Keller A, et al. Giant iliopsoas bursitis: sonographic findings with magnetic resonance correlations. *J Clin Ultrasound.* 2002;30:437–441.

The authors present a case of anterior hip mass that represented a large iliopsoas bursa seen at MRI and ultrasound.

Blankenbaker DG, De Smet AA, Keene JS. Sonography of the iliopsoas tendon and injection of the iliopsoas bursa for diagnosis and management of the painful snapping hip. *Skeletal Radiol.* 2006;35:565–571.

The authors show that steroid injection of the iliopsoas bursa can provide long-term relief and predict good outcome after surgical tendon release in patients with clinically suspected snapping iliopsoas tendon.

Carson BW, Wong A. Ultrasonographic guidance for injections of local steroids in the native hip. *J Ultrasound Med.* 1999;18:159–160.

The authors describe the use of ultrasound for guidance of steroid injection into the hip joint.

Choi YS, Lee SM, Song BY, et al. Dynamic sonography of external snapping hip syndrome. *J Ultrasound Med.* 2002;21:753–758.

The authors show that dynamic ultrasound was effective in the diagnosis of external snapping hip due to abnormal iliotibial band and gluteus maximus movement over the greater trochanter.

Cody DD, Mahesh M. AAPM/RSNA physics tutorial for residents: technologic advances in multidetector CT with a focus on cardiac imaging. *Radiographics.* 2007;27:1829–1837.

The authors review the development, radiation issues, and technical aspects of multidetector CT.

Cyteval C, Hamm V, Sarrabere MP, et al. Painful infection at the site of hip prosthesis: CT imaging. *Radiology.* 2002;224:477–483.

The authors show in a prospective study of 65 patients that CT findings of soft-tissue fluid was most sensitive and periostitis most specific in the diagnosis of hip prosthesis infection.

Durkee NJ, Jacobson J, Jamadar D, et al. Classification of common acetabular fractures: radiographic and CT appearances. *AJR Am J Roentgenol.* 2006;187:915–925.

The authors propose an algorithm to accurately classify the five most common acetabular fractures with CT correlation, including multiplanar reformatted images and 3D surface rendering.

Fairbairn KJ, Mulligan ME, Murphey MD, et al. Gas bubbles in the hip joint on CT: an indication of recent dislocation. *AJR Am J Roentgenol.* 1995;164:931–934.

The authors show in a retrospective study of 79 patients that in the absence of penetrating trauma, intracapsular gas bubbles on CT are reliable indicators of recent hip dislocation.

Feldman F, Staron RB. MRI of seemingly isolated greater trochanteric fractures. *AJR Am J Roentgenol.* 2004;183:323–329.

The authors show that MRI more accurately defines the extent of greater trochanteric fractures after acute trauma compared to radiography and bone scintigraphy.

Flohr TG, Schaller S, Stierstorfer K, et al. Multi-detector row CT systems and image-reconstruction techniques. *Radiology.* 2005;235:756–773.

The authors review the general technical principles of multidetector row CT and topics related to patient radiation exposure and dose management.

Greenspan A. Bone island (enostosis): current concept—a review. *Skeletal Radiol.* 1995;24:111–115.

The author reviews imaging of bone islands, which characteristically appear as a homogeneously dense, sclerotic focus in the cancellous bone with distinctive radiating bony streaks that blend with the trabeculae of the host bone.

Harcke HT. Screening newborns for developmental dysplasia of the hip: the role of sonography. *AJR Am J Roentgenol.* 1994;162:395–397.

The author proposes an ultrasound screening protocol for diagnosis of developmental hip dysplasia.

Jacobson JA, van Holsbeeck MT. Musculoskeletal ultrasonography. *Orthop Clin North Am.* 1998;29:135–167.

The authors review musculoskeletal applications of ultrasound.

Kassarjian A, Yoon LS, Belzile E, et al. Triad of MR arthrographic findings in patients with cam-type femoroacetabular impingement. *Radiology.* 2005;236:588–592.

The authors retrospectively describe three abnormal findings associated with cam-type femoroacetabular impingement as seen at MR arthrography, which include abnormal head–neck morphology, anterosuperior cartilage abnormality, and anterosuperior labral abnormality.

**Kim WY, Hutchinson CE, Andrew JG, et al. The relationship between acetabular retroversion and osteoarthritis of the hip.** *J Bone Joint Surg Br.* **2006;88:727–729.**

The authors retrospectively reviewed 117 hip CT exams and found that acetabular retroversion was associated with findings of hip osteoarthrosis.

**Kitamura N, Pappedemos PC, Duffy PR 3rd, et al. The value of anteroposterior pelvic radiographs for evaluating pelvic osteolysis.** *Clin Orthop Relat Res.* **2006;453:239–245.**

The authors show that although radiographs are useful to screen for clinically important pelvic osteolysis after total hip arthroplasty, computed tomography images are necessary to accurately measure lesion volumes.

**Koski JM, Anttila PJ, Isomaki HA. Ultrasonography of the adult hip joint.** *Scand J Rheumatol.* **1989;18:113–117.**

The authors measured the anterior hip joint capsule with ultrasound in 75 subjects and concluded that an ultrasonographic distance between the hip joint capsule and the femur of 7 mm or more, and a difference between the hips of 1 mm or more suggest an intracapsular effusion in the joint in adults.

**Leunig M, Beck M, Kalhor M, et al. Fibrocystic changes at anterosuperior femoral neck: prevalence in hips with femoroacetabular impingement.** *Radiology.* **2005;236:237–246.**

The authors retrospectively evaluated 117 hips with femoroacetabular impingement and showed a high prevalence of juxta-articular fibrocystic changes at the anterosuperior femoral neck suggesting an association and possible causal relationship between these alterations and femoroacetabular impingement.

**Lubovsky O, Liebergall M, Mattan Y, et al. Early diagnosis of occult hip fractures: MRI versus CT scan.** *Injury.* **2005;36:788–792.**

The authors assessed 13 elderly patients after trauma and found that MRI was more accurate than CT for obtaining early diagnosis of occult hip fractures.

**Mahesh M. Search for isotropic resolution in CT from conventional through multiple-row detector.** *Radiographics.* **2002;22:949–962.**

The author shows that the development of multiple-row detector helical CT scanners and isotropic imaging has the capability to produce 3D images that approach the ideal of a true 3D radiograph.

**Murphey MD, Vidal JA, Fanburg-Smith JC, et al. Imaging of synovial chondromatosis with radiologic-pathologic correlation.** *Radiographics.* **2007;27:1465–1488.**

The authors comprehensively review the radiologic and pathologic features of primary synovial chondromatosis.

**Nishii T, Tanaka H, Nakanishi K, et al. Fat-suppressed 3D spoiled gradient-echo MRI and MDCT arthrography of articular cartilage in patients with hip dysplasia.** *AJR Am J Roentgenol.* **2005;185:379–385.**

The authors evaluate 20 dysplastic hips and show that multidetector CT arthrography is a sensitive and reproducible method for assessing articular cartilage lesions.

**Nishii T, Tanaka H, Sugano N, et al. Disorders of acetabular labrum and articular cartilage in hip dysplasia: evaluation using isotropic high-resolutional CT arthrography with sequential radial reformation.** *Osteoarthritis Cartilage.* **2007;15:251–257.**

The authors show that isotropic CT arthrography with radial reformation technique allowed accurate assessment of labral and cartilage disorders, and that labral tear was associated with adjacent cartilage disorder in hip dysplasia.

**Park JS, Ryu KN, Hong HP, et al. Focal osteolysis in total hip replacement: CT findings.** *Skeletal Radiol.* **2004;33:632–640.**

The author reviewed the CT findings of osteolysis in 30 total hip arthroplasty patients, which appeared as multilobulated lucent areas with expansile periosteal reaction and cortical abnormalities mimicking infection or tumor. CT was useful for assessment of extent of focal osteolysis.

**Pateder DB, Hungerford MW. Use of fluoroscopically guided intra-articular hip injection in differentiating the pain source in concomitant hip and lumbar spine arthritis.** *Am J Orthop.* **2007;36:591–593.**

The authors evaluated the utility of fluoroscopic hip injection in 83 patients to determine the origin of atypical lower extremity pain differentiating hip versus spine origin with 97% positive predictive value and 100% negative predictive value.

**Pelsser V, Cardinal E, Hobden R, et al. Extraarticular snapping hip: sonographic findings.** *AJR Am J Roentgenol.* **2001;176:67–73.**

The authors found abnormal movement of 22 iliopsoas tendons and 2 iliotibial tracts with dynamic ultrasound in 26 cases of snapping hip, of which 14 were painful.

**Pfirrmann CW, Chung CB, Theumann NH, et al. Greater trochanter of the hip: attachment of the abductor mechanism and a complex of three bursae—MR imaging and MR bursography in cadavers and MR imaging in asymptomatic volunteers.** *Radiology.* **2001;221:469–477.**

The authors evaluated trochanteric anatomy with MRI, bursography, MR bursography, and anatomic analysis in 10 cadavers and 12 normal volunteers describing the gluteal tendon attachments and 3 bursae about the greater trochanter.

**Pourbagher MA, Ozalay M, Pourbagher A. Accuracy and outcome of sonographically guided intra-articular sodium hyaluronate injections in patients with osteoarthritis of the hip.** *J Ultrasound Med.* **2005;24:1391–1395.**

The authors show that needle placement in the hip joint using ultrasound was 100% accurate in 30 injections using CT as a standard of reference and that 80% of patients had less pain 6 months after the final injection.

**Rezig R, Copercini M, Montet X, et al. Ultrasound diagnosis of anterior iliopsoas impingement in total hip replacement.** *Skeletal Radiol.* **2004;33:112–116.**

The authors report a case of impingement between the iliopsoas tendon and the adjacent total hip replacement components diagnosed by ultrasound and confirmed by CT.

**Robben SG, Lequin MH, Diepstraten AF, et al. Anterior joint capsule of the normal hip and in children with transient synovitis: US study with anatomic and histologic correlation.** *Radiology.* **1999;210:499–507.**

The authors study the anterior hip joint capsule in 6 cadavers, 58 healthy children, and 105 children with transient synovitis and show that the increased thickness of the joint capsule in transient synovitis is caused by effusion with no evidence for capsule swelling or synovial hypertrophy.

**Rosenthal DI, Hornicek FJ, Torriani M, et al. Osteoid osteoma: percutaneous treatment with radiofrequency energy.** *Radiology.* **2003;229:171–175.**

The authors describe their experience in radiofrequency ablation of osteoid osteomas in 263 patients and report an initial treatment success rate of 91%, concluding that the technique is safe and effective.

**Rydberg J, Liang Y, Teague SD. Fundamentals of multichannel CT.** *Semin Musculoskelet Radiol.* **2004;8:137–146.**

The authors describe advantages of multichannel CT, such as thin slice acquisition allowing high resolution isotropic imaging, faster scanning decreasing motion artifact, and higher X-ray tube currents improving imaging around metal hardware.

**Strouse PJ, DiPietro MA, Adler RS. Pediatric hip effusions: evaluation with power Doppler sonography.** *Radiology.* **1998;206:731–735.**

The authors evaluated 30 hips in 29 consecutive patients showing that power Doppler did not depict increased flow in most patients with septic arthritis, and normal flow on power Doppler sonograms did not exclude septic arthritis.

**Tallroth K, Lepisto J. Computed tomography measurement of acetabular dimensions: normal values for correction of dysplasia.** *Acta Orthop.* 2006;77:598–602.

The authors retrospectively evaluated 70 hips with CT and recorded normal dimensions, angles, and other acetabular measurements, which are important when planning realignment of the osteotomized acetabulum.

**Tehranzadeh J, Mossop EP, Golshan-Momeni M. Therapeutic arthrography and bursography.** *Orthop Clin North Am.* 2006; 37:393–408.

The authors review the technique of arthrography in different joints and bursae and discuss the pros and cons of the use of corticosteroids versus viscosupplementation in therapeutic arthrography.

**van Holsbeeck MT, Eyler WR, Sherman LS, et al. Detection of infection in loosened hip prostheses: efficacy of sonography.** *AJR Am J Roentgenol.* 1994;163:381–384.

The authors studied 15 asymptomatic and 33 symptomatic hips with evidence for loosening after arthroplasty with ultrasound and found that the normal anterior pseudocapsule to proximal femur distance was less than 3.2 mm while in 6 infected hips the mean distance was 10.2 mm with extraarticular extension of joint fluid.

**Wank R, Miller TT, Shapiro JF. Sonographically guided injection of anesthetic for iliopsoas tendinopathy after total hip arthroplasty.** *J Clin Ultrasound.* 2004;32:354–357.

The authors report 2 patients with iliopsoas pain after total hip arthroplasty who had symptomatic relief from ultrasound-guided steroid and anesthetic injection, subsequently treated with tendon release.

**Weybright PN, Jacobson JA, Murry KH, et al. Limited effectiveness of sonography in revealing hip joint effusion: preliminary results in 21 adult patients with native and postoperative hips.** *AJR Am J Roentgenol.* 2003;181:215–218.

The authors prospectively evaluated the accuracy of ultrasound in diagnosis of hip joint effusion in 21 consecutive patients using arthrocentesis as the standard of reference and found that anterior recess distention and echogenicity could not be used indicators of adult hip joint effusion in native or postoperative hips.

**Wines AP, McNicol D. Computed tomography measurement of the accuracy of component version in total hip arthroplasty.** *J Arthroplasty.* 2006;21:696–701.

The authors prospectively compared intraoperative estimate of total hip arthroplasty version to CT measurements and found that 71% of femoral and 45% of acetabular components were within the expected clinical version range, and that the intraoperative estimation of acetabular and femoral version in a total hip arthroplasty is of limited accuracy.

# CHAPTER 6

# The Technique and Art of the Physical Examination of the Adult and Adolescent Hip

*Hal David Martin*

## INTRODUCTION

The hip is a complex joint that is surrounded by deep muscle and ligamentous tissues. Problems of the hip are often not recognized as the source of symptoms in a timely fashion. The time delay until treatment leaves patients in search of answers, which confounds and confuses the clinical picture after other treatments have been rendered. The modern understanding of other joints (e.g., knee, shoulder) developed rapidly as arthroscopic and clinical evaluations became structured, and the physical examinations became more inclusive as this understanding grew. At this time, the hip is being replaced, resurfaced, reconstructed, and reshaped as never before to provide improved patient function and to meet the expectations of both the patient and the surgeon.

The physical examination of the adult and adolescent hip continues to evolve as a product of biomechanical and surgical advancements, and it is a comprehensive assessment of three distinct tissue types that interrelate in a static and dynamic fashion. A thorough physical assessment is critical to the development of treatment options, interoperative considerations, and future diagnostic strategies. Hip motion occurs in 6 degrees of freedom in a symphony of musculotendinous, ligamentous, and osseous balance. To appreciate this achievement of function, it is important to understand the balance and interrelationship that each system has with the others. The hip will optimally be recognized early during the presentation of the complaint, but this is dependent on a consistent way of interpreting these interrelationships. The goal of this chapter is to do three things: 1) to identify key tests to be routinely performed during the physical examination of the hip; 2) to describe how these critical tests are performed, and to begin a discussion of the biomechanical importance of these assessments.

Ideally, orthopedic surgeons are familiar with an organized basic hip examination that can be performed quickly and efficiently to screen the hip, back, abdominal, neurovascular, and neurologic systems and to find the comorbidities that coexist with complex hip pathology. It is important that the physical examination of the hip is inclusive enough to rule out other joints as the primary cause of a complaint. Each examination or physical evaluation has a specific way of being performed, although interobserver consistency and practice are some of the most important aspects of the evaluation.

The order of the examination is one that is easy on the patient and on the flow of the physician and an assistant, if available. A physical examination is dictated by the pertinent history and especially by the age of the patient; any history of trauma or other related symptoms of the back; or neurologic, abdomen, or lower-extremity complaints. Some hint of the presence of an intra-articular cause versus an extra-articular one is assimilated by the presenting location. A review of the patient's history is obtained, which includes the history of the present condition, the date of the onset, the presence or absence of trauma, the mechanism of injury, the pain, the location, and factors that increase or decrease any associated pain. The presence or absence of popping is also beneficial to assess. Potential sources of disruption of the vascular supply of the femoral head are assessed, including metabolic disorders such as abnormalities that involve lipids, the thyroid, homocysteine, and clotting mechanisms. The patient's social history can also affect the blood supply to the femoral head; therefore, the presence of or exposure to tobacco, alcohol, steroids, and altitude issues are routinely recognized.

Past tests or evaluative studies are recorded, which may include magnetic resonance imaging or arthrography, x-rays, laboratory results, or previous consults. Current limitations that involve the activities of rotation (e.g., getting into or out of a bathtub or car, activities of daily living, jogging, walking, stairs) will help to detect and direct possible further intra- or extra-articular assessment. The presence of associated complaints (e.g., abdominal or back pain, numbness, weakness, cough or sneeze exacerbation) helps to rule out thoracolumbar issues, which are occasionally confused with the hip as a partial or dominant cause of complaint. Finally, the goals of treatment are discussed and reviewed with the patient.

A Modified Harris Hip Score is a general guide to establishing gross levels of function. Other hip scores have been outlined with quantifications in more specific patient populations, such as the Non-Arthritic Hip Score, the Hip Disability and Osteoarthritis Outcome Score, the Musculoskeletal Function Assessment, the Short Form 36, and the Western Ontario and McMaster University Osteoarthritis Index. An ongoing consensus score is under way by the Multicenter Arthroscopy of the Hip Outcomes Research Network (MAHORN) Group to add an internationally accepted score; this is in its final stages of testing. This test will help to compare outcomes and provide a consensus for comparison among examiners as well as among different centers. The use of a verbal analog score is also subjectively useful.

## THE TECHNIQUE OF PHYSICAL EXAMINATION

Hip complaints may present in a complex fashion that requires a thorough assessment to separate the comorbidities that frequently exist. The technique of physical examination is

**Table 6–1   MOST FREQUENT TESTS PERFORMED BY MAHORN GROUP SPECIALISTS**

| Standing Position | Supine Position |
|---|---|
| Gait | Flexion ROM |
| Single Leg Stance Phase Test | Flexion Internal Rotation |
| Laxity | Flexion External Rotation |
| **Lateral Position** | FADDIR Test |
| Palpation | Palpation |
| Passive Adduction Test | FABER Test |
| Abductor Strength | Straight Leg Raise Against Resistance |
| **Prone Position** | Strength Assessment |
| Femoral Anteversion Test | Passive Supine Rotation |
| | DIRI |
| | DEXRIT |

dependent on the examiner's experience and efficiency. Adequate time with the patient is scheduled to allow for a comprehensive assessment. Most hip examiners have a structured examination that is generally used in all cases and that helps to differentiate the specific pathologies upon presentation. The physical examination will be fine tuned and directed through the review of the history of present illness.

As with other extremity examinations, loose-fitting clothing around the waist that allows for access and patient comfort is helpful. An assistant to record the examination is useful for the accuracy and documentation of the examination. A standardized written form is helpful for thoroughness, especially when first starting a comprehensive hip evaluation or when the presentation is complex.

A vast number of tests exist for the examination of the hip, and it is not necessary to include them all in a single evaluation. Therefore, components of the examination can be classified as basic, which should always be included, and specific, which should be used as needed to define a specific diagnosis or combination of diagnoses. The most common examinations as determined by the MAHORN Group are shown in Table 6-1. This is a consensus among hip specialists to identify basic and specific components of the physical examination.

## THE STANDING EXAMINATION OF THE HIP

As the patient stands, a general point of pain is noted with one finger, and this can usually help to direct the examination. Pain in the groin region leads to the suspicion of an intra-articular problem, and lateral-based pain is primarily associated with both intra- and extra-articular aspects. Posterosuperior pain requires a thorough evaluation for differentiating hip and back pain; back issues are many times noted concomitantly with musculotendinous hip pathology. The shoulder height and iliac crest heights are noted to evaluate leg-length discrepancies. The general body habitus is assessed, and issues of ligamentous laxity are determined by the middle-finger test or hyperextension of the elbows or knees. Structural versus nonstructural scoliosis is differentiated by forward bending, and the degree of spinal motion is recorded.

Gait abnormalities often help to detect hip pathology as a result of the hip's role in supporting the body weight. Joint stability, preservation of the labrum and articular cartilage, and proper functioning of the hip joint involve three biomechanical and anatomic geometries of the femur and the acetabulum: fem-

oral head–neck offset, acetabular anteversion, and acetabular coverage of the femoral head. These relationships are important for the transfer of dynamic and static load to the ligamentous and osseous structures. Hip congruency (i.e., the rotation of the femoral head within the acetabular–labral complex) and articular stabilization (i.e., limiting translations of the femoral head within the acetabular–labral complex) are also regulated by the ligaments and muscles that cross the hip joint. The ligamentous capsule must maintain the stability of the hip, whereas the musculature of the lower limbs produces the forces that are required during ambulation. The patient is taken into the hallway so that a full gait of six to eight stride lengths can be observed (video). Key points of gait evaluation include foot rotation (i.e., the internal/external progression angle), pelvic rotation in the X and Y axes, stance phase, and stride length. The gait viewed from the foot-progression angle will detect the possibility of osseous or static rotatory malalignment that exists with increased or decreased femoral anteversion as compared with a capsular or musculotendinous issue. The knee and thigh are observed simultaneously to assess for any rotatory parameters. The knee may want to be held in either the internal or external rotation to allow for proper patellofemoral joint alignment, but this may produce a secondary abnormal hip rotation. This abnormal motion is usually present in cases of severe increased femoral anteversion that precipitates a battle between the hip and knee for a comfortable position, which will affect the gait.

Pelvic rotation is assessed by noting iliac crest rotation and terminal hip extension. On average, a normal gait requires 8 degrees of hip rotation and 7 degrees of pelvic rotation, for a total rotation of 15 degrees. The pelvic wink is demonstrated by an excessive rotation in the axial plane toward the affected hip, thus producing extension and rotation through the lumbar spine to obtain terminal hip extension. This winking gait is associated with laxity or hip-flexion contractures, especially when seen in combination with increased lumbar lordosis or a forward-stooping posture. Excessive femoral anteversion or retroversion can affect a wink on terminal hip extension, because the patient will try to create greater anterior coverage with a rotated pelvis. Injury to the anterior capsule can also contribute to a winking gait.

The normal gait can be broken down into two phases: the stance phase (60%) and the swing phase (40%). During the stance phase, the body weight must be supported by a single leg with the gluteus maximus, vasti, gluteus medius, and gluteus minimus providing the majority of the support forces. The maximum ground reactive force occurs during heel strike at 30 degrees of hip flexion. A shortened stance phase can be indicative of neuromuscular abnormalities, trauma, or leg-length discrepancies. The Abductor Deficient gait is an unbalanced stance phase that is attributed to abductor weakness and that is often referred to as an *abductor lurch*. The Abductor Deficient gait may present in two ways: with a shift of the pelvis away from the body (i.e., a "dropping out" of the hip on the affected side) or with a shift of the weight over the adducted leg (i.e., a shift of the upper body "over the top" of the affected hip). The antalgic gait is characterized by a shortened stance phase on the painful side, thus limiting the duration of weight bearing (i.e., a self-protecting limp caused by pain). A short leg gait is noted by the drop of the shoulder in the direction of the short leg.

In addition to body habitus and gait evaluation, the Single Leg Stance Phase test is performed during the standing evaluation of the hip. The Single Leg Stance Phase test is performed on both legs, with the nonaffected leg examined first to establish a baseline reference for the patient's function. As the patient lifts and holds one foot off the ground for 6 to 8 seconds, the contralateral hip abductor musculature and neural loop of proprioception are being tested. The pelvis will tilt toward the unsupported side if the musculature is weak or if

**Table 6–2**  STANDING EXAMINATION ASSOCIATIONS

| Test/Assessment | Association |
| --- | --- |
| Spinal Alignment | Shoulder height, iliac crest height, lordosis, scoliosis, leg length discrepancy, trunk flexion and side-to-side ROM |
| Ligamentous Laxity | Check for laxity in other joints: thumb, elbows, shoulders, or knee |
| Single Leg Stance Phase Test | Proprioception mechanism disruption, strength of abductor musculature |
| Gait | |
| Abductor Deficient Gait | Proprioception mechanism disruption, weak abductor strength |
| Pelvic Rotational Wink | Contracted hip flexor, excessive femoral anteversion, laxity of the hip capsule (anterior), intra-articular pathology |
| Foot Progression Angle with Excessive External Rotation | Femoral retroversion, excessive acetabular anteversion, abnormal torsional parameters, effusion, ligamentous injury |
| Foot Progression Angle with Excessive Internal Rotation | Excessive femoral anteversion, acetabular retroversion, abnormal torsional parameters |
| Short Leg Limp | Iliotibial band pathology, uneven leg lengths |

**Table 6–3**  SEATED EXAMINATION ASSOCIATIONS

| Test/Assessment | Association |
| --- | --- |
| Neurological Assessment | Symmetrical sensation of the sensory nerves originating from the L2-S1 levels, deep tendon reflexes: patellar and Achilles tendons |
| Straight Leg Raise | Symptoms of radicular neuropathy |
| Vascular Assessment | Dorsalis pedis pulse and posterior tibial artery pulse |
| Lymphatic Assessment | Inspection of the skin for swelling, scarring, or side to side asymmetry |
| Seated Piriformis Stretch Test | Deep gluteal syndrome, sciatic nerve entrapment, piriformis syndrome |
| Hip internal rotation ROM | Bilateral assessment noting any side-to-side differences. Normal between 20° and 35° |
| Hip external rotation ROM | Bilateral assessment noting any side-to-side differences. Normal between 30° and 45° |

the neural loop of proprioception is disrupted. Normal dynamic midstance translocation is 2 cm during a normal gait pattern; therefore, the rationale is that a shift of more than 2 cm constitutes a positive Single Leg Stance Phase test. Table 6-2 provides an outline of the standing examination.

## THE SEATED EXAMINATION OF THE HIP

The seated hip examination consists of a thorough neurologic and vascular examination (video). The need to check the fundamentals would appear obvious even in healthy individuals. Criteria exist for both the care of the patient and coding. The posterior tibial pulse is checked first, any swelling of the extremity is noted, and an inspection of the skin is performed at this time. A straight-leg raise test is then performed by having the patient extend the knee into full extension. This test is helpful for detecting radicular neurologic symptoms, such as the stretching of an entrapped nerve root.

The loss of internal rotation is one of the first signs of the possibility of an intra-articular disorder; therefore, an important assessment is the internal and external rotation in the seated position. The seated position ensures that the ischium is square to the table, thus providing sufficient stability at 90 degrees of hip flexion and a reproducible platform for accurate rotational measurement. Passive internal and external rotation testing is performed gently and compared between the two sides. Seated rotation range of motion is also compared and contrasted with the extended position of the hip. Table 6-3 provides normal internal and external rotation ranges of motion in these positions.

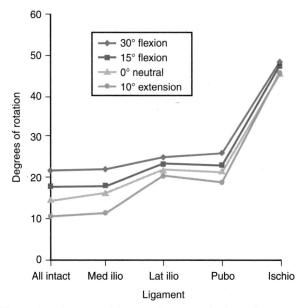

**Figure 6–1**  Summary of the internal rotation of cadaveric hip ligaments through ranges of motion from 30 degrees of flexion to 10 degrees of extension along a neutral swing path. After transection of the ischiofemoral ligament *(Ischio)*, internal rotation doubled. The lateral arm of the iliofemoral ligament *(Lat ilio)* was also noted to contribute to the stability of the hip in internal rotation. Med ilio, medial arm iliofemoral ligament; Pubo, pubofemoral ligament. *Reprinted from* Arthroscopy, 24, *The function of the hip capsular ligaments: a quantitative report. Martin HD, Savage A, Braly BA, Palmer IJ, Beall DP, Kelly B. 188-95, 2008, with permission from Elsevier.*

Musculotendinous, ligamentous, and osseous control of internal and external rotation is complex (Figure 6-1); therefore, any differences in seated positions as compared with extended positions may raise the question of ligamentous abnormality as compared with osseous abnormality. Sufficient internal rotation is important for proper hip function; there should be at least

10 degrees of internal rotation during the midstance phase of the normal gait. The loss of internal rotation at the hip can be related to diagnoses such as arthritis, effusion, internal derangements, slipped capital femoral epiphysis, and muscular contracture. Pathology related to femoroacetabular impingement or to rotational constraint from increased or decreased femoroacetabular anteversion can result in significant differences between the sides. An increased internal rotation in combination with a decreased external rotation may indicate excessive femoral anteversion, although the hip capsular function will require further assessment; this is correlated with the radiographic findings. Table 6-3 provides an outline of the seated examination.

## THE SUPINE EXAMINATION OF THE HIP

A battery of tests with the patient in the supine position helps to further distinguish internal from extra-articular sources of hip symptoms. The supine examination begins with the assessment of passive hip flexion. Both knees are brought up to the chest, and the degree of flexion is recorded. It is important to note the pelvic position; the hip may stop early in flexion, with the end range of motion being predominately pelvic rotation. From this position, the Hip Flexion Contracture test is performed by having the patient extend and relax one leg down toward the table. Any lack of terminal hip extension, which is noted by the inability for the thigh to reach the table, demonstrates a hip-flexion contracture. This exercise is performed on both sides to compare the differences. An important aspect of the Hip Flexion Contracture test is to obtain the zero set point for the lumbar spine. Patients with hyperlaxity or connective tissue disorders could have a false-negative result. In these patients, the zero set point can be established with an abdominal contraction. The Hip Flexion Contracture test could also be falsely negative if there is lumbar spine hyperlordosis as a result of a previous spinal fusion (video).

During the course of the supine examination, any pop in this plane can sometimes be related to a snapping iliopsoas tendon. A fan test (video) in which the patient circumducts and rotates the hip in a rotatory fashion can help to delineate the presence of the snapping iliopsoas tendon over the femoral head or the innominate. A hula-hoop maneuver in which the patient stands and twists can help to distinguish the pop internally from the external pop of coxa sultans externus as a result of the subluxing iliotibial band over the greater trochanter.

Tests—including those of flexion, adduction, and internal rotation—are useful for the detection of impingement or intra-articular pathology. The degree of flexion required in this position of adduction and internal rotation depends on the degree of impingement and the type and location of the impingement. The degree of hip flexion with the amount of pressure of the internal rotation is taken on a case-by-case basis, depending upon the function required of the patient as well as the patient's complaint. The traditional McCarthy test elicits a pop when the examined hip is circumducted in this flexed, adducted, internally or externally rotated position while the contralateral leg is held in flexion, as with the Hip Flexion Contracture test. The Dynamic Internal Rotatory Impingement test (DIRI) and Dynamic External Rotatory Impingement test (DEXRIT) (video) are performed as a traditional McCarthy test; however, a positive test is noted by recreation of the patient's pain. It is important that the zero set point of the pelvis is obtained by having the patient hold the nonaffected leg in flexion beyond 90 degrees. The DEXRIT (Figure 6-2) is performed passively by rotating the examined hip in a wide arc from the flexed position to an abducted, extended position while simultaneously externally rotating the femur. The DIRI test is performed by rotating the hip conversely in a wide arc from a slightly abducted, flexed position into a flexed, adducted, and internally rotated

position. The reproduction of these dynamic supine tests is interoperatively helpful for assessment and treatment.

The flexion/abduction/external rotation test or the *FABER test* (video) is helpful in for determining hip complaints as compared with non-hip complaints. A positive recreation of pain can be associated with musculotendinous or osseous posterior lateral acetabular incongruence.

Palpation of the abdomen is performed, and any abdominal tenderness is appreciated. Abdominal tenderness is differentiated from fascial hernia and adductor tendonitis. Resisted torso flexion with palpation of the abdomen will differentiate the fascial hernia from other complaints. Palpation of the adductor tubercle with active testing will detect adductor tendonitis.

Other useful tests may include the Tinel's test of the femoral nerve. The Tinel's test is found to be positive with hip-flexion contractures of more than 25 degrees. A heel strike test (video) is performed by striking the heel abruptly, which is indicative of some type of trauma or stress fracture. The Passive Supine Rotation test (video) involves passive internal and external rotation of the femur, with the leg lying in an extended or slightly flexed position. The Passive Supine Rotation test is performed bilaterally, and any side-to-side differences with regard to this maneuver can alert the examiner to the presence of laxity or effusion. Table 6-4 provides an outline of several supine examinations and their possible associations.

The importance of multiple examinations is recognized for the detection of intra-articular pathology. Even in the presence of normal internal and external rotation, there is a need for the further delineation of the relationships that exist between the musculotendinous, osseous, and ligamentous structure. Tests for impingement can have good specificity and reasonable predictive value for osseous abnormalities; however, no single test is sensitive enough to be used exclusively for the detection of subtle pathology. Furthermore, the ligamentous contribution to the range of motion varies with flexion and rotation.

## THE LATERAL EXAMINATION OF THE HIP

The lateral examination places the hip in an excellent position for further musculotendinous, ligamentous, and osseous evaluations. The lateral examination begins with the patient on the contralateral side for palpating the areas of the supra-SI and SI joints, the muscles of abduction, and, in particular, the origin of the gluteus maximus as it inserts along the lateral border of the sacrum and the most posterior aspect of the ilium. The next point of palpation is the ischium for detecting hamstring avulsions or tendonitis. Finally, the piriformis is palpated for any sign of tenderness, along with the abductor musculature, which includes the gluteus maximus, the gluteus medius, the gluteus minimus, and the tensor fascia lata. An active piriformis test (Figure 6-3; video) is performed by having the patient push the heel down into the table, thus abducting and externally rotating the leg against resistance, while the examiner monitors the piriformis. The Active Piriformis test is similar to Pace's sign performed in the seated position useful for evaluating deep gluteal syndrome.

Tests of Passive Adduction (Figure 6-4) are performed with the leg in three positions: extension (the tensor fascia lata contracture test), neutral (the gluteus medius contracture test), and flexion (the gluteus maximus contracture test). A traditional Ober test is performed with the hip in extension or neutral and then in adduction toward the table. Evaluation of gluteus medius tension is achieved by the release of the iliotibial band with knee flexion, and the hip should be able to be adducted down toward the table. Any restrictions of these motions are recorded. When performing the gluteus maximus contracture test, the shoulder is rotated toward the side of the table, with the hip flexed and knee extended. If adduction cannot occur in this position, the

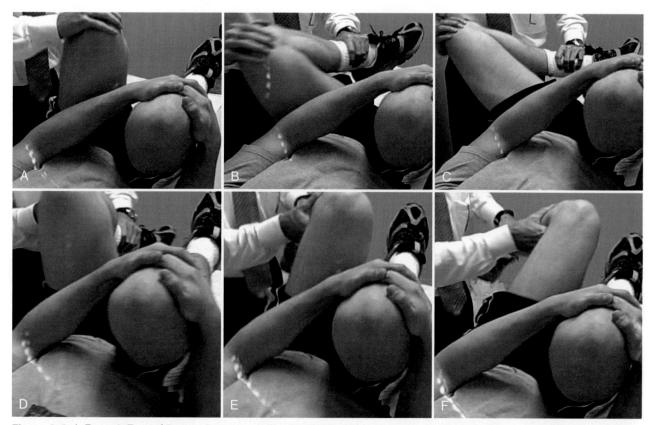

**Figure 6–2 A,** Dynamic External Rotatory Impingement Test (DEXRIT). Patient positioning is supine with the contralateral hip held in flexion by the patient. The examiner begins with the affected hip in flexion, slight adduction, and neutral rotation. **B, C,** The examiner passively brings the affected hip through a wide arc of abduction and external rotation. **D,** Dynamic internal rotatory impingement (DIRI) test. Patient positioning is supine with the contralateral hip held in flexion by the patient. **E, F,** The examiner passively brings the affected hip into flexion and through a wide arc of adduction and internal rotation. *Reprinted from* Arthroscopy, *26, The pattern and technique in the clinical evaluation of the adult hip: the common physical examination tests of hip specialists. Martin HD, Kelly BT, Leunig M, et al. 161-172, 2010, with permission from Elsevier.*

## Table 6-4   SUPINE EXAMINATION ASSOCIATIONS

| Test/Assessment | Association |
| --- | --- |
| Hip ROM (passive) | Hip flexion (normal 100-110°), abduction (normal 45°), and adduction (normal 20-30°), ROM until a firm endpoint or pain |
| Flexion, adduction, internal rotation (FADDIR) | FAI-anterior, anterior labral tear |
| Hip Flexion Contracture Test | Contracted hip flexor (psoas), neuropathy of the femoral nerve, intra-articular pathology, abdominal etiology |
| Flexion, abduction, external rotation (FABER) | Differentiation of hip pathology from lumbar or sacroiliac joint pathology |
| Dynamic Internal Rotatory Impingement Test (DIRI) | FAI—anterior, anterior labral tear |
| Dynamic External Rotatory Impingement Test (DEXRIT) | FAI—superior, superior labral tear |
| Posterior Rim Impingement Test | FAI—posterior, posterior labral tear |
| Passive Supine Rotation Test | Bilateral assessment noting any side-to-side differences, laxity, effusion, synovitis, internal derangement |
| Heel Strike | Trauma, femoral stress fracture |
| Straight Leg Raise Against Resistance | Intra-articular pathology as the psoas places pressure on the labrum, strength of the hip flexors and psoas |
| Palpation | |
|   Abdomen | Fascial hernia (also palpate with abdominal contraction), associated gastrointestinal/genitourinary pathology |
|   Pubic Symphysis | Osteitis pubis, calcification, fracture, trauma |
|   Adductor Tubercle | Adductor tendonitis |

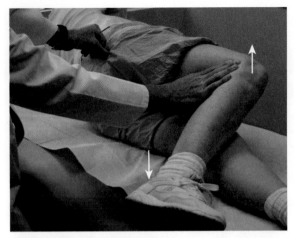

**Figure 6–3** The active piriformis test.

gluteus maximus portion is contracted. The hip should be able to freely come into a full adducted position, and any restriction of the gluteus maximus is recognized. The gluteus maximus is balanced with the tensor fascia lata anteriorly. If the hip does not come beyond the midline in the longitudinal axis of the torso, it is graded as 3+ restriction above the torso, 2+ at the midline, and 1+ restriction below. A clear delineation of the exact area of restriction will help to direct physical therapy and treatment options.

Strength is assessed with any type of lateral-based hip complaint. The gluteus medius strength test is performed with the knee in flexion. Each muscle group is graded in the traditional fashion on a 5-point scale.

Next is the passive assessment of flexion, adduction, and internal rotation, which is performed in a dynamic manner. The critical factor is the way in which the leg is held (Figure 6-5). The examiner holds the monitoring hand in and around the superior aspect of the hip, with the lower leg cradled on the forearm with the knee upon the hand. The hip is then brought

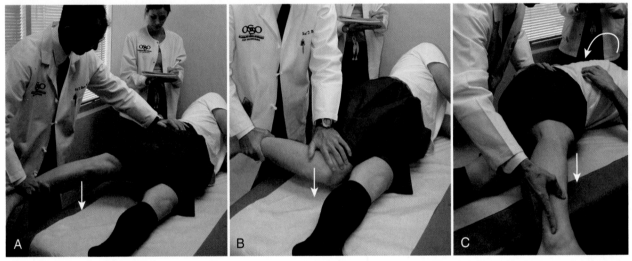

**Figure 6–4** Passive adduction testing. **A,** The tensor fascia lata contracture test is performed with knee extension. The examiner passively brings the hip into extension and then adduction. **B,** The gluteus medius contracture test is performed with the hip in a neutral position and the knee in flexion, thus eliminating contribution of the iliotibial band. The examiner passively adducts the hip toward the examination table. **C,** The gluteus maximus contracture test is performed with the ipsilateral shoulder rotated toward the examination table. The examined leg is held in knee extension as the examiner passively brings the hip into flexion and adduction. *Reprinted from* Arthroscopy, 26, *The pattern and technique in the clinical evaluation of the adult hip: the common physical examination tests of hip specialists. Martin HD, Kelly BT, Leunig M, et al. 161-172, 2010, with permission from Elsevier.*

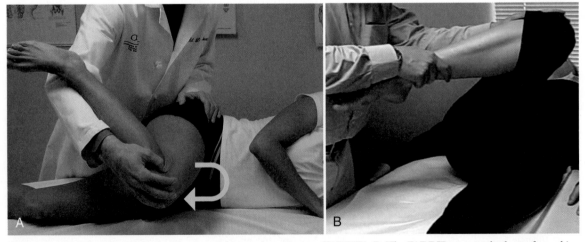

**Figure 6–5 A,** The lateral flexion, adduction, and internal rotation test (FADDIR). **B,** The FADDIR test can also be performed in the supine position. Figure 6-5B *reprinted from* Arthroscopy, 26, *The pattern and technique in the clinical evaluation of the adult hip: the common physical examination tests of hip specialists. Martin HD, Kelly BT, Leunig M, et al. 161-172, 2010, with permission from Elsevier.*

into flexion and adduction and internally rotated. Any reproduction of the patient's complaint and the degree of impingement are noted. FADDIR can also be performed in the supine position.

The lateral rim impingement test (video) is performed with the hip passively abducted and externally rotated. Any type of recreation of a posterior or lateral rim complaint or impingement can be precipitated in this position. Other tests may include the extension, abduction, and external rotation test (as with the apprehension test performed on the shoulder) for the detection of any type of anterior capsular laxity or injury. Forward pressure is applied to the posterior aspect of the hip, and the recreation of the patient's complaint pain is a positive test. Current research suggests that this position specifically releases the teres ligament. Table 6-5 provides an outline of several lateral examinations and their possible associations.

## THE PRONE EXAMINATION OF THE HIP

The prone examination is composed predominately of the palpation of four distinct areas: the supra-SI, the SI, the gluteus maximus origin, and the spine (facet); these different areas are used to identify the exact area of the complaint. Should the pain be identified in the supra-SI joint region in or around the facet, a lumbar hyperextension test (video) can help to identify the exact location of suspected pain. If this test is positive, the patient can then be placed into a supine position with the knees flexed. If this helps to alleviate the pain, the back should be further evaluated.

The Femoral Anteversion test will give the examiner a generalized idea of femoral anteversion and retroversion. With the patient in the prone position, the knee is flexed to 90 degrees, and the examiner manually rotates the leg while palpating the greater trochanter. The examiner positions the greater trochanter so that it protrudes most laterally, thereby placing

### Table 6-6   PRONE EXAMINATION ASSOCIATIONS

| Test/Assessment | Association |
|---|---|
| Rectus Contracture Test | Contracture of the rectus femoris muscle |
| Femoral Anteversion Test | Femoral anteversion (normal between 10-20°), ligamentous injury, increased laxity |
| Palpation | |
| Supra-SI | Mechanical conflict with the transverse process and ilium |
| SI | Inflammation of the SI joint |
| Gluteus Maximus Insertion | Tendonitis of the gluteus maximus insertion |
| Spine | Mechanical pathology related to the spine (facets) |
| With Lumbar Hyperextension | Help to identify location of spinal pain; if positive, place in supine position with knee flexion |

the femoral head into the center portion of the acetabulum. Femoral anteversion and retroversion are assessed by noting the angle between the axis of the tibia and an imaginary vertical line (video). Normally, femoral anteversion is between 8 and 15 degrees. If there is a significant difference of internal rotation in the extended and the seated flexed positions, an osseous cause versus a ligamentous one should be differentiated.

The Rectus Contracture test is performed with the patient in the prone position, and the lower extremity is flexed toward the gluteus maximus. Any raise of the pelvis or restriction of hip-flexion motion is indicative of rectus femoris contracture. Table 6-6 provides an outline of the prone examination.

## SPECIFIC TESTS

Further specific tests are useful for the assessment of complex hip pathology. Shown in the video are several tests performed by hip specialists. Dr. Marc Philippon (Figure

### Table 6-5   LATERAL EXAMINATION ASSOCIATIONS

| Examination | Assessment/Association |
|---|---|
| Flexion, Adduction, Internal Rotation (FADDIR) | FAI—anterior, anterior labral tear |
| Lateral Rim Impingement | FAI—lateral, lateral labral tear, instability |
| Tests of Passive Adduction | |
| Tensor Fascia Lata Contracture Test | Contracture of the tensor fascia lata muscle |
| Gluteus Medius Contracture Test | Contracture of the gluteus medius muscle, torn gluteus medius (decreased strength with knee flexion, suspect tear) |
| Gluteus Maximus Contracture Test | Contracture of the gluteus maximus, iliotibial band contribution, decreased abductor strength |
| Palpation | |
| Greater Trochanter | Greater trochanteric bursitis |
| Sacroiliac Joint | Differentiation of hip and back pathology |
| Maximus Origin | Tendonitis of the gluteus maximus origin |
| Ischium | Tendonitis of the biceps femoris muscle, avulsion fracture, ischial bursitis |

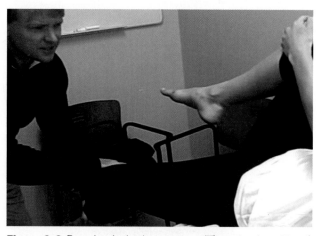

**Figure 6-6** Posterior rim impingement test. The patient is positioned at the edge of the examination table and holds the contralateral leg in flexion. The examiner passively brings the affected hip into extension, abduction, and external rotation. *Reprinted from* Arthroscopy, 26, *The pattern and technique in the clinical evaluation of the adult hip: the common physical examination tests of hip specialists. Martin HD, Kelly BT, Leunig M, et al. 161-172, 2010, with permission from Elsevier.*

6-6) demonstrates the posterior rim impingement test in which the recreation of pain is a positive test. Dr. Jon Sekiya performs the passive supine rotation bilaterally for detecting capsular laxity of the left leg. Also shown is the scour test, which the examiner performs similarly to DIRI test but that involves the placement of pressure on the knee during the assessment for detecting interarticular congruence. Dr. Michael Leunig has the patient perform a bicycle test while monitoring the iliotibial band for the detection of coxa saltans externus. The fulcrum test (performed by the author) is performed with the examiner's knee placed under the patient's knee, thus acting as the fulcrum. The patient then performs a straight-leg test against resistance. The importance of bilateral assessment is demonstrated by Dr. Bryan Kelly when performing the straight-leg test against resistance. RobRoy Martin, PhD, demonstrates the foveal distraction test. Interarticular pressure is alleviated by gently pulling the leg away from the body. Both the relief of pain and the recreation of pain will help to delineate an extra-articular pathology from an intra-articular pathology. Also shown is the FABER test, which is described in the section entitled "The Supine Examination of the Hip." The Seated Piriformis Stretch test is performed in the seated position with the hip at 90° of flexion. The examiner extends the knee and passively moves the flexed hip into adduction with internal rotation while palpating 1cm lateral to the ischium (middle finger) and proximally at the sciatic notch (index finger). A positive test is the recreation of the posterior pain and may indicate deep gluteal syndrome.

## SUMMARY

A general overview of the hip examination form is provided in Figure 6-7. Further diagnostic tests (e.g., x-ray, magnetic resonance imaging and arthrography, injection tests) will also aid in the diagnosis of hip pathology. The use of a formalized, reproducible examination will help identify the hip as the source of pain and comorbidities in a timely fashion.

The physical examination of the hip involves an assessment of the balance of osseous, ligamentous, and musculotendinous tissues and their interrelationships; these relationships are important for the development of diagnostic and treatment strategies. This chapter has opened a framework for discussion of clinically and biomechanically relevant physical examinations, and it has identified and described a battery of tests that is common in the physical examination of the adult and adolescent hip at this time.

---

**PHYSICAL EXAMINATION:** HT:        WT:        T:        R:        P:        BP:

**Gait/Posture:**
- Shoulder height:           Equal     Not equal
- Iliac crest height:        Equal     Not equal
- Active Forward Bend:                 Degrees
- Spine:          straight
                  scoliosis:    structural      non-structural
- Recurvatum: thumb test     elbows         knees              >5 degrees
- Lordosis:       normal       increased     paravertebral muscle spasms
- Gait:           normal       antalgic      abductor deficient (Trendelenburg)
                  pelvic wink  arm swing     short stride length      short stance phase
       Foot progression angle:   external    neutral        hyperpronation
- Single Leg Stance Phase Test (Trendelenburg Test):     R              L

**Seated Examination:**
- Neurologic Findings:
     Motor:
     Sensory:
     DTR:                Achilles          Patella
- Circulation:          DP                PT
- Skin Inspection:
- Lymphatic:          lymphedema     no lymphedema      pitting edema: 1+ 2+
- Straight Leg Raise:  R      L
- Range of Motion:    Internal Rotation:     External Rotation:
                       R      L           R      L

**Supine Examination:**
- Leg lengths:        R    cm          L    cm      equal/not equal
- ROM:                Right Leg                 Left Leg
     Flexion:         80 100 110 120 130 140     80 100 110 120 130 140
     Abduction:       10  20  30  45  50         10  20  30  45  50
     Adduction:       0  10  20  30              0  10  20  30
- Hip Flexion Contracture Test (Thomas Test):     R  +  −      L  +  −
     FADDIR:                                      R  +  −      L  +  −
- DIRI:                                           R  +  −      L  +  −
- DEXRIT:                                         R  +  −      L  +  −
     Posterior Rim Impingement Test:              R  +  −      L  +  −
       Apprehension Sign:                         R  +  −      L  +  −
- Abdomen:                                        Tender       Non-tender
- Adductor Tubercle:                              Tender       Non-tender
- Palpation pubic symphysis/Adductor             Tender       Non-tender
- Tinels – femoral nerve                          R  +  −      L  +  −
- FABER (Patrick Test):                           R  +  −      L  +  −
- Straight Leg Raise Against Resistance (Stitchfield Test):     R  +  −      L  +  −
- Passive Supine Rotation Test (Log Roll Test):   R  +  −      L  +  −
- Heel Strike:                                    R  +  −      L  +  −

**Figure 6–7** Physical Examination of the Hip Intake Form (from the upcoming Elsevier publication: Ch. 1 Clinical Examination and Imaging of the Hip. In C. Guanche & JWT Byrd (Eds.). *Advanced Hip Arthroscopy. Arthroscopy Association of North America.* Elsevier).

**Lateral Examination:**
- Palpation:

| | | |
|---|---|---|
| SI joint | Tender | Non-tender |
| Ischium | Tender | Non-tender |
| Greater trochanter | Tender | Non-tender |
| ASIS | Tender | Non-tender |
| Piriformis | Tender | Non-tender |
| Tinels – sciatic nerve | | |
| G. Max insertion into ITB | Tender | Non-tender |
| Sciatic nerve | Tender | Non-tender |
| Gluteus medius | Tender | Non-tender |

  Abductor strength:      Straight leg _____ Gluteus max _____ Gluteus medius _____
- Tensor Fascia Lata Contracture Test:      Grade (1–3)_____
- Gluteus Medius Contracture Test:      Grade (1–3)_____
- Gluteus Maximus Contracture Test:      Grade (1–3)_____
- Lateral Rim Impingement Test:      R + –      L + –
- FADDIR Test:      R + –      L + –

**Prone Examination:**
- Rectus Contracture Test (Ely's Test):   R + –      L + –
- Femoral Anteversion Test (Craig's Test): _____ degrees anteversion
- Palpation:
    - Spinous processes      + –
    - SI joints      R + –      L + –
    - Bursae ischium

**Specific Tests**

| | |
|---|---|
| Philippon Internal Rotation Test | Seated Piriformis Stretch Test |
| McCarthy's Sign | Pace Sign |
| Scours | ABDEER |
| Foveal Distraction | Dynamic Trendelenberg |
| Bicycle | Supine abduction external rotation |
| Fulcrum | |

**RADIOLOGY REVIEW:**
**Standing A/P**

| | | | | |
|---|---|---|---|---|
| 1. Leg Lengths: | Right long | Left long | | |
| 2. Neck Shaft Angle: | degrees | | | |
| 3. Trabecular Pattern: | Normal | Compression dominance | | |
| 4. Center Edge Angle: | degrees | | | |
| 5. Acetabular Inclination: | degrees | | | |
| Acetabular Dome Shape: | I  II | III  A.  B.  C. | | |
| 6. Joint Space Width: | | | | |
| Central: | 0 mm  2 mm | 3 mm  4 mm | 5 mm | |
| Lateral: | 0 mm  2 mm | 3 mm  4 mm | 5 mm | |
| 7. Lateralization: | mm | | | |
| 8. Head Sphericity: | Less than 2 mm | Greater than 2 mm | | |
| 9. Acetabular Cup Depth: | Profunda | Protrusio | | |
| 10. Anterior Posterior Wall Orientation: | Anteversion | Retroversion | High Retroversion | |
| Others: | | | | |
| Sclerosis | Herniation pit | | Thin inner table | |
| Osteophytes | Retained Hardware | | Teres insertion | |

**Lateral**

| | |
|---|---|
| Alpha Angle:      degrees | Head Sphericity: <2 mm   >2 mm |
| Herniation Pit | Anterior Margin Osteophytes |

**Biometrics**

| | | |
|---|---|---|
| Alpha Angle: | Femoral Version: | Acetabular Version: |
| degrees | degrees | degrees |

**MRI/Arthrogram**

| | | | | |
|---|---|---|---|---|
| Labrum: | Torn | Normal | | |
| Tear Type: | Grade | | | |
| Location: | Anterior | Superior | Lateral | Posterior |
| Iliopsoas tendon shape | Ligament teres | | | |
| Iliofemoral ligament on Axial | IT Band | | | |
| Bone Edema | Os Acetabuli | | | |
| AVN:   Grade | Cyst | | | |

**Figure 6–7   cont'd**

## ACKNOWLEDGEMENTS

The procedures and reasoning set forth in this chapter would not be possible without the dedication of many physicians whose works set the foundation for the physical examination of the hip. I owe them all a tremendous debt of gratitude for allowing me to build upon their works and to take the research of the hip another step forward.

## ANNOTATED REFERENCES AND SUGGESTED READINGS

McCarthy J, Noble P, Aluisio FV, Schuck M, Wright J, Lee JA. Anatomy, pathologic features, and treatment of acetabular labral tears. *Clin Orthop Relat Res.* 2003;38–47.

Hoppenfeld S, Hutton R. Physical examination of the hip and pelvis. In: Hoppenfeld S, Hutton R, eds. *Physical Examination of the Spine and Extremities.* Upper Saddle River: Prentice Hall; 1976:143–169.

Reider B. *The Orthopaedic Physical Examination*. Philadelphia, PA: Saunders; 1999.

Byrd J. *Operative Hip Arthroscopy*. 2nd ed. New York, NY: Springer; 2005.

Above references present the historical development of the physical examination of the hip by many generations of surgeons, therapists, and physicians and how the physical exam is designed to detect a wide variety of pathologies.

Braly BA, Beall DP, Martin HD. Clinical examination of the athletic hip. *Clin Sports Med*. 2006;25:199–210, vii.

Martin HD. Clinical examination of the hip. *Operative Techniques in Orthopaedics*. 2005;15:177–181.

Above references provide a succinct and complete method for the physical examination of the hip. Included are descriptions of the examination test as well as their relationships to the possible pathology of the hip.

Biering-Sorensen F. Physical measurements as risk indicators for low-back trouble over a one-year period. *Spine*. 1984;9:106–119.

Brown MD, Gomez-Marin O, Brookfield KF, Li PS. Differential diagnosis of hip disease versus spine disease. *Clin Orthop Relat Res*. 2004;280–284.

Giles LG, Taylor JR. Low-back pain associated with leg length inequality. *Spine*. 1981;6:510–521.

Above references help to guide the physician toward the differential diagnosis of hip versus back pain. Many clinicians find it difficult to differentiate between symptoms caused by a spine disorder or a hip disorder. If surgery is indicated, the order in which these operations take place is an important factor in the patient's long-term outcome. The presence of a limp, groin pain, or limited internal rotation of the hip can significantly predict the diagnosis of a disorder as originating primarily from the hip, as opposed to originating from the spine. These variables are of primary importance to the clinician when making a differential diagnosis between hip disease and spine disease. Muscle contracture of the hip flexors or extenders as well as the length discrepancy have also been identified as factors that can cause hip and low back pain to present together.

DeAngelis NA, Busconi BD. Assessment and differential diagnosis of the painful hip. *Clin Orthop Relat Res*. 2003;11–18.

Scopp JM, Moorman CT, 3rd. The assessment of athletic hip injury. *Clin Sports Med*. 2001;20:647–659.

Above references review the common problem of hip pain seen by orthopaedic surgeons and provide an approach to the patient with hip pain. Included is important information to be gained from the history and physical examination and relevant radiographic studies and laboratory tests. A differential diagnosis for patients presenting with the complaint of hip pain and indications for hip arthroscopy are provided.

Kim YT, Azuma H. The nerve endings of the acetabular labrum. *Clin Orthop Relat Res*. 1995;176–181.

Martin HD, Savage A, Braly BA, Palmer IJ, Beall DP, Kelly B. The function of the hip capsular ligaments: a quantitative report. *Arthroscopy*. 2008;24:188–195.

Torry MR, Schenker ML, Martin HD, Hogoboom D, Philippon MJ. Neuromuscular hip biomechanics and pathology in the athlete. *Clin Sports Med*. 2006;25:179–197, vii.

Above references provide an in-depth review of the musculotendinous, ligamentous, and osseous anatomy and biomechanics of the hip joint. A thorough and complete physical examination is dependent upon a comprehensive understanding of the balance between the musculotendinous, ligamentous, and osseous tissues.

Beall DP, Sweet CF, Martin HD, Lastine CL, Grayson DE, Ly JQ, et al. Imaging findings of femoroacetabular impingement syndrome. *Skeletal Radiol*. 2005;34:691–701.

Ganz R, Parvizi J, Beck M, Leunig M, Notzli H, Siebenrock KA. Femoroacetabular impingement: a cause for osteoarthritis of the hip. *Clin Orthop Relat Res*. 2003;112–120.

Ito K, Minka MA, 2nd, Leunig M, Werlen S, Ganz R. Femoroacetabular impingement and the cam-effect. A MRI-based quantitative anatomical study of the femoral head-neck offset. *J Bone Joint Surg*. 2001;83:171–176.

Martin HD, Kelly BT, Leunig M, Philippon MJ, Clohisy JC, Martin RL, Sekiya JK, Pietrobon R, Mohtadi NG, Sampson TG, and Safran MR. The pattern and technique in the clinical evaluation of the adult hip: the common physical examination tests of hip specialists. *Arthroscopy*. 2010;26:161–172.

Martin RL, Enseki KR, Draovitch P, Trapuzzano T, Philippon MJ. Acetabular labral tears of the hip: examination and diagnostic challenges. *J Orthop Sports Phys Ther*. 2006;36:503–515.

Above references provide reviews of the current concepts of femoroacetabular impingement. Discussed are radiographic techniques and analyses as well as clinical and intra-operative findings associated with femoroacetabular impingement and labral tears.

O'Leary JA, Berend K, Vail TP. The relationship between diagnosis and outcome in arthroscopy of the hip. *Arthroscopy*. 2001;17:181–188.

Above reference discusses the presence of mechanical symptoms having a positive predictive value in determining the possible outcome in hip arthroscopy related to internal derangement, such as a torn acetabular labrum.

Voos JE, Rudzki JR, Shindle MK, Martin H, Kelly BT. Arthroscopic anatomy and surgical techniques for peritrochanteric space disorders in the hip. *Arthroscopy*. 2007;23:1246, e5.

Above reference reviews the role of successful hip arthroscopy in peritrochanteric space disorders.

# CHAPTER 7

# Nonoperative Management and Rehabilitation of the Hip

*RobRoy L. Martin and Keelan R. Enseki*

## INTRODUCTION

The growing interest in musculoskeletal-related hip pathology is largely related to the evolution of hip arthroscopy and the recognition of previously unknown or underappreciated pathologies. Not only are new surgical interventions available for both intra- and extra-articular hip pathologies, but innovative conservative interventions have also been developed. An understanding of anatomic considerations, the recognition of pertinent clinical findings, and knowledge of available research are needed for the appropriate conservative management of individuals with hip pain. As compared with other body regions, there is a limited amount of information available regarding conservative management for individuals with musculoskeletal hip pathology. However, concepts that are commonly applied to the shoulder may prove to be useful in this area. The purpose of this chapter is to outline the evaluation process that we use to develop an intervention plan to conservatively manage individuals with musculoskeletal-related hip pathology.

Evaluation algorithms and classification-based treatment systems are commonly used in the orthopedic community to assist with determining a diagnosis, prognosis, and intervention plan. An algorithm implemented during the patient evaluation allows for the systematic collection of information, whereas classification-based treatment defines subgroups of patients who are likely to respond to a specific treatment approach. A number of evaluation algorithms and classification-based treatment systems have been developed for various body regions; however, there are few that are specific to the hip. We have integrated an evaluation algorithm and classification-based treatment to help conservatively manage individuals with hip pain; this plan includes the consideration of the lumbosacral spine, the extra-articular soft tissue, and the intra-articular structures. Intra-articular pathologies are further divided to consider the issues of impingement, hypermobility, and hypomobility. An outline of our proposed algorithm can be found in Figure 7-1.

## LUMBOSACRAL SPINE

Similar to the evaluation process for the shoulder, in which radiating symptoms from the cervical spine should first be ruled out, pain radiating from the lumbosacral spine should first be considered as a possibility for individuals with hip pain. In addition, because of the kinetic relationship between the hip and the lumbosacral complex, conditions in these areas commonly coexist. This holds particularly true for more chronic cases in which muscle dysfunction (e.g., gluteus medius) causes gait deviations that negatively affect

the lumbosacral spine. Therefore, the first step in our evaluation algorithm is to perform tests to rule out a lumbosacral spine contribution to the patient's symptoms. Many tests that assess the lumbosacral region have been described. Examples of such tests include lumbar range of motion, the palpating of pelvic landmarks, standing flexion, long sit, prone knee flexion, flexion abduction external rotation test (FABER), and hip internal rotation range of motion. If any of these tests is positive for a lumbosacral disorder, treatment may be directed toward this area. The effect of this treatment on hip pain can be evaluated and modified accordingly. In our evaluation and treatment of lumbosacral problems, we use a classification system that was initially described by Delitto and colleagues. This approach has been modified slightly by the results of subsequent research as summarized by Fritz and colleagues. This classification system includes the categories of manipulation and mobilization, stabilization, specific direction preference exercises (e.g., flexion, extension, lateral shift), and traction.

The mobilization classification makes use of a treatment technique that is thought to generally mobilize the lumbosacral complex. In our experience, however, the technique is often directed toward the sacroiliac joint. Tests to assess for sacroiliac joint abnormalities include assessing pelvic landmarks for symmetry, the seated flexion test, the long sit test, the Gillet test, and the FABER test. Childs and colleagues developed a clinical prediction rule for the mobilization category that involves the following five factors: 1) the duration of the current symptoms being less than 16 days; 2) a score on the work subscale of the fear-avoidance belief questionnaire of less than 19; 3) hypomobility of the lumbar spine (assessed with posterior-to-anterior pressure); 4) internal rotation of one hip of more than 35 degrees; and 5) symptoms that do not extend distal to the knee. When four of these five factors were present, the patient was very likely to improve with a mobilization treatment. However, when two or fewer factors were present, the mobilization treatment was almost always associated with failure. These findings are consistent with Brown and colleagues, who found that individuals with limited hip internal rotation were 3.63 times more likely to have a hip disorder than a spine disorder.

Examination and treatment with the mobilization of the lumbosacral complex are supported in the literature for individuals with hip pain. Cibulka and Delitto found that athletes with anterior or lateral hip pain and positive signs of sacroiliac joint dysfunction have a favorable treatment outcome with mobilization directed at the sacroiliac joint. The technique we use as an intervention for patients who we feel meet the criteria for the mobilization subgroup is depicted in Figure 7-2. The technique involves positioning the patient in a side-bending position toward and with rotation away from the painful

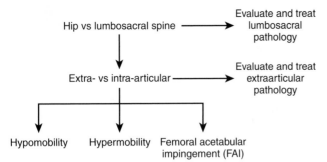

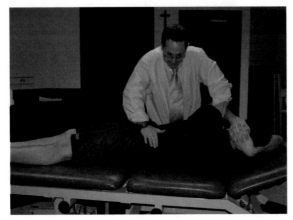

**Figure 7–1** The evaluation algorithm for individuals with musculoskeletal hip pathology.

**Figure 7–2** Sacroiliac joint mobilization performed with the patient in the supine position. The technique involves positioning the patient in a side-bending position toward and with rotation away from the painful side, with respect to the lumbar spine. A force directed anterior to posterior is applied to the ipsilateral anterior superior iliac spine with a Grade 5 thrusting maneuver.

side, with respect to the lumbar spine. A force directed anterior to posterior is applied to the ipsilateral anterior superior iliac spine with a Grade 5 thrusting maneuver. It should be noted that, before this manipulation is applied, contraindications for a thrust mobilization must be thoroughly cleared. The effect of this technique for reducing the patient's hip pain is assessed. Depending on the amount of pain reduction and the results of reassessing previously positive signs, the evaluation can continue accordingly. In general, patients who fall into this category are also given lumbopelvic range-of-motion and stabilizing exercises. We find that patients with hip pain commonly have signs and symptoms that are consistent with this category and that they often positively respond to some degree to this mobilization technique.

Stabilization classification describes treating patients who are thought to have instability of the lumbar spine. Therefore, patients in the stabilization category appear to be generally very flexible, to have increased segmental lumbar movement, and to have weakness in the muscles that support the spine. Hicks and colleagues identified predictors for improvement with this treatment that included being less than 40 years old, having an average straight-leg raise of more than 91 degrees, and having aberrant movements present with lumbar flexion and extension performed when standing. Treatment emphasizes spinal stabilization through muscle strengthening and includes exercises to target the lumbopelvic musculature. We emphasize that these exercises are not meant to aggravate the patient's symptoms and therefore will modify or omit them as appropriate.

Although the specific exercise and traction categories are not as commonly used as the mobilization and stabilization categories for individuals with hip pain, these categories are worthy of review. The specific exercise classification identifies subjects who preferentially respond to movements in one direction. Repeated or sustained lumbar flexion, extension, and side bending are performed to assess which of these movements produces a favorable response with regard to the patient's symptoms; the movements that produce a favorable response are then incorporated into the patient's intervention program. Those patients who best respond to an extension-specific exercise program are generally characterized by having symptoms that are distal to the buttocks, symptoms that centralize with lumber extension movements, and symptoms that spread distally down the lower extremity with lumber flexion. Those who may best respond to a flexion-specific exercise program are generally more than 50 years old, have imaging evidence of lumbar stenosis, and have pain that is relieved with sitting and increased with standing or walking. Those who may best respond to a side-bending–specific exercise program generally have a lateral shift in the frontal plane with visual deviation of the shoulder relative to the pelvis.

The traction classification seems to be the least common classification into which patients may fall, and it also has the least amount of evidence to support the interventions being used in treatment. The most common indication for this subgroup of patients is evidence of nerve root compression and symptoms that do not centralize with movements in one direction. When individuals meet the criteria for this subgroup, lumbar traction is applied as an intervention. This traction can be applied in the form of mechanical traction, deweighted treadmill, or aquatic exercises.

Individuals with symptoms below the knee are thought to primarily have lumbosacral disorders. These individuals are commonly categorized into either the exercise-specific or traction groups. Although hip pathology can occur concurrently with these groups, we find that the mobilization classification is the most common subgroup into which these patients fall, because the individual's hip pain is either entirely or partially reduced with the use of the mobilization technique. Because lumbopelvic and hip pathologies can coexist, individuals with hip pain and positive signs of lumbosacral involvement often require an examination to determine the contribution of intra- and extra-articular soft-tissue pathology.

## EXTRA-ARTICULAR SOFT-TISSUE DISORDERS

After the lumbosacral spine is evaluated and intervention applied as appropriate, extra-articular soft tissue and intra-articular structures need to be considered when the patient's symptoms are not satisfactorily resolved. Examination to determine if the patient's symptoms are of intra-articular origin includes the FABER, scour, and impingement tests. If these tests do not reproduce the patient's symptoms, we consider the symptoms to be primarily from the extra-articular soft tissue that surrounds the hip. Common muscles that are involved include the adductor longus, the gluteus medius, the proximal hamstring, the psoas, and the abdominal musculature (i.e., sports hernia). The trochanteric bursa is another extra-articular soft-tissue structure that can cause pain and thus should be included in this discussion. Musculotendinous disorders including muscle strains and tendon disorders should be painful with palpation, stretching, and resisted movements directed at the involved muscle or tendon. If the source of pain is solely intra-articular in origin, then palpable pain is rarely present.

When treating soft-tissue disorders around the hip, an injury treatment program will depend on the phase of the injury, which can be defined as acute/inflammatory, subacute, or chronic/remodeling. Acute injuries are treated with modalities to promote healing and to decrease pain and inflammation, such as massage, submaximal isometric exercises, passive range-of-motion exercises, and lumbopelvic stabilizing exercises. It is important to emphasize that all of these intervention techniques should be pain free for the patient. Concentric movement through a full range of motion can be used as the criterion to progress to the subacute phase. Subacute injuries are treated with concentric exercises, including functional closed chain and weight-bearing exercises. Progression includes the addition of lumbopelvic stabilization activities, general flexibility, and progressive balance and stability exercises. Criteria to progress to chronic/remodeling phase can include a range of motion equal to that of the uninvolved side and strength of approximately 75% of that of the uninvolved side. Pain with resistance testing should be minimal. The remodeling phase should emphasize eccentric exercises and sport-specific training. Throughout this rehabilitation process, the strengthening of the lumbopelvic stabilizing muscles should be encouraged. However, we find educating the patient to engage these muscles during sport-specific activity to be critical. Lower-extremity biomechanics and muscle imbalances need to be carefully evaluated and corrected as appropriate. Our program often includes the use of foot orthoses or heel or shoe lifts as well as education in proper training techniques.

This generic program can be used to treat any musculotendinous disorder, including those that involve the gluteus medius, the proximal hamstring, the psoas, and the abdominals. However, the adductor longus may be the most commonly treated musculotendinous disorder. Holmich and colleagues found that, as compared with passive physical therapy of massage, stretching, and modalities, an 8- to 12-week strengthening program produced better outcomes. The strengthening program consisted of progressive resistive adduction and abduction, balance training, abdominal strengthening, and skating movements on a slide board. Both strength and flexibility issues have been found to play a role in the onset of musculotendinous injuries; however, Tyler and colleagues found that strength deficits play a larger role.

Athletic pubalgia (i.e., sports hernia) should also be addressed when discussing the treatment of musculotendinous disorders that can cause hip pain. The condition is described as chronic inguinal or pubic pain caused by the disruption of the inguinal canal components. Athletic pubalgia is often difficult to diagnose. The symptoms may include lower abdominal or groin pain that is usually made worse with sudden movements such as sprinting, kicking, side stepping, sneezing, or coughing. The symptoms generally begin slowly. We find that muscle imbalances between the psoas and the abdominals contribute to this problem. A tight and strong psoas can cause a tilting of the pelvis anteriorly, thereby stretching the weaker lower abdominal muscles. This muscle imbalance may eventually lead to small tears in the abdominal wall muscles. Individuals who engage in a lot of activity that requires prolonged forward bending (e.g., soccer, ice hockey) may be at risk for this disorder. Objectively, we find tenderness in the lower abdomen and at the top of the groin. The treatment progression can be similar to that of the generic program outlined for musculotendinous disorders. However, an emphasis is placed on reducing excessive anterior pelvic tilt. Therefore, we include exercises to stretch tight hip flexors and to strengthen muscles that promote a posterior pelvic tilt, as indicated.

When discussing extra-articular soft-tissue disorders around the hip, trochanteric bursitis with proximal iliotibial band (ITB) syndrome should be included in the discussion. Trochanteric bursitis can be caused by direct trauma, although it is more commonly related to biomechanical issues that produce an adductor moment on the ITB. We find that the most common cause of

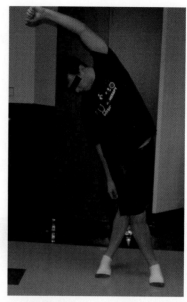

**Figure 7–3** Standing iliotibial band stretch for the left hip. Stretching is done with adduction, slight extension, slight external rotation, and side bending away.

bursitis at the hip is a tight ITB. Trochanteric bursitis can also be associated with excessive adduction (i.e., pelvic drop) that results from weak hip abductors. Other causes include training errors, tight adductors, increased pronation, worn shoes, and leg-length discrepancy.

When present at the hip, ITB syndrome frequently manifests itself as a "snap," and it is a subcategory of what has become known as *snapping hip syndrome*. Of course, there are other causes of snapping in the hip, and these must be entertained. First and foremost, it is necessary to determine whether the snapping sensation is intra- or extra-articular. Extra-articular snapping from a tight ITB commonly occurs during weight bearing with hip adduction and, internal and external hip rotation; this causes a taut ITB to move back and forth over the greater trochanter. Extra-articular snapping can also occur as a result of a tight iliopsoas as the tendon moves over the iliopectineal eminence during hip flexion and extension. The Ober and modified Thomas tests can be used to assess psoas and ITB flexibility. Intra-articular snapping or clicking that results from a labral tear may be reproduced during the FABER test.

The treatment of trochanteric bursitis with proximal ITB syndrome can involve a generic progression of therapy: decrease inflammation, improve the range of motion, increase strength, and return to activity. Proper ITB stretching is done with adduction, slight extension, and slight external rotation, as outlined in Figure 7-3. We also find benefit from the manual stretching depicted in Figure 7-4. It makes sense to incorporate components of both hip flexion and hip extension into the adduction stretch because of the attachments of both the tensor and gluteus maximus to the ITB. Other manual stretching, deep soft-tissue mobilization and massage, and other modalities may be indicated. We find that the most successful treatments include interventions that address more than the lateral hip pain and that also correct any biomechanical abnormalities and muscle imbalances.

## INTRA-ARTICULAR PATHOLOGY

We include the FABER, scour, and impingement tests, as previously noted, to help determine whether the patient's symptoms are of intra-articular origin. If these tests reproduce the patient's

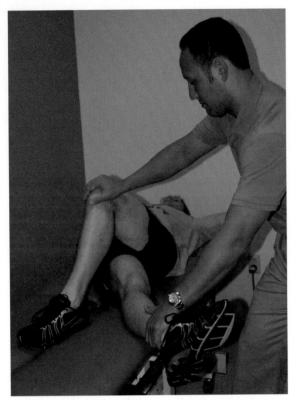

**Figure 7–4** Manual supine iliotibial band stretch. During this stretch, the patient's target hip is passively adducted under the flexed uninvolved extremity. Emphasis should be placed on keeping the pelvis immobile during the maneuver.

The logroll test typically demonstrates an increase in motion on the involved side as compared with the uninvolved side in these individuals. Treatment generally emphasizes strengthening the surrounding musculature and performing neuromuscular training and proprioceptive exercises. Patients with anterior hip laxity commonly elicit symptoms of instability with external rotation of the hip (e.g., when swinging a golf club). Exercises that reproduce these movements are avoided, whereas closed-chain activities with internal rotation are encouraged. We commonly use an exercise that incorporates the use of a resistive rubber cord, as depicted in Figure 7-5. During this exercise, it is important to maintain a neutral and stable pelvis to work the internal rotators and to engage the gluteus medius and the lumbopelvic stabilizers.

The symptoms of individuals with degenerative joint disease and hypomobility usually consist of pain in the groin that may be referred to the anterior thigh. Furthermore, patients typically report joint stiffness after immobility (i.e., first thing in the morning and lasting at least 60 minutes) and pain after too much weight-bearing activity. Physical findings include a loss of motion at the hip in a capsular pattern (particularly with hip internal rotation range of motion of 15 degrees or less and hip flexion range of motion of 115 degrees or less), positive intra-articular special tests (i.e., FABER, scour, and impingement), and antalgic gait often with associated Trendelenburg or compensated Trendelenburg deviations. Criteria to help with the diagnosis of hip osteoarthritis have been outlined by Altman and colleagues. Although individuals with isolated focal cartilage lesions may not present with signs and symptoms as severe as those with osteoarthritis, the intervention program that we use for both types of patients is similar.

The treatment approach for a patient with hypomobility and possible cartilage damage should incorporate several strategies, including education, the use of an assistive device, exercise, and joint mobilization. Exercises can include stretching,

symptoms, we consider the patient to have intra-articular pathology. After we determine that the origin of the patient's symptoms is intra-articular, we assess for possible associated factors. Identifying factors associated with an intra-articular hip pathology may be similar to the identifying factors associated with shoulder pathology. We include tests for femoral acetabular impingement (FAI), capsular laxity, and articular cartilage degeneration to consider the issues of impingement, hypermobility, and hypomobility in our conservative intervention. There is little information about the conservative treatment of intra-articular lesions, including labral tears. However, if the experience is similar to that of glenohumeral labral tears, surgical intervention may be required for individuals who fail 4 to 6 weeks of conservative therapy and who want to maintain a high level of activity.

FAI is a common cause of hip pain. Patients with FAI generally report a pinching pain in the groin that occurs with sitting. A positive flexion adduction, internal rotation impingement test may indicate potential FAI. The treatment of FAI may be analogous to that of shoulder impingement; therefore, treatment should avoid movements that cause the abutment of the femoral head–neck junction with the acetabulum and address the movement dysfunction caused by weakness, restricted range of motion, and muscle imbalance. Therefore, we recommend that sagittal- and frontal-plane activities be performed within a limited pain-free range of motion. Just as scapular stabilization is important with shoulder impingement conditions, lumbopelvic stabilization may be important for individuals with FAI; we therefore include exercises to address this area. Again, all activities should be pain free to avoid joint irritation.

Capsular laxity of the hip may be comparable with capsular laxity of the shoulder. Generally, individuals with this condition have engaged in repetitive forceful rotational activities. We commonly find that repeated forceful external rotation to the end of the range of motion causes iliofemoral ligament insufficiency.

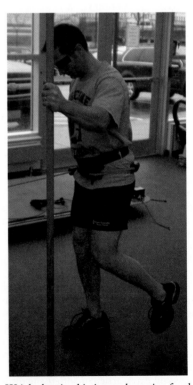

**Figure 7–5** Weight-bearing hip internal rotation for the right hip with the use of a resistance cord. A resistance cord is attached around the patient's waist to create a rotary moment at the hip. The patient assumes a single-limb stance position and keeps the pelvis level. The patient performs internal rotation with the weight-bearing hip against the force of the resistance cord.

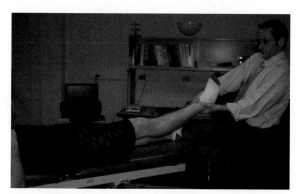

**Figure 7–6** Long-axis distraction of the hip joint. The patient is in the supine position. The clinician grasps the lower leg of the patient and places the hip in the open-pack position (30 degrees of flexion, 30 degrees of abduction, and 5 degrees of external rotation). A distraction force is created parallel to the axis of the femur.

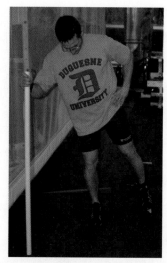

**Figure 7–7** Weight-bearing hip abduction that targets the muscles of the weight-bearing extremity. The patient stands on the targeted extremity while abducting the opposite hip. The hip abductors, the external rotators, and the lumbopelvic stabilizers are engaged to maintain neutral hip rotation and abduction.

strengthening, neuromuscular training, and proprioceptive activities. Strengthening exercises of the hip and lumbopelvic stabilizing should be included, and general stretching should be done to increase the range of motion and flexibility. Hinman and colleagues found that aquatic exercises produced favorable outcomes for those patients with osteoarthritis. The goal of exercises for individuals with arthritis is to help dissipate joint reaction forces. However, we use caution with weight-bearing activities in an effort to prevent further degradation of the cartilaginous surfaces. Therefore, we recommend that weight-bearing activities with internal rotation be avoided.

Patients should also be educated with respect to impact activities that negatively affect the disease process. Weight loss should also be discussed, when indicated. Messier and colleagues found that, for every pound of weight lost, there is a fourfold reduction in the load exerted per step at the knee during daily activities. In addition, an assistive device (e.g., a cane) for use on the contralateral (unaffected) side should be recommended to relieve joint pressure, if necessary. Youdas and colleagues found that 25% of the body weight can be offloaded from a lower extremity with the use of a cane.

The most compelling evidence for the treatment of hypomobility resulting from arthritic changes relates to the use of manual hip mobilization. We use a distraction technique that positions the hip in an open-pack position (30 degrees of flexion, 30 degrees of abduction, and 5 degrees of external rotation) while a traction force is applied, as shown in Figure 7-6. Increases in joint motion may be achieved by instituting a progressive series of joint mobilization techniques followed by stretching, as tolerated. We have found that improvements in motion allow the patient to perform daily activities at a higher level with less pain.

## SPECIFIC EXERCISES

### Hip Musculature

During rehabilitation, the muscles that surround the hip joint are commonly targeted for strengthening. These muscles include the gluteus maximus, the gluteus medius, the internal rotators, and the external rotators. We commonly use weight-bearing hip internal rotation (see Figure 7-5), weight-bearing hip abduction (Figure 7-7), resisted lateral walking, mini squats with resisted abduction and external rotation, and step-up exercises, as appropriate, in our strengthening program. There are a number of studies that have demonstrated the potential effectiveness of various exercises to strengthen the muscles that surround the hip joint. Bolgla and colleagues found that weight-bearing left hip abduction with the hip at

0 degrees and 20 degrees of flexion demonstrated significantly more right gluteus medius electromyographic activity as compared with similar non–weight-bearing exercises. Ayotte and colleagues demonstrated that unilateral wall squat, forward step-up, retro step-up, lateral step-up, and unilateral mini squat exercises all produced electromyographic activity within a strengthening range. The unilateral wall squat and the forward step-up produced significantly greater activity than the other three exercises. As the individual completes exercises that focus on the hip musculature, we emphasize trunk stabilization to engage the lumbopelvic stabilizers. We also modify or omit any exercise that aggravates patient symptoms.

### Lumbopelvic Musculature

Similar to scapulothoracic stabilization for patients with shoulder pathology, we feel that lumbopelvic stabilization exercises may need to be given to those patients with musculoskeletal conditions of the hip. We commonly use exercises to target the lumbar extensors, the abdominal musculature, and the quadratus laborum. These exercises include posterior pelvic tilting, bridging with resisted hip abduction and external rotation, quadruped alternating hip and shoulder lift (Figure 7-8), side

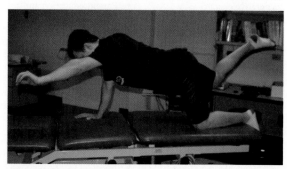

**Figure 7–8** Alternating elevation of the upper and lower extremities in the quadruped position (i.e., the bird dog exercise). One upper extremity and the opposite lower extremity are lifted until they are parallel with the table. The patient returns to the starting position, and then the movement is repeated with the opposite extremities. Emphasis is placed on maintaining pelvic stability throughout the exercise.

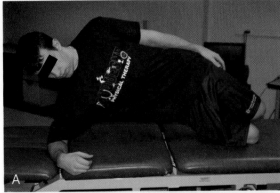

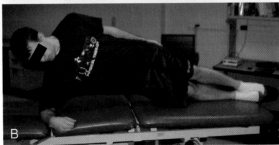

**Figure 7–9** The side plank progression. For these exercises, the patient laterally raises the body from a flat surface to a neutral position. **A**, The patient uses the knee for support. **B**, The patient progresses to using the feet for support.

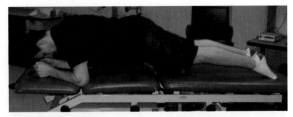

**Figure 7–10** The prone plank exercise. During this exercise, the patient supports the body weight with the elbows and toes by engaging the trunk musculature.

plank progressions (Figure 7-9), and prone plank (Figure 7-10). Again, we modify or omit any exercise that aggravates patient symptoms.

## CONCLUSION

This chapter outlines the evaluation process that we use to develop an intervention plan to conservatively manage individuals with musculoskeletal-related hip pathology. We have integrated a general evaluation algorithm and classification-based treatment that includes considerations of the lumbosacral spine, the extra-articular soft tissue, and the intra-articular structures. Intra-articular pathologies are further divided to consider the issues of impingement, hypermobility, and hypomobility. Table 7-1 presents a summary of the interventions

**Table 7–1** AN OVERVIEW OF INTERVENTIONS FOR COMMON MUSCULOSKELETAL HIP DISORDERS

| Diagnosis | Intervention Techniques |
|---|---|
| Femoral acetabular impingement | • Hip strengthening as tolerated<br>• Limiting activities in frontal and sagittal planes<br>• Lumbopelvic strengthening and stabilization |
| Hypermobility | • Closed-chain strengthening for hip musculature in the frontal and transverse (internal rotation) planes<br>• Avoiding activities that are commonly symptomatic (e.g., pelvic rotation, excessive external rotation of the hip)<br>• Proprioception and neuromuscular training<br>• Lumbopelvic strengthening and stabilization |
| Hypomobility: cartilage/degenerative changes | • Joint mobilization<br>• Patient education and activity modification<br>• Stretching as indicated<br>• Hip strengthening as tolerated with limited weight-bearing internal rotation<br>• Proprioception and neuromuscular training<br>• Lumbopelvic strengthening and stabilization<br>• Aquatic activities |
| Musculotendinous disorders: adductor longus, gluteus medius, proximal hamstring, psoas, and abdominal musculature (i.e., sports hernia/athletic pubalgia) | • Acute injuries: modalities to promote healing and decrease pain and inflammation, such as massage, submaximal isometric exercises, passive range-of-motion exercises, and lumbopelvic stabilizing exercises<br>• Subacute injuries: concentric exercises, including functional closed-chain and weight-bearing exercises, lumbopelvic stabilization activities, general flexibility exercises, and progressive balance and stability exercises<br>• Chronic/remodeling phase: eccentric exercises and sport-specific training<br>• Correct lower-extremity biomechanics and muscle imbalances as needed |
| Trochanteric bursitis/iliotibial band syndrome | • Iliotibial band stretching<br>• Hip strengthening that emphasizes the hip abductors<br>• Lumbopelvic strengthening and stabilization<br>• Correct lower-extremity biomechanics and muscle imbalances as needed<br>• Modalities to promote healing and to decrease pain and inflammation |

Specific exercises that can be used for patient home programs are included in the Expert Consult website.

that we commonly use to treat the various conditions outlined in this chapter. In addition, the CD that accompanies this book contains a user-friendly version of this table that will allow health care professionals to produce exercise programs; these programs contain pictures and instructions that can be given to patients in a clinical setting.

## ANNOTATED REFERENCES AND SUGGESTED READINGS

Altman R, Alarcon G, Appelrouth D, et al. The American College of Rheumatology criteria for the classification and reporting of osteoarthritis of the hip. *Arthritis Rheum.* 1991;34:505–514.

Ayotte NW, Stetts DM, Keenan G, Greenway EH. Electromyographical analysis of selected lower extremity muscles during 5 unilateral weight-bearing exercises. *J Orthop Sports Phys Ther.* 2007;37:48–55.

Bolgla LA, Uhl TL. Electromyographic analysis of hip rehabilitation exercises in a group of healthy subjects. *J Orthop Sports Phys Ther.* 2005;35:487–494.

Brown MD, Gomez-Marin O, Brookfield KF, Li PS. Differential diagnosis of hip disease versus spine disease. *Clin Orthop Relat Res.* 2004;419:280–284.

Childs JD, Fritz JM, Piva SR, Erhard RE. Clinical decision making in the identification of patients likely to benefit from spinal manipulation: a traditional versus an evidence-based approach. *J Orthop Sports Phys Ther.* 2003;33:259–272.

Cibulka MT, Delitto A. A comparison of two different methods to treat hip pain in runners. *J Orthop Sports Phys Ther.* 1993;17:172–176.

Delitto A, Erhard RE, Bowling RW. A treatment-based classification approach to low back syndrome: identifying and staging patients for conservative treatment. *Phys Ther.* 1995;75:470–485; discussion 485–489.

Fritz JM, Cleland JA, Childs JD. Subgrouping patients with low back pain: evolution of a classification approach to physical therapy. *J Orthop Sports Phys Ther.* 2007;37:290–302.

Hicks GE, Fritz JM, Delitto A, McGill SM. Preliminary development of a clinical prediction rule for determining which patients with low back pain will respond to a stabilization exercise program. *Arch Phys Med Rehabil.* 2005;86:1753–1762.

Hinman RS, Heywood SE, Day AR. Aquatic physical therapy for hip and knee osteoarthritis: results of a single-blind randomized controlled trial. *Phys Ther.* 2007;87:32–43.

Hoeksma HL, Dekker J, Ronday HK, et al. Comparison of manual therapy and exercise therapy in osteoarthritis of the hip: a randomized clinical trial. *Arthritis Rheum.* 2004;51:722–729.

This article asserts that effect of a manual therapy program on hip function is superior to an exercise therapy program for patients with osteoarthritis of the hip.

Holmich P, Uhrskou P, Ulnits L, et al. Effectiveness of active physical training as treatment for long-standing adductor-related groin pain in athletes: randomised trial. *Lancet.* 1999;353:439–443.

Messier SP, Gutekunst DJ, Davis C, DeVita P. Weight loss reduces knee-joint loads in overweight and obese older adults with knee osteoarthritis. *Arthritis Rheum.* 2005;52:2026–2032.

Nicholas SJ, Tyler TF. Adductor muscle strains in sport. *Sports Med.* 2002;32:339–344.

This review article describes treatment guidelines for adductor muscle strains.

Tyler TF, Nicholas SJ, Campbell RJ, McHugh MP. The association of hip strength and flexibility with the incidence of adductor muscle strains in professional ice hockey players. *Am J Sports Med.* 2001;29:124–128.

Whitman JM, Flynn TW, Childs JD, et al. A comparison between two physical therapy treatment programs for patients with lumbar spinal stenosis: a randomized clinical trial. *Spine.* 2006;31:2541–2549.

These authors find that those who may best respond to a flexion-specific exercise program are generally more than 50 years old and have imaging evidence of lumbar stenosis.

Youdas JW, Kotajarvi BJ, Padgett DJ, Kaufman KR. Partial weight-bearing gait using conventional assistive devices. *Arch Phys Med Rehabil.* 2005;86:394–398.

# CHAPTER 8

# Assessing Outcomes After Hip Surgery

*Nick G. Mohtadi, M. Elizabeth Pedersen, and Denise Chan*

## INTRODUCTION

The assessment of outcomes after any type of surgery can be categorized in a variety of different ways. Simply put, the outcome of a procedure can be anything that is measured or observed. It can range from something as simple as measuring the range of motion to a complex, multifaceted, disease-specific, health-related quality-of-life outcome questionnaire.

Outcomes can be considered objective; this means that they are undistorted by emotion or personal bias and based on observable phenomena. Outcomes can also be described as subjective, which means that the effect takes place within the mind and is modified by individual bias. The irony of the subjective categorization when it comes to measuring outcomes in medicine or surgery is that we consider something like an x-ray to demonstrate objective outcomes but visual analog pain assessments to show a subjective outcomes. However, the fact is that the interpretation of the x-ray is open to observer bias and therefore has a component of subjectivity. By contrast, a patient's response to a visual analog pain scale can be reproduced and assessed for error, and it therefore has the essential properties of an objective measurement. Whether the outcome is objective or subjective is not as important as whether the thing being measured represents the truth with respect to the outcome of a particular procedure.

With regard to hip outcome measures, several authors have addressed this area in the past. In 1972, Andersson compared 77 patients with the use of nine different methods and converted the final outcomes into a categoric scale of "good," "fair," and "bad." The results were very disparate, with good outcomes ranging from 97.5% to as low as 30%, depending on the outcome used. The author's final conclusion emphasized the importance of achieving agreement about what outcome should be used. In 1990, Callaghan and colleagues came to similar conclusions. In 1993, Bryant and colleagues used a statistical approach to analyze two separate groups of patients. They identified three core factors that were statistically independent: walking distance, hip flexion, and pain. These factors represented independent variables with respect to the outcome of hip arthroplasty. The authors' conclusion was that combining these variables into a composite score is "arbitrary and without scientific foundation." More recently, authors have recognized the need to assess health-related quality of life as a measure of health status of patients. Ethgen and colleagues performed a systematic review of outcomes related to hip and knee arthroplasty. They identified several important outcome measures, but their focus was on whether arthroplasty surgery improves quality of life. They stated the following: "If clinicians are interested in going beyond the pathophysiology…, if they seek to perceive the broader implications of diseases and strategies implemented to counter these diseases, it is necessary to consider outcomes that encompass several dimensions of health, as a health-related quality-of-life instrument does." With this compelling statement in mind, this chapter will focus on the quality and methodology of outcome measures that have been created or used by orthopedic surgeons to assess the management of traumatic and degenerative conditions of the hip. The essential information is based on a systematic review performed by the authors.

Forty-one clinical rating systems for the outcome measurement of orthopedic patients with hip disease were identified. We will start with a general statement about outcomes and present a historic perspective. We will then classify the tools according to whether they were clinician or patient based, their method of administration (i.e., clinician or self-administered), and their purpose (i.e., evaluative, discriminative, or predictive). In the next part, we will critically appraise each tool for its quality by evaluating its creation methodology, looking at its population of interest, and reviewing the psychometrics (i.e., reliability, validity, and responsiveness) of the outcome measures. The final part of the chapter will focus on the development of a new health-related quality-of-life instrument that focuses on young, active patients with hip problems.

## OUTCOME ASSESSMENT: GENERAL

The purpose of outcome measures can be classified as either disease specific, such as those tools created to assess osteoarthritis, or joint specific, such as those created to assess the outcome of any pathology of the hip. These measures can also be classified according to the person who completes the assessment. Traditionally, outcomes have been assessed by clinicians and include objective measures such as radiographic assessments. The clinician also asks the patient about pain and other subjective measures. These "clinician-based" or "clinician-administered" tools may not capture the patient's perceived outcomes. Therefore, more recently, "patient-based" or "patient-administered" tools have been created.

The objective of the tool must also be considered. If the goal is to follow patients over time and to assess changes, an evaluative index is necessary, because it can measure the magnitude of longitudinal change in an individual or a group of individuals. If the objective is to differentiate among patients to determine treatment, a discriminative index should be used, because it distinguishes among individuals or groups. Finally, to prognosticate, a predictive index can be used to classify individuals into a set of predefined measurement categories.

The second factor to consider when choosing an outcome measure is the quality of the tool, which is determined by the creation methodology. The creation of a questionnaire should follow a structured methodology that includes generating and reducing items. After it has been created, the tool must be tested for psychometric properties (i.e., reliability, validity, and responsiveness) within the target population.

*Reliability* refers to the ability of the tool to yield consistent and reproducible results. The questionnaire must be reproducible so that results will be the same for the same patient with the same amount of pathology on two separate occasions when measured by either the same or different raters. In addition, the items within the tool itself must be consistent so that all questions pertain to the concept that is being assessed.

*Validity* refers to how well an instrument fulfills the function for which it is being used. The different types of validity are face, content, construct, and criterion validity. *Face validity* ensures that the questionnaire "looks good" or appears to measure the intended content or trait. Without face validity, the tool will not be accepted. *Content validity* refers to the comprehensiveness of the instrument and how well the items represent all relevant concerns. *Construct validity* is the extent to which a particular tool can be shown to measure a hypothetical construct. Many of the factors that affect the ultimate outcome of a treatment (e.g., patient satisfaction) are intangible and therefore difficult to test. Construct validity tests these intangible qualities by proposing and testing logical relationships among different tools to measure similar or different outcomes. Construct validity can be tested with the use of convergent validity (when a high positive correlation is desired) and divergent validity (when a high negative correlation is desired). Finally, *criterion validity* is the validity of the questionnaire as compared with a gold standard. However, there is often no gold standard against which a particular questionnaire or tool can be compared.

*Responsiveness* refers to the ability of an instrument to measure change. However, this may be limited by ceiling or floor effects. *Ceiling effects* occur when the ability to record improvement is limited by the maximum obtainable value, and *floor effects* occur when the ability to record deterioration is limited by the minimum obtainable value.

## HISTORIC SUMMARY

There are many outcome measures that have been created for use in the population of orthopedic patients with hip disease. Most outcomes have been created for older patients who either require hip replacement or have a fracture.

The first published outcome tool for the hip was created by Ferguson and Howorth to assess the operative management of children with slipped capital femoral epiphysis. The authors measured the range of motion of the hip in all planes and multiplied each measurement by different modifiers to give the motions different weightings. This index of mobility was then modified by Gade, who changed the weighting of the actions for use in a total hip arthroplasty population. In 1954, Shepherd modified this index to use it as the mobility assessment for his tool, which also includes assessment of pain and function as well as the patient's own assessment. Shepherd's modification was further refined by Harris in 1969.

The first functional assessment appears to have come from France; it was published by Judet and Judet in 1952 and then in a different form by Merle D'Aubigné. The Merle d'Aubigné-Postel hip score was created in 1954 to grade the functional value of the hip in 405 patients who were treated with arthroplasty for the management of fractures of the femoral head or neck, osteoarthritis, or congenital dislocations. This score has subsequently been modified into other hip outcome measures: Charnley used the tool to assess low-friction total hip arthroplasties, Dutton and colleagues modified the tool for the assessment of patients with hip resurfacing, and Matta and colleagues adapted the score for patients with acetabular fractures. The Merle d'Aubigné-Postel score continues to be widely used for the assessment of hip arthroplasty in Europe. It has also been used by Letournel and Judet to assess acetabular fracture treatment, and it has since become the primary outcome measure for assessing the patient population with acetabular fractures.

In North America, the Harris Hip Score is more commonly used for the assessment of total hip arthroplasty. This score was created in 1969 "in an effort to encompass all the important variables into a single reliable figure, which is both reproducible and reasonably objective. The system was also designed to be equally applicable to different hip problems and different methods of treatment." This disease-specific measure was created to evaluate patients having a total hip arthroplasty after a hip dislocation or an acetabular fracture. In 1973, Ilstrup and colleagues modified the Harris Hip Score to create a computerized method of following the results of total hip arthroplasty. Over a 40-year period, many other scores were developed as clinician assessments of arthritis.

In 1968 Goodwin developed what was considered to be a predictive tool for patients with hip fracture treatment. In 1982 Keene and Anderson developed the Hip Fracture Functional Rating Scale as a predictive measure to help with patient discharge planning and placement. Other outcome measures were developed to assess traumatic hip dislocations and for patients with slipped capital femoral epiphysis.

Before 1985, all measures were clinician based, and none of these tools made use of a standardized methodologic process for its creation; rather, these tools were created by one or more clinicians on the basis of what was felt to be clinically relevant. Since 1987, the methodology for creating a tool has been described, and the newer tools have followed a structured creation format. Most tools have still been directed toward the patient population with arthritis, which generally includes patients with an average age of more than 70 years.

## CLASSIFICATION (TABLE 8-1)

All tools created before 1986 were clinician based, whereas all but two tools, created after 1986, are patient based. Of the patient-based tools, 10 are self-administered, 3 are meant to be administered by a clinician, and 1 can be either self- or clinician-administered. There are 3 predictive tools; all of the other tools are evaluative, and there are no discriminative tools. There are two main populations for which these scores have been created: middle-aged to elderly patients undergoing a hip replacement and elderly patients with fractures of the hip. Several other tools were created to be inclusive of all ages. One tool was created to capture higher activity levels among an older arthritic population, and two tools—the Non-Arthritic Hip Score and the Hip Outcome Score—were created specifically to capture the concerns of young, active patients with pre-arthritic hips.

### Creation Methodology

All patient-based tools were created in accordance with formal methodology. By comparison, none of the clinician-based tools made use of a formal process, other than reviewing older outcome measures. Of the tools that followed a formal creation process, four did not include patient input. The process of item generation was well described, and only some of the questionnaires included patient input as a critical step, including the Western Ontario and MacMaster University Osteoarthritis Index (WOMAC), the Musculoskeletal Function Assessment (MFA), and the Osteoarthritis Knee and Hip Health Quality of

**Table 8–1** HIP OUTCOME MEASURES

| Name | Author | Type | Purpose | Administrator | Population |
|------|--------|------|---------|---------------|------------|
| Ferguson and Howorth | A.B. Ferguson, M.B. Howorth (1931) | Disease: SCFE | Evaluative | Clinician | 8- to 17-year-old patients with SCFE |
| Gade Index | H.G. Gade (1947) | Joint: hip arthritis | Evaluative | Clinician | Patients with THA |
| Thompson and Epstein | V.P. Thompson, H.C. Epstein (1951) | Disease: hip dislocation | Evaluative | Clinician | 0- to 80-year-old patients with hip dislocation |
| Judet and Judet score | R. Judet, J. Judet (1952) | Joint: hip arthritis | Evaluative | Clinician | Patients with THA |
| Merle D'Aubigné-Postel | R. Merle d'Aubigné, M. Postel (1954) | Joint: hip arthritis | Evaluative | Clinician | Patients with THA |
| Shepherd | M.M. Shepherd (1954) | Joint: hip arthritis | Evaluative | Clinician | Patients with THA |
| Stinchfield | F.E. Stinchfield, B. Cooperman, C.E. Shea (1957) | Joint: hip arthritis, AVN, or OA | Evaluative | Clinician | Patients with hemiarthroplasty for fracture, AVN, or OA |
| Iowa/Larson Hip Chart | C.B. Larson (1963) | Joint: hip | Evaluative | Clinician | Patients of any age with any hip condition |
| Danielsson | L.G. Danielsson (1964) | Disease: OA | Evaluative | Clinician | Patients of any age with hip OA |
| Lazansky | M.G. Lazansky (1967) | Joint: hip arthritis | Evaluative | Clinician | Patients of any age with bilateral hip OA or THA |
| Goodwin | R.A. Goodwin (1968) | Disease: femoral neck fracture | Evaluative | Clinician | Patients with hemiarthroplasty for femoral neck fracture |
| Harris Hip Score | W.H. Harris (1969) | Joint: posttraumatic hip arthritis | Evaluative | Clinician | Patients with THA after acetabular fracture (mean age, 47 years) |
| Öhman | U. Öhman, N.-Å. Björkegren, G. Fahlström (1969) | Disease: hip fracture | Evaluative | Clinician | Patients with hip fracture (mean age, 71.5 years) |
| Charnley | J. Charnley (1972) | Joint: hip arthritis | Evaluative | Clinician | Patients between 30 and 80 years old with THA |
| Andersson and Möller–Nielsen | G. Andersson, J. Möller–Nielsen (1972) | Joint: hip arthritis, AVN, and trauma | Evaluative | Clinician | Patients of any age with hemiarthroplasty for OA or AVN |
| McKee | G.K. McKee, S.C. Chen (1974) | Joint: hip arthritis | Evaluative | Clinician | Patients with THA |
| Hospital for Special Surgery Hip Rating System | P.D. Wilson (1972) | Joint: hip arthritis | Evaluative | Clinician | Patients between 35 and 70 years old with cemented THA |
| Ilstrup | D.M. Ilstrup, D.R. Nolan, R.D. Beckenbaugh, and M.B. Coventry (1973) | Joint: hip arthritis | Evaluative | Clinician | Adults with THA |
| Hip Fracture Functional Rating Scale | J.S. Keene, C.A. Anderson (1982) | Disease: hip fracture | Predictive | Clinician | Patients with hip fracture (mean age, 76 years) |
| University of California Los Angeles Score | R.O. Dutton, H.C. Amstutz, B.J. Thomas, and A.K. Hedley (1982) | Joint: hip arthritis | Evaluative | Clinician | Patients who are less than 65 years old with AVN with hip resurfacing |
| Mayo Clinical Hip Score | B. Kavanagh, R. Fitzgerald (1985) | Joint: hip arthritis | Evaluative | Clinician | Patients with THA |
| Hospital for Special Surgery Rating system for Revision Total Hip Replacement | P.M. Pellicci, P.D. Wilson Jr., C.B. Sledge et al. (1985) | Joint: hip arthritis | Evaluative | Clinician | Patients with primary or revision hip arthroplasty |
| Western Ontario and McMaster Arthritis Index (WOMAC) | N. Bellamy and W.W. Buchanan (1986) | Disease: OA | Evaluative | Patient: self-administered | Patients with OA |

Continued

**Table 8–1** HIP OUTCOME MEASURES—Cont'd

| Name | Author | Type | Purpose | Administrator | Population |
|---|---|---|---|---|---|
| McMaster Toronto Arthritis patient preference questionnaire (MACTAR) | P. Tugwell, C. Bombardier, W.W. Buchanan et al. (1987) | Disease: RA | Evaluative | Patient: clinician-administered | Patients with RA |
| Japanese Orthopedic Association hip score | H. Yano, S. Sano, Y. Nagata et al. (1990) | Joint: hip arthritis | Evaluative | Clinician | Patients with rotational acetabular osteotomy for OA |
| Total Hip Arthroplasty Outcome Evaluation | M.H. Liang, J.N. Katz, C. Phillips et al. (1991) | Joint: hip arthritis | Evaluative | Patient: self- or clinician-administered | Patients with THA |
| Lequesne Algofunctional Index | M.G. Lequesne, M. Samson (1991) | Disease: OA hip and knee (separate index for each joint) | Evaluative | Clinician | Patients with OA |
| Hip Rating Questionnaire | N.A. Johanson (1992) | Joint: hip arthritis | Evaluative | Patient: self-administered | Patients scheduled to have THA (mean age, 65 years) |
| Parker and Palmer Mobility Score | M.J. Parker, C.R. Palmer (1993) | Disease: hip fracture | Predictive | Clinician | Patients with hip fracture |
| Patient Specific Index (PASI) | J.G. Wright, S. Rudicel, A.R. Feinstein (1994) | Joint: hip arthritis | Evaluative | Patient: self-administered | Patient scheduled to have THA (mean age, 64 years) |
| Musculoskeletal Functional Assessment (MFA) | D.P. Martin, R. Engelberg, J. Agel et al. (1996) | Disease: extremity MSK complaint | Evaluative | Patient: self-administered | Patients with MSK disorders of the extremities |
| Oxford Hip Score | J. Dawson, R. Fitzpatrick, A. Carr, and D. Murray (1996) | Joint: hip arthritis | Evaluative | Patient: self-administered | Patients with THA |
| Functional Recovery Score | J.D. Zuckerman, K.J. Koval, G.B. Aharonoff et al. (2000) | Disease: hip fracture | Predictive | Patient: clinician-administered | Patient with hip fractures (mean age, 76 years) |
| Lower Extremity Measure | S. Jaglal, Z. Lakhani, J. Schatzker (2000) | Disease: hip fracture | Evaluative | Patient: clinician-administered | Patients with hip fractures |
| Non-Arthritic Hip Score (NAHS) | C.P. Christensen, P.L. Althausen, M.A. Mittleman et al. (2003) | Joint: hip pain | Evaluative | Patient: self-administered | 10- to 40-year-old patients with hip disability with or without OA |
| Hip disability and Osteoarthritis Outcome Score (HOOS) | M. Klassbo, E. Larsson, E. Mannevik (2003) | Disease: hip OA | Evaluative | Patient: self-administered | Patients with hip OA and no surgical management |
| American Academy of Orthopedic Surgeons Lower Limb Instruments | N. Johanson, M.H. Liang, L. Daltroy et al. (2004) | Disease: hip or knee MSK complaint | Evaluative | Patient: self-administered | Patient with hip or knee arthritis or both |
| Osteoarthritis Knee and Hip Quality of Life questionnaire (OAKHQOL) | A.C. Rat, J. Coste, J. Pouchot et al. (2005) | Disease: hip or knee OA | Evaluative | Patient: self-administered | Patients with hip or knee OA or both |
| Hip Outcome Score (HOS) | R.L. Martin, B.T. Kelly, and M.J. Philippon (2006) | Joint: hip acetabular tears | Evaluative | Patient: self-administered | Patients scheduled to have arthroscopy for labral tears |

*SCFE*, slipped capital femoral epiphysis; *THA*, total hip arthroplasty; *AVN*, avascular necrosis; *OA*, osteoarthritis; *RA*, rheumatoid arthritis; *MSK*, musculoskeletal.

Life (OAKHQOL) assessment. In some other cases, outcome items were added to existing questionnaires from the literature. The remaining outcomes made use of clinician input, the existing literature, or both. Item reduction varied among the existing hip outcomes. Some made use of formal testing by calculating the frequency and importance of the items generated, others made use of factor analysis, and others involved a group consensus to determine which items should be retained. Three outcomes did not make use of a formal process of reducing items. Only four tools pretested new measures to ensure that both the wording and the format were appropriate.

## Psychometrics (Table 8-2)

Table 8-2 shows the evaluative tools that have been tested for reliability, validity, and responsiveness. Of the clinician-based tools, only the Harris Hip Score and Lequesne Index have been tested for reliability and shown to have internal consistency. Ten of the patient-based measures have demonstrated internal consistency. Two others—the Total Hip Arthroplasty Outcome Evaluation and the Hip Rating Questionnaire—have also been tested for internal consistency, but the results were poor. The majority of the questionnaires have demonstrated adequate reproducibility or test/retest reliability. All tools in Table 8-2 were presumed to have both face and content validity because patients and clinicians were involved in their creation or because they have been used by other surgeons in clinical practice or research. All have been tested for construct validity against other questionnaires. Only three tools have been tested for criterion validity: the Hip Rating Questionnaire was compared with the 6-minute walk test; the MFA was compared with stair climbing and walking speed; and the Lower-Extremity Measure was compared with the timed up-and-go test.

## Recommendations

### General Musculoskeletal Complaints

There are two outcome measures that have been well designed for general musculoskeletal complaints of the lower extremity: the MFA and the American Academy of Orthopedic Surgeons Outcomes Questionnaires (AAOS Outcomes Questionnaires) The MFA was developed in 1996 to detect differences in function among patients with musculoskeletal disorders of the extremities. It is an evaluative, self-administered, patient-based tool that is appropriate for adult patients (i.e., an average age of 40) with various disorders, including upper-extremity injuries (45%), lower-extremity injuries (45%), repetitive-motion disorders (6%), osteoarthritis (3%), and rheumatoid arthritis (2%). It was created by a group of clinicians that included academic and community orthopedic surgeons as well as rehabilitation medicine specialists, physical therapists, and occupational therapists. It was developed with a formal methodology that included item generation. Items were identified by a review of existing scores and by interviews with patients and clinicians. Item reduction followed a formal process of determining the items that were prevalent, important, representative, and measurable. The MFA is consistent and reproducible, and face and content validity were ensured during its creation. Good construct validity was shown by comparing MFA scores with physicians' ratings of patient functioning. When tested for criterion validity against stair climbing and self-selected walking speed, the tool showed poor agreement. This lack of correlation likely reflects the fact that the MFA was designed for a broad range of musculoskeletal disorders, including upper-extremity injuries.

The AAOS Outcomes Questionnaires were "designed for the efficient collection of outcomes data from patients of all ages with musculoskeletal conditions." The outcome tools were separated into a Lower Limb Core Scale, a Hip and Knee Core

Scale, a Sports/Knee Module and a Foot, and Ankle Module. The Lower Limb Core and the Hip and Knee Core Scales are essentially identical instruments with seven questions. The essential difference between the two questionnaires is that the words "lower limb" is substituted with "hip/knee." This self-administered, patient-based, evaluative tool was created in 2004 with the use of a modified group technique that involved surgeons and health-services researchers. The group identified items after a review of the literature and then reduced these items by consensus. It is appropriate for adult patients around 48 years old with hip or knee complaints. It is reliable, with good internal consistency and reproducibility, as demonstrated by a test followed 24 hours later by a retest. Although patients were not involved in the generation or reduction of items, patients were asked if the questionnaires addressed their concerns to ensure face and content validity. The AAOS tool has shown good to excellent construct validity against the WOMAC (Pearson value, 0.89), the Medical Outcomes Study 36-Item Short-Form Health Survey (SF-36; Pearson value, 0.7), physician assessments of pain (Pearson value, 0.69), and physician assessments of function (Pearson value, 0.73). The AAOS is responsive, but it may show slight ceiling effects.

### Osteoarthritis of the Hip

The best tool for general osteoarthritis of the hip is the Hip Disability and Osteoarthritis Outcome Score (HOOS). The HOOS is a patient-based, self-administered, evaluative tool created from the WOMAC. The WOMAC is a patient-based self-assessment tool that was initially developed in 1988 for patients with symptomatic osteoarthritis of the hip or knee. The items on the WOMAC were generated from interviews with 100 patients with osteoarthritis. It was tested with a group of patients with an average age of 71 years who were undergoing total hip arthroplasty. The WOMAC has been found to be both consistent and reproducible, and face and criterion validity were ensured during its development. Construct validity was determined by testing it against the SF-36. This tool is also responsive; however, the WOMAC does not capture the concerns of more active patients.

The HOOS was developed in part to capture the higher activity levels of patients with hip osteoarthritis. The questions for the HOOS were generated by interviewing more than 100 patients with hip disability and with or without hip osteoarthritis. Items were reduced by factor analysis to 40 items and include all of the items from the WOMAC in unchanged form. This tool has high reliability for all components of the questionnaire and high internal consistency. Content validity was ensured by having a subgroup of 26 patients rate the relevance of the importance of each item on a Likert scale, with "1" indicating that the item was irrelevant and unimportant and "3" indicating that the item was very relevant and very important. Construct validity was evaluated by comparing HOOS scores with those of the SF-36 general health status questionnaire. Responsiveness to clinical change was evaluated by calculating standardized response means and comparing the results with those of the WOMAC. This tool is good for patients with an average age 65 to 70 years with primary hip osteoarthritis who are having total hip replacements.

### Hip Arthroplasty

The best clinician-based tool for the evaluation of hip arthroplasty is the Harris Hip Score. This tool was created in 1969 to evaluate pain, activity, and function after total hip arthroplasty. The average age of patients involved in the original study was 47 years (range, 22 to 71 years). The development of this outcome tool did not follow a defined methodology. The small number of patients (n = 30) involved in the creation of this tool and the absence of group consensus among orthopedic experts suggests

**Table 8-2** TOOLS THAT HAVE BEEN TESTED FOR RELIABILITY, VALIDITY, AND RESPONSIVENESS

| Name | Reliability | | Validity | | Responsiveness |
| | Internal Consistency | Reproducibility | Construct | Criterion | |
|---|---|---|---|---|---|
| Merle d'Aubigné-Postel | Not tested | Inter-rater Kendall-Tau, 0.74 to 0.81; intra-rater Kendall-Tau, 0.64 (Bach et al., 2003) | Versus Harris Kendall-Tau, 0.85; versus Charnley Kendall-Tau, 0.88 (Bach et al., 2003); versus Harris Spearman, 0.82; versus Harris Kappa, 0.49 (Ovre et al., 2005) | N/A | Ceiling effects (Ovre et al., 2005) |
| Harris Hip Score (HHS) | Not tested | Inter-rater Kendall-Tau 0.75 to 0.8; intra-rater Kendall-Tau, 0.64 (Bach et al. 2003); inter-rater ICC, 0.69 to 0.83; intra-rater ICC, 0.55 (Wright and Young, 1997) | Versus Merle D'Aubigné Kendall-Tau, 0.85; versus Charnley, 0.83 (Bach et al., 2003); versus Merle d'Aubigné Spearman, 0.82; versus Merle d'Aubigné Kappa, 0.49 (Ovre et al., 2005); versus MACTAR, PASI Spearman, 0.50 to 0.81; versus MACTAR, 0.50 (Wright and Young, 1997) | N/A | SRM, 1.8 (Wright and Young, 1997); ceiling effects (Ovre et al., 2005); responsiveness ratio, 2.9 (Wright and Young, 1997) and 1.7 (Hoeksma et al., 2003) |
| Charnley | Not tested | Inter-rater Kendall-Tau, 0.71 to 0.79, intra-rater Kendall-Tau not tested (Bach et al., 2003) | Versus Merle D'Aubigné Kendall-Tau, 0.88; versus HSS Kendall-Tau, 0.81 (Bach et al., 2003) | N/A | Not tested |
| Hospital for Special Surgery (HSS) | Not tested | Inter-rater Kendall-Tau, 0.73 to 0.8; intra-rater Kendall-Tau, 0.58 (Bach et al., 2003) | Versus Merle D'Aubigné Kendall-Tau, 0.85 (Bach et al., 2003); versus Harris Kendall-Tau, 0.81 (Bach et al., 2003) | N/A | Not tested |
| Lequesne Algofunctional Index | Cronbach alpha, 0.83 overall (Stucki et al., 1998) | Intra-rater ICC, 0.94 (Stucki et al., 1998) | Versus WOMAC Spearman, 0.82; versus Kellgren OA, 0.37 (Stucki et al, 1998) | N/A | Not tested |
| McMaster Toronto Arthritis Patient Preference Questionnaire (MACTAR) | Total score correlated with partitions Pearson, 0.82 to 0.92 (Verhoeven et al., 2000) | Intra-rater ICC, 0.78; inter-rater Kendall-Tau not tested (Wright and Young, 1997) | Versus Harris Spearman, 0.5; versus PASI Spearman, 0.65 (Wright and Young, 1997); versus HAQ Pearson, 0.73; versus AIMS Pearson, 0.61 (Verhoeven et al., 2000) | N/A | SRM, 4.9 (Wright and Young, 1997) and 2.2 (Verhoeven et al., 2000) |
| Western Ontario McMaster Arthritis Index (WOMAC) | Tested and found to be consistent but no alpha values reported (Bellamy et al., 1988) | Kendall-Tau, 0.68, 0.48, and 0.68 for pain, stiffness, and function subscales, respectively (Bellamy et al., 1988) | Versus Spearman PASI, 0.51 to 0.83; versus MACTAR, 0.37 to 0.66; versus Harris, 0.56 to 0.79 (Wright and Young, 1997) | N/A | SRM, 1.26 for stiffness, 2.25 for physical function (Boardman, 2000), 2.4 for global score (Theiler, 1999) |
| Total Hip Arthroplasty Outcome Evaluation | Domains compared, Spearman 0.11 to 0.5 (Katz) | Test/retest Spearman, 0.76 to 0.91 | Versus SIP Spearman, 0.32 (pain), 0.43 (walking), and 0.56 (activity) | N/A | Not tested |
| Hip Rating Questionnaire | Domains compared, correlation coefficients 0.34 to 0.41 | Test/retest kappa, 0.7 | Versus AIMS correlation coefficient, 0.615 | Versus 6-minute walk test correlation coefficient, 0.6 | Responsiveness ratio, 1.09 (Johanson et al., 1992) |
| Patient Specific Index (PASI) | Not tested | Inter-rater ICC, 0.80 to 0.88; intra-rater ICC, 0.92 (Wright and Young, 1997) | Versus Harris Spearman, 0.5 to 0.81; versus MACTAR Spearman, 0.65 (Wright and Young, 1997) | N/A | SRM, 1.0 (Wright and Young, 1997) |

| Instrument | Internal consistency | Test/retest reliability | Construct validity | Validity versus other measures | Responsiveness |
|---|---|---|---|---|---|
| Musculoskeletal Functional Assessment (MFA) | Cronbach alpha, 0.85 (Martin et al., 1996) | Test/retest Spearman, >0.7 (Martin et al., 1996) | Versus scales from other measures Pearson, 0.43 (Engelberg et al., 1999) | Versus stair climb Spearman, 0.34; versus walking speed Spearman, 0.35 (Engelberg et al., 1999) | No ceiling or floor effects (Martin et al., 1996) |
| Oxford Hip Score | Cronbach alpha, 0.84 preoperatively and 0.89 postoperatively (Dawson et al., 1996) | Test/retest Bland-Altman, 7.27 (Dawson et al., 1996) | Versus Charnley Pearson, 0.15 to 0.58 (Dawson et al. 1996), versus EQ5D Pearson, 0.67 preoperatively and 0.77 postoperatively | N/A | Effect size, 2.75 (Dawson et al., 1996) |
| Lower Extremity Measure | Cronbach alpha, 0.94 (Jaglal et al., 2000) | Test/retest ICC, 0.85 (Jaglal et al., 2000) | Versus physical function of SF-36 Pearson, 0.78 (Jaglal et al., 2000) | Versus timed up-and-go Pearson, 0.56 (Jaglal et al., 2000) | SRM from prefracture to 6 weeks, 1.9; effect size, 2.6 (Jaglal et al., 2000) |
| Non-arthritic Hip Score | Cronbach alpha, 0.68 to 0.92 (Christensen et al., 2003) | Test/retest Pearson, 0.96 (Christensen et al., 2003) | Versus Harris Pearson, 0.82; versus SF-12 Pearson, 0.59 (Christensen et al., 2003) | N/A | Not tested |
| Hip disability and Osteoarthritis Outcome Score (HOOS) | Cronbach alpha, 0.77 to 0.93 | Test/retest ICC 0.78 to 0.91 by domain (Klassbo et al., 2003) | Versus SF-36 Spearman, 0.49 to 0.66 by domain (Nilsdotter et al., 2003) | N/A | SRM, 1.64 to 2.11, depending on domain (Nilsdotter et al., 2003) |
| American Academy of Orthopedic Surgeons Lower Limb Instruments | Cronbach alpha, 0.8 (Johanson et al., 2004); Cronbach alpha 0.89 to 0.93 on norms (Hunsaker et al., 2002) | Test/retest Pearson, 0.91 (Johanson et al., 2004) | Versus WOMAC Pearson, 0.89; versus SF-36 Pearson, 0.7; versus physician-assessed pain Pearson, 0.69; versus physician-assessed function, 0.73 (Johanson et al., 2004) | N/A | SRM, 1.7 (Marx et al., 2005) |
| Osteoarthritis knee and hip quality of life questionnaire (OAKHQOL) | Cronbach alpha, 0.73 to 0.96 (Rat et al., 2005) | Test/retest ICC, 0.36 to 0.88 (Rat et al., 2005) | Versus WOMAC Spearman, 0.84 to 0.88; versus Lequesne, 0.60 to 0.66; versus Harris, 0.48; versus SF-36, 0.32 to 0.77 (Rat et al., 2006) | N/A | SRM, 0.13 to 1.25, depending on domain (Rat et al., 2006) |
| Hip Outcome Score (HOS) | Cronbach alpha, 0.95 to 0.96 (Martin et al., 2006) | Not tested | Versus SF-36 physical function Pearson, 0.72 to 0.76; versus SF-36 physical component summary score, 0.68 to 0.74; versus SF-36 mental health Pearson, 0.23 to 0.27; versus SF-36 mental component summary score Pearson, 0.10 to 0.18 (Martin et al., 2006) | N/A | Able to differentiate at a minimum of 2 years of follow up between groups of patients with good versus excellent results (Martin and Philippon, 2007) |

*SRM*, standardized response mean; *ICC*, intra-class correlation coefficient; *SF-36*, short form-36 health status survey; *SF-12*, short form-12 health status survey; *HAQ*, health assessment questionnaire; *EQ5D*, euroQOL 5D; *SIP*, sickness impact profile.

that this tool lacks face validity. At the time of development, the Harris Hip Score was compared with two existing tools: the Shepherd system and the Larson system; however, comparability with these scales is limited. There were no detailed statistical analyses performed to determine construct validation.

The Harris Hip Score has been tested against the SF-36 and the WOMAC, and it has been shown to have high validity, reliability, and responsiveness. It has also been compared with the original and modified Merle D'Aubigné-Postel Scores, and it has demonstrated high overall correlation among acetabular fracture patients. The Harris Hip Score has been shown to be effective for evaluating changes in hip function; however, when it was tested among patients with acetabular fractures, the outcome demonstrated ceiling effects, which suggests a limitation in the clinical use of this outcome.

With only 12 questions, the Oxford Hip Score is the simplest outcome assessment tool. This self-administered, evaluative, patient-based outcome measure was created in 1996 to assess the perception of pain and function among patients undergoing total hip arthroplasty. This evaluative tool is good for patients who are between 35 and 90 years old with primary or secondary osteoarthritis. The methodology for developing the Oxford Hip Score involved item generation and reduction on the basis of a review of the WOMAC, the Patient-Specific Index, Charnley Hip Score, and the Harris Hip Score as well as on interviews with patients. The Oxford Hip Score has high internal consistency and satisfactory reproducibility. Face and construct validity were ensured by involving patients and reviewing the literature during item generation. Construct validity was established by testing this outcome measure against the Charnley Hip Score, the SF-36, and the Arthritis Impact Measurement Scale. It has also been shown to be responsive and sensitive to change as compared with the EuroQoL.

For young patients with arthritis of the hip and knee, a better tool is the OAKHQOL outcome measure. This is a self-administered, patient-based, evaluative tool that was created to fulfill the need for a "disease-specific instrument with good content, construct validity, and responsiveness in assessing the [quality of life] of patients with lower limb [osteoarthritis] RAT, 2005." The development of the OAKHQOL followed a structured methodology to ensure content validity. Items were generated and reduced with the use of focus groups that involved patients, rheumatologists, orthopedic surgeons, physiotherapists, and occupational therapists. The OAKHQOL was found to have high internal consistency with factor analysis and dimensional analysis; in addition, it is reproducible as demonstrated by testing followed by retesting after 10 to 21 days. This outcome measure has demonstrated adequate face and construct validity as compared with the SF-36 and a pain visual analog scale. Responsiveness was not tested, and there is no information regarding the scoring or the interpretation of the scores.

### Nonarthritic, Young, Active Patients With Hip Pathology

A population that has recently been identified as a group that requires orthopedic services is the young population with hip pain but no evidence of osteoarthritis. Unfortunately, a well-developed outcome for this population is lacking. Although the Non-Arthritic Hip Score has been administered to assess this specific population, it is not a robust tool. The Non-Arthritic Hip Score was created in 2003 to assess pain and function among young, active patients with activity-limiting hip pain, both pre-operatively and postoperatively. This tool is a patient-based, self-administered questionnaire that was developed as a modification of the WOMAC. The Non-Arthritic Hip Score is intended for patients between 20 and 40 years old who are experiencing hip pain without an obvious radiographic diagnosis. The items were generated through pilot test interviews with patients of varying

educational levels as well as with health professionals. The tool has been shown to be reproducible, but retesting occurred at any time between 1 and 16 days after the original testing. The tool has internal consistency as assessed with the use of the Cronbach coefficient alpha. Construct validity was determined by comparing the Non-Arthritic Hip Score to the Harris Hip Score and the Short Form-12 for 48 patients.

Although this tool attempts to capture a younger population that has not been previously represented by other hip outcome assessments, the methodology is not ideal because the total number of questions (n = 20) was arbitrarily determined, which may result in a misrepresentation of items that are relevant to a young, active patient with nonarthritic hip problems. In addition, the items were taken directly from the WOMAC index, which was generated for an older, more sedentary population; therefore, the tool may be predisposed to ceiling effects, thus limiting its use for a younger, more active population. In addition, the sections that address pain, mechanical symptoms, and physical function ask the patient to consider problems that have occurred during the previous 48 hours, which may be too short of a time line to be truly representative of the problems that these patients are experiencing.

Most recently, the Hip Outcome Score (HOS) has been developed for younger, more active patients between the ages of 13 and 66 years. This is a self-administered, patient-based tool that is designed specifically to evaluate patients with labral tears who are functioning throughout a wide range of ability. Therefore, the HOS includes only two subscales: activities of daily living and sports. Items were generated by physicians and physical therapists and reduced by factor analysis; no patients were involved with item generation. The tool does show internal consistency as determined by Cronbach coefficients, but it has not been tested for reproducibility. The HOS demonstrated good construct validity as measured by convergent and divergent validity with the SF-36 questionnaire with the use of Pearson correlation coefficients. The items in the HOS were evaluated for their potential to be responsive with the use of an item-response theory analysis; however, testing in patients for sensitivity to change over time was not conducted. Although this tool followed a formal creation methodology and includes an analysis of the questionnaire's content (which was not done for other outcome tools), it is limited by the specific nature of the population of interest. It may also underrepresent other areas of concern for these patients (e.g., symptoms, work-related issues), because the questionnaire only focuses on two subscales. More recently, the tool has been tested for validity in a group of hip arthroscopy patients with a minimum of 2 years of follow up. It was compared with the SF-36, and it was found to correlate well with measures of physical function. In addition, patients known to have better results scored higher on the tool, thus indicating that it is also likely to be responsive.

### Creation of a Health-Related Quality-of-Life Outcome Measure for Young and Active Patients With Hip Disease

For the past 3 years, the authors—in combination with the Multicentre Arthroscopy of the Hip Outcomes Research Network, the Canadian Orthopaedic Trauma Society, and local hip arthroplasty surgeons—have been developing a new outcome measure. There was a perceived need for a more appropriate way to assess patients who are young and active that would differ from existing outcome assessment tools, which were created for the older population with arthritis and fracture. This outcome has proceeded through the Item Generation, Item Reduction, and Pre-testing phases of development. This outcome has been formulated using modern methodological principles. This international collaboration has utilized the input from over 400 active patients between the ages of 18 and 60. All patients were screened to be active based on the modified Tegner Activity Scale of 4 or higher. In its current form the questionnaire has 33 questions that are divided into four domains: symptoms and functional limitations (16 questions), job-related concerns (4 questions), sports and recreational physical activities (6 questions), and social, emotional, and lifestyle concerns (7 questions). This distribution of questions into the domains was determined through an assessment of redundancy, standard and item total correlations, factor analysis, and test/re-test reliability. The questionnaire has no demonstrable floor or ceiling effects, has an overall Pearson correlation of 0.96 on test/re-test analysis, with an error of 5%. The questionnaire has been shown to be qualitatively responsive over time. Face validity has been established by incorporating the patient input at the item generation and reduction phases. Content validity has been confirmed by ensuring that all domains are represented and that experts have been included in the development of the questionnaire. Construct validation has been shown by comparing this questionnaire to the non-arthritic hip score. The two questionnaires were highly correlated at 0.81. The intention of this outcome measure is to evaluate patients who are young and active with traumatic and other hip diseases who are being treated with newer techniques such as arthroscopy and hip resurfacing.

## CONCLUSION

As the orthopedic care of patients with hip pathology continues to evolve, it is important that new therapies be assessed with the use of an appropriate outcome measure. Although there have been many tools developed, few of these have been created with the use of sound methodology or tested for reliability, validity, and responsiveness. Therefore, care must be taken when choosing an outcome measure for use in standard clinical practice research studies. Existing tools provide the clinician or researcher with a select number of options for assessing hip osteoarthritis and other hip-related conditions. There is promise that the newly developed outcome measure (HipQOL) for young active patients will fulfill this role. Future research and development is under way to address this concern.

## ANNOTATED REFERENCES AND SUGGESTED READINGS

**Amstutz HC, Thomas BJ, Jinnah R, Kim W, Grogan T, Yale C. Treatment of primary osteoarthritis of the hip. A comparison of total joint and surface replacement arthroplasty. *J Bone Joint Surg Am*. 1984;66(2):228–241.**

**Andersson G. Hip assessment: a comparison of nine different methods. *J Bone Joint Surg Br*. 1972;54B:621–625.**

This publication was the first to review the previously published hip outcome measures. Nine were available. Andersson compared the results of 77 patients who had been treated by Moore arthroplasty. Patients were classified as good, fair, or bad. Each outcome was used to classify the patients into the three categories. It was very evident from the results that depending on which outcome was used provided a very different distribution of patients. The conclusion was that it would be important to achieve agreement on how patients were to be assessed.

**Bach CM, Feizelmeier H, Kaufmann G, Sununu T, Gobel G, Krismer M. Categorization diminishes the reliability of hip scores. *Clin Orthop Relat Res*. 2003;411:166–173.**

**Bellamy N, Buchanan WW. A preliminary evaluation of the dimensionality and clinical importance of pain and disability in osteoarthritis of the hip and knee. *Clin Rheumatol*. 1986;5(2):231–241.**

**Bellamy N, Buchanan WW, Goldsmith CH, Campbell J, Stitt LW. Validation study of WOMAC: a health status instrument for measuring clinically important patient relevant outcomes to antirheumatic drug therapy in patients with osteoarthritis of the hip or knee. *J Rheumatol*. 1988;15(12):1833–1840.**

This publication established the final dimensions (Pain; Stiffness; Physical Function) of the WOMAC. The authors established face, content and construct validity, reliability, responsiveness, and relative efficiency of the instrument. The WOMAC is a disease-specific outcome designed to be used in clinical trials.

**Boardman DL, Dorey F, Thomas BJ, Lieberman JR. The accuracy of assessing total hip arthroplasty outcomes: a retrospective correlation study of walking ability and 2 validated measurement devices. *J Arthroplasty*. 2000;15(2):200–204.**

**Bryant MJ, Kernohan WG, Nixon JR, Mollan RAB. A statistical analysis of hip scores. *J Bone Joint Surg Br*. 1993;75–B(5): 705–709.**

These authors used a factor analytical approach to evaluate variables which were part of 13 methods of hip scoring. They identified three essential variables to assess patients who had a hip arthroplasty. These three variables were walking distance, hip flexion, and pain. The authors concluded that a three-factor hip score should be used to assess the results of hip arthroplasty. However, they suggested that each variable be recorded separately, because combining them into a composite score would be an arbitrary process without scientific foundation.

**Callaghan JJ, Dysart SH, Savori CG, Hopkinson WJ. Assessing the results of hip replacement: a comparison of five different rating systems. *J Bone Joint Surg Br*. 1990;72 B:1008–1009.**

The authors compared the results of measuring outcomes in 100 patients who had received an uncemented total hip arthroplasty. They compared the five most frequently used rating systems (Hospital for Special Surgery; Mayo Clinical Hip Score; Iowa/Larson Rating scale for hip disabilities; Harris Hip Score; Merle d'Aubiné-Postel) to the patient's impression of their hip in categories of excellent, good, fair, and poor. They stated that the Hospital for Special Surgery rating produced the most optimistic and the Merle d'Aubigné-Postel rating the most pessimistic.

They also compared the rating to Charnley's functional classes to which no meaningful relationship was demonstrated. The authors concluded that functional class should be included in all rating systems and that descriptive words such as *limp* or *pain* should be used in precisely the same way, but provided no good evidence for this statement.

**Charnley J. The long-term results of low-friction arthroplasty of the hip performed as a primary intervention. *J Bone Joint Surg Br*. 1972;54(1):61–76.**

**Christensen CP, Althausen PL, Mittleman MA, Lee JA, McCarthy JC. The nonarthritic hip score: reliable and validated. *Clin Orthop Relat Res*. 2003;406:75–83.**

This outcome, which is based on the WOMAC, was specifically designed to address a younger and more active population of patients. This 20-item questionnaire incorporated 10 questions directly from the WOMAC measuring pain and physical function. The remaining 10 questions include 4 questions pertaining to mechanical symptoms and 6 questions related to levels of activity. The psychometric properties of the Nonarthritic Hip Score (NAHS) questionnaire were evaluated in a group of 65 patients with an average age of 32.5 years. The NAHS demonstrated excellent reliability and compared favorably to the Harris Hip Score and the SF-12. However, ceiling effects are likely present since the NAHS overall score was very similar to the Harris Hip Score, which was developed for older patients undergoing arthroplasty surgery.

**Danielsson LG. Incidence and prognosis of coxarthrosis. *Acta Orthop Scand*. 1964;66(Suppl):1–114.**

D'Aubigné RM, Postel M. Functional results of hip arthro-plasty with acrylic prosthesis. *J Bone Joint Surg Am.* 1954; 36-A(3):451–475.

Dawson J, Fitzpatrick R, Carr A, Murray D. Questionnaire on the perceptions of patients about total hip replacement. *J Bone Joint Surg Br.* 1996;78(2):185–190.

The Oxford Hip Score demonstrated in this article represents a very simple and validated way of assessing patients with hip arthritis. It primarily addresses pain and functional complaints with a 5-point descriptive scale for each question.

Dawson J, Fitzpatrick R, Frost S, Gundle R, McLardy-Smith P, Murray D. Evidence for the validity of a patient-based instrument for assessment of outcome after revision hip replacement. *J Bone Joint Surg Br.* 2001;83(8):1125–1129.

Dutton RO, Amstutz HC, Thomas BJ, Hedley AK. Tharies sur-face replacement for osteonecrosis of the femoral head. *J Bone Joint Surg Am.* 1982;64(8):1225–1237.

Engelberg R, Martin DP, Agel J, Swiontkowski MF. Musculoskeletal function assessment: reference values for patient and non-patient samples. *J Orthop Res.* 1999;17(1):101–109.

Ethgen O, Bruyere O, Richy F, Dardennes C, Reginster JY. Health-related quality of life in total hip and total knee arthro-plasty. A qualitative and systematic review of the literature. *J Bone Joint Surg Am.* 2004;86-A(5):963–974.

These authors focused on summarizing the literature on the use of health-related quality-of-life instruments to evaluate patients treated with hip or knee arthroplasty surgery. They emphasized the importance of measuring a broader concept of health rather than the more traditional approach of the pathophysiology of hip and knee problems. They identified seven generic and eleven specific instruments that focused on the dimensions of health-related quality of life that were specific to arthritic diseases or total hip and total knee arthroplasty. The Short Form-36 (generic) and the Western Ontario and McMaster University Osteoarthritis Index were the most frequently used.

Ferguson AB, Howorth AB. Slipping of the upper femoral epiphy-sis. *JAMA.* 1931;97(25):1867–1872.

Gade HG. A contribution to the surgical treatment of osteoarthri-tis of the hip joint. A clinical study: comments on the follow up examinations and the evaluation of the therapeutic results. *Acta Chir Scandinavica.* 1947; Supplementum 120:37–45.

Goodwin RA. The Austin Moore prosthesis in fresh femoral neck fractures (A review of 611 post operative cases). *Am J Orthop Surg.* 1968;10(2):40–43.

Guyatt GH, Bombardier C, Tugwell PX. Measuring disease-specific quality of life in clinical trials. *Cmaj.* 1986;134(8): 889–895.

Guyatt GH, Feeny DH, Patrick DL. Measuring health-related quality of life. *Ann Intern Med.* 1993;118(8):622–629.

Harris WH. Traumatic arthritis of the hip after dislocation and acetabular fractures: treatment by mold arthroplasty. An end-result study using a new method of result evaluation. *J Bone Joint Surg Am.* 1969;51(4):737–755.

This article represents the origin of the Harris Hip Score that is currently used today based on the results of 30 patients treated for traumatic arthritis. Harris proposed a new clinician-based evaluation tool that was based on 100 points. This scale is made up of 44 points attributed to pain, 47 points to function, 5 points for range of motion, and 4 points for the absence of deformity. The amount of pain is graded from disabled (0 points—i.e., bedridden) to none (44 points). Function is divided into "daily activities," which is weighted with 14 points, and "gait," which has 33 points

assigned to it. The range of motion score is determined by a composite measurement of flexion, abduction, external rota-tion in extension, internal rotation in extension, adduction, and extension. Each measurement is multiplied by an index factor from a table to give the maximal possible score for each motion. They are added together and multiplied by 0.05 to get the final point value out of the 5 available points. The range of motion part was originally described by Ferguson and Howorth in 1931 and modified by Gade in 1947. The final 4 points are given for an absence of a deformity (i.e., per-manent flexion contracture of >30 degrees; fixed adduction of >10 degrees; fixed internal rotation of >10 degrees or a limb-length discrepancy of >3.2 cm.) At the time of this publi-cation there was no information on the measurement proper-ties of the scale.

Hoeksma HL, Van Den Ende CH, Ronday HK, Heering A, Breedveld FC. Comparison of the responsiveness of the Harris Hip Score with generic measures for hip function in osteoarthritis of the hip. *Ann Rheum Dis.* 2003;62(10): 935–938.

Hopkins KD. *Educational and psychological measurement and evaluation.* 8th ed. Toronto: Allyn and Bacon; 1998.

Hunsaker FG, Cioffi DA, Amadio PC, Wright JG, Caughlin B. The American Academy of Orthopaedic Surgeons outcomes instruments: normative values from the general population. *J Bone Joint Surg Am.* 2002;84-A(2):208–215.

Ilstrup DM, Nolan DR, Beckenbaugh RD, Coventry MB. Factors influencing the results in 2,012 total hip arthroplasties. *Clin Orthop Relat Res.* 1973;(95):250–262.

Jaglal S, Lakhani Z, Schatzker J. Reliability, validity, and respon-siveness of the lower extremity measure for patients with a hip fracture. *J Bone Joint Surg Am.* 2000;82-A(7):955–962.

Johanson NA, Charlson ME, Szatrowski TP, Ranawat CS. A self-administered hip-rating questionnaire for the assessment of outcome after total hip replacement. *J Bone Joint Surg Am.* 1992;74(4):587–597.

Johanson NA, Liang MH, Daltroy L, Rudicel S, Richmond J. American Academy of Orthopaedic Surgeons lower limb outcomes assessment instruments. Reliability, validity, and sensitivity to change. *J Bone Joint Surg Am.* 2004;86-A(5): 902–909.

Judet R, Judet J. Technique and results with the acrylic femoral head prosthesis. *J Bone Joint Surg Br.* 1952;34-B(2):173–180.

Keene JS, Anderson CA. Hip fractures in the elderly. Discharge predictions with a functional rating scale. *AMA.* 1982;248(5):564–567.

Kirkley A, Griffin S. Development of disease-specific quality of life measurement tools. *Arthroscopy.* 2003;19(10):1121–1128.

Kirshner B, Guyatt G. A methodological framework for assessing health indices. *J Chronic Dis.* 1985;38(1):27–36.

This publication outlines the different types of health status mea-sures including discriminative, predictive, and evaluative indices. They emphasize that the requirements for maximizing the func-tions of discrimination, prediction, or evaluation may impede the others. They describe the process of developing a measure of qual-ity of life and the importance of each of the steps. The process and major issues with respect to the construction and validation of a measurement tool are discussed and provide the framework for assessing outcome measures.

Klassbo M, Larsson E, Mannevik E. Hip disability and osteoar-thritis outcome score. An extension of the Western Ontario and McMaster Universities Osteoarthritis Index. *Scand J Rheumatol.* 2003;32(1):46–51.

The Hip disability and Osteoarthritis Outcome Score (HOOS) was derived from the WOMAC and followed the same process as the equivalent Knee Osteoarthritis Outcome Score (KOOS). The authors added questions that were taken directly from the KOOS, which was derived from the WOMAC and the Anterior Cruciate Ligament Quality of Life outcome questionnaire. The HOOS is a self-rated evaluative instrument for patients with hip problems. It should be pointed out that there were no new items or questions generated to create the HOOS.

Larson CB. Rating scale for hip disabilities. *Clin Orthop Relat Res.* 1963;31:85–93.

Lazansky MG. A method for grading hips. *J Bone Joint Surg Br.* 1967;49(4):644–651.

Letournel E, Judet R. *Fractures of the acetabulum.* New York, London, Berlin, Heidelberg: Springer-Verlag; 1993.

Lequesne MG, Samson M. Indices of severity in osteoarthritis for weight bearing joints. *J Rheumatol Suppl.* 1991;27:16–18.

Liang MH, Katz JN, Phillips C, Sledge C, Cats-Baril W. The total hip arthroplasty outcome evaluation form of the American Academy of Orthopaedic Surgeons. Results of a nominal group process. The American Academy of Orthopaedic Surgeons Task Force on Outcome Studies. *J Bone Joint Surg Am.* 1991;73(5):639–646.

Martin RL. Hip Arthroscopy and Outcome Assessment. *Operative Techniques in Orthopaedics.* 2005;15:290–296.

Martin DP, Engelberg R, Agel J, Snapp D, Swiontkowski MF. Development of a musculoskeletal extremity health status instrument: the musculoskeletal function assessment instrument. *J Orthop Res.* 1996;14(2):173–181.

This generic musculoskeletal instrument was developed to be patient based and self reported. The authors created an outcome that avoided the problems of other generic measures used to assess patients with musculoskeletal disorders. They created a 100-item questionnaire that was reliable and internally consistent with content validity.

Martin DP, Engelberg R, Agel J, Swiontkowski MF. Comparison of the Musculoskeletal Function Assessment questionnaire with the Short Form-36, the Western Ontario and McMaster Universities Osteoarthritis Index, and the Sickness Impact Profile health-status measures. *J Bone Joint Surg Am.* 1997;79(9):1323–1335.

Martin RL, Kelly BT, Philippon MJ. Evidence of validity for the hip outcome score. *Arthroscopy.* 2006;22(12):1304–1311.

Martin RL, Philippon MJ. Evidence of reliability and responsiveness for the Hip Outcome Score. *Operative Techniques in Orthopaedics.* 2005;15:290–296.

This publication introduces the Hip Outcome Score (HOS), which was developed to address the deficiency in preexisting outcomes for young patients undergoing arthroscopy. The HOS has two subscales: Activities of Daily Living (ADL) and Sports. The psychometrics of this instrument have been determined subsequent to this publication. The main problem with this outcome is that no patients were directly involved in the determination of the items included in the two subscales.

Martin RL, Philippon MJ. Evidence of validity for the hip outcome score in hip arthroscopy. *Arthroscopy.* 2007;23(8):822–826.

Martin RL, Philippon MJ. Evidence of reliability and responsiveness for the hip outcome score. *Arthroscopy.* 2008;24(6):676–682.

Marx RG, Jones EC, Atwan NC, Closkey RF, Salvati EA, Sculco TP. Measuring improvement following total hip and knee arthroplasty using patient-based measures of outcome. *J Bone Joint Surg Am.* 2005;87(9):1999–2005.

Matta JM, Mehne DK, Roffi R. Fractures of the acetabulum. Early results of a prospective study. *Clin Orthop Relat Res.* 1986;(205):241–250.

McDowell I, Newell C. *Measuring health: a guide to rating scales and questionnaires.* New York: Oxford University Press; 1987.

Mohtadi N. Development and validation of the quality of life outcome measure (questionnaire) for chronic anterior cruciate ligament deficiency. *Am J Sports Med.* 1998;26(3):350–359.

Mohtadi NG, Pedersen ME, Chan D. The creation of a hip outcome measure for young patients with hip disease. *In: World Congress of Sports Trauma.* Hong Kong; 2008.

Mohtadi N, Pedersen ME, Mahorn D, Chan, Fredine J. *Validation of the Hip Quality of Life Questionnaire.* New York: International Hip Arthroscopy Association; 2009.

Nilsdotter AK, Lohmander LS, Klassbo M, Roos EM. Hip disability and osteoarthritis outcome score (HOOS)–validity and responsiveness in total hip replacement. *BMC Musculoskelet Disord.* 2003;4:10.

Ohman U, Bjorkegren NA, Fahlstrom G. Fracture of the femoral neck. A five-year follow up. *Acta Chir Scand.* 1969;135(1):27–42.

Ovre S, Sandvik L, Madsen JE, Roise O. Comparison of distribution, agreement and correlation between the original and modified Merle d'Aubigne-Postel Score and the Harris Hip Score after acetabular fracture treatment: moderate agreement, high ceiling effect and excellent correlation in 450 patients. *Acta Orthop.* 2005;76(6):796–802.

Parker MJ, Palmer CR. A new mobility score for predicting mortality after hip fracture. *J Bone Joint Surg Br.* 1993;75(5):797–798.

Pedersen ME, Chan D, Mohtadi NG. Hip outcome measures: A systematic review of the literature. In: *Alberta Orthopaedics Residents Day; 2006;* Red Deer, Alberta; 2006.

Pellicci PM, Wilson Jr. PD, Sledge CB, Salvati EA, Ranawat CS, Poss R, et al. Long-term results of revision total hip replacement. A follow up report. *J Bone Joint Surg Am.* 1985;67(4):513–516.

Rat AC, Coste J, Pouchot J, Baumann M, Spitz E, Retel-Rude N, et al. OAKHQOL: a new instrument to measure quality of life in knee and hip osteoarthritis. *J Clin Epidemiol.* 2005;58(1):47–55.

The Osteoarthritis of Knee and Hip Quality of Life questionnaire is a step beyond the WOMAC in that it addresses the full dimensions of quality of life. This well-developed questionnaire has 40 questions divided into 5 dimensions (Pain; Physical activities; Mental health; Social support; Social functioning). In addition, there are three questions that relate to relationships, sexual activity, and professional life. This questionnaire was developed in France and although published in English has not been validated from a cross-cultural perspective.

Rat AC, Pouchot J, Coste J, Baumann C, Spitz E, Retel-Rude N, et al. Development and testing of a specific quality-of-life questionnaire for knee and hip osteoarthritis: OAKHQOL (OsteoArthritis of Knee Hip Quality Of Life). *Joint Bone Spine.* 2006;73(6):697–704.

Schmalzried TP, Silva M, de la Rosa MA, Choi ES, Fowble VA. Optimizing patient selection and outcomes with total hip resurfacing. *Clin Orthop Relat Res.* 2005;441:200–204.

Shepherd MM. Assessment of function after arthroplasty of the hip. *J Bone Joint Surg Am.* 1954;36B(3):354–363.

Shields RK, Enloe LJ, Evans RE, Smith KB, Steckel SD. Reliability, validity, and responsiveness of functional tests in patients with total joint replacement. *Phys Ther.* 1995;75(3):169–176; discussion 176–179.

Shimmin AJ, Bare J, Back DL. Complications associated with hip resurfacing arthroplasty. *Orthop Clin North Am.* 2005;36(2):187–193, ix.

Soderman P, Malchau H. Is the Harris hip score system useful to study the outcome of total hip replacement? *Clin Orthop Relat Res.* 2001;384:189–197.

Stucki G, Sangha O, Stucki S, Michel BA, Tyndall A, Dick W, et al. Comparison of the WOMAC (Western Ontario and McMaster Universities) osteoarthritis index and a self-report format of the self-administered Lequesne-Algofunctional index in patients with knee and hip osteoarthritis. *Osteoarthritis Cartilage.* 1998;6(2):79–86.

Sullivan M, Karlsson J. The Swedish SF-36 Health Survey III. Evaluation of criterion-based validity: results from normative population. *J Clin Epidemiol.* 1998;51(11):1105–1113.

Tegner Y, Lysholm J. Rating systems in the evaluation of knee ligament injuries. *Clin Orthop Relat Res.* 1985;198:43–49.

Theiler R, Sangha O, Schaeren S, Michel BA, Tyndall A, Dick W, et al. Superior responsiveness of the pain and function sections of the Western Ontario and McMaster Universities Osteoarthritis Index (WOMAC) as compared to the Lequesne-Algofunctional Index in patients with osteoarthritis of the lower extremities. *Osteoarthritis Cartilage.* 1999;7(6):515–519.

Thompson VP, Epstein HC. Traumatic dislocation of the hip: a survey of two hundred and four cases covering a period of twenty-one years. *J Bone Joint Surg Am.* 1951;33(3):746–778.

Treacy RB. To resurface or replace the hip in the under 65-year-old: the case of resurfacing. *Ann R Coll Surg Engl.* 2006;88(4):349–353; discussion 349–353.

Tugwell P, Bombardier C, Buchanan WW, Goldsmith CH, Grace E, Hanna B. The MACTAR Patient Preference Disability Questionnaire—an individualized functional priority approach for assessing improvement in physical disability in clinical trials in rheumatoid arthritis. *J Rheumatol.* 1987;14(3):446–451.

Verhoeven AC, Boers M, van der Liden S. Validity of the MACTAR questionnaire as a functional index in a rheumatoid arthritis clinical trial. The McMaster Toronto Arthritis. *J Rheumatol.* 2000;27(12):2801–2809.

Ware Jr. J, Kosinski M, Keller SD. A 12-Item Short-Form Health Survey: construction of scales and preliminary tests of reliability and validity. *Med Care.* 1996;34(3):220–233.

Wilson Jr. PD, Amstutz HC, Czerniecki A, Salvati EA, Mendes DG. Total hip replacement with fixation by acrylic cement. A preliminary study of 100 consecutive McKee-Farrar prosthetic replacements. *J Bone Joint Surg Am.* 1972;54(2):207–236.

Wright JG, Rudicel S, Feinstein AR. Ask patients what they want. Evaluation of individual complaints before total hip replacement. *J Bone Joint Surg Br.* 1994;76(2):229–234.

Wright JG, Young NL. A comparison of different indices of responsiveness. *J Clin Epidemiol.* 1997;50(3):239–246.

Yano H, Sano S, Nagata Y, Tabuchi K, Okinaga S, Seki H, et al. Modified rotational acetabular osteotomy (RAO) for advanced osteoarthritis of the hip joint in the middle-aged person. First report. *Arch Orthop Trauma Surg.* 1990;109(3):121–125.

Zuckerman JD, Koval KJ, Aharonoff GB, Hiebert R, Skovron ML. A functional recovery score for elderly hip fracture patients: I. Development. *J Orthop Trauma.* 2000;14(1):20–25.

# Arthroscopic Management

# CHAPTER 9

# Supine Approach to Hip Arthroscopy

*Zackary D. Vaughn and Marc R. Safran*

## INTRODUCTION

Two standard positions have been used for hip arthroscopy: lateral and supine. The supine approach is often favored for its familiar positioning with easy reference to the anatomic landmarks to which most surgeons are accustomed. The maneuverability and functionality of the arthroscopic equipment are also most similar to that used for other arthroscopic procedures with patients in the supine position. The anatomic orientation required for this position appears to be easier to attain from the surgeon's standpoint than that required for the lateral position. With the patient in the supine position, the operative extremity can be mobilized (i.e., dynamic testing in hip flexion–extension and rotation) during the procedure, and it also allows for capsular relaxation and the dynamic visualization of the joint and the peripheral compartment. With the supine approach, traction may be applied with the use of a standard hip fracture table or other device, whereas the lateral position requires a more specialized setup. In addition to the position being more familiar to classic total joint surgeons, the main benefit of the lateral position is that it uses gravity more effectively to allow the soft tissue to fall away from the greater trochanter as the primary landmark for instrumentation. This is most significant for the larger, moderately obese patient. However, some feel that the lateral approach is more time consuming and that using fluoroscopic imaging with a C-arm may be insufficient to get around an obese patient under the operating room table. In the end, both of these positions are effective, with surgeon preference and patient comfort being the determining factors as far as which one is chosen. Our preferred method is the supine position for the reasons outlined previously. This chapter describes our general surgical technique for patients in the supine position.

## GENERAL CONSIDERATIONS

The hip joint is not a true space. To perform hip arthroscopy of the central compartment, which is the area within the acetabulum, traction must be applied. Usually 8 mm to 12 mm of joint space opening is required to perform hip arthroscopy safely. If there is too little traction, then iatrogenic injury to the articular cartilage may occur while trying to travel through the joint. If there is too much traction, then there is increased potential risk of injury to the neural structures around the joint and the perineum as well as risk to the knee, foot, and ankle. Traction may be applied with the use of a standard fracture table or with the use of other commercially available attachments that have been devised for regular operating room tables, although some authors have reported using weight over the end of a standard

operating room table as a means of applying traction. Usually 25 lb to 50 lb of force is needed to apply adequate traction for hip arthroscopy.

To facilitate traction, we prefer the use of general anesthesia with paralysis. This allows for adequate traction without undue force to reduce the risk of injury to the nerves and the perineum. Arthroscopy of the hip may be performed with spinal anesthesia if there is adequate muscle relaxation. As an adjunct to general anesthesia, we have also used a lumbar plexus block to reduce the amount of narcotic intraoperatively, thereby reducing the amount of nausea postoperatively and the amount of pain during the immediate postoperative period (usually 12 to 18 hours). We prefer hypotensive anesthesia to reduce bleeding within the joint, thereby allowing for better visualization.

Hip arthroscopy is facilitated by the use of specialized instrumentation. Although extra-long arthroscopes and cannulas may be used, there is a risk of damage to these instruments. A standard-length hip arthroscope with a cannula that has a modified bridge is most commonly used, and this has been used almost exclusively by the senior author for the past 15 years. Only in the particularly obese patient is the extra-long arthroscopic lens needed. Cannulated hip arthroscopy systems that make use of Nitinol wires and blunt trochars have significantly reduced complications and aided in the development of arthroscopy portals. Many specialized extra-long instruments have been developed to perform therapeutic hip arthroscopy, including longer arthroscopic motorized shavers and burrs. Some shavers are curved to help facilitate access to areas around the femoral head. Other instruments include modified hand instrumentation, such as arthroscopic knives, rongeurs, meniscal biters (i.e., forward and backward, straight and upbiting), curettes, and even microfracture awls. Radiofrequency devices that are narrow and that bend at the tip are quite useful for tissue ablation and tissue shrinkage. In addition, instrumentation for labral repair (e.g., suture anchors that fit through narrow cannulas) is also available.

The senior surgeon generally uses 5.0-mm cannulas for the three central compartment portals, although, in tight hips with limited distraction, a 4.5-mm cannula may be used. However, when using gravity inflow for fluid, the fluid dynamics with the 4.5-mm cannula are suboptimal, and the cannula is changed, when possible. Alternatively, the introduction of irrigation fluid with a pump may overcome the limited dynamics of the smaller cannula. Frequently, 5.5-mm or 5.6-mm cannulas are necessary for the introduction of many instruments, including labral repair instruments, curettes, microfracture awls, and some labral biters. Alternatively, a slotted cannula (i.e., half-pipe) can allow for the maintenance of the portal while allowing larger instruments to be introduced (e.g., curved shaver, microfracture awl).

Saline or lactated Ringer's solution with epinephrine is usually used during hip arthroscopy as irrigation fluid. Irrigation fluid is introduced with the use of a gravity inflow system to reduce the risk of clinically significant fluid extravasation, because there have been reported cases of intra-abdominal fluid extravasation that have resulted in cardiac arrest. Visualization is enhanced with the use of hypotensive anesthesia and 5.0-mm or larger cannulas. However, on occasion, a pump is needed to perform arthroscopy (in the senior author's experience, this happens with less than 1% of cases).

To ensure the adequate visualization of the entire joint, the senior author prefers using three portals for central compartment arthroscopy on all patients and using both the 30-degree and 70-degree lenses in all three central compartment portals. To help with the maneuverability of both the arthroscope and the instrumentation, capsulotomies made with an arthroscopic knife or a radiofrequency probe do allow for significant freedom for access and visualization.

## SURGICAL TECHNIQUE

For the supine position technique, the patient is given a general anesthetic that provides muscle relaxation. Paralysis is recommended, because this allows less force to be used to distract the hip, with the purpose of reducing the risk of pudendal nerve injury from pressure between the pelvis and the perineal post of the traction table. The patient is placed supine on the fracture table with both feet secured to traction boots or mobile spars, depending on the specific table used. A well-padded perineal post is placed, and the patient is brought into position so that the post is firmly situated against the perineum and lateralized toward the operative hip, with care taken to protect the genitalia. The operative leg is positioned in 10 degrees of abduction, neutral flexion–extension, and neutral rotation. The nonoperative extremity is positioned in 45 degrees to 60 degrees of abduction, neutral flexion–extension, and neutral rotation to serve as countertraction for lateralization. Gentle traction is applied to the abducted nonoperative leg, which lateralizes the patient's pelvis and results in the perineal post resting on the inner upper thigh of the operative extremity (Figure 9-1). This allows for the pressure of the perineal post to be diverted away from the perineum itself to minimize the risk of neuropraxia to the pudendal nerve as traction is applied to the operative leg. In addition—and quite important—this also helps to generate the appropriate vector of force for a uniform distraction both laterally and distally (Figure 9-2). Traction to the operative leg straight distally would be met with unnecessary resistance to overcome the inferior transverse acetabular ligament. Lateralization of the hip with the use of the post helps to pull the femoral head laterally and distally from the socket without having to overcome the ligament as a barrier to distal translation.

After the patient has been positioned appropriately and slight traction has been applied to the nonoperative extremity, traction on the operative limb can be applied. This should be incremental, and it can be monitored with serial images from an image intensifier (i.e., C-arm). A tensiometer can also be used; however, the senior author has not found this to be useful. Jim Glick has shown that the risk of nerve injury as assessed by somatosensory evoked potentials is associated with the duration of traction rather than the amount of traction (Glick, personal communication). Thus, the absolute amount of traction is apparently not important. Some surgeons use the tensiometer to evaluate any changes in tension. We use the fluoroscopic image intensifier routinely; we bring the base of the machine in from the foot of the table in between the patient's abducted legs, and we center the column over the operative hip (see Figure 9-1). Incremental traction is then applied until approximately

8 mm to 10 mm of femoroacetabular joint distraction is generated. The area of the proposed anterolateral portal is identified and marked; the area around this proposed portal site is prepared with Betadine solution; and a spinal needle is then used to enter the hip joint to verify the correct path of the anterolateral portal, to ease joint access, and to perform an air arthrogram to release negative intra-articular pressure. In a cadaver study, Dienst and colleagues demonstrated that positioning the hip in 20 degrees of flexion and performing an air arthrogram (i.e., disrupting the vacuum seal and distending the hip joint) reduced the amount of traction required to distract the joint for safe entry, thereby further reducing the risk of neuropraxia. The needle is placed from the intended anterolateral portal with the guidance of the fluoroscopic image intensifier (Figure 9-3). The needle needs to enter the central compartment to effectively reduce the intra-articular pressure. We have shown that placing the needle onto the femoral neck does not release the negative intra-articular pressure within the joint. Care is taken to keep the spinal needle close to the femoral head (to reduce the risk of injury to the labrum) and to keep the longer part of the tip away from the femoral head. When the suction seal is broken, the joint will open more widely. The needle position relative to the femoral head is evaluated before and after the seal is broken. If the needle moves proximally when the negative pressure is released, the labrum may have been violated by the needle. If the needle moves with the femoral head, the labrum has likely not been injured.

## CENTRAL COMPARTMENT

The anterolateral portal (Figure 9-4) is started approximately 1 cm anterior to the superior aspect of the anterior border of the greater trochanter. The needle is placed nearly parallel to the floor and angled toward the sourcil of the acetabulum, between the labrum and the distracted femoral head (see Figure 9-3, B). Avoiding the labrum is the key aspect of this part of the procedure. This can be optimized by careful visualization with the C-arm and by trying to keep the needle closer to the femoral head. The apex of the needle is kept away from the femoral head to help avoid injury to the femoral head articular cartilage. If the needle is near the acetabulum and does not pass easily after the puncture of the capsule, then it is likely within the substance of the labrum; it must be withdrawn and carefully redirected. After the needle is placed appropriately, the obturator of the spinal needle may be removed to allow for the inflow of air. This air arthrogram will verify appropriate placement, reduce the amount of traction required, and further increase the joint space produced by the traction with the same amount of force (see Figure 9-3, B and C). When this procedure is completed, the spinal needle is removed, the traction is released, and the patient's hip can then be prepped and draped from the pelvis to the knee.

When the patient has been draped, the traction can be reapplied and verified with the C-arm, and then the anterolateral portal is created. Once again, place the spinal needle into the hip joint by following the same format and path. After the needle has been verified with the arthroscope to be intra-articular within the capsule and not damaging the labrum or articular cartilage, a guidewire is placed through the spinal needle. The spinal needle is then removed, leaving the guidewire in the place. A scalpel with a No. 11 blade is used to make a 5-mm incision over the guidewire. The cannulated trocar system is then used to place the arthroscope. Slowly and with controlled pressure and twisting to pierce the hip capsule, the blunt cannulated trocar is then introduced over the guidewire; this will provide moderate resistance (Figure 9-5). Care

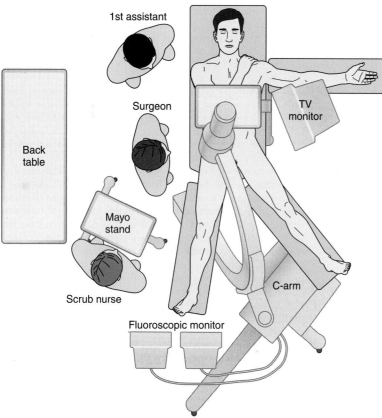

1st assistant

Surgeon

Back table

Mayo stand

Scrub nurse

Fluoroscopic monitor

TV monitor

C-arm

**A**

**Figure 9–1 A,** Schematic representation of the setup for supine hip arthroscopy. **B,** Typical setup for supine approach for hip arthroscopy. Note that the perineal post is lateralized toward the affected side. The nonoperative leg is abducted, and mild traction is applied to help with lateralization and countertraction. The operative leg is in slight abduction, neutral rotation, and neutral flexion–extension. *Part A redrawn from Safran, MR. Hip Arthroscopy—The Basics. In: Weisel S ed.* Operative Techniques in Orthopaedic Surgery. *Lippincott Williams and Wilkins; Philadelphia; 2010.*

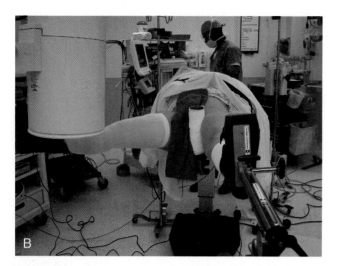

**B**

must be taken to not advance the guidewire too far or to bend the guidewire when inserting the cannula, because this may fracture the guidewire. Sharp trochars are discouraged, because this may cause iatrogenic injury to the joint. Trochar and sheath entry into the joint can be visualized with the C-arm. After getting inside of the joint, the blunt obturator and guidewire are removed, and an arthroscope with a 70-degree lens is introduced. When a clear picture is obtained, a cursory visualization of the hip joint may be conducted. The anterior portal is usually made right after the anterolateral portal is achieved. The anterior portal is made with the guidance of arthroscopic visualization to reduce the risk of iatrogenic injury to the acetabular or labral cartilage. Some surgeons insufflate fluid into the joint after the spinal needle for the anterolateral portal is intro-

duced to allow for joint distention. The senior author does not do this and in fact does not run fluid into the joint until the spinal needle for the second portal has been established. There is often blood in the joint after distraction and capsular injury from the entry into the joint. With no outflow of fluid, insufflation of the joint will result in cloudy visualization or obstructed visualization through the bloody fluid. Thus, the second portal is created while the joint is dry.

Generally, we create the second (anterior) portal before performing a complete evaluation of the hip. The second portal is made under arthroscopic and fluoroscopic visualization to ensure that the labral and articular cartilage is not damaged with the introduction of the needle, trochar, and cannula for the second portal. After the second portal is made (usually the

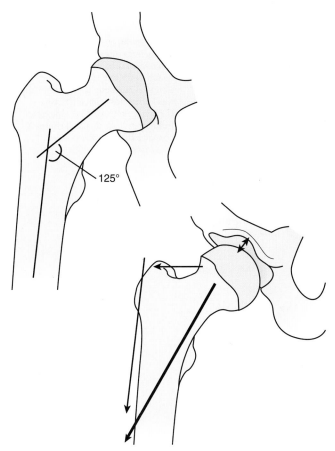

**Figure 9–2** Schematic representation of the effect of perineal post lateralization. The vector of pull is more in line with the femoral neck, thereby reducing the risk of injury and the need to overcome the transverse acetabular ligament. *From Byrd JWT. The supine position. In: Byrd JWT ed. Operative hip arthroscopy. New York; Thieme Publishers; 1998: Figure 9.2, page 125.*

during the introduction of the first portal, then the cannula is repositioned with the use of arthroscopic and fluoroscopic guidance.

Next, the second portal is created; this is an anterior working and visualization portal. There are several described locations for the introduction of the anterior portal. One of the more common places for the anterior portal is at the intersection of a line drawn caudally from the anterior superior iliac spine and a perpendicular line drawn from the tip of the greater trochanter (see Figures 9-4 and 9-5). This portal carries the risk of injury to the lateral femoral cutaneous nerve (because of this superficial nerve's intimate proximity to the portal) and to the rectus femoris. Our current preferred location for the anterior portal was described by Philippon (personal communication, 2007) and can be considered a mid-anterior portal. This portal is located 6 cm to 8 cm distal and anteromedial to the anterolateral portal at a 45-degree angle (Figure 9-6). This portal minimizes the risk of injury to the lateral femoral cutaneous nerve and the rectus femoris. In general, the different anterior portals are very near the arborization of the lateral femoral cutaneous nerve. Therefore, care must be taken when making this portal so that the skin incision remains superficial, with the No. 11 scalpel blade being used to reduce the risk of injury to the lateral femoral cutaneous nerve. The method for creating this portal is identical to that of creating the anterolateral; however, now the spinal needle may be visualized with the arthroscope in the anterolateral portal when the needle enters the joint, and care must be taken to pierce the capsule while avoiding injury to the labrum and the chondral surface (Figure 9-7). The spinal needle, the guidewire, and the subsequent trochar with cannula sheath all can be visualized with the arthroscope during entry to help avoid injury to the labrum and the articular cartilage. With this portal established, the arthroscope may be exchanged in this anterior portal to visualize the anterolateral portal placement to verify that no iatrogenic damage has occurred to the labrum. If the anterolateral portal is disrupting the labrum, it can now be redirected with the help of visualization from the anterior portal.

The posterolateral portal is the third and final standard portal for visualizing the central intra-articular compartment. Some surgeons do not routinely make a posterolateral portal, or, if they do, it serves as an inflow portal. The senior author prefers to use all three central compartment portals routinely to allow for the complete visualization of all structures in the hip joint from multiple perspectives. This portal is created in the same fashion as the other portals, and it is started 1 cm posterior to the posterosuperior border of the greater trochanter and in line with the anterolateral portal. The spinal needle can be directly

anterior portal), the arthroscope is placed into the cannula of the second portal to allow for the visualization of the initial (anterolateral) portal to ensure that the labrum was not injured with the creation of this first portal, which was placed under fluoroscopic visualization only. If the labrum was not injured, the arthroscope is replaced in the anterolateral portal cannula, and attention is turned to making the third portal and starting the complete diagnostic arthroscopy. If the labrum was injured

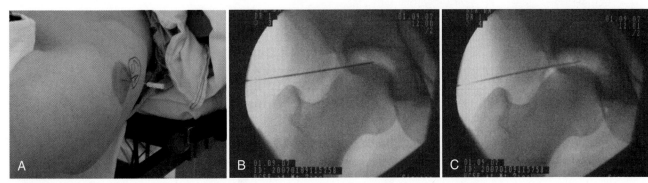

**Figure 9–3 A,** Spinal needle introduced at the proposed anterolateral portal to remove the negative intra-articular pressure to help ensure that appropriate distraction may be obtained during surgery. **B** and **C,** Fluoroscopic view of the hip with the needle introduced into the joint. In **B,** the needle is in the joint before the removal of the stylet and thus before air is introduced into the joint. In **C,** the stylet has been removed. By removing the stylet, air rushes into the joint, thereby removing the negative intra-articular pressure within the joint and allowing for more distention and distraction of the joint without adding more traction force.

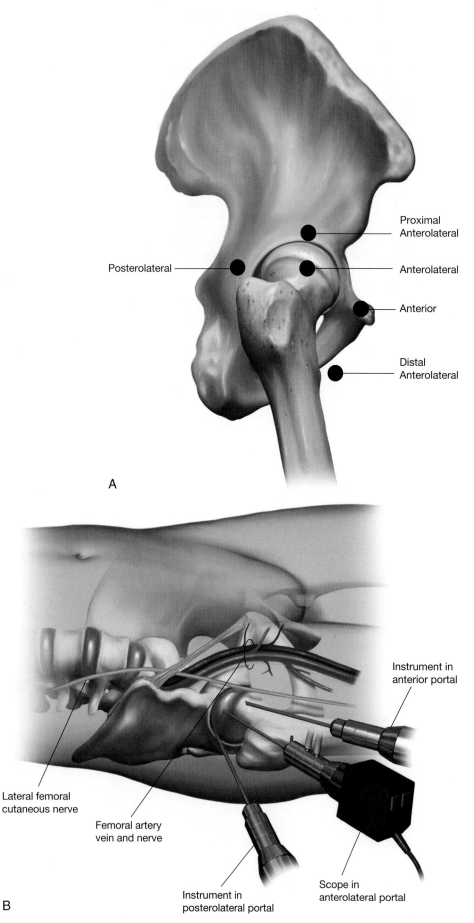

**Figure 9–4 A,** Schematic representation of where the three portals for hip arthroscopy begin. **B,** Schematic representation of the pathways of these three portals. **C,** The operating theater after the anterolateral portal has been established. *Redrawn from Safran MR. Hip Arthroscopy—The Basics. In: Weisel S ed.* Operative Techniques in Orthopaedic Surgery. *Lippincott Williams and Wilkins; Philadelphia; 2010.*

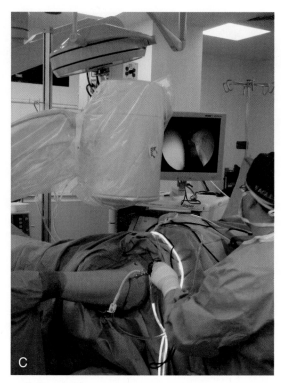

**Figure 9–4**—cont'd

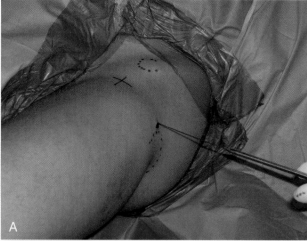

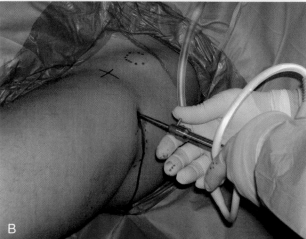

**Figure 9–5** **A,** After the guidewire has been placed into the joint through the spinal needle and the spinal needle has been removed, the blunt trochar and sheath are introduced into the joint over the guidewire. **B,** The arthroscope is then placed into the cannula to begin the visualization of the joint.

visualized arthroscopically when it enters the joint through the joint capsule, and it should be placed in a convergent fashion with the arthroscope in the anterolateral portal. Leg position is important when making this portal. If the lower extremity is in external rotation, the posteriorly positioned greater trochanter results in a sharper angle for the spinal needle, thereby increasing the risk of injury to the sciatic nerve. Flexion of the hip also draws the sciatic nerve closer to the joint, which also increases risk of injury. With this final portal established, the arthroscope may be used to visualize the central compartment from each portal and to treat the observed pathology.

The 70-degree arthroscope lens is best used for examining the peripheral aspect of the central compartment (i.e., labrum, labral–chondral interface, acetabular rim, and peripheral femoral head), whereas the 30-degree arthroscope lens will provide better visualization of the central femoral head, the deep acetabular fossa, and the ligamentum teres. The 30-degree arthroscope lens is the senior author's preferred lens to use in the peripheral extra-articular compartment for the treatment of such conditions as femoroacetabular impingement, synovial chondromatosis, and the removal of loose bodies.

## PERIPHERAL COMPARTMENT

The peripheral compartment can be accessed through a variety of portals. The senior author prefers to use the same anterolateral portal incision and one additional portal to access the peripheral compartment and to treat any pathology. For the majority of problems in the peripheral compartment, the senior author prefers flexing the patient's hip 20 degrees to 45 degrees to reduce tension from the anterior capsule and ligaments to assist with access and the mobility of the instrumentation in this area. The scope can be brought into the peripheral compartment via the anterior or anterolateral portal while the traction is removed from the extremity. Alternatively, a new capsulotomy may be made with the use of the spinal needle–guidewire–

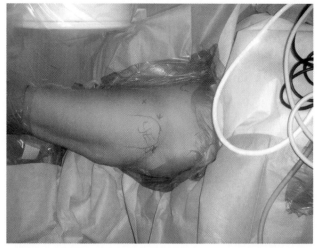

**Figure 9–6** The position of the modified anterior portal as described by Philippon (personal communication). This portal is 7 cm distal and medioanterior to a 45-degree angle from the anterolateral portal. This portal reduces risk to the lateral femoral cutaneous nerve, and it is a better angle for the placement of labral repair anchors.

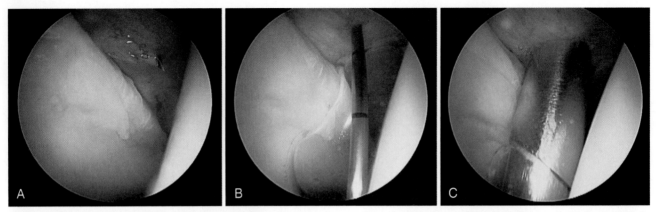

**Figure 9–7** Making the anterior portal. **A,** An arthroscopic view from the anterolateral portal of the right hip with the use of a 70-degree angled lens. The acetabulum is to the left and the femoral head to the right. The red at the top of the image is the anterior capsule, and the anterior torn labrum is seen at the upper left. The needle can be seen just penetrating the capsule. **B,** The needle is in the joint, away from the articular cartilage and the labrum, protected from iatrogenic damage. **C,** The trochar and the sheath are brought into the joint without causing injury to the articular or labral cartilage to make the anterior portal safely, under arthroscopic visualization.

cannulated trochar system. With the use of the same anterolateral portal, the blunt obturator and arthroscope cannula are redirected inferiorly to the anterior femoral neck, which can be guided by feel and with the assistance of the C-arm. After the arthroscope is in place, it can be introduced, and the peripheral compartment can then be visualized. A second accessory working portal can be created in line with the anterolateral portal, approximately 4 cm to 7 cm distal. This typically requires the introduction of the spinal needle that enters the peripheral compartment capsule laterally; the needle is then exchanged for the guidewire, which is then exchanged for the cannulated trochar with sheath.

The senior author accesses the peripheral compartment for femoral acetabular impingement differently. The anterolateral portal skin incision is used, and the blunt trochar with cannula sheath is introduced to the lateral apex of the femoral head; this spot is outside of the joint capsule. A proximal anterolateral portal is then made, 4 cm proximal to but in line with the anterolateral portal. A 5.0-mm or 5.5-mm aggressive shaver is introduced through this proximal anterolateral portal. The tip of the shaver and the tip of the arthroscope should be next to each other at the lateral aspect of the femoral head outside of the capsule, as described in the senior author's chapter about the arthroscopic management of cam impingement. The aggressive oscillating shaver is used to penetrate the lateral aspect of the capsule with the use of fluoroscopic and then arthroscopic visualization. Ultimately, with the help of arthroscopic visualization, a 1-cm to 1.5-cm window can be created in the lateral capsule; the peripheral compartment can be accessed through this opening.

Loose bodies may be removed from this accessory portal, or a high-speed burr may be placed for the performance of an osteoplasty for femoral head–neck junction lesions associated with femoroacetabular impingement. From this compartment, structures such as the labrum, the medial synovial fold, the capsular reflection, and the zona orbicularis can be visualized. These landmarks are useful for identifying other areas of pathology, such as the iliopsoas bursa and the tendon.

## CONCLUSION

Diagnostic and therapeutic hip arthroscopy may be easily performed with the patient in the supine position for central compartment, peripheral compartment, or even greater trochanteric space arthroscopy. With the surgeon paying attention to detail, limiting traction to less than 2 hours, making capsulotomies, and using the myriad of available instruments for hip arthroscopy, this procedure is reliable and reproducible, with a low risk of complications.

## ANNOTATED REFERENCES

**Byrd JWT. Hip arthroscopy utilizing the supine position.** *Arthroscopy.* **1994;10:275–280.**

Twenty patients treated for mechanical hip pain with arthroscopic procedures are described, including a technique for hip arthroscopy in the supine position and portal positioning. Excellent visualization was achieved in all cases and no major complications were encountered. Two transient neuropraxias of the pudendal nerve are reported.

**Byrd JWT. The supine position. In: Byrd JWT, ed. *Operative hip arthroscopy.* Thieme Publishers, New York, 1998:123–138.**

The supine positioning technique is described in this comprehensive textbook covering the evaluation and arthroscopic treatment of non-arthritic hip pathology. Safe positioning, portal placement, and basic arthroscopic technique is described.

**Byrd JWT, Pappas JN, Pedley MJ. Hip arthroscopy: an anatomic study of portal placement and relationship to extra-articular structures.** *Arthroscopy.* **1995;11:418–423.**

Eight fresh cadaveric paired hip specimens were dissected after placing Steinmann pins into the hip joint to simulate placement of portal sites. Neurovascular structures potentially at risk were evaluated for proximity to the portals. The anterior portal was found to be on average 0.3 cm from at least one of the branches of the lateral femoral cutaneous nerve. The superior gluteal nerve and sciatic nerves averaged 4.4 cm and 2.9 cm away from their respective portals.

**Dienst M, Seil R, Gödde S, Brang M, Becker K, Georg T, Kohn D. Effects of traction, distention, and joint position on distraction of the hip joint: an experimental study in cadavers.** *Arthroscopy.* **2002;18(8):865–871.**

Eight cadaveric hip joints were evaluated in the supine position on a fracture table with applied traction. Joint distraction was improved up to a 2.25-fold increase in distraction for the same amount of applied force by allowing distention of the hip joint from disrupting the negative pressure seal and allowing distention with air. Better distraction was also identified at 20 degrees of flexion. The authors concluded that air distention can avoid excessive traction forces and reduce the risk of neurologic injuries.

# Lateral Approach to Hip Arthroscopy

*Thomas G. Sampson*

## INTRODUCTION

Hip arthroscopy was first performed in our practice with the use of the supine approach on a fracture table for distraction. During our early experiences, problems of getting into the hip joint and complications such as the scuffing of articular cartilage, poor maneuverability, and the inability to achieve the result before extensive extravasation made the procedure difficult. Specific instruments were not developed, and distraction parameters were not established. As a result, the procedure was not predictable for entering the intra-articular space that is now known as the central compartment. In 1931, Burman was the first to use an arthroscope in the hip in a cadaveric study. However, he was unable to enter the central compartment, even with distraction. Our associate James M. Glick, MD, performed 11 procedures between 1977 and 1982, and he had difficulty getting in on two occasions. Because of our experience with the lateral decubitus positioning in total hip replacements, the idea of approaching hip arthroscopy in a similar way was developed. We dissected a cadaver hip to determine the most direct access to the intra-articular space, and we then described the anterior–peritrochanteric and posterior–peritrochanteric trochanteric portals (Figure 10-1); these have subsequently been referred to as the anterolateral and posterolateral portals. In 1986, distraction was introduced by Erikkson with the use of a fracture table to facilitate entry into the central compartment. We developed a rope-and-pulley system with weights as we used for shoulder arthroscopy as our first hip distractor (Figure 10-2). The first patient in whom we performed arthroscopy with the lateral approach was a massively obese woman with hip pain in whom Dr. Glick had previously performed arthroscopy without success in the supine position. In the lateral decubitus position, the obese portions of her thigh drooped down to expose a prominent greater trochanter. The neurovascular structures are safely away from the portals, and the surgeon is very familiar with their location; these portals offer a direct shot into the femoroacetabular joint. Many of the surgeons interested in hip arthroscopy at that time adopted the technique and continue to use it today.

In response to industry's interest in developing arthroscopic instruments and distractors, the supine approach was once again used and described by Byrd. There have been editorials, journal articles, and book chapters that argue the benefits of one as compared with the other, and it is my opinion that the approach that is used should be based on the training and comfort level of the surgeon. All procedures that involve hip arthroscopy are done with the use of both techniques in equal measure, and complications are not technique specific. A distractor (Hip Positioning System; Smith & Nephew, Andover, MA 01810)

has been designed to be used on any operating room table for both techniques, and all instruments designed for hip arthroscopy can be used for patients who are in either position.

The major advancements in getting into the central compartment were a result of distraction and the use of Nitinol wire cannulated trochars (Figure 10-3). Later, the development of longer arthroscopes, slotted (half-pipe) cannulas, and curved and flexible instruments allowed for advanced techniques that have followed a similar path as those used for knee and shoulder arthroscopy.

## INDICATIONS

As Thomas Byrd said, "the key to successful results most clearly is proper patient selection." In our practice, we believe that the patient's expectations should match the surgeon's. Hip arthroscopy during the early 1980s was felt to be a procedure looking for indications. Clearly, the list of indications has grown with the advancements of the technique.

### Loose and Foreign Bodies

Originally hip arthroscopy was performed for the removal of loose and foreign bodies. Today, this has been the clearest indication for the procedure, and arthroscopy has essentially replaced arthrotomy as a much less invasive alternative. The loose bodies may be from synovial chondromatosis (i.e., rice-like or osseocartilaginous), bullets, or loose cement or wires used in total hip replacements.

### Osteochondral Fracture Fragments

Articular cartilage injury from a younger patient falling directly onto the side of a hip may result in an osteochondral fracture and loose fragments, with the reaction of the head resembling aseptic necrosis. The removal of the fragment and the microfracture of the base have been shown to be beneficial.

### Labral Lesions

Labral lesions represent the most common indication for hip arthroscopy; however, their treatment has resulted in a dearth of new procedures. In the past, partial or total excision was the treatment of choice. However, the outcome was not predictable, especially in the presence of articular cartilage damage or arthritis. Primary labral repair was equally controversial and

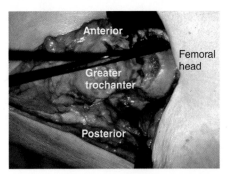

**Figure 10–1** The original cadaver dissection performed by James M. Glick and Thomas G. Sampson to develop the portals for the lateral approach.

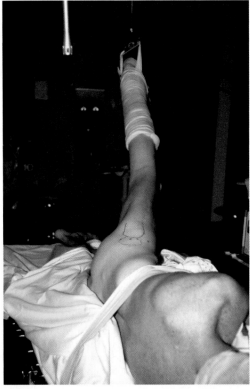

**Figure 10–2** The first hip distractor design. This design makes use of Buck's traction as a leg holder that is suspended with ropes and pulleys from the ceiling and the wall, with more than 45 lb of weight.

also had unpredictable outcomes. Recently, femoroacetabular impingement has helped to explain the cause of atraumatic labral tears; its treatment with head–neck osteoplasty, rim trimming, and labral debridement or refixation has become more common when labral tears are treated.

### Developmental Dysplasia

In the past, developmental dysplasia of the hip was a contraindication for hip arthroscopy, and osteotomy was recommended. Today, if the dysplasia is borderline (i.e., a center-edge angle of 20 degrees to 25 degrees) or in combination with femoroacetabular impingement, then the patient may benefit from

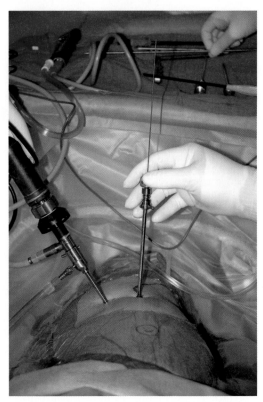

**Figure 10–3** The arthroscope has a shortened hub, and the hip trochar is cannulated for a Nitinol wire. Note that the Mayo stand is above the patient's shoulder and that it is used to keep the instruments organized for easy access by the surgeon.

arthroscopic treatment. The intra-articular pathology includes labral tears, articular cartilage damage, and the disruption of the ligamentum teres. The peripheral compartment pathology may have a lax capsule and an anterior rim osteophyte. Techniques to treat this condition arthroscopically have had favorable outcomes that have obviated arthrotomy. Capsulorrhaphy for laxity can be performed more successfully and with less biomechanical instability.

### Synovial Disease

The treatments of synovial diseases with biopsy for rheumatic diseases or synovectomy for pigmented villonodular synovitis (PVNS), synovial chondromatosis, or infection are very effective. The problem has been getting to all of the synovial surfaces within the central and peripheral compartments, but this issue has been improved with capsulotomy.

### Adhesive Capsulitis

Adhesive capsulitis has been recognized as a cause of hip pain similar to that seen in the shoulder. Debridement and synovectomy for primary or revision cases have shown benefit.

### Sepsis

Sepsis has clearly been successfully treated with hip arthroscopy. Arthroscopy with washout and debridement is now the primary treatment for acutely infected total hips.

### Femoroacetabular Impingement

Femoroacetabular impingement is a mismatch between the shape of the head–neck junction and the acetabulum that causes an overload to the labrum and the articular cartilage that results in damage to both. The arthroscopic technique has evolved from the open technique and today is accepted as a treatment for the condition. Labral refixation and bone reshaping of both the head–neck junction and the acetabular rim are performed to correct the defects.

### Hip Arthritis

The treatment of hip arthritis has had an upsurge with the use of hip arthroscopy as a bridge technique before total hip replacement. With the advent of bone reshaping techniques being performed arthroscopically, the results of debridement, microfracture, and resection osteoplasty have improved the outcomes as compared with debridement alone. Of course, moderate to severe osteoarthritis with a loss of joint space and a limited range of motion are contraindications.

### Staging Aseptic Necrosis

The treatment of end-stage aseptic necrosis has met with poor results; however, staging for open techniques (e.g., vascularized fibular grafts) has employed hip arthroscopy.

### Coxa Sultans

Coxa sultans (i.e., snapping hip syndrome) can be treated arthroscopically with releases. The iliopsoas tendon is accessible at the lesser trochanter and in the transcapsular region near the inferior synovial fold for an arthroscopically facilitated release. The peritrochanteric region is the latest frontier in hip arthroscopy. Release of the iliotibial band for the external snapping and repair of gluteus medius ruptures (i.e., the rotator cuff of the hip) has been performed with success.

## SURGICAL TECHNIQUE

### Anesthesia

Most commonly, we use general anesthesia. If regional anesthesia is used, there must be muscle relaxation. Antibiotic prophylaxis is warranted with the use of one of the cephalosporins. Deep vein thrombosis prophylaxis is performed with the use of compression stockings and a sequential pump on the downside leg.

### Patient Positioning

The patient is placed on a well-padded operating room table in the lateral decubitus position (Figure 10-4). An axillary roll is positioned, and hip positioners are used to support the pelvis. By preventing the pelvis from rolling back on the perineal post, the risk of pudendal neuropraxias may be reduced.

The foot is wrapped with padding, and the foot holder is applied, with care taken to avoid skin pinching by the device. The leg is held in abduction by the assistant during the careful placement of the well-padded perineal post. We have determined that the post should have an outer diameter of more than 9 cm for safety; commercially available hip distractors all exceed this size. The genitalia are inspected to ensure that they are free from compression. The foot holder is applied to the distraction arm, and only enough traction is applied to support the leg.

The fluoroscopic C-arm is brought in with the apex under the table and centered at the level of the greater trochanter. Preoperative x-rays are performed to check positioning and hip anatomy. A trial of distraction will be of benefit for two reasons: 1) to check for the distractibility of the joint and 2) to ensure that the foot is properly secured in the foot holder. If the hip does not distract well, this may be the result of a tight or hypertrophic capsule, and a few minutes of traction may allow the hip to relax. Failure to distract may require greater forces of distraction, or it may necessitate capsulotomy. If the foot slips out of the holder during the trial, less padding may help to prevent slippage. Adequate security of the foot in the holder is imperative to prevent an accidental release of the distraction when the instruments are in the central compartment, which may result in iatrogenic articular cartilage damage.

Sticky towels or drapes are placed from the iliac crest to 6 inches below the greater trochanter and from a sagittal line lateral to the anterior superior iliac spine anterior and the sciatic notch posterior.

The anesthesiologist is at the head of the table, the surgeon stands anterior, and the assistant stands posterior. The scrub technician stands next to the surgeon, with the C-arm in between them. A Mayo stand is placed above the patient's shoulder for easy accessibility to the instruments and for the organization of the arthroscopic cords.

We typically drape with split sheets, and we use a large plastic pouch to catch fluids.

### Distraction

For optimal viewing and safe surgery, at least 1.2 cm of distraction is required before the femoroacetabular joint (central compartment) is entered. Three commercially available distractors for the lateral approach are available from Mizuho OSI (Union City, CA 94587-1234), Innomed, Inc. (Savannah, GA, 31404), and Smith & Nephew. The Mizuho OSI and the Smith & Nephew distractors have the advantage in that hip mobility is adjustable during surgery (Figure 10-5).

Not all distractors have a tensiometer to measure the force of distraction. Distraction should be thought of in the same way as a tourniquet. James M. Glick, MD, demonstrated that, with the use of evoked potentials, forces of less than 75 lb for less than 2 hours were safe and did not cause permanent neuropraxias. In our practice, we have performed more than 750 procedures without a tensiometer, with care taken to keep the distraction time to a minimum; we have had no neuropraxias. We try for traction of less than 50 lb and for less than 1 hour to allow for a large margin of safety. It is important to realize that complications may occur from too little or too much traction and that, to accomplish the procedure, the joint surfaces must be separated for the introduction of instruments.

The perineal post should have padding of at least 9 cm in diameter, and it should be positioned eccentrically over the pubic symphysis, with little to no compression to the downside thigh (Figure 10-6).

We initiate the operative distraction after the case is entirely set up and after all of the equipment has been turned on and is functioning. We record the traction time, which may be entered in the operative record. The assistant or the circulating nurse announces the distraction time at 15-minute intervals.

After the intra-articular portion of the surgery is finished, all of the distraction forces are released, and the periarticular work in the peripheral compartment can be performed without distraction concerns.

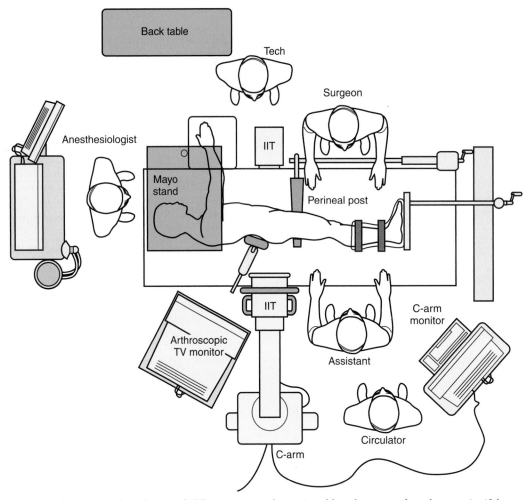

**Figure 10–4** The room setup for the lateral approach. The surgeon stands anterior, although some prefer to be posterior if they perform total hip procedures from the posterior approach. The assistant works from the opposite side, and the scrub technician is to the side of the surgeon. The C-arm lies below the table throughout the case, and a Mayo stand is placed above the patient's shoulder for instruments. *IIT*, image intensifier.

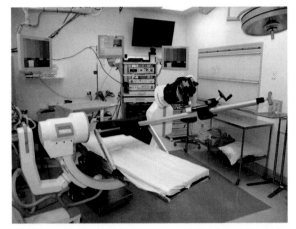

**Figure 10–5** A commercially available lateral hip distractor made by Smith & Nephew.

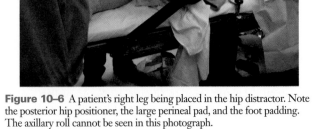

**Figure 10–6** A patient's right leg being placed in the hip distractor. Note the posterior hip positioner, the large perineal pad, and the foot padding. The axillary roll cannot be seen in this photograph.

## OPERATING ROOM SETUP

### Leg Position

With the patient in traction, the hip capsule is maximally relaxed in 15 degrees of flexion, neutral rotation, and 15 degrees of abduction. We use this as a starting position, and we make positional adjustments during the procedure to facilitate the ability to get into different areas. In addition, the perineal post may be elevated laterally to add an abduction moment for better viewing.

## Instruments

The 30-degree arthroscope is best for central viewing. It is easier to get oriented with this angle, and it is the best for getting started with the use of the lateral approach. The 70-degree arthroscope is best for peripheral viewing, for use around the femoral head and deep in the fossa, for viewing the fovea, and for creating additional portals. For thin patients, standard arthroscopic equipment may be used if the sheath has a short hub. The advantage of commercially available hip kits is that they contain the proper sheath lengths and cannulated systems. The option for longer arthroscopes should be available for larger patients and for those cases in which excessive swelling occurs in the thigh during the procedure.

Both straight and curved graspers are necessary, and so are straight and curved shavers. To insert curved instruments, a slotted cannula or a flexible plastic sheath is used.

Radiothermal probes are used for coagulation and for the cutting and ablation of tissues (e.g., capsule, labrum). Many of these probes are curved or bendable, and they can reach lesions that are not accessible to straight shavers. Flexible wands for hips can be manually maneuvered with a trigger handle.

Angled neurocurrettes and picks are used to treat arthritic defects and to remove attached and loose bodies that are located in areas that are difficult to reach, such as the medial acetabular fossa and the anteromedial acetabulum.

### The Pump

It is generally accepted to use a pump system because the exact pressure and flow can be controlled and monitored. We recommend using an outflow-dependent pump, which lowers the amount of extravasation into the soft tissues. The pump pressure is set in the same way that it is for shoulder settings or slightly above diastolic pressure.

### The Tower

The arthroscopic tower with the monitor and instrument boxes should be placed posterior and slightly cephalad adjacent to the C-arm for optimal viewing of all the settings by the surgeon. The cords from the tower are brought onto the Mayo stand and organized for the surgeon to easily reach for the shaver and wands. It is more efficient and safe for the Mayo stand to act as neutral ground that only one person accesses to avoid accidental glove punctures or lacerations (Figure 10-7, *A* and *B*).

## THE PROCEDURE

The portals for the lateral approach are nearly identical to the supine approach, except the anterior portal is located approximately 2 cm lateral to the anterior superior iliac spine (ASIS) line. As a result, the anterior portal courses in an intermuscular plane between the sartorius and the tensor fascia lata (Figure 10-8).

Distraction can only be initiated after everything is set up; the patient is prepped and draped; all of the instruments, the camera, and the shaver sets have been plugged in; the foot controls have been positioned; and it has been determined that everything is functioning correctly. For small and flexible patients, start with 25 lb to 50 lb of force. With large and stiff patients, start with 50 lb to 75 lb if you are using a tensiometer; if you are not using a tensiometer, apply weight until you observe at least 1 cm to 2 cm of separation between the head and the acetabulum on the fluoroscopic view.

Viewing with the C-arm fluoroscope and starting with the anterolateral portal, a long 17-gauge needle is inserted, and it is observed passing between the head of the femur and the acetabulum (but closer to the femur to avoid puncturing the labrum). Listen for a hiss of sound as the joint suction seal is broken and room air is sucked into the joint. Observe for the

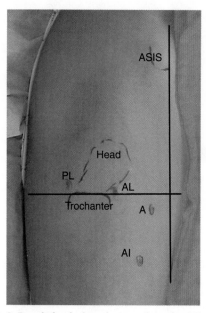

**Figure 10–8** Portals for the lateral approach on the right hip. *A,* Anterior; *AI,* anteroinferior; *AL,* anterolateral; *ASIS,* anterosuperior iliac spine; *PL,* posterolateral.

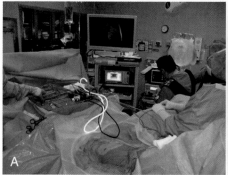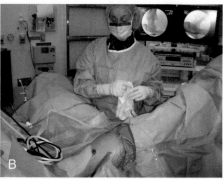

**Figure 10–7** The surgeon's view from the front of the patient. **A,** There is a clear view of the tower's instrument boxes, the monitor, and the outflow-dependent pump. The Mayo stand is above the patient's shoulder, and it is used for organization and for easy access to the instruments. **B,** A view of the fluoroscopic monitor toward the foot of the table.

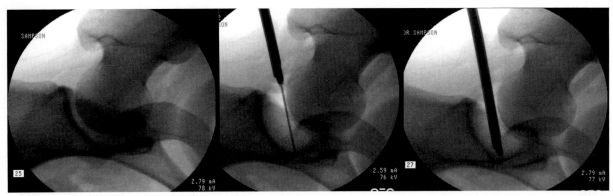

**Figure 10–9** Fluoroscopic view of the distraction of the hip joint and the insertion of the cannulated trochar over the Nitinol wire.

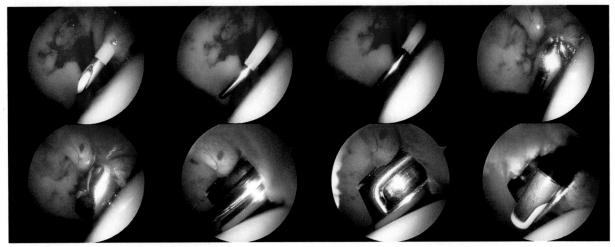

**Figure 10–10** Arthroscopic view from the anterolateral portal of the progression of steps of inserting the needle, the Nitinol wire, the cannulated trochar, the switching stick, the slotted (half-pipe) cannula, and, finally, the radiofrequency (RF) probe through the anterior portal.

traction forces to reduce on the tensiometer or for a sudden distal subluxation of the hip. Obtain the desired distraction, which is usually more than 1.2 cm. Insert a Nitinol wire through the needle, and incise the skin with a No. 11 blade. Push the cannulated arthroscopic sheath over the wire and into the joint while advancing it concentrically over the wire to prevent kinking and wire breakage. Backing the wire out slightly will reduce cartilage trauma.

If it is difficult to advance into the joint, suspect that the wire is going through the labrum. In such instances, it is best to start over and to reposition the needle to avoid labral avulsions or tears. In some cases, with stiff hips, the anterior capsule is very thick and very difficult to penetrate. In that situation, it is best to begin with the posterolateral portal or to gently cut the capsule with a long Beaver blade through the arthroscopic sheath before advancing into the joint. Entry into the joint should always be controlled to avoid damaging the labrum or scuffing the cartilage. However, pushing a cannula through the anterior hip capsule is difficult and requires a lot of force as compared with any other joint in the body (Figure 10-9).

Introduce a 30-degree arthroscope, and visually sweep the joint under air or fluid. Next, create the anterior and posterolateral portals with the use of the same technique and with the added benefit of viewing the entry of the needle, the Nitinol wire, and the instruments under direct vision to prevent injury to the cartilage and the labrum. We feel that this approach is

much safer and that iatrogenic injury is reduced. When creating the anterior portal, take care to only incise the skin superficially to avoid the laceration of a branch of the lateral femoral cutaneous nerve. Spreading through the subcutaneous tissue with a clamp is also advised for this portal (Figure 10-10).

After the arthroscope and the instruments are in place, the central compartment should be inspected in a methodic fashion to plan the necessary treatment. Attention to time is imperative to allow for the sufficient management of the pathology.

## THE VISUAL SWEEP AND ANATOMY

The acetabulum and its structures are viewed first. Initially, the femoral head cannot be entirely viewed with the hip distracted. However the hidden portions will be observed when the peripheral compartment is inspected later during the procedure (Figure 10-11).

With the 30-degree scope, start by observing the acetabular fossa and the fat pad. Petechial hemorrhage is normal as a result of the traction forces that are pulling negative pressure on the vessels. However, atrophy of the fat pad is abnormal. Look for loose bodies, rice bodies, notch osteophytes, and masses. Advance the scope deep to view the ligamentum teres to look for tears or avulsions. The transverse acetabular ligament is very hard to see unless the patient has hyperlaxity.

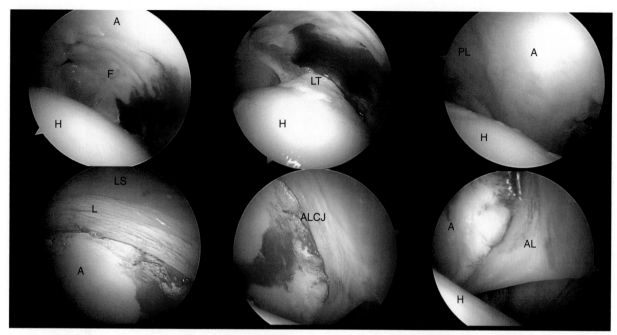

**Figure 10–11** Arthroscopic view of a right hip in room air. *A*, Acetabulum; *AL*, anterior labrum; *ALCJ*, anterior labrocartilaginous junction; *F*, fossa; *H*, head; *L*, labrum; *LS*, lateral sulcus; *LT*, ligamentum teres; *PL*, posterior labrum.

Rotate the scope posterior and inferior, and pick up the posterior labrum at the articular margin, noting the posterior third. Look behind the labrum for loose bodies, and then follow the labrum lateral and anterior, noting a normal cleft in the posterior articular margin with a small labral cartilage sulcus. The sulcus is not an old avulsion fracture nor from a posterior subluxation. Note any labral fraying or tears and articular changes.

Look at the middle third, and note any labral cartilage separations, fraying, or degenerative changes. The surface may be smooth, or it may have a cobblestone appearance during the early stages of degeneration.

As the scope is rotated to the anterior area, look for hypertrophy of the labrum in patients with dysplasia. The acetabular cartilage may be soft, or it may appear blistered or delaminated in dysplastic patients with anterior groin pain, instability, or popping. Look anterior beyond the labrum in the sulcus for synovitis and loose bodies. Move the scope to the superior sulcus of the joint to see the nonarticular side of the labrum in the pericapsular space from anterior to posterior. Look for evidence of cysts, spurring, and labral tears. All the while, a probe or a switching stick is used to probe.

Next, observe as much of the femoral head as possible with the same method, and, if necessary, rotate the leg while it is in traction. At this point, we switch to a 70-degree scope to look deeper into the notch and to have a better view of the femoral head fovea with its ligamentum teres insertion.

After viewing this area from the anterolateral portal, the same procedure is carried out from the posterior portal if we are not satisfied with the initial viewing.

If getting into the central compartment is very difficult or if the surgical plan is to remove bone in patients with femoroacetabular impingement, a capsulotomy is performed first. The capsule is viewed by sweeping the muscle with a switcher stick and removing the interval bursa with the shaver. Using a radiofrequency (RF) cutting probe and positioning the tool near the base of the neck anterior to the lateral neck to avoid damage to the lateral epiphyseal branch of the medial femoral circumflex artery, the capsule is incised along the neck. Care is taken as the labrum is approached to avoid cutting it. Many times, the zona orbicularis looks like the labrum, and it is distinguished by its more distal position on the neck as seen on the C-arm x-ray. If the capsule is excessively thick, a partial capsulectomy is then performed.

Corrective surgery is performed, depending on the diagnosis, and the distraction is completely released to allow the hip to be moved in rotation and flexion.

With the hip in slight flexion and neutral rotation, the 17-gauge needle is inserted through the anterolateral portal along the femoral neck toward the head–neck junction. While this procedure is observed under fluoroscopy, a small pop is felt as the needle passes through the capsule, and the effusion dribbles out of the needle (Figure 10-12). A Nitinol wire is passed and bounced off of the medial capsule to confirm that it is intra-articular. The arthroscopic sheath is advanced over the wire, and then the anterior, medial, inferior, and posterior peripheral spaces can be viewed.

First, note that the femoral head is seated in the labrum as it transforms into the transverse acetabular ligament. The zona orbicularis crosses the field, and one may see the vincula-like vessel in the lateral synovial fold going into the femoral neck. Push the scope deep and posterior to view the sulcus, and look for loose bodies.

As the scope is withdrawn, rotate it, and then advance it anterior medial and inferior to appreciate the reflection of the iliopsoas tendon on the capsule. The tendinous bulge on the capsule

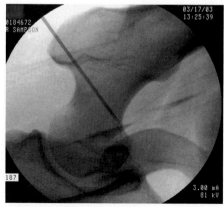

**Figure 10–12** Fluoroscopic view of a left hip with a Nitinol wire in the peripheral compartment touching the medial capsule from the anterior portal.

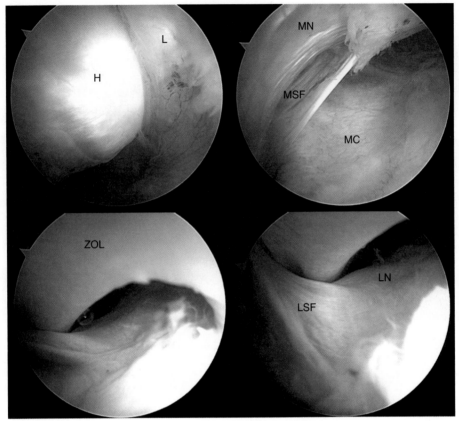

**Figure 10–13** Arthroscopic view of a right hip in the peripheral space. *H*, Head; *L*, labrum; *LN*, lateral neck; *LSF*, lateral synovial fold; *MC*, medial capsule; *MN*, medial neck; *MSF*, medial synovial fold; *ZOL*, zona orbicularis lateral portion.

is usually opposite the inferior synovial fold at the head–neck junction; it should not be mistaken for the zona orbicularis. Flexing the hip will relax the capsule for a larger field of view, and this improves the mobility of the scope and the operative instruments (Figure 10-13). An anteroinferior portal may be created at the level of the femoral neck midway between the head–neck junction and the lesser trochanter for both the arthroscope and the operative instruments. A far anteroinferior portal may be used at the level of the lesser trochanter for iliopsoas release.

At the completion of the procedure, close the wounds, and apply a standard dressing. An intra-articular injection of a long-acting local anesthetic (e.g., bupivacaine) will make recovery and the trip home from the surgical center more tolerable.

In the recovery room, have the patient begin both passive and active range-of-motion exercises of the hip. Crutches are used, with the amount of weight bearing being dependent on the patient's diagnosis and treatment.

## TECHNICAL PEARLS

- Position the patient on the table closer to the side on which the surgeon is working for better ergonomics and less surgeon fatigue.
- Pad down the bony prominences on the side, the perineal nerve, and the foot.
- Carefully place the axillary roll.
- Check the part of the genitalia against the perineal post.
- Pad the foot that is going into the distractor, and double check that it is well seated and securely strapped in.
- Test the distractor before scrubbing to prevent inadvertent foot slippage.
- Keep the C-arm fluoroscope under the table throughout the case for instrument positioning and for checking the surgical progression.
- Always use a C-arm x-ray to confirm needle and cannula placement.
- Choose special instruments ahead of the procedure (e.g., spinal curettes and heavy graspers for large, loose bodies and osteophytectomy; labral refixation anchors).
- If there is a lot of resistance during needle placement, it may be because the needle is hitting the acetabular rim (not seen on x-ray) or the labrum. Back out, and reposition the needle.
- When distracting the hip, if there is poor excursion of the head (i.e., less than 0.5 cm), try to break the suction seal of the labrum with the spinal needle.
- If distraction does not separate the head from the acetabulum despite any amount of distraction in any position, getting into the central compartment may be facilitated by extra-articular capsulotomy and rim trimming of the acetabulum.
- Intra-articular capsulotomy facilitates instrument mobility.
- When working in the anterior portion of the central compartment, bringing the leg into additional extension will open up the space.
- Any instrument may be placed with the use of a slotted cannula.

### TECHNICAL PEARLS—Cont'd

- Use distraction judiciously and only when it is necessary to work in the central compartment. All peripheral compartment work should be done without distraction.
- Flex and externally rotate the hip when accessing the medial and posteromedial peripheral space.
- Do a wide capsulotomy when taking out loose bodies and when treating femoroacetabular impingement (Figure 10-14, *A* through *C*).
- Make a new portal if the current portal is not working well.

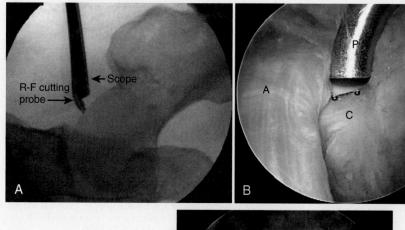

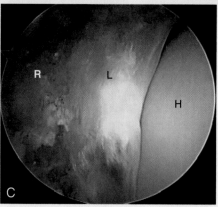

**Figure 10–14**   A capsulotomy that starts in the extracapsular region is used to get into tight hips and for bone resection for femoroacetabular impingement. **A,** Fluoroscopic view that places the radiofrequency (RF) cutting probe on the anterolateral capsule. **B,** The RF cutting probe *(P)* on the capsule *(C)*. Note the reflected head of the rectus femoris *(A)*. **C,** Arthroscopic view after capsulotomy; note the acetabular rim *(R)*, the labrum *(L)*, and the head of the femur *(H)*.

The dressings are removed after 24 hours, and the patient is then allowed to shower. Therapy is started within a week to help the patient to regain motion and strength.

## POSTOPERATIVE REHABILITATION

Aggressive physical therapy is not necessary after most hip arthroscopic procedures. In some cases, moving too quickly with rehabilitation may cause unnecessary pain, which impedes progress. If a therapist is used, he or she must have full knowledge of the procedures performed and the precautionary restrictions imposed.

We have found that instructions to the patient for self-therapy during the first month have eliminated the complications that can result from physical therapy. After a month, prescribed therapy may be used. We initiate the patient on stationary bike and elliptical trainer exercises that are followed by swimming and pool exercises. The idea is to allow for early range of motion and weight bearing for better joint mobility and proprioception.

In most cases, repetitive joint percussion (e.g., running) is avoided until pain and swelling are gone and the patient has good hip stability, which usually happens approximately 3 months after the procedure.

## RESULTS

The success of the lateral approach cannot be measured by a double-blind prospective study, but it should be judged by the facilitation of the ability to get into the central compartment of the hip. In that sense, it was the first, most reproducible, and widely used technique before the development of specific hip kits or hip distractors. The outcomes of treating specific conditions with the use of either the lateral or the supine approaches are the subject of other chapters in this book.

## COMPLICATIONS

There are many potential complications; however, with experience and attention to detail, they may be eliminated. In our first 60 cases, we had complications 15% of the time; in our most recent 1000 cases, we have had a complication rate of only 0.4%. We have never had a deep infection; however, there have been four superficial infections that have involved the anterior portal. It is not uncommon to have instruments pass in and out of the portals numerous times during a case, which can irritate and injure the skin around the portal.

During the early years of the development of this procedure, there were more extravasations into the thigh and, in nine cases, into the retroperitoneal space; the latter required an intensive care unit stay with the patient intubated and, in one case, a paracentesis to drain the fluid. This complication was virtually eliminated with the modern outflow-dependent pumps and with careful attention paid to the operative time.

Neuropraxia of the pudendal nerve was common before the use of more than 9 cm of padding on the perineal post and before its position was offset from the pubic symphysis. Damage to the major nerves has rarely occurred, and, with the use of modern distractors and keeping distraction time to less than 2 hours, it is even more rare. Scope trauma to the articular cartilage occurs even by the most experienced surgeons, and it is generally underreported. Instrument breakage does occur, but most of these broken instruments are retrieved. Infections are very rare. We have never had a patient develop deep sepsis after hip arthroscopy, but, if this did occur, the treatment is arthroscopic lavage, synovectomy, and parenteral antibiotics.

## ANNOTATED REFERENCES AND SUGGESTED READINGS

Burman MS. Arthroscopy or the direct visualization of joints: an experimental cadaver study. *J Bone Joint Surg*. 1931; 13:5–9.

This is a classic article and perhaps the first on hip arthroscopy in the English literature. He described a method of arthroscoping large joints including hips using cadavers. His drawings essentially documented the parts of the peripheral space of the hip as it was essentially impossible for getting onto the central compartment.

Byrd JW, Chern KY. Traction versus distension for distraction of the joint during hip arthroscopy. *Arthroscopy*. 1997;13(3):346–349.

This study shows that distention may facilitate distraction but the degree is variable.

Byrd JW. Hip arthroscopy utilizing the supine position. *Arthroscopy*. 1994;10(3):275–280.

Byrd showed a method and merits for the supine approach to hip arthroscopy. He described how to reproducibly place the first portal anterolateral with a 70-degree arthroscopy, angling the instrument precisely at a 30-degree angle cephalad from the trochanteric line and watching from within the joint as the posterior and anterior portals are created. He showed a new line of cannulated instruments to facilitate exchange of the scope and instruments between portals. The indications, early results, and complications were presented.

Byrd JW, Pappas JN, Pedley MJ. Hip arthroscopy: an anatomic study of portal placement and relationship to the extra-articular structures. *Arthroscopy*. 1995;11(4):418–423.

The purpose of this study is to accurately describe the relationship of the major neurovascular structures to standard portals used in hip arthroscopy. This is a cadaver study in which the portal placements are compared to the normal surrounding anatomy. They showed that avoidance of vital structures depended on good portal placement.

Eriksson E, Arvidsson I, Arvidsson H. Diagnostic and operative arthroscopy of the hip. *Orthopedics*. 1986;9(2):169–176.

Eriksson described a method of hip arthroscopy on patients with hip pain using the supine approach. He used a fracture table to distract the hip joint to get into the central compartment. He studied the forces necessary to adequately distract the hip for arthroscopy.

Farjo LA, Glick JM, Sampson TG. Hip arthroscopy for acetabular labral tears. *Arthroscopy*. 1999;15(2):132–137.

Glick JM, Sampson TG, Gordon RB, et al. Hip arthroscopy by the lateral approach. *Arthroscopy*. 1987;3(1):4–12.

Glick and Sampson et al. presented a new method using the lateral decubitus position for hip arthroscopy. The anterior and posterior portals are described and their advantage for a direct approach to enter the central compartment (intra-articular space) safely and with reproducible results. A method of distraction using skin traction with ropes, wall pulleys, and traction weights was used to distract the hip joint to facilitate getting into the hip joint. The indications, early outcomes, and complications are discussed.

Glick JM, Sampson TG. Hip arthroscopy by the lateral approach. In: McGinty JB, ed. *Operative arthroscopy*. Philadelphia and New York: Lippincott-Raven; 1996:1079–1090.

This chapter describes the lateral approach to hip arthroscopy. The setup with patient position, protection with padding, and the perineal post to be greater than 9 cm are shown. Details for placing the x-ray image C-arm under the table and the use of a moble hip distractor and cannulated instruments for getting the arthroscope and instruments are presented in detail. The indications are presented with examples of each. The outcomes and complications are discussed as well as how to reduce complications.

Griffin DR, Villar RN. Complications of arthroscopy of the hip. *J Bone Joint Surg Br*. 1999;81(4):604–606.

Ilizaliturri Jr V, Villalobos Jr F, Chaidez P, et al. Internal snapping hip syndrome: treatment by endoscopic release of the iliopsoas tendon. *Arthroscopy*. 2005;21(11):1375–1380.

Sampson TG, Glick JM. Indications and surgical treatment of hip pathology. In: McGinty JB, ed. *Operative arthroscopy*. Philadelphia and New York: Lippincott-Raven; 1996:1067–1078.

Sampson TG. Complications of hip arthroscopy. *Clin Sports Med*. 2001;20(4):831–835.

Sampson TG. Arthroscopic iliopsoas release for coxa saltans interna (snapping hip syndrome). In: Byrd JW, ed. *Operative hip arthroscopy*. New York: Springer; 2005:189–194.

Sampson T. Hip morphology and its relationship to pathology: dysplasia to impingement. *Operative Techniques in Sports Medicine*. 2005;13(1):37–45.

Sampson TG. The lateral approach. In: Byrd JW, ed. *Operative hip arthroscopy*. New York: Springer; 2005:129–144.

Sampson TG. Arthroscopic treatment of femoroacetabular impingement: a proposed technique with clinical experience. *Instr Course Lect*. 2006;55:337–346.

Thomas Byrd JW. Indications and contraindications. *Operative hip arthroscopy*, 2nd edition, Springer 2005.

Villar R. Hip arthroscopy. *J Bone Joint Surg Br*. 1995;77(4):517–518.

# CHAPTER 11

# Peripheral Compartment Approach to Hip Arthroscopy

*Michael Dienst*

## INTRODUCTION

Arthroscopy without traction of the peripheral compartment (PC) has become an integral part of hip arthroscopy. It has contributed to a better understanding of the functional anatomy and pathogenesis of new concepts such as femoroacetabular impingement and other pathologic conditions of the hip joint. With the tremendous improvement of its technique and the development of better instrumentation, a completely new field of therapeutic options has evolved.

The acetabular labrum is the key structure during portal placement and therapeutic arthroscopy within the hip joint. The labrum seals the joint space between the lunate cartilage and the femoral head by maintaining a vacuum force of about 120 N to 200 N, which keeps the femoral head within the socket. To overcome the vacuum force and the passive resistance of the soft tissues, traction is needed to separate the head from the socket, to elevate the labrum from the head, and to allow the arthroscope and other instruments access to the narrow "artificial space" between the weight-bearing cartilage of the femoral head and the acetabulum. However, if traction is applied, the joint capsule with the iliofemoral, ischiofemoral, and pubofemoral ligaments is tensioned, and the joint space peripheral to the acetabular labrum decreases. Thus, to maintain the space of the PC for better visibility and maneuverability during arthroscopy, traction should be avoided.

The hip is divided arthroscopically into two compartments that are separated by the labrum (Figure 11-1). The first is the central compartment (CC), which comprises the lunate cartilage; the acetabular fossa; the ligamentum teres; and the loaded articular surface of the femoral head. This part of the joint can be visualized almost exclusively with traction. The second is the PC, which consists of the unloaded cartilage of the femoral head; the femoral neck, with the medial, anterior, and posterolateral synovial folds (i.e., Weitbrecht ligaments); and the articular capsule with its intrinsic ligaments, including the zona orbicularis. This area can be better seen without traction.

In addition to its importance in therapeutic hip arthroscopy, the PC can be used as an intermediate space to control the placement of portals to the CC. In our practice, we have been using this technique successfully for more than 4 years; it has a smaller risk of iatrogenic lesions of the acetabular labrum and the femoral head cartilage.

## INDICATIONS

Arthroscopy without traction of the PC should be performed in all cases. For the treatment of unclear hip pain, the PC needs to be scanned for pathologic changes. Most hip disorders present with primary or secondary lesions in the PC, such as the following:
- Peripheral lesions of the acetabular labrum, such as intralabral or perilabral ossifications, labral cysts, and ganglia
- Primary (e.g., rheumatic) or reactive synovitis within the perilabral sulcus and gutters
- Loss of head–neck offset in femoroacetabular impingement
- Impinging osteophytes at the head–neck junction
- Hypertrophy of the synovial folds at the head–neck junction
- Loose bodies in degenerative joint disease or after trauma
- Tumor-like lesions or benign tumors such as chondromas and osteochondromas with synovial chondromatosis or pigmented villonodular synovitis

In addition, the PC allows access to periarticular structures such as the following:
- The psoas tendon sheath and the psoas tendon
- Periarticular cysts
- Heterotopic ossifications of the periarticular muscles

## HISTORY AND PHYSICAL EXAMINATION

There are no symptoms or functional tests during physical examination that are specific for pathologies within the PC. In addition, most hip disorders present with primary or secondary changes of the PC rather than of the CC only.

The most important thing to do during the primary preoperative workup is to determine whether the source of pain is intra-articular or extra-articular. This determination can be made by going through a thorough diagnostic checklist (see Chapter 3: Imaging: Plain Radiographs and Chapter 6: The Technique and Art of the Physical Examination of the Adult and Adolescent Hip).

## IMAGING AND DIAGNOSTIC STUDIES

Radiologists and surgeons need to consider that the hip joint is not limited to the direct articulation between the cartilage of the femoral head and the lunate cartilage of the acetabulum. The PC joint extends to the intertrochanteric line anteriorly

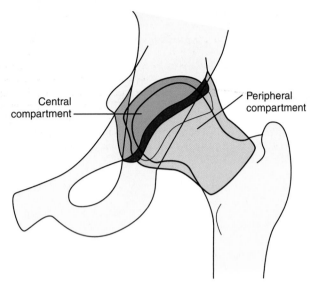

**Figure 11–1**  Arthroscopic compartments of the hip joint. *With permission from Michael Dienst, MD.*

and to the femoral neck posteriorly. Thus, the assessment of roentgenograms, computed tomography scans, and magnetic resonance images has to include this part of the joint.

Consequently, radiographs need to be evaluated for the contour of the head–neck junction, the overcoverage of the anterolateral acetabular rim, and perilabral ossifications in cases that involve femoroacetabular impingement. Here, one has to differ between the primary signs of impingement (i.e., loss of offset) and osteophytes, which are signs of osteoarthritis and secondary changes. In general, the removal of osteophytes does not lead to the same good results as the reshaping of the head–neck junction in femoroacetabular cam impingement. In addition, osteophytes are indicators of cartilage degeneration within the CC, which is important for the patient's prognosis. The soft tissues around the femoral neck have to be analyzed for subtle or more prominent ossifications that indicate osteochondromas within the PC. With magnetic resonance imaging, the space underneath the articular capsule needs to be scanned for an effusion; inflammation; thickening; villous or nodular hypertrophy of the synovium; loose bodies; and chondromas. The latter often accumulate in the pouch underneath the transverse ligament and in the gutter medially to the femoral neck. Depending on their cartilaginous or bony structure, size, and location, one has to decide whether to perform the removal through the arthroscope or via open surgery. The labrum needs to be analyzed for the degree of degeneration, tears at the labrum–cartilage junction, intralabral or perilabral cysts, and ossifications. These are important indicators for determining whether the labrum can be saved, trimmed or resected, or temporarily detached for the trimming of the bony rim. Some of this intra-articular work can be done under traction from the CC, and some can be done without traction via the PC. Radial magnetic resonance cuts can be helpful for the better imaging of the contour of the head–neck junction in different positions. For cases in which the loss of offset extends posterolaterally, only very experienced arthroscopic surgeons are capable of reshaping the head–neck junction sufficiently.

Diagnostic injections of the hip joint with local anesthetics are very helpful for the differentiation of intra-articular causes of pain from those that are extra-articular. Under fluoroscopy or ultrasound, the needle is introduced via the proximal anterolateral portal to the anterolateral head–neck junction and into the PC. Here, the space between the capsule and the bone allows for safe and effective fluid aspiration or injection. The straight anterior puncture or injection without imaging has a high risk of periarticular misplacement.

## SURGICAL TECHNIQUE

### Positioning and Switching Between the Compartments

Hip arthroscopy with and without traction can be performed with the patient in the lateral or supine position. From our experience, the decision of whether to use the lateral or supine position is more a matter of individual training and habit of use. However, because of the almost exclusive use of the proximal and distal anterolateral and anterior portals during hip arthroscopy without traction, we prefer the supine position.

To allow for a complete diagnostic arthroscopic examination of the hip, both techniques with and without traction are combined for arthroscopy of the CC and the PC; this requires specific attention to positioning, table equipment, and draping. The order of arthroscopy with and without traction depends on different parameters (Figure 11-2). In "standard" cases with good distraction and visibility, we prefer to access the PC first to control portal placement to the CC. However, there are cases in which the distraction of the hip is insufficient and visibility in the PC decreased. Here, a release of different parts of the joint capsule can be performed to increase the PC space and improve distraction. We usually start with a release of the zona orbicularis that extends into the iliofemoral ligament in cases of severe capsular thickening or fibrosis, and this is followed by therapeutic procedures such as the reshaping of the head–neck junction. At this point, traction is again applied. If distraction is improved, portals to the CC can be placed under arthroscopic control. However, if distraction is still not sufficient, arthroscopy of the PC only should be considered to avoid iatrogenic damage of the acetabular labrum and the femoral head cartilage during portal placement to the CC.

For arthroscopy of the PC, a good range of movement is important to relax parts of the capsule and to increase the intra-articular volume of the area that needs to be inspected and addressed. In addition, only without traction can the impingement maneuver and other functional tests be reproduced under various degrees of flexion, rotation, and abduction. Another advantage of the nontraction technique is the possibility of "hiding" the hyaline cartilage of the femoral head under the socket by flexion to avoid damage when working in the PC.

During the past several years, we have removed the foot from the traction module to allow for the maximum range of movement. However, this technique is time consuming and strenuous for the assistant who is holding the leg. In addition, switching back into the CC under traction is difficult, because the foot needs to be readapted to the traction module. Especially for femoroacetabular impingement cases, there is a need to alternate between both compartments with and without traction. Thus, we changed our technique. For arthroscopy of the PC, the foot is kept in the traction module. The traction is released, and the traction module with the foot is slid in with the extension bar. With this technique, the hip and knee can be flexed up to 90 degrees, abducted to about 30 degrees, and rotated 20 degrees internally and externally (Figure 11-3). When reentering the CC, the extension boom is drawn out, and the hip and knee are extended. Before traction is applied, the room nurse has to check for possible soft-tissue entrapment at the perineum.

### Portals to the Peripheral Compartment

Basically, portals are established where they are needed. With our current knowledge, most pathology in the PC can be addressed via anterior and lateral portals. It is still difficult to access the posteromedial parts of the PC for both viewing and working. The posteromedial peripheral space is significantly

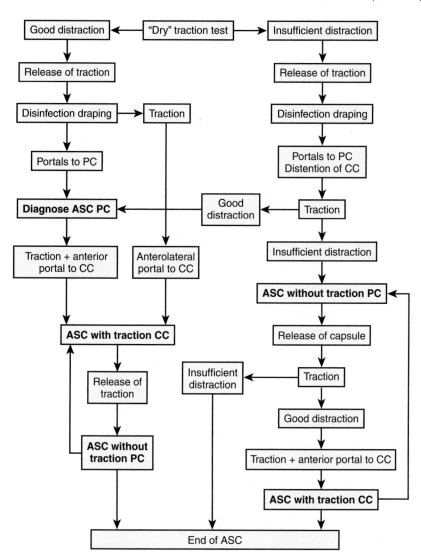

**Figure 11–2**   Flowchart for switching between the central compartment and the peripheral compartment. *ASC*, arthroscopy; *CC*, central compartment; *PC*, peripheral compartment. *With permission from Michael Dienst, MD.*

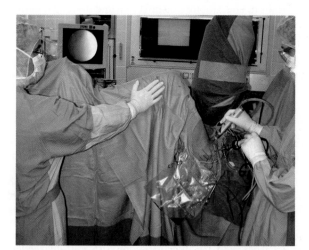

**Figure 11–3**   Supine position for hip arthroscopy without traction. Flexion and rotation in the hip can be achieved by shortening the extension boom and unlocking the rotation jig; abduction can be achieved by unlocking the jig at the base of the extension boom. The assistant is supporting the position. *With permission from Michael Dienst, MD.*

smaller and additionally hidden from the posterior part of the greater trochanter. Thus, this part of the PC can sometimes be better seen and accessed via the CC under traction. The distal part of the posteromedial space of the PC cannot be seen from the CC but rather from the perilabral sulcus and the space directly peripheral to the posterior part of the transverse ligament. Here, loose bodies and chondromas can be reached via the posterolateral portal.

A comprehensive overview of the PC can be obtained from the proximal anterolateral portal only (Figure 11-4). At this level, the soft-tissue mantle is relatively thin, and the position of the portal is near the lateral cortex of the femoral head. Therefore, the maneuverability of the arthroscope is sufficient for moving it into the medial recess, gliding over the anterior surface of the femoral head to the lateral recess, and passing the lateral cortex of the femoral neck for the inspection of the posterolateral recess. With the need for better access to the lateral and posterolateral head and neck area for therapy of the cam type of femoroacetabular impingement and the removal of chondromas from the medial area underneath the transverse ligament in patients with synovial chondromatosis, a two-portal technique for the PC is usually preferred.

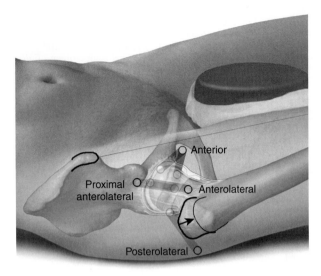

**Figure 11–4** Portals to the peripheral compartment of the hip. *From Dienst M (Ed).* Hip arthroscopy. *Elsevier Urban & Fischer, Munich; 2009.*

### Proximal Anterolateral Portal

The position and direction of the proximal anterolateral portal are different for the anterolateral portal to the CC in that the incision lies more proximally and anteriorly. Usually the perfect spot for the skin incision can be found by palpating a soft spot one third of the distance along a line drawn from the anterior superior iliac spine to the tip of the greater trochanter. Here, one can feel the anterior margin of the gluteus medius. On its way to the joint capsule, the needle only penetrates the tensor fasciae latae. Under fluoroscopy, the needle is directed perpendicular to the femoral neck axis to the anterolateral transition from the femoral head to the neck (Figure 11-5). The

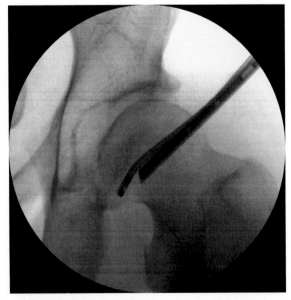

**Figure 11–5** Fluoroscopic view of the position of the arthroscope introduced over the femoral head–neck junction perpendicular to the neck axis via the proximal anterolateral portal. A radiofrequency probe is inserted via the anterior portal. *With permission from Michael Dienst, MD.*

proximal anterolateral portal is predominantly used as a viewing portal. However, in patients with femoroacetabular cam impingement, this portal becomes important for the removal of the lateral and posterolateral extension of the head–neck bump.

### Anterior Portal

With the use of the same skin incision as was used for the anterior portal to the CC, the needle is directed more inferiorly and not so far medially, aiming for the anterior junction of the femoral head and neck. It is important to perforate the anterior capsule lateral to the psoas tendon and proximal to the zona orbicularis to stay away from the femoral nerve and to have sufficient mobility of the instrument, respectively. The anterior portal is mostly used for the introduction of instruments. The mediolateral position of the skin incision for the anterior portal to the PC depends on the localization of the pathology. In femoroacetabular cam impingement, it is beneficial to place this portal 2 cm to 3 cm lateral to the vertical line from the anterosuperior iliac spine. Thus, the more lateral extension of the head–neck bump can be better accessed. For chondromatosis cases, we prefer a more medial position on the line of the anterosuperior iliac spine to reach the medial recess underneath the transverse ligament, where chondromas often hide.

## Special Equipment for Arthroscopy of the Peripheral Compartment

### Operating Table and Devices

The PC can be viewed with an arthroscope on a regular basic operating table with the patient in the supine or the lateral position. However, the need for arthroscopy of the CC in many cases requires the option of distracting the hip joint. The big advantage of a standard fracture table is its stable application of traction. For the combination with arthroscopy without traction, the extension booms must have the option of gliding in and out during arthroscopy to flex and extend the hip and knee joints (see Figure 11-3). The position of abduction and rotation needs to be adjustable. In particular, the option for lengthening and shortening the extension booms depends on the height of the patient. It is important to check before disinfection and draping if enough hip flexion can be achieved or if additional lengthening or shortening adapters are needed. During the past several years, alternative devices have been developed. In general, they provide similar functions with somewhat less effective traction but somewhat better motion during the nontraction part of the procedure.

### Lenses and the Arthroscopy Shaft System

With respect to the thicker soft-tissue mantle, it is beneficial to use regular-length arthroscopes with shafts that have additional working length. This is usually achieved by mounting the water inflow farther backward. Extra-long arthroscopes are more sensitive to torque, and replacements are often not immediately available if intraoperative damage occurs. The more experienced the surgeon is, the more frequently the 70-degree lens is used. The PC is usually completely visualized with an arthroscope with a 70-degree lens; however, when working in the acetabular fossa with traction, the 30-degree lens often has advantages. The 70-degree lens offers the great advantage for inspection from different perspectives.

## Access System

For the PC, the same principles apply as those used for the CC. The key to successful hip arthroscopy is a precise and atraumatic access system. This can be managed with cannulated, specific hip arthroscopy instrumentation only. Shafts, closed/slotted/half-pipe cannulas, and possibly also shaver systems need to be cannulated and compatible with the basic guidewire access system. In particular, the half-pipe cannulas provide for the atraumatic and rapid introduction and exchange of instruments. Aiming devices are beneficial for both beginning and advanced arthroscopic hip surgeons to reduce access trauma and operating time.

## Instruments

Diagnostic and therapeutic hip arthroscopy can be effective only if specific hip arthroscopy instrumentation is available. Unstable cartilage or labrum flap tears can often be identified with extra-long straight and curved probes only. For synovectomy and a capsular release within the PC, short and extra-long shaver blades of different sizes and tip configurations are necessary. Thus, only with extra-long curved blades can the medial gutters beneath the transverse ligament or the posterolateral perilabral sulcus be accessed and freed of loose bodies or synovial hypertrophy. Particularly for the treatment of femoroacetabular cam impingement, special extra-long burrs are required to address the anterolateral head–neck junction. Extra-long straight, curved, and potentially movable radiofrequency tips are mandatory for effective synovectomy and control of bleeding.

## Diagnostic Round and Arthroscopic Anatomy of the Peripheral Compartment

To increase the mobility of instruments and to improve inspection and access to the medial and lateral areas of the femoral neck, a release of the anterolateral articular capsule and mainly of the zona orbicularis is often necessary. We prefer to resect the zona orbicularis only, from medial to lateral. In narrow compartments and in patients with a significant loss of rotation, parts of the iliofemoral ligament are also removed.

Similar to arthroscopies of other joints, the key to an accurate and complete diagnosis of lesions within the hip joint is a systematic approach. A sequence of examination should be developed and carried out in the same way in every hip, progressing from one part to another of the joint cavity.

The PC can be divided into seven zones: 1) the anterior neck area; 2) the medial neck area; 3) the medial head area; 4) the anterior head area; 5) the lateral head area; 6) the lateral neck area; and 7) the posterior area. During a diagnostic round trip, the PC can best be viewed starting from the anterior surfaces of the femoral neck (Figure 11-6).

### The Anterior Neck, Medial Neck, and Medial Head Areas

The anteromedial part of the zona orbicularis and the anterior and medial synovial folds are inspected. The medial synovial fold, which is not adherent to the femoral neck, can be found very consistently, and it represents a helpful landmark, especially if visibility within the PC is limited by synovial disease or loose bodies.

By rotating the scope cranially, the anterior capsular recess and the anterior margin of the femoral head can be inspected. Here, in line with the medial synovial fold, the psoas tendon is lying anterior to the capsule. Sometimes the tendon shines through a thin articular capsule, or it may even be accessed

directly via a hole that connects the hip joint and an iliopectineal bursa. Caudally, a complete view of the inferior reflexion of the articular capsule can be achieved. Moving the scope medially over the medial synovial fold, the medial neck area can be examined. By rotating the 70-degree lens, the medial margin of the femoral head, the medial transition from the anterior horn of the labrum to the transverse ligament, the medial wall of the capsule with the zona orbicularis, and the medial recess can be inspected. Rotating the lens downward, the zona orbicularis vanishes posterior to the femoral neck. Instrument access to the medial area is possible via the anterior portal to search for loose bodies and chondromas underneath the transverse ligament. In addition, changes in hip position, a short period of high-flow irrigation, and the use of a suction forceps or manual ballottement from a posterior position may be necessary to bring loose bodies from the posterior area into the medial or anterior recess.

### The Anterior Head, Lateral Head, and Lateral Neck Areas

Further rotation and gentle sliding over the cartilage of the femoral head allow for the viewing of the mostly unloaded cartilage of the femoral head and the labrum from the medial to the anterior and lateral areas. This movement can be hindered by a tight zona orbicularis and extensive synovitis but facilitated by flexion of the hip up to 90 degrees and variations of abduction and rotation. Here, anterior portal placement to the CC can be achieved under direct arthroscopic control. The anterior and anterolateral labrum–head junction needs to be assessed for femoroacetabular impingement with flexion and internal rotation. With regard to other joints, arthroscopy offers the advantage of direct inspection under functional testing. With positive cam or pincer impingement, the depression of the labrum or the early contact of the labrum with the femoral neck with flexion and internal rotation can be observed. In these cases, the labrum frequently shows a significant synovial injection with prominent vessels on its peripheral side as well as a dull, round, free edge. The head–neck transition presents with a loss of offset (i.e., a bump). Frequently, a more extensive lateral synovectomy and the release of the zona orbicularis are necessary to improve the viewing of this region. When sliding laterally over the femoral neck and turning the scope backward, the lateral part of the femoral neck with the zona orbicularis running posteriorly and the posterolateral synovial fold containing the end branches of the medial femoral circumflex artery may be seen. The posterolateral synovial fold is sometimes adherent to the posterolateral neck, and it is not as prominent as the medial fold. In opposition with the medial synovial fold, which can be resected when the fold is inflamed and thickened, any lesion to the lateral fold must be avoided to not compromise the vascular supply of the femoral head.

### Posterior Area

Access to the posterior region may be hindered in cases with capsular thickening and capsular fibrosis. It can be achieved by moving the arthroscope posteriorly between the zona orbicularis and the posterolateral synovial fold. With the 70-degree lens, the posterolateral part of the head, neck, and labrum can be inspected. Parts of the posterior area can be viewed and accessed from the medial neck and head area, as indicated previously. In addition, during arthroscopy of the CC with traction, parts of the posterior area can be inspected with the 70-degree arthroscope introduced via the anterolateral portal rotated posteriorly.

Slow withdrawal of the arthroscope to the anterior neck surface finishes the diagnostic round trip of the PC.

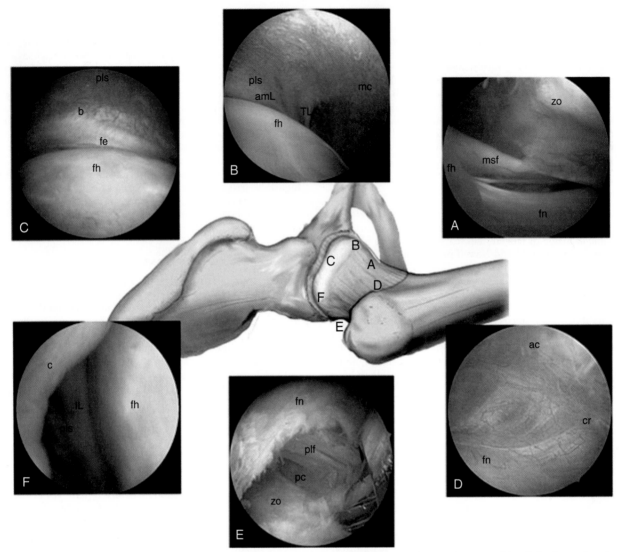

**Figure 11–6**   Diagnostic round trip of the peripheral compartment. **A,** Anteromedial neck area. *fh,* Femoral head; *fn,* femoral neck; *msf,* medial synovial fold; *zo,* anteromedial capsule with the zona orbicularis. **B,** Medial head area. *aml,* Anteromedial horn of the labrum; *fh,* femoral head; *mc,* medial capsule; *pls,* perilabral sulcus; *TL,* transverse ligament. **C,** Anterior head area. *b,* Base of the labrum; *fe,* free edge of the labrum; *fh,* cartilage of the femoral head; *pls,* perilabral sulcus. **D,** Anteroinferior neck area. *ac,* Anterior capsule; *cr,* anteroinferior reflection of the capsule; *fn,* anterior surface of the femoral neck. **E,** Posterolateral area. *fn,* Lateral border of the femoral neck; *pc,* posterior capsule; *plf,* posterolateral synovial fold with the end vessels of the medial circumflex artery; *zo,* lateral zona orbicularis. **F,** Lateral head area. fh, Cartilage of the femoral head; IL, lateral portion of the labrum; pls, perilabral sulcus; c, capsule. *With permission from Michael Dienst, MD.*

### The Peripheral Compartment as an Intermediate Space for Safe Access to the Central Compartment

Direct arthroscopic access to the CC is technically demanding. In addition, particularly for the arthroscopic surgeon who is less experienced with this procedure, the acetabular labrum and cartilage of the femoral head are at risk for iatrogenic injury. Thus, we prefer to access the PC first and to then control the first portal placement to the CC via arthroscopic means from the PC (Figure 11-7).

The hip is placed in 10 degrees of flexion, neutral rotation, and 0 degrees to 10 degrees of abduction, with the knee straight. Without traction, the PC is accessed via the proximal anterolateral portal. The anterior head area is inspected. Under arthroscopic control, the anterior portal to the CC is placed. As soon as the guidewire is passed underneath the labrum (see Figure 11-7), traction is applied, and the wire is advanced into the acetabular fossa. The arthroscope is exchanged with an irrigation cannula via the proximal anterolateral portal, and the arthroscope is introduced via the anterior portal into the CC. At this point, additional portal placement to the CC (anterolateral and posterolateral) can be controlled arthroscopically.

### COMPLICATIONS

A review of the literature reveals that most complications associated with hip arthroscopies are caused by traction. The nontraction technique for arthroscopy of the PC avoids complications such as soft-tissue damage of the perineum and foot or neurologic deficits from the compression of the pudendal nerve and the superficial nerves at the ankle or from the tension of the femoral and sciatic nerve palsies around the hip joint. In addition, if arthroscopy is limited to the PC, there is no risk of damage to the

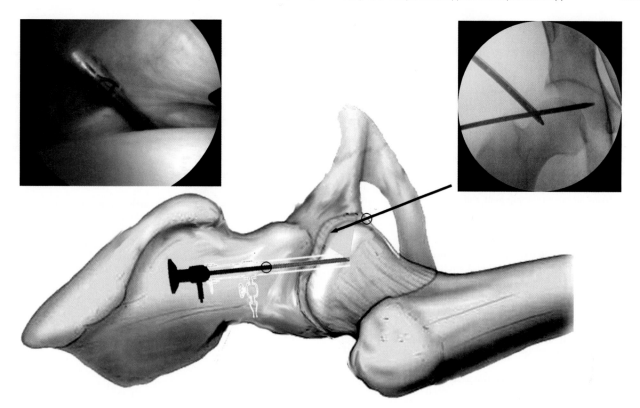

**Figure 11–7**   Anterior portal placement to the central compartment via arthroscopic control from the peripheral compartment. The left upper insert shows the arthroscopic view; the right upper insert shows the fluoroscopic view. *With permission from Michael Dienst, MD.*

## TECHNICAL PEARLS

*Hip Arthroscopy Without Traction of the Peripheral Compartment*

**Positioning**

- Supine position
- No traction
- Table or device should allow for traction, no traction, and motion

**Access and Portals**

- Main viewing portal should be proximal to the anterolateral portal
- Main working portal should be the anterior portal
- Ability to switch between portals, if necessary

**Diagnostic Round**

- Always include the peripheral compartment
- Establish a systematic sequence of viewing
- Consider variations from the normal anatomy

**Therapeutic Arthroscopy**

- Release of the zona orbicularis and eventually of the iliofemoral ligament
- Play with flexion and rotation to increase visibility and access

Here, the labrum and the cartilage need to be avoided during the maneuvering of mechanical and radiofrequency probes. Frequently, it is beneficial to flex and externally or internally rotate the hip joint to "hide" the femoral head cartilage underneath the labrum and socket and to thus increase a certain area of the PC for better inspection and maneuverability.

Depending on the skin incision sites and the direction of the portals, similar risks apply as those associated with arthroscopy of the CC. The standard anterolateral and proximal anterolateral portal are within the safest zone during hip arthroscopy; neurovascular structures are far away. By contrast, the anterior portal is always very close to a branch of the lateral cutaneous femoral nerve. It is recommended to avoid a deep skin incision, because the nerve or one of its branches runs close to the skin level. We prefer to choose a portal site that is 2 cm to 3 cm lateral to the vertical line from the anterior superior iliac spine and not too distal. On its way to the PC, the direction of the anterior portal should not be too far medial to avoid contact with the femoral nerve. However, the tendency is usually the opposite. The medial direction of the anterior portal should be about 30 degrees, depending on the skin entry site, and the soft-tissue mantle should be a bit more or less. Because the femoral nerve runs farther medially on its course to the distal thigh, the distance to the capsular entry site of the anterior portal at the level of the PC is even bigger as for access to the CC. We prefer to control the direction and capsular perforation of the anterior portal by arthroscopic means via the proximal anterolateral portals. The needle should enter the joint lateral to the psoas tendon (i.e., lateral to the medial synovial fold with the hip in neutral rotation).

Working within the PC requires specific attention to fluid management. In contrast with arthroscopy in the CC, the space in the PC can significantly decrease with the extravasation of

acetabular labrum and the hyaline cartilage of the weight-bearing area of the femoral head as long as the arthroscope and the other instruments are not too close to the articulating joint space. However, in cases of femoroacetabular impingement and synovial disease, the arthroscopist has to work directly at the acetabular rim, within the perilabral sulcus, and at the head–neck junction.

fluid into the periarticular space. Thus, big incisions or resections of the capsule should be avoided during the early phase of the operation. We prefer to limit the capsular release of the zona orbicularis. Operations in the lateral and posterolateral peripheral spaces are performed at the end of the procedure. Here, a release of the iliofemoral ligament may be necessary.

## ANNOTATED REFERENCES

**Byrd JWT, Pappas JN, Pedley MJ. Hip arthroscopy: an anatomic study of portal placement and relationship to the extra-articular structures.** *Arthroscopy.* **1995;11:418–423.**

This is an important anatomic study of the relationship of the standard portals to the hip joint and neurovascular structures. If the recommendations for portal placement are followed, the three standard portals are a safe distance away from the femoral and sciatic neurovascular bundles.

**Dienst M, Gödde S, Seil R, et al. Hip arthroscopy without traction: in vivo anatomy of the peripheral hip joint cavity.** *Arthroscopy.* **2001;17:924–931.**

This article describes the arthroscopic anatomy of the PC. The technique of arthroscopy without traction for the PC with a sequence of systemic viewing is suggested.

**Dienst M, Seil R, Kohn D. Safe arthroscopic access to the central compartment of the hip joint.** *Arthroscopy.* **2005;21: 1510–1514.**

This is author's preferred operative technique for accessing the PC first to control portal placement to the central compartment.

**Dorfmann H, Boyer T. Arthroscopy of the hip: 12 years of experience.** *Arthroscopy.* **1999;15:67–72.**

This article describes the experience Parisian rheumatologists with arthroscopy of the CC and PC. Information about 413 arthroscopies over the course of 12 years is reported. The main indication for these hip arthroscopies was the removal of loose bodies.

**Dorfmann H, Boyer T, Henry P, DeBie B. A simple approach to hip arthroscopy.** *Arthroscopy.* **1988;4:141–142.**

On the basis of experience with 60 hip arthroscopies, French rheumatologist Henri Dorfmann first publishes a description of the arthroscopic separation of the hip joint into the CC and the PC.

**Gautier E, Ganz K, Krügel N, et al. Anatomy of the medial femoral circumflex artery and its surgical implications.** *J Bone Joint Surg Br.* **2000;82-B:679–683.**

This is an important anatomic study of the vascular supply of the femoral head. The end vessels of the medial circumflex femoral artery run along the posterolateral surface of the femoral head–neck junction and must not be injured during arthroscopy to avoid the avascular necrosis of the femoral head.

**Klapper RC, Silver DM. Hip arthroscopy without traction.** *Contemp Orthop.* **1989;18:687–693.**

These authors report about their experience with hip arthroscopy without traction for the treatment of eight patients. The authors recommend draping the leg free for flexion and rotating the lower extremity to increase exposure and maximize the visualization of the joint.

**Wettstein M, Jung J, Dienst M. Arthroscopic psoas tenotomy.** *Arthroscopy.* **2006;22:907.e1–907.e4.**

This article describes an operative technique that makes use of the PC to access the psoas tendon sheath.

# CHAPTER 12

# Complex Therapeutic Hip Arthroscopy With the Use of a Femoral Distractor

*Hassan Sadri*

## INTRODUCTION

Hip pain in young adults is often characterized by nonspecific symptoms, normal imaging studies, and vague findings from the history and physical examination. As such, identifying the source and mechanism of the pain can be difficult. At the same time, treatment needs to be specific, because its effects will be experienced longer in this population. Emphasis will be placed on a newly established frequent cause of hip pain in the young adult called *femoroacetabular impingement*, which is a subtle form of early degenerative hip disease. A thorough arthroscopic correction of this pathology will be presented. The technique treats the acetabular component as well as the head component. This also includes labral suturing and cartilage transplantation, when necessary.

However, for such complex arthroscopic reconstructive surgery, longer traction times are necessary. It has been reported that traction times of more than 90 to 120 minutes on a traction table can provoke severe neurologic and perineal skin lesions in up to 15% of cases. The most frequent neurologic lesions reported are pudendal nerve lesions that result in clinical impotence as a result of the compression of the nerve on the perineal post of a traction table. Sciatic and femoral nerves are also at risk because of the overstretching that occurs during longer periods of time. Because these reconstructive procedures are time consuming, have a steep learning curve, and, above all, can provoke fearful complications, we have used invasive hip distraction (DR hip distractor, DR Medical, Solothurn, Switzerland) for these indications (Figure 12-1, *A*). Thus, by avoiding the need for traction against a perineal post with a traction table, we have not encountered the previously mentioned complications that occur with the use of the invasive hip distraction technique. The hip distractor allows the surgeon to perform these time-consuming surgical steps without the pressure of time to attain the same degree of perfection as occurs with open surgery. The results obtained are therefore identical to those of the open surgical technique. This is also a wonderful teaching tool, because beginners can also perform these more complex procedures without worrying about distraction time and the related complications.

## BASIC SCIENCE

Sufficient hip distraction involves traction forces of about 250 N to 500 N. After the suction seal is broken, the force needed diminishes significantly. However, on a traction table, much of the traction force is lost by uselessly distracting the knee (about 5 mm) and ankle joints (another 5 mm). After the invasive hip distractor has been installed, it produces a traction force of 500 N exclusively on the hip joint; this force is calculated in the elasticity of the dedicated Schanz screws. After this traction force is attained, the dedicated Schanz screws will be seen on the image intensifier to start bending (Figure 12-2, *A* through *D*).

In addition, on a traction table, the femoral head has a tendency to slide anteriorly and to reduce the anterior joint space because of the acetabular anteversion. However, most often, the lesions are in the anterior and superior regions, and most surgeons prefer to internally rotate the lower extremity to avoid this anterior joint space narrowing on a traction table. Internal rotation moves the sciatic nerve anteriorly and thus puts it at risk if the surgeon chooses a posterolateral portal approach. Invasive hip distraction avoids this by allowing for a controlled anterior-to-posterior traction vector in neutral rotation (Figure 12-3, *A* and *B*). A posterolateral portal approach is thus very safe without putting the sciatic nerve at risk.

## INDICATIONS

- Complete femoroacetabular impingement correction (i.e., head–neck junction correction, labral suturing, and cartilage transplantation)
- Labral suturing
- Acetabular cartilage transplantation
- Osteochondromatosis and chondromatosis
- Keen hip arthroscopy beginner who wants to progress to more complex surgery
- Senior hip arthroscopy surgeons who are teaching procedures to beginners
- Other complex hip arthroscopy procedures in which more than 90 minutes of hip distraction time is needed
- "Nondistractable" hips on traction tables
- When traction on the lower limb is not desirable (e.g., ipsilateral lower limb fracture, knee prosthesis)
- Obese patients in whom powerful distraction is needed (Invasive hip distraction has been used successfully in patients who weigh up to 160 kg.)

## SURGICAL TECHNIQUE

We have tried the lateral and supine approaches for this indication. We are largely in favor of the lateral decubitus position, and the setup is in a way that is similar to that of the classic lateral

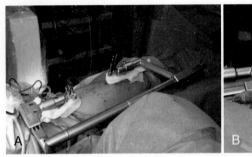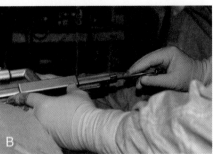

**Figure 12–1 A,** Posterior view of right hip with the invasive hip distractor installed. Note the anterior-to-posterior precision screw mechanism *(left)*, which allows for an increase in the anterior-to-posterior traction vector, thus opening the anterior joint space. The proximal-to-distal traction is controlled by the distal *(right)* precision screw mechanism. **B,** The proximal-to-distal controlled traction mechanism.

approach, with some differences. Three standard arthroscopy portals are used: the posterolateral portal, the anterolateral portal, and the anterior portal (Figure 12-4).

We have abandoned the use of a traction table for hip arthroscopy as a result of a high associated neurologic complication rate. Although we followed the standard recommendations to avoid the neurologic complications of hip arthroscopy that were found in the literature (e.g., the use of a very large perineal post), of our first 20 cases, two slowly regressive pudendal nerve lesions with clinical impotence were encountered. These complications were likely the result of the fact that more than 90 minutes of traction were used to correct complex acetabular anomalies. We now have experience with more than 1000 cases of hip arthroscopy, and, sadly, our operative and traction times have not changed; this is because more and more complex cases are operated on arthroscopically and because labral suturing is necessary in about a third of cases. In the case of labral suturing, an average of four anchors is necessary, with some cases requiring eight anchors; this anchoring is of course time consuming, and it puts the nerves at risk. For this reason, since 2000, we have been using an invasive hip distraction device (see Figure 12-1, *A* and *B*), which is still in use at our institution. The device avoids the use of the perineal post, which is responsible for the pudendal nerve lesions. For more than 1000 cases, we have not documented a single nerve lesion as a result of traction with this type of hip distraction. Neurologic complication rates from procedures that involve the use of traction tables can be as high as 10% to 15%. These complications are certainly also related to experience with the technique and thus also to traction times. However, as mentioned previously in the case of complex surgery, the acetabular corrective surgery can be time consuming, particularly if labral reattachment or autologous cartilage transplantation is involved.

We prefer the lateral approach and invasive hip distraction for the following practical reasons:

- For the beginner, it is always possible if technical difficulties are encountered to convert to mini open or open surgery

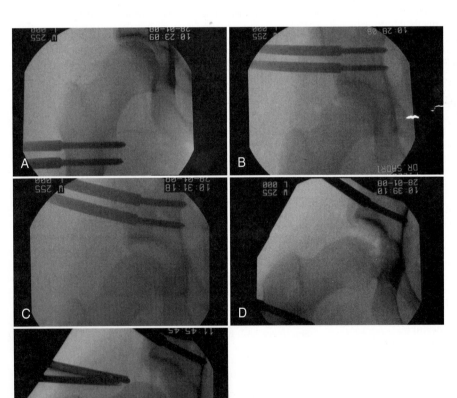

**Figure 12–2 A,** Image intensifier view. Two distal Schanz pins in place at the level of the lesser trochanter. **B,** Two proximal Schanz screws 1 cm above the acetabular sourcil. **C,** Lower limb in neutral position with same view as that seen in part B but with traction applied. Note that 12 mm of joint space distraction is already visible in this young and muscular patient. The proximal Schanz screws have started to bend, thus signaling a sufficient 500 N of distraction force. **D,** Lower limb in 30 degrees of abduction. Note 18 mm of distraction (i.e., three times the diameter of the 6-mm Schanz screws). **E,** Same view as that seen in part D but after cam (i.e., pistol grip head) component correction with a burr.

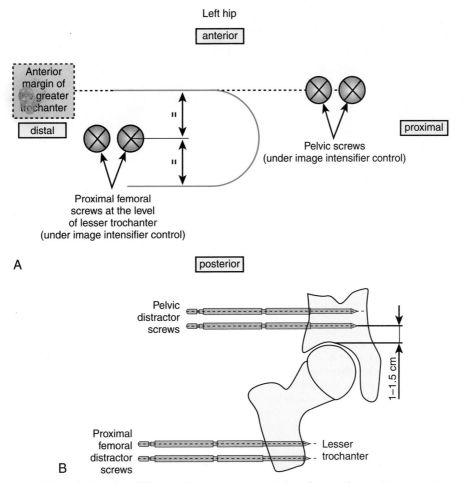

**Figure 12–3   A,** Schematic view of a left hip with four Schanz screws in place showing the anterior-to-posterior traction forces that open the anterior joint space without the need for internal rotation. **B,** Anteroposterior schematic view of a right hip with the proximal acetabular and distal femoral Schanz screws.

without redraping; this would not easily be the case if a standard traction table were being used. If necessary, conversion to a mini posterior approach is always possible with the patient in the lateral position rather than the supine position. We can compare this with the beach-chair position used for shoulder arthroscopy. An example of when this would occur would be in case of instrument breakage. Indeed, instruments

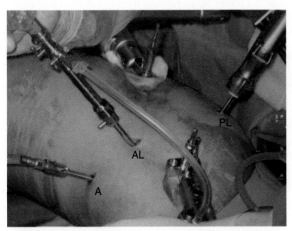

**Figure 12–4**   Proximal view of the setup of a right hip with invasive distraction and posterolateral *(PL)*, anterolateral *(AL),* and anterior *(A)* portals.

tend to slide on the posterior horn of the acetabulum in the direction of the ligamentum transversum, and extraction can be difficult. With the patient in the lateral decubitus position, instruments fall into the pulvinar and are stopped by fatty tissue from sliding farther, and extraction is thus easier.

- Invasive hip distraction avoids the dreadful neurologic complications caused by lengthy distraction times in difficult or complex reconstructive hip arthroscopies. Thus, beginners feel no time pressure, and more complex hip reconstructions (e.g., labral detachment, described later in this chapter) and suturing are possible.
- Invasive hip distraction can be easily freed to dynamically test impingement-free motions of the hip during and after surgery (i.e., maximum flexion, 90 degrees of flexion, maximum internal rotation, and maximum abduction). These can be tested without difficulty (and in the same manner in which they are tested in open surgery) to ascertain that no impingement is present. Another advantage of this approach is that there is no compromise of surgical sterility unlike with a traction table where sterility may be compromised with a non-sterile traction boot.
- Finally, with the patient in the lateral decubitus position, bubbles that come from radiofrequency devices are easily evacuated through incisions; this is in contrast with having patients in the supine position, where such bubbles tend to accumulate anteriorly.

The lower extremity is draped so that it can be moved freely (Figure 12-5, *A* and *B*). The C-arm fluoroscope is brought

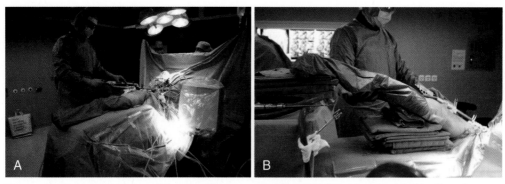

**Figure 12–5**    **A,** General view of the setup. The procedure is being performed on the right hip. Note the image intensifier is in the horizontal position. The surgeon is dorsal to the patient. Note also that the fluid drains into the pouches of the drapes, thus keeping the patient and the floor dry. **B,** The same view that is shown in part A but with 30 degrees of abduction and 10 degrees of flexion relaxing the capsule and permitting for much better distraction.

under the table and draped, thus providing a good anterior-to-posterior view (see Figure 12-2, *A* through *E,* and 12-5, *A* and *B*). The invasive hip distractor is set up with the patient in slight hip flexion. One dedicated Schanz screw is placed 1 cm above the acetabular sourcil under image intensifier control, and another is placed at the level of the lesser trochanter. The proximal screws are in line with the anterior trochanteric margin (see Figure 12-3, *A* and *B,* and 12-6, *B*). The relative positions of the proximal and distal Schanz screws produce an anterior-to-posterior traction vector that optimizes the anterior joint space opening, even if no lower limb internal rotation is applied. The invasive hip distractor is installed on the inserted Schanz screws (see Figure 12-6, *A* through *C*). The device has a precision screw mechanism that can move the tubes precisely so that they fit onto the Schanz screws. After the distractor is installed, two other Schanz screws—one proximally in the acetabulum and one distally in the femur—are applied through the distractor's guiding tubes (see Figure 12-6, *C*). This stabilizes the rotational forces and allows for a better anterior-to-posterior distraction vector. Bolts are then put on every Schanz screw to push the tubes around the screws down onto the bone. The whole hip distractor is thus an angularly stable construct that improves traction forces. After the invasive hip distractor is installed, distraction is applied on the hip by turning the axial distraction screw (see Figure 12-1, *A* and *B*). The lower extremity is then set in abduction of approximately 30 degrees to 45 degrees (see Figure 12-5, *A* and *B*). This maneuver and the previously mentioned slight flexion of about 10 degrees will relax the superior and anterior hip capsule, including the iliofemoral ligament, and this will permit better distraction (see Figure 12-5, *B*). With adequate distraction (ideally 12 mm), the hip joint is decompressed with a large

spinal needle, and the suction seal is broken. However, about 5% of hips are considered not distractable or insufficiently distractable on traction tables. In these cases, invasive hip distraction can be useful by permitting for controlled capsular releases, which is described later in this chapter. With the use of a cannulated system, the arthroscope is first introduced into the anterolateral portal (see Figure 12-4). We prefer using the 70-degree scope, which provides a better view initially, especially in tighter joints. The posterolateral and anterior portals are then created under direct visual control, with the labrum and the femoral head being avoided. The hip is first viewed under air, and this is followed by fluid.

The following description is for the treatment of femoroacetabular impingement with the correction of the head–neck junction, acetabular lesions (including labral debridement or sutures), and acetabular cartilage transplantation. It is not the purpose of this chapter to describe femoroacetabular impingement and its treatment principles. However, we have kept the same treatment principles that their originators, Ganz and Beck, described for open surgery. Thus, the final treatment will depend on the types of lesions encountered and the type of impingement.

The joint is evaluated with the arthroscope in the usual way. The lesions are identified on the acetabular side. Typical findings are fraying or complex tears of the acetabular labrum in the anterior and superior quadrants. In patients with cam impingement, tears of the articular side of the labrum are frequent and associated with adjacent labral cartilage damage.

After the lesions are identified, a capsulotomy is performed with a dedicated beaver blade, typically from 9 o'clock to 4 o'clock for a right hip. This is essential because it enables the surgeon to freely move the instruments and not be limited by the capsular resistance.

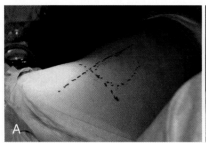 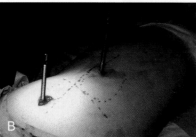 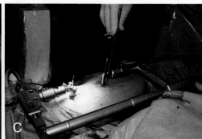

**Figure 12–6**    **A,** Installation of the invasive hip distractor; posterior view of a right hip in lateral decubitus. The greater trochanter is drawn, where the posterolateral, anterolateral, and anterior portals will be approximately established. **B,** The proximal Schanz screw *(left)* is placed on the anterior trochanteric margin line 1 cm above the acetabular sourcil under image intensifier control, and the distal *(right)* screw is at the level of the lesser trochanter in the middle of the anteroposterior diameter of the proximal femur. **C,** The invasive hip distractor is placed on the two initial Schanz screws, and a second distal Schanz screw *(shown)* is placed distally to stabilize the rotation of the device. A second proximal Schanz screw will be placed proximally.

On the acetabular side, complex labral tears are debrided with an adequate shaver or an angulated radiothermal device (30 degrees or 60 degrees). The articular cartilage lesions are similarly debrided or smoothed to a stable area, and microfracture is performed when necessary. If the cartilage lesions of the acetabulum are larger than 3 cm², we believe that cartilage transplantation techniques can be considered. We have used three-dimensional matrix-based transplantations, such as autologous chondrocyte transplantation with the use of a three-dimensional scaffold (M-ACT), autologous membrane-induced chondrogenesis, and scaffold-augmented microfracture. When M-ACT (Figure 12-7, A and B) is applied, we use the head–neck junction as the donor site for chondrocytes.

If the labrum can be preserved, which it typically can be in the case of articular longitudinal partial tears, it is detached from the acetabular rim to create a bucket-handle tear (Figure 12-8, A through D), as would be done during open surgery. Often, this reveals labral ossifications (see Figure 12-8, A). In the case of acetabular retroversion or labral ossifications, these are resected with a burr. Rarely, if no acetabular version anomaly or labral ossification is present, the acetabular bone rim is freshened with a burr. In the former and the latter cases, the labrum is then reinserted (see Figure 12-8, A through D) with the use of impacted bioabsorbable small anchors with high-traction–resistant nonabsorbable sutures (2.4-mm and 3.0-mm Bio-SutureTak or knotless 2.5-mm and 3.0-mm PushLock [Arthrex, Karlsfeld, Germany]). We prefer bioabsorbable anchors because they do not influence magnetic resonance imaging signals in case this type of imaging technique is needed in the future. In the case of future total hip arthroplasties, these anchors will not interfere with the implantation. Highly resistant sutures such as FiberWire (Arthrex, Germany) are essential because of the 360-degree angulation that is usually needed in the hip when suture management is required; absorbable sutures tend to break in this situation. In our experience, suture passers (Hip Low Profile Suture Lasso [Arthrex, Germany]) and shuttle techniques are the least aggressive methods of labral suturing. Indeed, the labrum is very thin in some cases, and bird-beak–type instruments are too bulky. Usually a minimum labral width of 5 mm seems to be the reasonable limit for reinsertion. It is essential to tie the knots on the extra-articular side of the joint (2.4-mm and 3.0-mm Bio-SutureTak [Arthrex, Germany]) so that they do not interfere with hip mechanics and thus preserve the cartilage. Knotless anchors can also be an advantage in that they avoid the presence of knots (2.5-mm and 3.0-mm PushLock [Arthrex, Germany]). Typically, the joint is viewed from the posterolateral portal, the drill comes in from the anterolateral portal, and shuttling (Hip Low Profile Suture Lasso [Arthrex, Germany]) is performed between the anterolateral and anterior portals or vice versa, depending on the region in which the suture is placed. Two long 8.25 mm × 90 mm or 8.25 mm × 110 mm transparent cannulas (hip disposable kits [Arthrex, Karlsfeld, Germany]) are used in the anterolateral and anterior portals.

After the labrum is treated by either resection or suture, the cartilage lesions are addressed. Depending on the size of the lesion, a decision is made to use a matrix-based treatment. Appropriate sized cannulas are also used with the same dimensions as previously mentioned. The matrix is then sutured to the labrum or placed on anchors at the rim with similar techniques (see Figure 12-7, A and B).

The traction is then reduced, and the head is viewed from the posterolateral portal. An anterior and superior capsulectomy is performed with the use of a punch and a very aggressive, large-diameter shaver (5.0 or 7.0 PITBULL shaver [DR Medical, Solothurn, Switzerland]) to visualize the anterior and superior portion of the head. Instruments are brought in through the anterolateral portal. The head–neck junction is inspected, and the fatty pars reflecta, which contains the nutrient vessels of the femoral head, is visualized. This is essential because this area contains the terminal branches of the medial circumflex artery, and it is thought to be the major blood supply of the femoral head. Typically, the impingement areas of the head–neck junction caused by the nonspheric portion of the femoral head are marked by chondral damage (Figure 12-9, A and B). This area will be resected with a burr in the anterolateral portal, which will render it concave (see Figure 12-9, B). After the resection is completed while viewing from the posterolateral portal, the viewing portal is switched to the anterolateral portal, the burr is brought in through the anterior portal, and the fluid outflow is changed to the posterolateral portal. The most important anterosuperior head correction is then initiated while viewing in this position. Medially, it is the medial synovial fold that usually marks the end of the head osteoplasty. This anterior area of the head–neck junction is indeed the major area in which impingement occurs, and it typically impinges during flexion and internal rotation.

During the procedure, fluoroscopy helps to quantify the head–neck junction resection. A depth of resection of 7 mm to 10 mm is usually required. However, the final dynamic testing of the hip is the most important step of the surgery. Typically, for a test of extreme flexion, extreme abduction, 90 degrees of flexion, and maximum internal rotation are necessary; this will detect whether the resection is sufficient or not. If the resection is not sufficient, it must be continued until impingement-free motion can be visually documented (Figure 12-10, A through C).

The case mentioned previously regarding nondistractable or insufficiently distractable hips needs to be further discussed. These hips are difficult to visualize either on a traction table or with the invasive distraction device. If the joint space opening is less than 12 mm, we do not recommend blind and forceful intra-articular penetration. After the invasive distractor is in place, the posterolateral portal is established. The arthroscope is brought into the hip capsule, and the two other anterolateral and anterior portals are made. While viewing from the posterolateral portal, the superior and anterosuperior capsule are freed from the attachment of the gluteus

**Figure 12–7   A,** Right hip. Posterolateral view of the anterosuperior acetabulum with Outerbridge grade IV triangular cartilage lesion. **B,** The same view that is shown in part A with M-ACT cartilage transplantation.

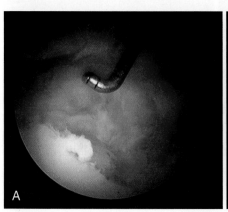
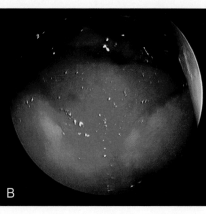

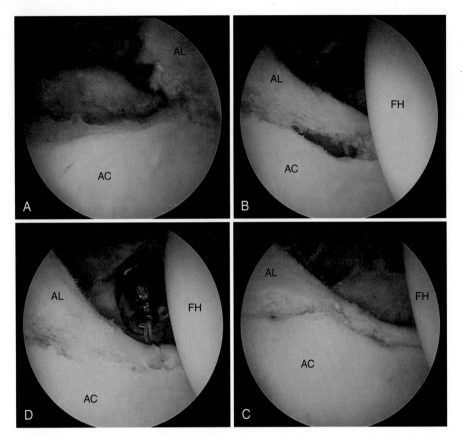

**Figure 12–8** **A,** Posterolateral arthroscopy view of a right hip with pincer impingement, acetabular ossification, and retroversion. *AC,* Anterior acetabulum; *AL,* labrum; *LO,* labral ossification and retroversion. **B,** Ossification removal and labral repair. *FH,* Femoral head. **C,** Cutting the suture after labral repair. **D,** Final result after labral repair.

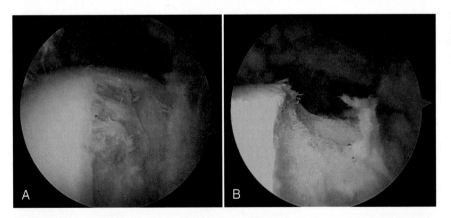

**Figure 12–9** **A,** Posterolateral view of the head and neck junction of a cam impingement correction before correction. **B,** After correction.

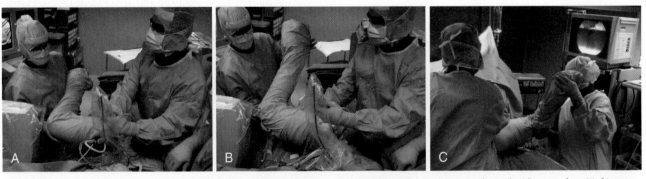

**Figure 12–10** **A,** Proximal view of a right hip in lateral decubitus position. Impingement-free testing is performed with more than 90 degrees of hip flexion and adduction. Here the hip is in neutral rotation. **B,** The same view that is shown in part A with maximal internal rotation. **C,** A distal view of what is shown in part B with maximal internal rotation and with the surgeon viewing an impingement-free motion with the arthroscope.

minimus fibers via extra-articular arthroscopy. An anterosuperior capsulectomy is then made until the head–neck junction is visible. Progressively, this capsulectomy is made in the direction of the acetabular rim until the labrum is visualized. The joint space will open slowly as a function of the extent of the superior and anterior capsulectomy. When this joint space is deemed sufficient, a Nitinol guidewire and a cannula are inserted between the labrum and the femoral head through the anterolateral portal. The other portals are then established in a similar way, as mentioned previously, under direct vision.

### TECHNICAL PEARLS

- Place the patient in the lateral decubitus position.
- Drape the lower limb so that it can be moved freely.
- Place the two proximal Schanz screws anteriorly in line with the anterior trochanteric margin 1 cm above the acetabular sourcil.
- Place the two distal Schanz screws in the middle of the femur at the level of the lesser trochanter.
- Apply distraction.
- Apply 10 degrees of flexion and 30 degrees to 45 degrees of abduction.
- A minimum of 12 mm of distraction should be visible after abduction is applied; if it is not (which occurs in 5% of cases), use the capsular release technique.

## POSTOPERATIVE REHABILITATION

The postoperative program described here is essentially for complex arthroscopic reconstructive surgery, such as femoroacetabular impingement correction. The patients are placed on crutches, and partial weight bearing of 5 kg to 10 kg is authorized during the first 6 weeks after the procedure. We have been voluntarily overcautious with regard to weight bearing, because most of the cases involved major head–neck junction osteoplasty. No neck fractures or other proximal femoral fractures around the Schanz screw holes have been observed in more than 1000 cases. After 6 weeks, abductor strengthening exercises are prescribed. Inline sports such as swimming and cycling are allowed when the patients feel comfortable, but no pivot contact sports or competitions are allowed for 6 months. If labral suturing or cartilage transplantation is performed, maximum hip flexion is limited to 70 degrees for 4 weeks. In the case of minor arthroscopic surgery such as labral resection, weight bearing is allowed as tolerated, and strengthening exercises are introduced as soon as pain regresses, which is often about 1 week after the procedure.

## RESULTS AND OUTCOMES

### RESULTS

- 1000 cases of femoroacetabular impingement correction with a minimum of 1 year of follow up
- Neurologic complication rate: 0.3%
- Patient satisfaction rate: 86%

For the first 1000 cases of femoroacetabular impingement with no joint space narrowing (Tönnis grade 0) that we treated with invasive hip distraction, the following results were obtained:

- Average operation duration: 175 minutes (range, 75 to 240 minutes)
- Mean age: 30 years (range, 19 to 54 years)
- 81% had mixed impingement correction with both cam and pincer components
- 86% patient satisfaction rate at 1 year

## COMPLICATIONS

In our experience, we have not had any fractures of the proximal femur or of the head-neck junction. We think that this is partially the result of the strict partial weight-bearing protocol that we apply, which means that we treat every patient as if he or she suffered a nondisplaced neck fracture. We have observed three (0.3%) lateral femoral cutaneous nerve neuropraxias; two resolved after 48 hours, and the other resolved after 6 weeks. This is probably a result of the use of the anterior portal, which is very close to the branches of this nerve. Vigorous instrumentation usually occurs through this portal, because most hip pathology is in the anterosuperior region. We usually try to move the anterior portal as laterally as possible, leaving 3 cm between the anterolateral portal and the anterior portal in an attempt to minimize the irritation of this nerve. No pudendal, sciatic, or femoral nerve lesions and no perineal skin lesions were observed. Five hematomas at the level of the distal Schanz screws that resolved spontaneously were documented. Overall, invasive hip distraction for complex reconstructive surgery with more than 90 to 120 minutes of traction time is very safe as compared with the reported complication rates of hip arthroscopy on traction tables.

## ANNOTATED REFERENCES

Beck M, Leunig M, Parvizi J, et al. Anterior femoroacetabular impingement: part II. Midterm results of surgical treatment. *Clin Orthop*. 2004;67–73.

This study present results after correction with open femoroacetabular surgery at 4.8 years; about 80% good results were reported when no hip joint space narrowing was present.

Byrd JW, Pappas JN, Pedley MJ. Hip arthroscopy: an anatomic study of portal placement and relationship to the extra-articular structures. *Arthroscopy*. 1995;11:418–423.

Precise portal placement is described as a function of anatomy.

Espinosa N, Rothenfluh DA, Beck M, et al. Treatment of femoroacetabular impingement: preliminary results of labral refixation. *J Bone Joint Surg A*. 2006;88:925–935.

This retrospective study compares two cohorts: one with labral resection and the other with labral fixation. Labral fixation seems to provide superior results.

Funke EL, Munzinger U. Complications in hip arthroscopy. *Arthroscopy*. 1996;12:156–159.

Neurologic and perineal skin complication rates of 10% are reported as a result of traction on a traction table.

Ganz R, Parvizi J, Beck M, et al. Femoroacetabular impingement: a cause for osteoarthritis of the hip. *Clin Orthop*. 2003;417:112–120.

Principles for treating femoroacetabular impingement are reported by the originator of the open technique.

Gautier E, Ganz K, Krugel N, et al. Anatomy of the medial femoral circumflex artery and its surgical implications. *J Bone Joint Surg Br*. 2000;82:679–683.

The importance of the medial circumflex artery in femoral head vascularization is shown.

Glick JM. Complications of hip arthroscopy by the lateral approach. In: Sherman OH, Minkoff J, eds. *Current management of complications in orthopaedics: arthroscopic surgery*. **Baltimore: Williams & Wilkins; 1990:193–201.**

An incidence of complications of up to 15% is reported, including eight neuropraxias, four sciatic complications, and four pudendal complications.

**Langlais F, Lambotte JC, Lannou R, et al. Hip pain from impingement and dysplasia in patients aged 20-50 years. Workup and role for reconstruction.** *Joint Bone Spine.* **2006;73:614–623.**

The favorable French experience with invasive hip distraction for the arthroscopic treatment of femoroacetabular hip impingement is reported.

**Lavigne M, Parvizi J, Beck M, et al. Anterior femoroacetabular impingement: part I. Techniques of joint preserving surgery.** *Clin Orthop.* **2004;418:61–66.**

Principles for the treatment of femoroacetabular impingement are reported.

**Sadri H. Eingriffe am Hyalinen Knorpel. In: Dienst M, ed.** *Hüftarthroscopie.* **Munich: Elsevier Urban & Fischer; 2009.**

Arthroscopy techniques and results for treating cartilage lesions are reported: cartilage transplantation (autologous membrane-induced chondrogenesis and scaffold-augmented microfracture) and microfractures.

**Sadri H, Menetrey J, Fritchy D, et al. Femoro-acetabular impingement: arthroscopic treatment compared with open surgery, a prospective randomized study.** *Clin Orthop.* **(accepted for publication)**

A prospective, randomized study of 63 patients with 2 years of follow-up. No significant differences were noted clinically between open surgery and arthroscopic surgery. However, postoperative pain, rehabilitation time, and time before going back to work significantly favored the arthroscopic technique.

**Sadri H, Menetrey J, Kraus E, et al. Arthroskopische Behandlung des femoroazetabulären Impingements.** *Arthroskopie.* **2006; 19:67–74 (German).**

Arthroscopic techniques for and the results of treating femoroacetabular impingement are reported.

**Sampson TG. Complications of hip arthroscopy.** *Clin Sports Med.* **2001;20:831–835.**

A complication rate of 6.4% for 530 hip arthroscopies is reported by a very experienced hip arthroscopy surgeon.

**http://www.dr-medical.ch**

This is the URL of the Web site of the creator of invasive hip distraction.

# CHAPTER 13

# Arthroscopic Labral Debridement

*Joseph C. McCarthy and Jo-Ann Lee*

## INTRODUCTION

Advances in technology have allowed for the arthroscopic treatment of an evolving series of conditions in and around the hip joint. Labral tears are the most common pathologies that are treated with hip arthroscopy, and they may contribute to the progression of degenerative arthritis. Patients who are at increased risk for developing arthritis in the presence of labral tears are those with developmental dysplasia, those with full-thickness chondral lesions, and those who have had tears present for more than 5 years. The key point to be emphasized is that surgical outcomes are significantly correlated with the extent of articular surface involvement and the degree of damage.

The labrum is innervated with all types of nerve fibers, including pain fibers, and thus tears of the labrum can result in hip pain in addition to mechanical symptoms of locking, catching, and buckling. The limited capacity of the labrum to heal in combination with the relative ease of the partial labrectomy procedure (as compared with labral repair) explains why partial labrectomy is currently the most commonly performed hip arthroscopy procedure.

## BASIC SCIENCE AND RATIONALE FOR TREATMENT

Microvascular studies have confirmed that the vascular supply of the acetabular labrum comes via the obturator artery, the superior gluteal artery, and the inferior gluteal artery, which are the same vessels that supply the bony structure of the acetabulum. These studies also showed no evidence of the penetration of vessels from the underlying acetabular bone into the labral substance. Labral tears most frequently occur on the articular nonvascular white zone, and they will not heal with conservative treatment. These tears are often delaminating tears that are not amenable to suture repair (Figure 13-1).

Labral tears are most frequently seen in the anterior acetabular quadrant (more than 90% in most series), and they are common in patients with degenerative hip disease or acetabular dysplasia. A common finding even with mild acetabular dysplasia is hypertrophy of the anterior labrum, which makes this area more susceptible to tearing. Because of the avascularity and degenerative nature of these lesions, they too are usually not amenable to suture repair (Figure 13-2). Posterior labral tears are most frequently seen after a posterior hip dislocation. Lateral tears are usually associated with additional labral and acetabular lesions.

When a labral tear occurs at the watershed zone, over time, it destabilizes the adjacent acetabular cartilage. When the destabilized cartilage is subjected to repetitive loading, joint fluid is pumped beneath the delaminating acetabular cartilage, thus accelerating the wear. Eventually, the fluid burrows beneath the subchondral bone to form a subchondral cyst. Thus, most labral tears have a limited capacity to heal, and the resultant treatment is a partial labrectomy.

## HISTORY AND PHYSICAL EXAMINATION

Labral tears most often present with mechanical symptoms such as buckling, clicking, or catching and a painful and restricted range of joint motion. Mechanical symptoms (i.e., catching, locking, or buckling) usually persist despite normal radiographic findings and failed conservative therapy. Positive examination findings include a positive McCarthy sign. (The hip is flexed, externally rotated, and then brought into extension. This may be repeated with internal rotation.) Most often, the painful click will accompany extension. The patient may also experience pain or a sensation of blocked range of motion with abduction or external rotation. Often patients will experience inguinal pain with resisted straight leg raising. Labral tears can also be associated with other intra-articular disorders. Degenerative labral tears, as mentioned previously, are seen with erosive changes in the acetabulum, the femoral head, or both. Anterior acetabular chondral injuries are frequently seen with anterior labral tears.

## IMAGING AND DIAGNOSTIC STUDIES

Radiologic studies including plain radiographs, arthrography, bone scintigraphy, computed tomography, and magnetic resonance imaging often have a poor diagnostic yield for intra-articular lesions. Although the addition of contrast agents in conjunction with computed tomography and magnetic resonance imaging may increase their sensitivity for evaluating intra-articular lesions of the acetabular labrum, these studies still have a limited ability to accurately evaluate chondral lesions of the acetabulum and the femoral head.

Occasionally an intra-articular joint injection with a steroid and Marcaine that is performed under fluoroscopic control may help to clarify whether the source of pain is intra-articular.

## SURGICAL TECHNIQUE

The lateral approach requires that the patient be positioned in the lateral decubitus position with the affected hip up. Most intra-articular lesions are found anteriorly, and these can easily be treated via the two primary portals of the lateral approach.

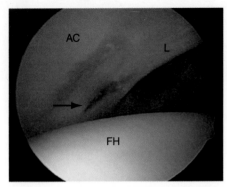

**Figure 13–1** Intraoperative photo of a delaminating tear (*arrow*) of the anterior acetabular labrum. Articular cartilage, AC; labrum, L; femoral head, FH.

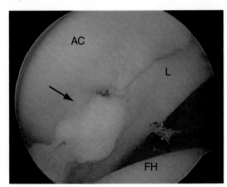

**Figure 13–2** Intraoperative photo of a hypertrophied (*arrow*), degenerative, torn anteromedial labrum. Articular cartilage, AC; labrum, L; femoral head, FH.

A modified fracture table or a dedicated hip distractor can be used for lateral positioning. Adequate distraction is required to lift the femoral head away from the acetabulum to allow for the passage of instruments without scuffing the chondral surfaces. Fluoroscopic images determine the relative distraction of the femoral head from the acetabulum. General anesthesia with adequate skeletal muscle relaxation also reduces the force that is required to distract the hip. Meticulous attention to detail can help to prevent an inadvertent loss of traction while instruments are in the joint, which may result in harm to the articular cartilage or instrument breakage within the joint.

The intra-articular structures in the hip joint can most often be visualized with a standard 30-degree arthroscope; however, there are times when a 70-degree lens may be needed. The arthroscope can be exchanged among the portals to facilitate the visualization of the existing pathology. Instruments should always be passed through long, tapered cannulas to protect the surrounding tissues and to provide safe entry into the joint. A variety of probes and hooks are first used to evaluate the intra-articular structures. Labral tears can be resected with a variety of long suction punches that have been designed specifically for hip arthroscopy. Extra-long mechanical shavers can also be useful for the debridement of labral tears. Flexible thermal devices that provide precise control of temperature and coagulation are extremely useful for debriding the torn labral rim. Although these tools are beneficial, they must be used judiciously to avoid the over-resection of tissue or the thermal injury of bone. Inflamed, redundant synovial tissue can also be resected and coagulated.

The arthroscopic treatment of these tears involves careful and conservative debridement back to a stable base and to tissue that appears to be healthy. The resection should never approach the rim, because this could result in an unstable hip. This procedure will eliminate the source of the mechanical symptoms that result from labral lesions.

Bony resection should not accompany the labral resection unless it has been dynamically proven at the time of surgery that bony collision is the source of the labral injury, which is done at the time of surgery by releasing the traction. The hip is then flexed and rotated under the arthroscopic vision of the peripheral compartment. Most bony impingement labral lesions occur superolaterally, whereas isolated labral lesions occur anteromedially. If the labral lesion is congruous with bony collision, then microresection of the labrum and judicious bone resection are appropriate. For noncongruous labral lesions, microresection is sufficient.

## CONTRAINDICATIONS

**TECHNICAL PEARLS**

- The femoral head must be distracted 8 mm to 10 mm from the acetabular chondral surface.
- Distraction time should be minimized to avoid neuropraxias and ankle strain.
- The most conservative means of resecting or stabilizing the labral tear should be emphasized, and the over-resection of the labral tissue should be avoided.

Moderate dysplasia is a contraindication for labral debridement or resection, because it may result in accelerated wear and instability. Pain in the absence of mechanical symptoms (e.g., catching, locking, buckling) is also a contraindication for labral surgery, especially for patients who are more than 30 years old. Advanced degenerative joint disease, protrusion, and a marked and limited range of motion are also contraindications.

## POSTOPERATIVE REHABILITATION

Hip arthroscopy is outpatient surgery, and most patients require crutches for 2 to 7 days postoperatively. Patients may progress to full weight bearing as soon as comfort allows. Most patients are able to drive within 24 to 48 hours after the surgery. Aspirin is prescribed as an anticoagulant for the first 4 weeks after surgery.

Activity is gradually increased as comfort permits. This includes walking (not on a treadmill), using a stationary bike, or swimming after the stitches are removed. High-impact activity and twisting and pivoting motions should be avoided for the first 6 weeks, because they may produce sharp pain until postoperative swelling has subsided. Other activities to be avoided include the NordicTrack, StairMaster leg-press machines, and deep squats. Depending on the job and the type of physical labor required, most patients return to work after 4 to 7 days.

Formal physical therapy is not encouraged for the first 6 weeks after surgery while joint effusion persists. Therapy protocols for patients with high demand (e.g., competitive athletes) also begin after the first 6 weeks. These patients begin with general conditioning and lower-body resistance training and then progress to more sport-specific activities.

## OUTCOMES

Surgical outcomes are directly dependent on the extent of articular surface involvement. More than 90% of patients will have an excellent result if the labral tear is addressed and if the femoral and acetabular chondral surfaces are intact. If there is a grade I or II chondral lesion of either the adjacent acetabular chondral

## Table 13-1 RESULTS

| Total No. of Hips: 170 | Total No. of Anterior Labral Tears: 113 | Anterior Acetabular Chondral Defects With Outerbridge Criteria | Outerbridge Grade | Anterior Femoral Head Chondral Defects With Outerbridge Criteria | Required Total Hip Arthroscopy Within 6 Years (Mean, 2.5 Years) |
|---|---|---|---|---|---|
| | 7 | 13 | I | 13 | |
| | 16 | 23 | II | 16 | |
| | 20 | 21 | III | 15 | 7 |
| | 35 | 43 | IV | 10 | 10 |

surface or the femoral head, 70% to 80% will have a good to excellent result. Conversely, if the articular cartilage involvement is full thickness and diffuse on the femoral head and the acetabulum, 70% to 80% of cases are associated with a poor result during follow up, and 40% to 50% will require total joint arthroplasty within 2 years of arthroscopy. Table 13-1 shows arthroscopic results at 2 to 5 years of follow up for 170 patients with hips with mild to moderate dysplasia.

## ANNOTATED REFERENCES

**Glick JM. Hip arthroscopy using the lateral approach. *Instr Course Lect.* 1988;37:223–231.**

Hip arthroscopy provides for complete visualization of the joint space with the use of a direct lateral approach over the greater trochanter, with the patient in the lateral decubitus position. The involved leg is held in an abducted and flexed position, with traction provided by pulleys hung overhead.

**McCarthy J, Noble P, Aluisio FV, Schuck M, Wright J, Lee JRN. Anatomy, pathologic features, and treatment of acetabular labral tears. *Clin Orth Rel Res.* 2003;406(1):38–47.**

Labral tears are most frequently anterior, and they are often associated with sudden twisting or pivoting motions. Labral tears that occur at the watershed zone may destabilize the adjacent acetabular conditions. Arthroscopic observations support the concept that labral disruption, acetabular chondral lesions, or both are frequently a part of a continuum of degenerative joint disease.

**McCarthy JC, Lee J. Hip arthroscopy: indications and technical pearls. *Clin Orthop Relat Res.* 2005;441:180–187.**

The development of hip-specific distraction equipment and instruments has allowed for the treatment of many conditions, especially loose bodies and labral and chondral injuries. The procedure can be performed safely and reproducibly, with minimal morbidity, and in a cost-efficient manner as outpatient surgery. Symptom relief and functional improvement can be achieved, but additional research is necessary to determine long-term outcomes. Level of Evidence: Level V (expert opinion).

**McCarthy JC, Lee JA. Acetabular dysplasia: a paradigm of arthroscopic examination of chondral injuries. *Clin Orthop.* 2002;122–128.**

The mild uncovering of the anterior femoral head subjects the labrum to increased load and potential susceptibility to tearing, most frequently anteriorly. The findings of the current study support the concept that labral disruption is frequently a predecessor in the continuum of degenerative joint disease.

**McCarthy JC, Lee JA. Hip arthroscopy: indications, outcomes, and complications. *Instr Course Lect.* 2006;55:301–308.**

Hip arthroscopy is technically demanding and requires special distraction tools and operating equipment. With proper patient selection, hip arthroscopy can successfully manage numerous intra-articular conditions, such as labral and chondral injuries, loose and foreign bodies, and synovial conditions.

**McCarthy JC, Noble PC, Schuck MR, Wright J, Lee J. The Otto E. Aufranc Award: the role of labral lesions to development of early degenerative hip disease. *Clin Orthop.* 2001;25–37.**

Arthroscopic and anatomic observations support the concept that labral disruption and degenerative joint disease are frequently part of a continuum of joint disease.

**Sampson TG. Complications of hip arthroscopy. *Clin Sports Med.* 2001;20(4):831–835.**

Complications associated with hip arthroscopy occur in between 1.6% and 5% of cases. Fortunately, with a greater understanding of causes and advancements in techniques and equipment, the incidence is declining. Most of the complications were transient neuropraxias and fluid extravasations that resulted in no permanent damage.

# CHAPTER 14

# Arthroscopic Labral Repair

*Carlos A. Guanche*

## INTRODUCTION

Our understanding of hip labral pathology as a cause of hip pain is evolving, and the various treatment interventions available are also in flux. The exact prevalence of acetabular labral tears in the general population is unknown. However, when investigating the incidence of these injuries among athletes who present with groin pain, a clinical assessment of 18 patients who presented to a sports clinic with complaints of groin pain and an age range of 17 to 48 years revealed that, in 4 of the 18 athletes (22%), a labral tear was documented with the use of magnetic resonance arthrography. On the basis of this analysis, it appears that an acetabular labral tear is certainly not uncommon and that treatment algorithms need to be delineated.

The current indications for labral repairs are somewhat variable. Although the labral tear as a result of a single traumatic event is the clearest indication for repair, this is a rare entity in clinical practice. More often, the inciting event is not obvious and chronic repetitive injuries leading to attritional tears are at fault, whereas in other cases femoroacetabular impingement or other bony variants may be at fault. It is important to realize not only that the labral tear should be treated but also that the underlying problems need to be addressed, or else the long-term outcomes will be poor.

## BASIC SCIENCE

The hip labrum is a fibrocartilaginous structure that surrounds the rim of the acetabulum in a nearly circumferential manner. It is contiguous with the transverse acetabular ligament across the acetabular notch inferomedially. The labrum is widest in the anterior half and thickest in the superior half, and it merges with the articular hyaline cartilage of the acetabulum through a transition zone of 1 mm to 2 mm. It is attached to the edge of the bony acetabulum via a thin tongue of bone that extends into the tissue via a zone of calcified cartilage, and it adheres directly to the outer surface of this bony extension without a zone of calcified cartilage. A group of three or four vessels are located in the substance of the labrum on the capsular side of this extension. The structure is separated from the hip capsule by a narrow synovial-lined recess, which is variable in size. In general, the vascular supply of the adult hip labrum is poor, and regional differences in vascularity exist. Kelly and colleagues used cadaveric injection studies to define the vascularity of this area, and they demonstrated that the capsular portion of the labrum is significantly more vascular than the articular side, with only the peripheral third

of the labrum having nutrient vessels. Extrapolating from our understanding of the healing capacity of the meniscus, repair strategies should be considered for tears that involve only the peripheral labrum.

The labrum functions to enhance the stability of the hip by maintaining the negative intra-articular pressure within the joint as well as by increasing congruity. With the use of a poroelastic finite element model, it has been determined that the labrum functions to provide structural resistance to the lateral motion of the femoral head within the acetabulum. Furthermore, it has been demonstrated that the labrum also functions to decrease contact pressures within the hip and to decrease cartilage surface consolidation. This effect is a result of maintaining the articular fluid in contact with the weight-bearing cartilage via a joint-sealing effect.

## INDICATIONS

- Mechanical symptoms with rotational activities
- Unremitting pain in the groin with weight-bearing activities
- Concomitant femoroacetabular impingement with healthy, repairable tissue
- Traumatic dislocation or subluxation with ongoing mechanical symptoms
- Subluxation episodes in high-performance athletes
- Tissue with obvious vascularity in the proper (capsular) anatomic zone
- Tear of larger than 1 cm

## DIAGNOSIS OF LABRAL TEARS OF THE HIP

The clinical presentation of patients with a tear of the labrum is variable, and, as a result, the diagnosis is often missed initially. Burnett and colleagues reported about a series of 66 patients in whom the diagnosis of a labral tear had been made by arthroscopy. In this series, the mean time from the onset of symptoms to diagnosis was 21 months. An average of 3.3 health care providers had seen each patient before the diagnosis of a labral tear was made. Groin pain was the most common complaint (92%), with the onset of symptoms most often being insidious. A positive "impingement sign" occurred in 95% of patients in this series; this sign consists of groin pain with flexion, adduction, and internal rotation of the symptomatic hip (Figure 14-1). Therefore, in young, active patients who present with complaints of groin pain, with or without a history of trauma, the diagnosis of a labral tear of the hip should be suspected and investigated further.

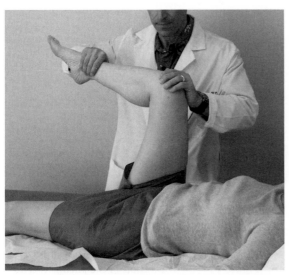

**Figure 14–1** Physical examination of a patient with a hip labral tear. The maneuver of hip flexion, adduction, and internal rotation (called the *impingement sign* in some descriptions) should elicit frank mechanical catching and a reproduction of the pain associated with a labral tear.

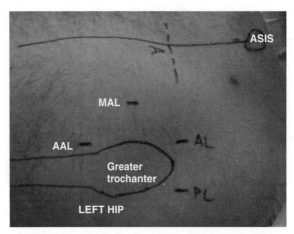

**Figure 14–2** The standard arthroscopic portals employed for access to the hip joint (in this case, the left hip) with the patient in the supine position. The accessory mid-anterolateral portal is useful as a result of its appropriate angle of approach to the acetabular bone. *A,* Anterior portal; *AAL,* accessory anterolateral portal; *AL,* anterolateral portal; *ASIS,* anterosuperior iliac spine; *PL,* posterolateral portal; *MAL,* mid-anterolateral portal.

## IMAGING AND DIAGNOSTIC STUDIES

Standard radiographs (weight-bearing anteroposterior pelvis and frog-leg lateral) are critical as part of the initial assessment to evaluate the patient for arthritis and femoroacetabular impingement and also for more subtle dysplasias. Multiple studies have demonstrated the superior accuracy of magnetic resonance arthrography (MRA) as compared with standard magnetic resonance imaging for the diagnosis of labral tears. Intra-articular gadolinium has been shown to improve the sensitivity of diagnosing labral pathology from 25% to 92% with the use of a small field of view. Therefore, when clinical suspicion of a hip labral tear exists, MRA with a small field of view is the study of choice.

An intra-articular lidocaine injection is useful for situations in which the diagnosis of labral pathology is equivocal or in which a tear has been diagnosed by MRA but it is uncertain whether symptoms are related to this finding. Similar to its use for diagnosing external impingement of the shoulder, if patients experience relief from symptoms after the injection, the diagnosis of pain as a result of hip intra-articular pathology is more certain. Although this does not confirm that the labral tear is the problem, it certainly makes the case that intra-articular pathology is at least somewhat responsible for the symptomatology.

## SURGICAL TECHNIQUE

The decision to proceed with operative intervention should be heavily weighed with regard to refractory mechanical symptoms. The majority of labral tears are treated with debridement; however, some tears are amenable to arthroscopic repair. Because the blood supply to the labrum enters from the adjacent joint capsule, peripheral tears have healing potential, and repairs should be considered if this pattern is encountered.

### Technique for Arthroscopic Labral Debridement

The procedure can be performed with the patient in either the supine or lateral position, depending on the level of comfort of the surgeon. The procedure should employ both a 30-degree and a 70-degree arthroscope for a thorough assessment of both the labrum and associated pathology. Modified arthroscopic flexible instruments, extended shavers, and hip-specific instrumentation should be available to improve access to all areas of the hip joint. In addition, the positioning of instruments should be done in the proper portals, with consideration for the anatomic structures near the hip joint (Figure 14-2).

A diagnostic arthroscopic examination of the central compartment can be performed systematically to evaluate not only the labrum from anterior to posterior but also to locate possible cartilage lesions on both the acetabular and femoral sides. In addition, the integrity of the ligamentum teres should be assessed; this area can be a source of pain as a result of impingement of the soft tissues between the femoral head and the acetabulum. Any loose bodies should be noted and their source identified. Finally, an assessment should be made of any obvious capsular redundancy or laxity.

Many patients will have a significant synovitis associated with the labral tearing, and an effort should be made to resect some of the inflamed tissue to improve visualization of the joint and to decrease the associated pain. This should be undertaken with a radiofrequency probe to decrease the potential for bleeding and the subsequent compromise of the surgical field.

The goal of the surgical procedure should be to preserve as much native tissue as is technically feasible while resecting the degenerative or damaged material. This is important to maintain the labrum's role as a secondary joint stabilizer and to minimize the potential for arthrosis. Frayed tissue should be debrided with the use of either motorized shavers or radiofrequency probes. It is important to delineate the areas of abnormal tissue that are identified both on radiographs (in the form of perilabral calcifications) and with magnetic resonance imaging or MRA (abnormal signal intensity) to thoroughly address the labral pathology.

Adjacent cartilage damage should be searched for and thoroughly addressed. Superficial lesions can be gently debrided with mechanical shavers and perhaps stabilized with the use of radiofrequency probes. Grade IV Outerbridge lesions should be managed with a thorough debridement down to a bleeding bed and by preparation with microfracture awls (Figure 14-3).

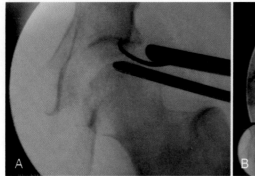
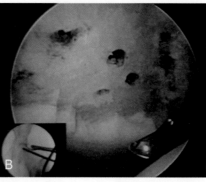

Figure 14–3 Chondroplasty of an articular cartilage lesion. **A,** Chondroplasty awl used for the preparation of significant chondral injuries of the acetabular and femoral cartilage. **B,** Final area of preparation with an obvious bleeding bed.

### Technique for Arthroscopic Labral Repair

The decision to perform a labral repair is still a process in its infancy. The current indications include tears that are symptomatic and that have either obvious vascularity within their substance or are repairable to the acetabular bony wall or the adjacent capsule. In general, a tear that is less than 1 cm in length does not require repair because there is minimal associated instability and mechanical symptomatology. In addition, the decision to perform a repair should be predicated on having the appropriate instrumentation and adequate technical ability.

The arthroscopic techniques include the use of routine anterior and anterolateral portals as well as an accessory mid-anterior portal that is halfway between the two portals and about 2 cm distal (see Figure 14-2). The routine use of several accessory portals is supported by the fact that the anterior anatomy allows for safe portal establishment anywhere between the standard anterior portal and the posterolateral portal.

As described previously, the surgical procedure includes a diagnostic arthroscopy with the treatment of any associated pathology. In addition, most labral tears that are repaired will also require at least a partial debridement of the avascular and often degenerative tissue. After the completion of the debridement, preparation is made for the repair. Similar to the concept of arthroscopic labral repair in the shoulder, the use of suture anchors has been shown to be effective for fixation for those cases in which a bony detachment exists. In situations in which the tear is in the labrocapsular junction, the repair can be performed with the use of suture material that is placed around the labrum and repaired to the adjacent capsular tissue.

When the labral tear involves a detachment from the acetabulum either as a result of trauma or attritional tearing, a suture anchor is required for the stabilization of the tear.

The area of the tearing is abraded and prepared with the use of either an aggressive shaver or a small burr. Fibrinous tissue is typically present at the bone–labrum interface, and an attempt is made to prepare the bed with a healthy vascular supply (Figure 14-4). The position of the anchor is critical to reestablishing the normal anatomy of the labrum. It should be placed on the acetabular rim to achieve an appropriate angle of approach while not penetrating into the articular cartilage. Avoiding chondral injury both in the head (upon delivery of the anchor) and with respect to acetabular penetration is important, because it can become a factor in joint degeneration. Both endoscopic and fluoroscopic visualization are essential (Figure 14-5). Options for repair include traditional suture anchors, which include knot tying or, more recently, the use of knotless anchors that allow for relatively easier technical maneuvers within the tight confines of the hip joint (Figure 14-6).

After the anchor is placed, a suture-passing device should be employed for the penetration of the labrum. A variety of devices exist for this purpose, with some employing shuttle devices and some simply penetrating through the tissue (Figure 14-7). Most of the instruments have been adapted from shoulder arthroscopy instrumentation. When the suture anchor is in place and the sutures have been passed, standard knot-tying techniques are employed (Figure 14-8).

For cases in which an intrasubstance split is to be addressed, the cleavage plane in the labrum should be fully defined and debrided of all nonviable tissue. A suture shuttle device can be used to deliver a looped monofilament suture between the junction of the articular cartilage and the fibrocartilage labrum. A suture penetrator is then employed through the capsule to grasp the loop of monofilament. The looped suture is then used to shuttle a monofilament suture around the labral tearing and through the capsule. At this point, the suture is tied in an extra-articular position with the use of tactile feel and an automatic suture cutter (Figure 14-9).

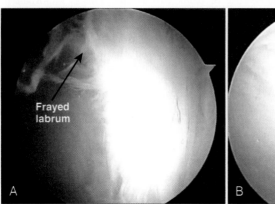
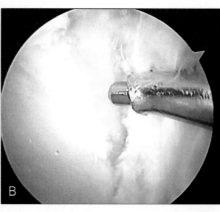

Frayed labrum

Figure 14–4 **A,** Labral tear in a left hip, viewed from the anterolateral portal. Note the frayed and devitalized tissue. **B,** Prepared bony bed in preparation for anchor delivery.

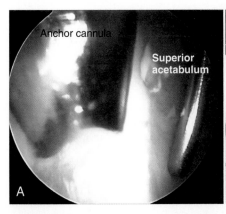
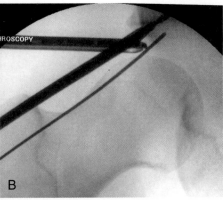

**Figure 14–5** Arthroscopic and endoscopic visualization of suture anchor insertion. **A,** Endoscopic view of suture anchor cannula before anchor delivery. This is a right hip viewed from the anterolateral portal. The metal anchor delivery cannula is placed in the anterior portal, and it rests on the anterior acetabular wall. **B,** Fluoroscopic image of the cannula with its angle of approach diverging from the articular margin.

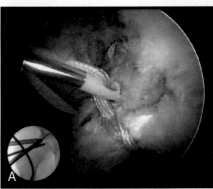
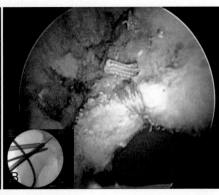

**Figure 14–6** Knotless anchor technique. **A,** The insertion of the knotless anchor in the superior acetabulum (PushLock anchor [Arthrex, Inc., Naples, FL]). **B,** Final anchor position with suture well away from the articular margin.

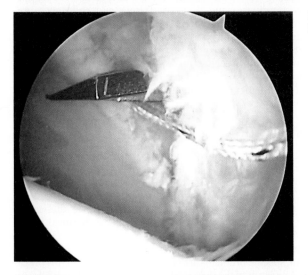

**Figure 14–7** Suture penetrator in place within the substance of a labrum that is detached from the acetabular bony wall.

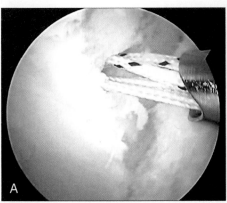
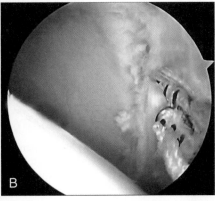

**Figure 14–8** Labral repair with the use of a suture anchor with penetrator devices. **A,** Anchor in place. **B,** Final repair.

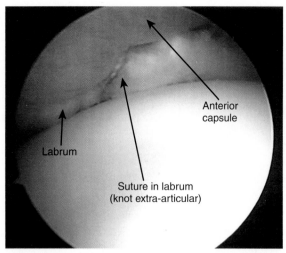

**Figure 14–9** Repair of a labrum with extracapsular suture positioning.

## REHABILITATION AFTER DEBRIDEMENT

> ### TECHNICAL PEARLS
>
> - Ensure that proper equipment is available, including longer instruments for anchor placement.
> - Ensure the proper orientation of suture anchor insertion by confirming the insertion angle both endoscopically and fluoroscopically.
> - Address the primary problem that caused the tear (i.e., look for impingement).
> - Use repair strategies that maximize the healing potential.
> - Prepare a bony bed.
> - Attempt to approximate the labrum to the capsule to increase the vascular supply.
> - Use accessory portals for anchor insertion if the available portals do not allow for an appropriate angle of insertion.

Formal therapy for range of motion and strengthening of the operative hip is begun 7 to 10 days after surgery. Weight bearing after an isolated arthroscopic labral debridement should be unrestricted, with the use of crutches limited to the early postoperative period only (i.e., 3 to 5 days). The standard protocol includes a gradual progression from increasing the range of motion to unrestricted strengthening. Aggressive hip flexor strengthening should be limited until full range of motion is obtained and until hip mechanics are relatively normal. For cases in which abnormal mechanics substitute the psoas or the hip flexors abnormally, a refractory tendonitis can develop. Explosive and rotational activities should be limited for at least 6 weeks. The return to unrestricted activity is predicated on a full, painless range of motion and the normal strength of the pelvic, abdominal, and lower-extremity musculature.

## REHABILITATION AFTER LABRAL REPAIR

Formal therapy for range of motion and strengthening of the operative hip should begin by 7 to 10 days postoperatively. Early range of motion is initiated to limit the scarring in the joint associated with the surgical trauma. Weight bearing after an isolated arthroscopic labral repair should be restricted to toe touching with the use of crutches for the first 4 weeks. The most important principle is to limit the rotational stresses that the repaired labrum experiences during the first few weeks. The ranges that

put the repair at risk include flexion past 90 degrees, abduction past 25 degrees, and internal or external rotation limited to 25 degrees. Limitations are placed on flexion past 90 degrees for 10 days, whereas abduction and adduction are limited to 25 degrees for 4 weeks. Beginning at 4 weeks, a gradual progression from increasing the range of motion to unrestricted strengthening is begun. The use of stationary bicycling is encouraged and instituted during the first 10 days. Aggressive hip flexor strengthening should be limited until full range of motion is obtained and hip mechanics have normalized. For cases in which abnormal mechanics substitute the psoas or the hip flexors abnormally, a significant tendonitis can develop. Explosive and rotational activities should also be limited for at least 12 weeks. The return to unrestricted activity is predicated on a full, painless range of motion and the normal strength of the pelvic, abdominal, and lower-extremity musculature; this typically occurs approximately 4 to 6 months postoperatively.

## RESULTS

There are numerous studies that detail the use of arthroscopy for treating lesions of the hip labrum. However, collective interpretation is confounded by the nonuniform use of outcome measures and a lack of validated outcomes for nonarthritic hip pain. Further complicating the matter is the fact that many published series contain heterogeneous study populations in which subjects have associated hip pathology (e.g., arthritis, dysplasia, femoroacetabular impingement) in addition to labral tearing.

To date, there are no published series about the long-term outcomes of the arthroscopic repair of hip labral tears. Indications for the lesions that are considered to be repairable are currently evolving. Recently, Hines and colleagues presented outcome results with a mean follow up of 9 months for a series of 52 patients who underwent arthroscopic hip labral repair. Another study by Ross, which looked at the results of 19 patients, has also recently been published. The results of these studies and of those that have documented the outcomes of labral debridements are summarized in Table 14-1.

## COMPLICATIONS

Hip arthroscopy has been shown to be relatively safe in several studies that have documented its effectiveness as well as the number of resulting complications. In one large series, there was a 1.6% complication rate, with problems that included transient palsy of either the sciatic or the femoral nerve, paresthesias as a result of lateral femoral cutaneous nerve palsy, perineal injury, and instrument breakage.

Although this study was not specific to the repair of the hip labrum, specific problems are certainly associated with this procedure. As a result of the tight confines and the multiple instruments that are inserted into the joint, the possibility of serious articular cartilage damage exists. Care should be taken while working within the joint to ensure that cartilage damage is minimal. In addition, with the insertion of suture anchors, there is the possibility of joint penetration. The liberal use of fluoroscopy to document the position of the anchor insertion instrument before committing to a specific angle is critical to a successful procedure.

## SUMMARY

The mechanical effects of the labrum appear to substantiate the need to preserve as much tissue as possible. The effects of a decrease in synovial fluid within the weight-bearing dome of the acetabulum as a result of labral resection are probably

**Table 14-1** SUMMARY OF STUDIES OF THE RESULTS OF ARTHROSCOPIC DEBRIDEMENT AND THE REPAIR OF TEARS OF THE HIP LABRUM

| Study | Labral Treatment | No. of Patients | Mean Length of Follow Up | Results |
|---|---|---|---|---|
| Byrd et al., 2000 | D (Debridement) | 35 | 2 years | Significant improvements in Harris Hip Scores, especially with regard to labral tears or loose bodies |
| Farjo et al., 1999 | D | 28 | 13 to 100 months | 71% good/excellent without arthritis; 21% good/excellent with degenerative joint disease (djd) |
| O'Leary et al., 2001 | D | 86 | 30 months | 91% improvement with labral tears; 40% improvement with osteonecrosis; 44% improvement with djd |
| Potter et al., 2005 | D | 40 | 13 to 55 months | 70% overall patient satisfaction |
| Santori et al., 2000 | D | 76 | 24 to 61 months | 67% overall satisfaction; mean Modified Harris Hip Score (MHHS), 89.8 |
| Hines et al., 2007 | R (Repair) | 52 | 9 months | 85% good/excellent results |
| Ross et al., 2006 | R | 19 | 6 months | Significant improvement in MHHS, Short Form-36 (SF-36), nonarthritic hips, and Visual Analog Score (VAS); 67% satisfied |

detrimental on a long-term basis. Therefore, the treatment of patients who have mechanical symptoms with underlying labral pathology needs to be undertaken in a conservative fashion to alleviate symptoms while also preventing (or at least delaying) the development of degenerative changes.

There are key questions that remain to be answered with regard to the use of hip arthroscopy to treat lesions of the hip labrum. First, what are the long-term results of the arthroscopic debridement of tears of the hip labrum? The results of the procedure as compared with those of the natural history of tears are unknown. Second, and in conjunction with the first question, how do the short- and long-term results of the arthroscopic repair of the torn hip labrum compare with those of arthroscopic debridement?

The available literature supports the concept that the labrum is important for both stability and cartilage homeostasis. The long-term effects of repair or excision clearly need to be further analyzed. It is intuitively apparent that the preservation of as much relatively normal labral tissue as possible—with any surgical procedure—is critical to the long-term preservation of the native hip joint.

## ANNOTATED REFERENCES AND SUGGESTED READINGS

Burnett RS, Della Rocca GJ, Prather H, et al. Clinical presentation of patients with tears of the acetabular labrum. *J Bone Joint Surg Am.* 2007;88A:1448–1457.

Byrd JW, Jones KS. Prospective analysis of hip arthroscopy with 2-year follow-up. *Arthroscopy* 2000;16:578–587.

Crawford MJ, Dy CJ, Alexander JW, et al. The biomechanics of the hip labrum and the stability of the hip. *J Orthop Res.* 2007;465:16–22.

This article is an analysis of the stability given to the hip by the labrum as well as of the clinical implications of disruption.

Espinosa N, Rothenfluh DA, Beck M, et al. Treatment of femoroacetabular impingement: Preliminary results of labral refixation. *J Bone Joint Surg.* 2006;88A:925–935.

This is a clinical study with more than 2 years of follow-up regarding patients who underwent open femoral neck resection with labral refixation and who are compared with a group that underwent labral excision.

Farjo LA, Glick JM, Sampson TG. Hip arthroscopy for acetabular labral tears. *Arthroscopy* 1999;15:132–137.

Ferguson SJ, Bryant JT, Ganz R, et al. The influence of the acetabular labrum on hip joint cartilage consolidation: a poroelastic finite element model. *J Biomech.* 2000;33:953–960.

This is a finite element model description of the structure and function of the labrum. The implications of a disrupted labrum are also discussed.

Griffin DR, Villar RN. Complications of arthroscopy of the hip. *J Bone Joint Surg.* 1991;81B:604–606.

This article includes a summary of 640 consecutive hip arthroscopies and the documentation of common complications.

Hines SL, Philippon MJ, Kuppersmith D, et al. Early results of labral repair. Presented at 2007 annual AANA meeting. April 27, San Francisco, CA; 2007.

This article presents the early clinical results of a group of patients undergoing hip labral repairs.

Kelly BT, Shapiro GS, Digiovanni CW, et al. Vascularity of the hip labrum: a cadaveric investigation. *Arthroscopy.* 2005;21(1):3–11.

Kelly BT, Weiland DE, Schenker ML, et al. Current concepts: arthroscopic labral repair in the hip: surgical technique and review of the literature. *Arthroscopy.* 2005;21:1496–1504.

This article depicts the current understanding of hip labral repairs as well as various surgical techniques.

Lage LA, Patel JV, Villar RN. The acetabular labral tear: an arthroscopic classification. *Arthroscopy.* 1996;12:269–272.

This is a descriptive classification of the commonly encountered types of labral tears.

McCarthy JC, Noble PC, Schuck MR, et al. The watershed labral lesion: its relationship to early arthritis of the hip. *J Arthroplasty.* 2001;16(8 Suppl 1):81–87.

This article provides an analysis of the senior author's patients and the description of a pathomechanical model that leads to chondral delamination in the absence of bony impingement.

Murphy KP, Ross AE, Javernick A, et al. Repair of the adult acetabular labrum. *Arthroscopy.* 2006;22:e3.

This article presents the result of a small series of patients with short-term follow-up after the labral repair of the hip.

O'Leary JA, Bernard K, Vail TP. The relationship between diagnosis and outcome in arthroscopy of the hip. *Arthroscopy* 2001;17:181–188.

Potter BK, Freedman BA, Andersen RC, et al. Correlation of short form-36 and disability status with outcomes of arthroscopic labral debridement. *Am J Sports Med* 2005;33:864–870.

Ross AE, Javernick M, Freedman B, et al. Arthroscopic hip labral repair. *Arthroscopy.* 2006;22:e30.

Santorini N, Villar RN. Acetabular labral tears: result of arthroscopic partial limbectomy. *Arthroscopy* 2000;16:11–15.

Seldes RM, Tan V, Hunt J, et al. Anatomy, histologic features, and vascularity of the adult acetabular labrum. *Clin Orthop.* 2001;382:232–240.

This descriptive classification correlates the type of tear encountered with the type of clinical pathology. The classification is based on the histologic analysis of tears.

Toomayan FA, Holman WR, Major NM, et al. Sensitivity of MR arthrography in the evaluation of acetabular labral tears. *AJR Am J Roentgenol.* 2006;186(2):449–453.

This article compares plain magnetic resonance imaging with MRA and includes a discussion of some of the standard techniques.

# CHAPTER 15

# Arthroscopic Capsular Plication and Thermal Capsulorrhaphy

*Anil S. Ranawat and Jon K. Sekiya*

## INTRODUCTION

The hip is an inherently stable articulation between the femoral head and the acetabulum. Unlike the shoulder, the primary component of hip stability is determined by its constrained osseous anatomy. Although traumatic hip subluxations and dislocation are well documented, recently there has been heightened interest in atraumatic instability as a source of recalcitrant hip pain and symptoms. In these cases, redundant or incompetent capsular–labral structures lead to microinstability. There is a dynamic and transient incongruency or subluxation within the femoroacetabular articulation that results in abnormal force distributions across the hip joint and ultimately in worsening capsular redundancy and injury, chondrolabral injuries, and femoral neck impingement at high flexion angles (i.e., secondary impingement). This ignites clinical symptoms and starts a cascade of pathologic events that result in hip pain, stiffness, flexion contractures, labral pathology, and degeneration of the hip. The causes of hip instability and capsular laxity are multifactorial and include such things as intrinsic ligamentous laxity, connective tissue diseases, overuse or repetitive activities, iatrogenic injuries, subtle hip subluxation injuries, and prior dislocations.

The mainstay of treatment for capsular laxity and atraumatic instability has been conservative. There have been a few reports of open capsular plication as a method of treatment, but these have mostly been for posttraumatic instability. Recently, improved understanding and imaging of the prearthritic hip has led to the development of arthroscopic treatment approaches. Early experience was primarily focused on arthroscopic thermal capsular shrinkage and capsulorrhaphy, which produced promising early results. However, because thermal capsulorrhaphy has recently fallen out of favor for addressing shoulder instability because it can result in collagen disruption, chondrolysis, and high long-term failure rates, there has been gradual movement toward arthroscopic hip capsular plication. This burgeoning technique provides the advantages of a reproducible and durable capsulorrhaphy with the desired amount of plication controlled by the surgeon without the potentially adverse affects of thermal shrinkage. We present here a review of atraumatic hip instability and capsular laxity, and we will discuss their relevant anatomy, evaluation, imaging studies, and management principles as well as arthroscopic techniques of capsular plications in both the central and peripheral compartments.

## BASIC SCIENCE

The hip is a constrained diarthrodial joint. The femoral head is an approximation of a sphere, and, under normal osseous parameters, the acetabulum covers approximately 170 degrees of the femoral head. The labrum is a fibrocartilage structure that further deepens the acetabulum. It functions to enhance stability by establishing a negative intra-articular pressure within the hip joint, preserving joint congruity, and limiting the fluid expression that acts as an important sealing function. The labrum also plays a role in helping to contain the femoral head in extremes of range of motion, especially in flexion. Its role in providing rotational stability is still unknown.

The surrounding capsular envelope consists of three ligaments: the iliofemoral ligament (i.e., the Y ligament of Bigelow), the pubofemoral ligament, and the ischiofemoral ligament (Figure 15-1). The iliofemoral ligament has a medial and lateral limb proximally, and distally it forms a deep circular band that surrounds the femoral neck in a leash-like fashion; this area is called the *zona orbicularis*. This "Y ligament" is the strongest, and it prevents the anterior translation of the hip during extension and external rotation when its fibers tighten. In flexion, these fibers loosen, which leads to a "screw home" effect in full extension. The pubofemoral ligament is slightly inferior to the iliofemoral ligaments, and it also controls external rotation in extension. The ischiofemoral ligament is a posterior structure that controls internal rotation in flexion and extension. Other secondary hip stabilizers include the ligamentum teres and the psoas tendon, which may provide important stability in cases of dysplasia or static ligament deficiencies.

The causes of chronic atraumatic hip instability and capsular laxity are multifactorial. Primary causes include milder forms of intrinsic ligamentous laxity as well as more extreme cases of connective tissue diseases such as Marfan syndrome or Ehlers-Danlos syndrome, with which patients may be able to voluntarily or habitually dislocate their hips. The more common (but less well-recognized) secondary causes are overuse and repetitive activities such as golf, dancing, gymnastics, and martial arts. In these cases, there is repetitive hip rotation with an axial load. Other secondary causes include iatrogenic injuries and subtle forms of trauma, including hip subluxations and even prior dislocations.

The last type of atraumatic hip instability involves osseous anatomic abnormalities on either the acetabular side or the femoral side. Inclination, version, and other osseous parameters of the weight-bearing surface affect the soft-tissue structures that surround the hip. For cases in which there is a deficiency of the bony acetabulum (dysplasia) or excessive femoral anteversion or valgus, there is more reliance on the surrounding soft-tissue structures. McKibbin has quantified this with an index of combined femoral and acetabular version that predicts increased stress to the anterior capsulolabral structures. He defined the McKibbin index as the sum of the angles of femoral and acetabular anteversion, with a total of more than 60 denoting severe instability.

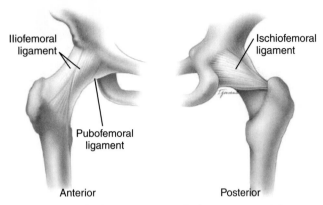

**Figure 15–1** The three primary capsular ligaments around the hip. The anterior ligamentous constraints of the hip are seen in the anterior view and include the iliofemoral and pubofemoral ligaments. The ischiofemoral ligament is the primary posterior restraint. *With permission from AJSM, Vol. 31, No. 6.*

## BRIEF HISTORY AND PHYSICAL EXAMINATION

The diagnosis of traumatic hip injuries has improved with increased attention and a heightened index of suspicion; however, the diagnosis of atraumatic hip instability remains difficult and confusing. Because the differential diagnosis of hip pain is quite broad, an accurate history is critical. Any overuse activities with repetitive stresses should heighten awareness, because these activities may injure the iliofemoral ligament or labrum and alter the balance of forces in the hip. In addition, a thorough family history and a review of systems should be performed to rule out connective tissue disorders.

During the physical examination, the patient's spine should first be examined to rule out other causes of hip pain. This should be followed by an examination of the elbows, hands, and knees to look for signs of hypermobility. Attention should also be paid to the patient's skin and eyes. Next, the range of motion of both hips should be assessed. These patients often have an increased range of motion as a result of capsular laxity, but any significant increase in internal rotation should heighten one's suspicion of increased femoral anteversion or other osseous abnormalities. This is followed by a thorough neurovascular examination that includes the reflexes. Next, specific hip testing should be performed, including the Ober test, the bicycle test, the psoas test, and the impingement test. In many cases, this process alters dynamic stabilizers (e.g., the iliopsoas) and leads to psoas and flexion contractures, internal coxa saltans, low back pain, and sacroiliac joint pain. Finally, hip-specific testing for capsular laxity should be performed. Patients with this condi-

tion will usually experience anterior hip pain while in the supine position with passive hip extension and external rotation (Figure 15-2, *A*). Patients may also have increased external rotation in full extension and distraction on the affected side (see Figure 15-2, *B*). Philippon and colleagues classified capsular laxity on the basis of these physical examination findings from grade 1 (mild) to grade 4 (severe), with grade 4 representing collagen vascular diseases.

## IMAGING AND DIAGNOSTIC STUDIES

The radiologic workup begins with plain radiographs, including an anteroposterior view of the pelvis, a weight-bearing anteroposterior view, and a cross-table lateral view of the affected hip. Additional studies that may be necessary include Judet oblique films to further assess the acetabulum. False-profile views are used to assess for dysplasia, and computed tomography scans with spot views of the distal femoral epicondyles can be used to assess for acetabular and femoral anteversion. Various radiographic indices have been described to assess osseous undercoverage; these include but are not limited to the Tönnis angle, the center-edge angle of Wiberg, the anterior center-edge angle of Lequesne and de Seze, the femoral head extrusion, and the subluxation index. Acetabular version can also be estimated on radiographs by assessing the relationship of the anterior and posterior walls. A crossover sign and a prominent ischial spine both represent a retroverted acetabulum. The degree of retroversion can be estimated by the location of the crossover of the anterior wall, with more inferior crossing suggesting increased retroversion.

Magnetic resonance imaging (MRI) is critical for the evaluation of atraumatic instability. In the acute setting of traumatic hip injuries, numerous studies have demonstrated that MRI may aid in the diagnosis of chondral injuries, loose bodies, labral tears, femoral head contusions, sciatic nerve injuries, and ligament disruptions. Likewise, in the setting of chronic atraumatic injuries, MRI is also very useful to find subtle derangements in capsulolabral structures (Figure 15-3) as well as osteonecrosis.

## INDICATIONS

Capsular laxity and atraumatic instability are difficult entities to assess, define, and ultimately treat; their management is still being developed. With the advent of better diagnostic and therapeutic capabilities, it is becoming increasingly clear that these pathologies exist. If a patient has a physical examination and history that are consistent with capsulolabral injury and instability and if appropriate imaging studies corroborate the clinical suspicion, then a trial of physical therapy and anti-inflammatory medication may be appropriately

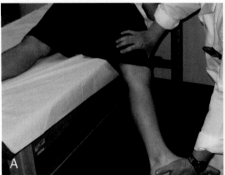
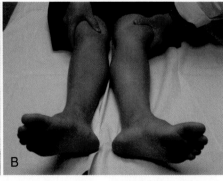

**Figure 15–2 A,** Apprehension test performed with the hip in extension, abduction, and external rotation, which can be positive in patients with both acetabular dysplasia and capsular laxity. **B,** Increased external rotation in extension of the affected limb in a patient with capsular laxity.

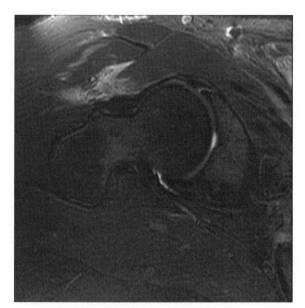

**Figure 15–3** Sagittal fat suppressed magnetic resonance arthrogram of a patient with capsular laxity and a labral tear from probable neck impingement or secondary impingement from an extreme range of motion.

administered in an attempt to break the cycle of painful capsulolabral pathology. If conservative management fails and the patient has significant pain relief after an intra-articular anesthetic injection, then hip arthroscopy can be considered; however, because of the dearth of literature and unclear outcomes of this therapy, the mainstay of treatment for capsular laxity should still be conservative.

The anatomic restoration of the labrum (i.e., labral repair) and a reduction in capsular laxity either by capsular plication or ther-

INDICATIONS

- Physical examination consistent with capsular laxity (i.e., ligamentous laxity signs, increased external rotation in extension, apprehension)
- Failure of conservative management
- No significant evidence of acetabular dysplasia or excessive femoral anteversion
- MRI evidence of chondrolabral injury
- Significant pain relief after intra-articular anesthetic injection

mal capsulorrhaphy have been described, with favorable preliminary results. In most cases, we perform capsular plication, because it is a reliable and measured reduction in capsular volume that is similar to the treatment of the shoulder. On rare occasions, when there is minimal capsular redundancy, we perform a thermal capsulorrhaphy; however, in most cases, we use the thermal device primarily as an adjunct. For cases in which atraumatic instability is a result of poor osseous coverage (e.g., acetabular dysplasia, excessive femoral valgus, increased femoral anteversion), hip arthroscopy should be approached with extreme caution, and redirectional osteotomies should be considered.

## SURGICAL TECHNIQUE

The arthroscopic technique begins with adequate and appropriate anesthesia. Most often a general anesthetic is used with muscle relaxation, but regional anesthesia is also a possibility. With the patient supine on the operating room table, an examination under anesthesia is performed. Internal and external rotation is noted in full extension and in flexion and then compared with the nonoperative side. A flexion, abduction, and external rotation (FABER) test is then performed, with the distance from the lateral side of the affected knee being to the top of the operative table. As with external rotation, the affected limb often exhibits an increased amount of external rotation. Next, the hip is distracted, and a subjective evaluation of the necessary force needed to distract the hip joint is performed. Finally, if there is any concern regarding frank anterior instability, the limb is placed in extension, abduction, and external rotation, and a fluoroscopic image is performed to document this.

At this point, both of the patient's feet are well padded, and the patient's extremities are well secured to the fracture table. A well-padded perineal post is placed in between the patient's extremities. The nonoperative limb is placed in full extension and mild abduction and then in minimal traction. The operative limb is put through a traction maneuver, which consists of abduction around the perineal post, axial traction, and adduction. Appropriate traction is then confirmed fluoroscopically. In cases of capsular laxity, minimal traction is usually needed to adequately distract the joint (Figure 15-4). The limb is then placed in internal rotation, which decreases the amount of hip distraction, reduces femoral anteversion, and subluxes the femoral head anteriorly, which enables the easy instrumentation of the joint. At this point, traction time is noted and documented.

The operative side is then prepped and draped in a sterile fashion. After confirming that preoperative antibiotics have

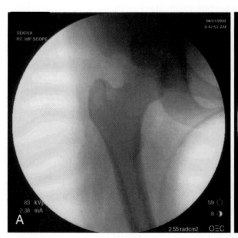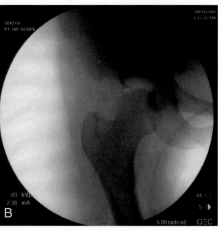

**Figure 15–4** With minimal traction, patients with capsular laxity with or without labral tears require little force to have adequate distraction. **A,** Before traction. **B,** After minimal traction.

been administered, a standard anterolateral arthroscopic portal is established under fluoroscopic guidance, which is then followed by an anterior portal, which is established under direct visualization with a 70-degree scope. At this point, a thorough diagnostic arthroscopy is performed, with careful attention paid to the capsulolabral structures in the central compartment. Any obvious peripheral labral tears are addressed surgically to enhance stability.

We currently perform three different arthroscopic techniques for atraumatic hip instability: central plication, peripheral plication, and thermal capsulorrhaphy. In many cases, a combination of techniques is performed. As stated previously, in most cases, we perform thermal capsulorrhaphy as an adjunct; rarely do we still use it as a primary mode of treatment. The technique begins as described previously. The capsule is then probed, and, if excessive laxity is present, a focal thermal capsulorrhaphy is performed. A flexible probe (Smith & Nephew, Andover, MA) is used at a temperature of 67°C and a power of 40 W. We use a technique that is similar to that described by Philippon and colleagues, who used a three-pass cornfield pattern. Care is taken to avoid any charring of tissue, but capsular contraction should be visualized (Figure 15-5). If capsular redundancy is still present after this procedure, a plication may also be performed, which is described later in this chapter.

For the central compartment technique, a minimal capsulotomy is performed anteriorly around the anterior portal in the medial limb of the iliofemoral ligament with either a beaver blade or an arthroscopic shaver to create some working room, to improve visualization, to create bleeding edges to help with healing. Then an 8.25 mm × 9 cm cannula (Arthrex, Naples, FL) is placed through the anterior working portal. A soft-tissue penetrator (Spectrum Suture Hook, Largo, FL) is then inserted through the anterior cannula. The penetrator pierces the medial portion of the iliofemoral ligament at the most medial extent of the intended plication. A No. 1 polydioxanone (PDS) suture (Ethicon, Somerville, NJ) is then shuttled into the joint as the penetrator is removed. Next, a soft-tissue penetrator/grasper (Bird Beak; Arthrex, Naples, FL) is inserted through the working portal and used to penetrate the lateral aspect of the iliofemoral ligament at the level of the desired plication. The PDS suture that was previously passed through the capsule and into the joint is grasped and removed from the joint through the cannula. The PDS suture is then used to shuttle a FiberWire suture (Arthrex, Naples, FL) through the capsule as the working suture.

A suture grasper is run along the length of the suture to ensure that no tangles exist. The FiberWire suture is checked to verify that it slides. Under direct visualization, the amount of tension and the ultimate plication are observed. Multiple passes, each being a separate plication, can be performed if more reduction in volume or a greater plication is desired. If not, then a blind, extracapsular, locking, sliding knot is tied with a knot pusher and followed by three half-hitch knots to back up the locking sliding knot; the suture is then cut (Figure 15-6, *A* through *E*).

For the peripheral compartment technique, traction is unnecessary, and the operative limb is placed in approximately 20 degrees to 30 degrees of flexion. The arthroscope is retracted from its intra-articular position into a position just under the capsule in the peripheral compartment, which can be performed from either the anterolateral portal or the anterior portal. A prior skin portal can be used (either anterolateral or anterior), or a new distal accessory portal can be established with a spinal needle under direct visualization. In unique situations, an osteoplasty is performed in addition to a capsular plication as a result of secondary impingement or neck impingement from an extreme range of motion. In these cases, a small capsulotomy may be established with an arthroscopic shaver in the anterior capsule to aid visualization.

An arthroscopic cannula (Arthrex, Naples, FL) is placed in the anterior working portal. In an identical manner to the intra-articular plication technique, a curved soft-tissue penetrator (Spectrum Suture Hook, Largo, FL) passes a No. 1 PDS suture (Ethicon, Somerville, NJ) after piercing the medial portion of the iliofemoral ligament at the most medial extent of the intended plication. This is most commonly performed from an "outside-in" vantage point, unlike the central technique, which is "inside out." Next, a Bird Beak (Arthrex, Naples, FL) captures the most lateral extent of intended plication, and a FiberWire (Arthrex, Naples, FL) is shuttled into position. As before, this process may be repeated through the same working portal until the desired amount of plication is achieved. Multiple configurations of capsular sutures can also be used, including a linear series of plications or even a crossing configuration like a "multi-pleat" technique. The plication is completed by tying a locking, sliding knot and backing it with three half-hitch knots. After sufficient capsular tension is achieved, stability is tested with gentle rotational testing. A technique similar to that of capsular plication may be used for posterior plication that involves the use of the appropriate posterior portals, but the posterior neurovascular structures must be carefully considered (Figure 15-7, *A* through *E*).

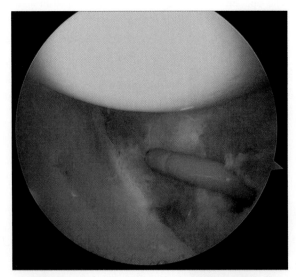

**Figure 15-5** Intraoperative photo of a thermal capsulorrhaphy being performed with a flexible probe with minimal charring.

**TECHNICAL PEARLS**

- Demonstrate appropriate patient selection.
- Capsular plication is favored over thermal capsulorrhaphy.
- If thermal capsulorrhaphy is performed, there should be no charring of tissue and a low threshold for supplementing with a plication.
- Both central and peripheral techniques are possible, with the latter not requiring traction.
- Plication techniques involve the use of both basic and advanced arthroscopic principles.
- Plication is performed under direct visualization; it can be measured, and it allows for the "multi-pleat" technique.

## POSTOPERATIVE REHABILITATION

The focus of the early postoperative period is on a gradual return of pain-free hip motion while protecting the capsular plication. For anterior plications, no external rotation or extension

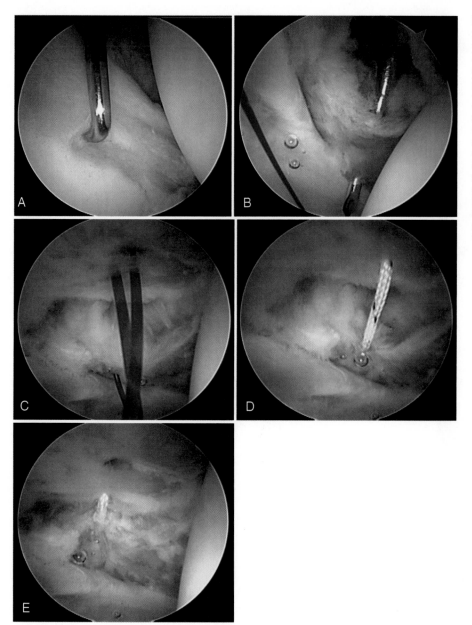

**Figure 15–6** Arthroscopic technique for the central compartment plication of a right hip. **A,** The arthroscope is in the lateral portal, and the camera is directed anteriorly as a nerve hook shows some labral fraying as a result of hypermobility. **B,** A small capsular window is made to create edges for the capsule to heal, and a polydioxanone (PDS) suture is passed through the medial limb of the anterior capsule. **C,** After a tissue penetrator device grabs the PDS suture and pulls it out through the lateral limb, the PDS suture now incorporates both limbs of the plication. **D,** The limbs of the PDS are then shuttled for a FiberWire suture (Arthrex, Naples, FL). **E,** An extracapsular locking arthroscopic knot is tied to plicate the tissue.

beyond neutral or abduction beyond 20 degrees of the involved hip is allowed. For patients with posterior capsular plications, internal rotation, flexion of more than 60 degrees, and adduction of more than 10 degrees are not allowed during the first 3 weeks after surgery. Patients are restricted to 30% partial weight bearing with crutches for the first few weeks and then gradually advanced. If a femoral osteoplasty is performed, patients may be protected longer. Patients may ride a stationary bicycle with no resistance, perform gluteal and quadriceps sets, and participate in heel slides and calf pumps. For those who underwent a posterior capsular plication, flexion is limited to 60 degrees when using the stationary bicycle for the first 6 weeks after the procedure. Although we routinely use continuous passive motion devices, for these patients we usually do not.

For the first 3 to 6 weeks, light resistance may be added to the stationary bicycle. Straight-leg raises may begin, and crutches should be weaned slowly, with the goal of full weight bearing by 6 weeks. Pool exercises of walking, jogging, and swimming with a buoy may begin. From 6 weeks to 3 months postoperatively, increased resistance is added to the stationary

bicycle, plyometrics is incorporated into the pool regimen, and seated rowing and elliptical machine use can begin. Hip flexor stretches should start along with toe raises with weights. After 3 months, slow jogging may begin on even ground, and closed-chain exercises should be initiated. After 5 months, patients may begin strengthening exercises and functional training. Full return to sport begins when normal strength is attained, when the patient can run at full speed without a limp, and when the patient regains the full range of motion.

## RESULTS

Overall, the literature is quite limited with regard to atraumatic instability and capsular laxity (Table 15-1). In terms of thermal capsulorrhaphy, the trend has been to move away from this modality because of the high rate of associated complications. Although the use of thermal energy as a means of shrinking redundant or lax connective tissues by collagen denaturation has been extensively studied in the shoulder, there are only a

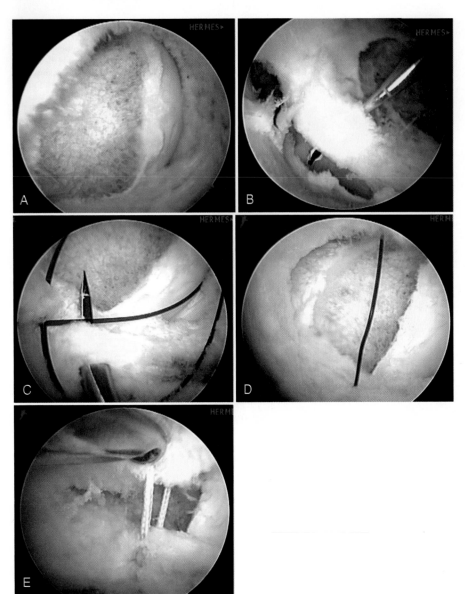

**Figure 15–7** Arthroscopic technique for the peripheral compartment plication of a left hip. **A,** The arthroscope is in the anterolateral portal, and the camera is directed proximally to visualize the two limbs of the anterior capsule that will be plicated. **B** and **C,** A tissue penetrator is used to shuttle a polydioxanone (PDS) suture into the capsule through the medial limb and then the lateral limb of the plication. **D,** The PDS suture then incorporates both limbs of the plication. **E,** The PDS is exchanged for a FiberWire suture (Arthrex, Naples, FL), and both limbs of the plication are brought together with an arthroscopic knot.

**Table 15-1** CLINICAL OUTCOMES

| Study | Arthroscopic or Open | Technique | No. of Patients | Results |
|---|---|---|---|---|
| Lieberman et al. (1993) | Open | Posterior bony Bankart | 1 | Good |
| Bellabarba et al. (1998) | Open | Posterior capsular imbrication | 1 | Good |
| Philippon et al. (2001) | Arthroscopic | Thermal capsulorrhaphy and labral debridement | 10 | Good |

few available studies in the hip. Philippon reported about 10 patients who had intractable hip pain with subtle signs of instability on examination in combination with the visualization of redundant capsular tissue during arthroscopy and labral tears. These patients underwent labral tear debridement with thermal capsulorrhaphy. They were allowed to bear weight as tolerated, and they had rotation and extension precautions for 18 days. Preliminary results showed excellent outcomes with regard to the first 8 patients resuming their preinjury athletic activities with minimal or no pain.

The literature about capsular plications is even more sparse. Bellabarba and colleagues described a group of patients that had

long-standing painful groin pain and snapping with no history of trauma. With the use of traction under fluoroscopy, these patients were diagnosed with idiopathic hip instability, but they also had mild evidence of acetabular dysplasia on radiographs. The authors postulated that the main pathologic process in these patients was capsular laxity rather than the dysplasia. One of these patients was treated with a posterior imbrication capsulorrhaphy, and her symptoms improved. However, it must be stressed that osseous deficiencies usually supersede soft-tissue abnormalities in the majority of cases.

In the literature, capsular laxity and instability secondary to post-traumatic injury are better defined. Open anatomic restoration of the capsulolabral structures has controlled symptoms and instability. These repairs have been performed for both anterior and posterior instability. For posterior instability, a soft-tissue Bankart-type repair has been performed. For anterior instability, an osseous repair of the anterior inferior iliac spine has been used as a means to repair the iliofemoral ligament.

## COMPLICATIONS

There are three groups of complications related to these techniques. The first are the general complications that are associated with hip arthroscopy, which include but are not limited to infection, nerve injuries, and vascular injuries; these are relatively minor. The unique complications associated with capsular plications are recalcitrant pain, recurrent capsular laxity, and overt instability or dislocation. The last set of complications is related to thermal capsulorrhaphy and includes chondrolysis, capsular injury and degeneration, and higher failure rates.

## SUMMARY

Recently, a growing understanding of atraumatic instability and capsular laxity of the hip joint has evolved as an underappreciated cause of hip pain. The burgeoning field of hip arthroscopy and the application of advanced arthroscopic techniques have provided the ability to address hip instability in a minimally invasive fashion. Thermal capsular shrinkage is a described technique for the treatment of capsular laxity; however, as a result of the growing concern about its associated complications in shoulder surgery results, its use has generally fallen out of favor.

We present our techniques for arthroscopic capsular plication to address capsular laxity. Our techniques are similar and adapted from those used successfully to address glenohumeral instability. The advantages of these techniques are that they enable the surgeon to determine the amount of capsule to be plicated, they provide a durable construct that provides adequate stability until the capsule heals, and they avoid any of the potential complications associated with thermal procedures. The central compartment technique allows for capsular plication without violation of the peripheral compartment, whereas the peripheral compartment technique allows for plication in a traction-free environment while the iliofemoral ligament is not under tension. The disadvantages of arthroscopic capsular plication include a requirement of proficiency with advanced arthroscopic techniques, motion around the hip being protected until the capsule is fully healed, and the potential for recurrent capsular laxity and instability. Overall, this method of addressing capsular laxity is useful because it may be used for both traumatic and atraumatic conditions. It provides a relatively easy, predictable, and durable method for the plication of pathologic tissue.

## ANNOTATED REFERENCES

Arnoczky SP, Aksan A. Thermal modification of connective tissues: basic science considerations and clinical implications. *Instr Course Lect.* 2001;50:3–11.

Description of when and how much thermal energy as a stimulant for tissue shrinkage should be used in surgery.

Bellabarba C, Sheinkop MB, Kuo KN. Idiopathic hip instability. An unrecognized cause of coxa saltans in the adult. *Clin Orthop.* 1998;355:261–271.

Study of five patients with no prior history of trauma were evaluated, all of whom had long-standing painful snapping in the groin. Simple manual longitudinal traction under fluoroscopy showed subluxation with appearance of a vacuum sign in the symptomatic hip, whereas no such finding was observed on the asymptomatic side.

Braly BA, Beall DP, Martin HD. Clinical examination of the athletic hip. *Clin Sports Med.* 2006;25(2):199–210, vii.

This paper describes a succinct and complete method for the clinical evaluation of the athletic hip including descriptions of examination tests as well as their relationships to possible pathology of the hip.

Clarke MT, Arora A, Villar RN. Hip arthroscopy: complications in 1054 cases. *Clin Orthop Relat Res.* 2003;406:84–88.

This prospective study of 1054 consecutive hip arthroscopies reports an overall complication rate of 1.4%, which included neurapraxia, portal wound bleeding, portal hematoma, trochanteric bursitis, and instrument breakage.

Dall D, Macnab I, Gross A. Recurrent anterior dislocation of the hip. *J Bone Joint Surg Am.* 1970;52(3):574–576.

A case report of a recurrent traumatic anterior dislocation of the hip in an adult male.

Elkousy HA, Sekiya JK, Stabile KJ, McMahon PJ. A biomechanical comparison of arthroscopic sliding and sliding-locking knots. *Arthroscopy.* 2005;21(2):204–210.

This study provides a biomechanical basis for the clinical use of arthroscopic sliding and sliding-locking knots and the square knot, all used in open surgery. All knot configurations maintained high loop security. Additionally, this study confirms that all knots, even the sliding-locking Weston knot, are best backed up with 3 half-hitches alternating posts and directions of the throws.

Ferguson SJ, Bryant JT, Ganz R, Ito K. An in vitro investigation of the acetabular labral seal in hip joint mechanics. *J Biomech.* 2003;36(2):171–178.

A study confirming the hypothesis that the labrum seals the hip joint, creating a hydrostatic fluid pressure in the intra-articular space, and limiting the rate of cartilage layer consolidation.

Ferguson SJ, Bryant JT, Ganz R, Ito K. The influence of the acetabular labrum on hip joint cartilage consolidation: a poroelastic finite element model. *J Biomech.* 2000;33(8):953–960.

A study using a devised model to investigate the influence of the acetabular labrum on the consolidation, and hence the solid matrix strains and stresses, of the cartilage layers of the hip joint. The model demonstrated that the labrum adds an important resistance in the flow path of the fluid being expressed from the cartilage layers of the joint.

Good CR, Shindle MK, Kelly BT, Wanich T, Warren RF. Glenohumeral chondrolysis after shoulder arthroscopy with thermal capsulorrhaphy. *Arthroscopy.* 2007;23(7):797, e1–e5.

A retrospective review of eight patients in which glenohumeral chondrolysis developed after shoulder arthroscopy in which thermal energy was used. Open surgical stabilization has not been known to have this complication, and it is speculated that heating of the joint fluid at the time of arthroscopy from any source plays a role in cartilage death.

Hawkins RJ, Krishnan SG, Karas SG, Noonan TJ, Horan MP. Electrothermal arthroscopic shoulder capsulorrhaphy: a minimum 2-year follow-up. *Am J Sports Med.* 2007;35(9):1484–1488.

A Level IV case series following the first 100 patients with glenohumeral instability treated with thermal capsulorrhaphy. Because of the high failure rates, the authors now augment thermal capsulorrhaphy with capsule plication and/or rotator interval closure in cases of posterior and multidirectional instability and have lengthened the initial immobilization period to improve outcomes.

Hewitt JD, Glisson RR, Guilak F, Vail TP. The mechanical properties of the human hip capsule ligaments. *J Arthroplasty.* 2002;17(1):82–89.

A study discussing information about the mechanical properties of the ligaments that form the hip capsule. Cadaver bone–ligament–bone specimens of the iliofemoral, ischiofemoral, and femoral arcuate ligaments were tested to failure in tension. The hip capsule was found to be an inhomogeneous structure and should be recognized as being composed of discrete constituent ligaments.

Kelly BT, Williams RJ 3rd, Philippon MJ. Hip arthroscopy: current indications, treatment options, and management issues. *Am J Sports Med.* 2003;31(6):1020–1037.

This paper describes the current clinical and radiographic methods to detect early hip joint disease and the current indications and surgical techniques of hip arthroscopy.

Larson CM, Guanche CA, Kelly BT, Clohisy JC, Ranawat AS. Advanced techniques in hip arthroscopy. *Instr Course Lect.* 2009;58:423–436.

A review of hip instability and peritrochanteric disorders.

Leunig M, Siebenrock KA, Ganz R. Rationale of periacetabular osteotomy and background work. *Instr Course Lect.* 2001;50:229–238.

This paper discusses the rationale and descriptions of different hip osteotomy procedures including "Bernese periacetabular osteotomy."

Liebenberg F, Dommisse GF. Recurrent post-traumatic dislocation of the hip. *J Bone Joint Surg Br.* 1969;51(4):632–637.

Two cases of recurrent post-traumatic dislocation of the hip are reported followed by a literature review emphasizing the rarity of the condition. Facts from each case lead the authors to make some tentative deductions including a proposed capsular pressure mechanism as the cause of dislocation.

Lieberman JR, Altchek DW, Salvati EA. Recurrent dislocation of a hip with a labral lesion: treatment with a modified Bankart-type repair. Case report. *J Bone Joint Surg.* 1993;75A(10):1524–1527.

A case report of a 17-year-old girl who sustained a posterior fracture-dislocation of the right hip and a description of the specific technique used to repair it. This demonstrates the importance of the capsule and labrum in the stability of the hip.

Martin HD, Savage A, Braly BA, Palmer IJ, Beall DP, Kelly B. The function of the hip capsular ligaments: a quantitative report. *Arthroscopy.* 2008;24(2):188–195.

Twelve matched pairs of fresh-frozen cadaveric hips were measured in internal and external rotation through ranges of motion from 30 degrees flexion to 10 degrees extension along a neutral swing path to analyze the anatomy and quantitative contributions of the hip capsular ligaments. It concluded that the ischiofemoral ligament controls internal rotation in flexion and extension.

McKibbin B. Anatomical factors in the stability of the hip joint in the newborn. *J Bone Joint Surg Br.* 1970;52(1):148–159.

The findings detail the relationship between the orientation of the femoral neck's anteversion and anteversion of the acetabulum to create an instability index in dysplasia of the hip.

Mintz DN, Hooper T, Connell D, Buly R, Padgett DE, Potter HG. Magnetic resonance imaging of the hip: detection of labral and chondral abnormalities using noncontrast imaging. *Arthroscopy.* 2005;21(4):385–393.

A Level II retrospective review of patients showed that noncontrast MRI of hip using an optimized protocol can noninvasively identify labral and chondral pathology.

Moorman CT 3rd, Warren RF, Hershman EB, et al. Traumatic posterior hip subluxation in American football. *J Bone Joint Surg Am.* 2003;85-A(7):1190–1196.

This study outlines the injury mechanism, pathoanatomy, clinical and radiographic findings, and treatment of traumatic hip subluxation in an athletic population. The pathognomonic radiographic and magnetic resonance imaging triad of posterior acetabular hip fracture, iliofemoral ligament disruption, and hemarthrosis defines traumatic posterior hip subluxation. It also recommends hip aspiration for acute hemarthrosis.

Nelson CL. Traumatic recurrent dislocation of the hip. Report of a case. *J Bone Joint Surg.* 1970;52A(1):128–130.

A case report of traumatic recurrent dislocation of the hip is presented that details a method of repair.

Philippon MJ. Debridement of acetabular labral tears with associated thermal capsulorrhaphy. *Operative Techniques in Sports Medicine.* 2002;10(4):215–218.

This paper discusses the operative treatment of capsular laxity.

Philippon MJ. New frontiers in hip arthroscopy: the role of arthroscopic hip labral repair and capsulorrhaphy in the treatment of hip disorders. *Instr Course Lect.* 2006;55:309–316.

This article describes hip pain and its causes, specifically labral tears, in younger patients and how they contribute to hip instability as well as certain management techniques.

Philippon MJ. The role of arthroscopic thermal capsulorrhaphy in the hip. *Clin Sports Med.* 2001;20(4):817–829.

This article review traumatic and atraumatic reasons for hip instability as well as the anatomic features that are important in hip stability.

Philippon MJ, Schenker ML. Athletic hip injuries and capsular laxity. *Operative Techniques in Orthopaedics.* 2005;15(3):261–266.

This early paper discusses the diagnosis of capsular laxity.

Ranawat AS, McClincey M, Sekiya J. Anterior hip dislocation after hip arthroscopy in a patient with capsular laxity of the hip: a case report. *JBJS Am.* 2009;91(1):192–197.

The first report of a complication of anterior instability after hip arthroscopy but also the successful surgical management of this complication.

Sekiya JK. Arthroscopic labral repair and capsular shift of the glenohumeral joint: technical pearls for a multiple pleated plication through a single working portal. *Arthroscopy.* 2005;21(6):766.

The author presents a new arthroscopic technique for shoulder stabilization that makes use of already known techniques by sequentially repairing the labral tear and performing a capsular shift through multiple separate pleated plications through a single working portal.

Sherlock DA. Traumatic anterior dislocation of the hip. *J Trauma.* 1988;28(3):411–413.

A case report of traumatic anterior dislocation of the hip discussing reduction which was unstable because of disruption of the iliofemoral ligament by detachment of the anterior inferior iliac spine. A stable reduction was achieved by operative reattachment of the anterior inferior iliac spine.

Shindle MK, Ranawat AS, Kelly BT. Diagnosis and management of traumatic and atraumatic hip instability in the athletic patient. *Clin Sports Med.* 2006;25(2):309–326, ix-x.

This article reviews the spectrum of traumatic and atraumatic hip instability; discusses the relevant anatomy, history, and physical examination findings, imaging studies, and treatment options with a focus on hip arthroscopy; and reviews the literature.

Shindle MK, Voos JE, Heyworth BE, et al. Hip arthroscopy in the athletic patient: current techniques and spectrum of disease. *J Bone Joint Surg Am.* 2007;89-A(suppl 3):29–43.

A lengthy detailed review with the purpose of helping readers 1) have a basic understanding of the intra-articular and extraarticular hip disorders that commonly occur in athletes; 2) be able to generate a differential diagnosis for hip pain; 3) have a basic understanding of the relevant anatomy, patient history, and physical examination findings for an athlete who presents with hip pain; and 4) be able to identify normal and abnormal findings on radiographic and magnetic resonance imaging studies.

Tonnis D, Heinecke A. Acetabular and femoral anteversion: relationship with osteoarthritis of the hip. *J Bone Joint Surg Am.* 1999;81(12):1747–1770.

A review of hip conditions including impingement, anteversion, and torsional deformities. It describes normal and abnormal ranges of anteversion/deformities and finally addresses surgical treatment options for them.

# CHAPTER 16

# Arthroscopic Iliotibial Band Lengthening and Bursectomy for Recalcitrant Trochanteric Bursitis and Coxa Saltans Externa

*Champ L. Baker III and Champ L. Baker, Jr.*

## INTRODUCTION

Pain over the lateral aspect of the hip can be attributed to a number of conditions. The differential diagnosis includes degenerative joint disease of the hip, avascular necrosis of the femoral head, stress fracture of the femoral neck, infection, entrapment neuropathies, referred pain from lumbar disc disease, sciatica, snapping hip, and trochanteric bursitis. Trochanteric bursitis is a very common condition that is treated by both orthopedic surgeons and general practitioners and can be a source of disabling lateral hip pain. A dull, intermittent, aching pain in the region of the greater trochanter characterizes the condition. Occasionally, the pain radiates to the lateral thigh or the buttocks. The condition is thought to be a result of repetitive microtrauma and friction between the iliotibial band (ITB) and the greater trochanter, with subsequent inflammation of the interposed bursa. Degeneration of the gluteal tendons at the trochanteric attachment can also occur.

Some patients present with complaints of pain and an audible snapping sensation near the lateral aspect of the hip. External snapping hip or *coxa saltans* is caused by a tight ITB sliding over the greater trochanter with repetitive flexion and extension of the hip. The condition must be differentiated from an internal snapping hip, which is commonly attributed to the sliding of the iliopsoas tendon over the femoral head or the iliopectineal eminence, and from intra-articular causes of snapping hip, such as loose bodies, labral tears, and synovial chondromatosis. Asymptomatic external coxa saltans does not require treatment, but occasionally patients develop associated trochanteric bursitis with resultant pain and disability.

Most patients with trochanteric bursitis respond to nonoperative treatment that typically consists of activity modification, nonsteroidal anti-inflammatory medications, the stretching of a tight ITB, physical therapy with modalities (e.g., heat, ultrasound), and local injections of corticosteroids and anesthetics directly into the bursa. For the small group of patients whose symptoms fail to resolve with nonoperative therapy, the excision of the trochanteric bursa is recommended. Historically, this procedure has been performed with the use of an open approach; however, several authors have recently reported similar success when performing the bursectomy arthroscopically. In patients who have a tight ITB and associated external snapping hip, an ITB lengthening should be performed concurrently with the bursectomy.

## HISTORY

Patients with trochanteric bursitis are typically middle aged, although the condition can also be seen in younger athletes, most often in young runners. The incidence is higher among females. The pain is characteristically located directly over the greater trochanter, with occasional radiation to the lateral thigh and buttocks. A select number of individuals may report a history of traumatic onset, but it is more commonly associated with repetitive microtrauma. Patients often complain of being unable to lie on the affected side because of the direct painful compression of the bursa. As a result of the sensation of the ITB sliding over the greater trochanter (which is often audible) with repeated hip flexion and extension, individuals with concurrent external snapping hip often state that they can dislocate the hip.

## PHYSICAL EXAMINATION

Tenderness to palpation over the greater trochanter is invariably present. Pain elicited with deep palpation over the greater trochanter when the affected hip is up and adducted with the patient in the lateral decubitus position is known as the *Little sign*. Pain is commonly elicited with active abduction and passive adduction of the hip. Patients may demonstrate a positive Ober test because of increased tension in the ITB. A response to a local injection in the bursa can be diagnostic as well as therapeutic. Individuals with an associated snapping ITB can often reproduce the snapping in the office, such as that which occurs with a running motion. Hip flexion flips the thickened posterior portion of the ITB anteriorly over the greater trochanter, and hip extension brings the affected ITB posteriorly over the trochanter; these movements are accompanied by an audible, palpable snapping sensation.

## IMAGING AND DIAGNOSTIC STUDIES

The diagnosis of trochanteric bursitis is a clinical one. Plain radiographs of the hip and pelvis are primarily used to rule out other disorders, but they may also reveal calcifications around the greater trochanter in 20% to 40% of patients. Coxa vara has been reported to be a predisposing anatomic factor among patients with external snapping hip. Although magnetic resonance imaging of the hip is not necessary for the diagnosis, it can show bursal inflammation and increased signal in the tendinous attachments to the greater trochanter. Plain radiographs and magnetic resonance imaging are useful primarily as exclusionary tools.

## INDICATIONS

Operative intervention is indicated for the following patients:
- Patients who exhibit a lack of response to an extended course (i.e., more than 6 months) of nonoperative therapy that consists of activity modification, physical therapy, nonsteroidal anti-inflammatory medications, and local injections of corticosteroids and anesthetics
- Patients who have a diagnosis confirmed by a good pain relief response to an anesthetic injection into the trochanteric bursa

## SURGICAL TECHNIQUE

Our preferred surgical technique for recalcitrant trochanteric bursitis is an arthroscopic trochanteric bursectomy. Patients are positioned in the lateral decubitus position with the affected extremity facing up. A deflatable beanbag is used to stabilize the patient, and all bony prominences are well padded. The leg is draped freely so that the hip can be taken through a full range of motion (Figure 16-1). The greater trochanter is palpated and outlined on the skin with a marker. A spinal needle is then inserted directly onto the trochanteric prominence. The needle is then withdrawn slightly by several millimeters, and approximately 30 mL to 40 mL of normal saline is injected into the bursa, thus creating a space underneath the ITB. We prefer to leave the needle in for the purpose of localization. Next, a proximal portal is created 2 cm to 3 cm proximal to the trochanter, and a distal portal is created 2 cm to 3 cm distal to the trochanter. The skin is incised in line with the long axis of the femur. A 4-mm, 30-degree arthroscope is introduced directly into the subcutaneous tissues above the ITB. A 4.5-mm shaver is placed in the other portal and localized to the arthroscope with a triangulation technique (Figure 16-2). The fat directly above the ITB is removed to allow for full visualization of the ITB (Figure 16-3). An arthroscopic ablation probe can also be used to maintain hemostasis and concurrently to remove adherent tissues.

After the ITB is clearly identified, the arthroscopic ablator is used to create a longitudinal incision approximately 7 cm to 8 cm in length in line with the fibers of the ITB just slightly posterior to its midline and the trochanteric prominence; this exposes the trochanteric bursa (Figure 16-4). The surgical assistant abducts the leg to further relax the incised ITB (Figure 16-5) and to allow

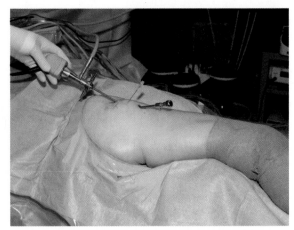

**Figure 16–2** The 4-mm, 30-degree arthroscope and 4.5-mm, full-radius shaver are inserted into the proximal and distal portals, respectively, in the subcutaneous tissues overlying the iliotibial band.

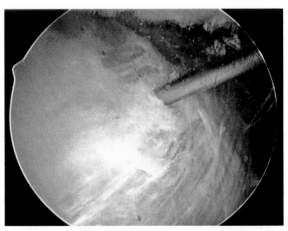

**Figure 16–3** The fat overlying the ITB is removed to allow for the visualization of the iliotibial band. The localizing needle is seen at the top of the photograph.

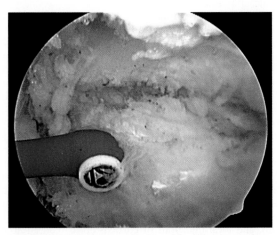

**Figure 16–4** To gain access to the bursa, the ablator is used to create a longitudinal incision in the iliotibial band just slightly posterior to the midline.

the surgeon to advance the arthroscope and instruments underneath the ITB. Next, the shaver and the ablator are used to thoroughly debride the bursa and its thick, fibrous adhesions. Having the assistant slowly internally and externally rotate the leg brings the posterior and anterior portions of the bursa, respectively, into

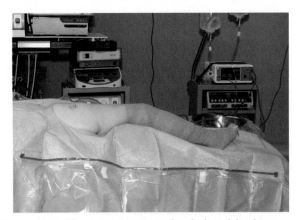

**Figure 16–1** The patient is positioned in the lateral decubitus position, with the entire hip and leg draped free.

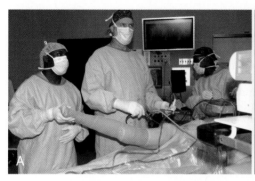

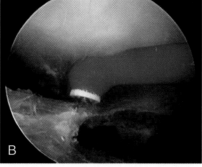

**Figure 16–5 A,** The assistant abducts the leg to relax the iliotibial band. **B,** With the use of the ablator, the surgeon debrides the bursa and its dense adhesions.

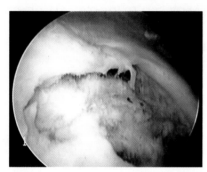

**Figure 16–6** A tear of the tendinous insertion of the abductor muscle.

view. Extreme internal rotation is avoided, because this maneuver places the posteriorly located sciatic nerve at risk. Coagulation is frequently necessary to maintain hemostasis and visualization.

After the bursa has been completely excised, the tendinous attachments of the gluteus minimus and the gluteus medius to the greater trochanter can be seen. Occasionally, irritation and scuffing of the tendinous insertions are noted, and, infrequently, tears and avulsions of the tendons (so-called *rotator cuff tears* of the hip) are present (Figure 16-6). Early in our experience, we treated the tears with gentle debridement, but, more recently, we have repaired these tears with nonabsorbable sutures with the use of a technique that is similar to the marginal convergence repair technique used for rotator cuff tears in the shoulder. After bursal excision has been completed and hemostasis is ensured, the instruments are withdrawn, and excess fluid is expressed from the portals. The portals are then closed with nylon suture, and a compression dressing and ice pack are applied.

In patients with associated external coxa saltans, an ITB lengthening procedure is necessary in addition to the standard trochanteric bursectomy. After the usual slightly posterior longitudinal incision is made in the ITB, the arthroscopic ablator is used to gently resect its anterior and posterior edges. Additional tissue is removed near the center of the midline cut to create an elliptical

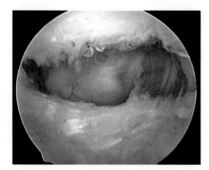

**Figure 16–7** An elliptical resection of the iliotibial band has been performed for the correction of external coxa saltans.

resection of the ITB (Figure 16-7). The posterior resection is slightly greater than the anterior resection, because the snapping usually results from the thickened posterior portion of the ITB flipping over the greater trochanter. An alternative method is to perform a crisscross secondary transverse incision, thereby effectively creating a cruciate-type release. The hip is taken through a range of motion to ensure adequate decompression and resection. The bursa is then resected as previously described.

## TECHNICAL PEARLS

- Sterilely prepare and drape the entire leg on the affected side to allow the assistant to freely abduct and rotate the hip. It is helpful to abduct the leg 20 degrees to 30 degrees before the horizontal split is made in the ITB to ensure that the split is not so far posterior that it makes it difficult to enter the bursa properly.
- The use of the ablator and the radiofrequency probe is extremely helpful to control bleeding, thereby allowing for a more complete and technically easier bursectomy. The 18-gauge needle should be left in place for orientation. It can be centered over the bony prominence of the tuberosity.
- If concomitant hip arthroscopy is performed, there are two choices for the bursectomy. If the hip arthroscopy is performed with the patient supine, then the bursectomy can be performed with the patient in the lateral decubitus position before turning the patient supine. The other alternative is to perform the entire procedure with the patient in the supine position, if that is the surgeon's preference; the bursa can then be addressed after the hip is evaluated. Alternatively, the entire procedure can be performed with the patient in the lateral decubitus position, if that is the surgeon's preference for the hip arthroscopy.
- After the endoscopic procedure is completed and excess fluid is expressed, a local anesthetic can be injected into the portal to help with postoperative pain relief. A compressive wrap with a cooling pad should be added to control edema.

## POSTOPERATIVE REHABILITATION

All of these surgeries are performed on an outpatient basis. Patients are allowed to be weight bearing as tolerated with the assistance of crutches or a walker. The first postoperative visit is at 48 to 72 hours after surgery. If patients exhibit an independent gait at that time, the assistive devices are discontinued. Sutures are removed 2 to 5 days after surgery, and the wounds are checked for excessive bleeding or swelling. Physical therapy is then begun to strengthen the hip musculature and to ensure the restoration of the full range of motion.

Because trochanteric bursitis can be caused by an abnormal gait, weakness of the hip flexors, or chronic low back pain, emphasis should be placed on correcting the cause of the problem. After the immediate postoperative regimen has been completed, attention should be focused on increasing the flexibility of the lumbar spine and correcting any weakness of the hip abductors.

## RESULTS AND OUTCOMES

In general, both open and arthroscopic treatments of trochanteric bursitis result in a high percentage of good outcomes (Table 16-1). Physicians agree that, in the majority of patients with this condition, a conservative approach will be successful; only a select few patients will require operative intervention. For a successful result in patients with external coxa saltans, the ITB should be effectively lengthened by one of several open or arthroscopic methods, such as a Z-plasty, an ellipsoidal-shaped or diamond-shaped resection, a cruciate or cross-shaped incision, or a simple longitudinal release.

## COMPLICATIONS

In the senior author's published series of 25 patients with refractory trochanteric bursitis who were treated with arthroscopic bursectomy and longitudinal ITB release, 1 patient developed a seroma that required an operative incision and drainage, and 1 patient continued to have postoperative pain and was treated with an open bursectomy that resulted in the successful resolution of symptoms. The most frequently reported complication in the literature has been the incomplete relief of symptoms after operative intervention. This can be minimized with an accurate preoperative diagnosis, a thorough bursectomy, and a

**Table 16-1** OUTCOMES OF THE TREATMENT OF TROCHANTERIC BURSITIS AND EXTERNAL SNAPPING HIP

| Author | Number of Patients (Hips) | Procedure | Length of Follow Up (Range) | Outcomes |
|---|---|---|---|---|
| **Arthroscopic Treatment of Trochanteric Bursitis** | | | | |
| Baker et al., 2007 | 25 (25) | Arthroscopic bursectomy with longitudinal release of ITB | 26 months (13.8 to 41 months) | Significant improvements in pain on VAS, mean Harris Hip Score, and SF-36 scores; 1 open revision required |
| Bradley and Dillingham, 1998 | 1 (2) | Arthroscopic bursectomy | 7 months | Able to return to collegiate basketball |
| Farr et al., 2007 | 2 (2) | Arthroscopic bursectomy with longitudinal release of ITB | 41 months (32 to 50 months) | Resumption of pain-free activities without recurrences |
| Fox, 2002 | 17 (27) | Arthroscopic bursectomy | 12-month minimum | 23 of 27: good to excellent results; 26 of 27: satisfied |
| **Open Treatment of Trochanteric Bursitis** | | | | |
| Brooker, 1979 | 5 (5) | Open bursectomy with trochanteric debridement and cruciate release of ITB | 12-month minimum | All patients satisfied with pain relief; mean Harris Hip Score improved from 46 to 88 |
| Govaert et al., 2003 | 10 (12) | Open trochanteric reduction osteotomy | 23.5 months (6 to 77 months) | Mean Merle d'Aubigné and Postel scores improved from 15.8 to 27.5 |
| Slawski and Howard, 1997 | 5 (7) | Open bursectomy with longitudinal release of ITB | 20 months (12 to 30 months) | Mean Harris Hip Score improved from 51.7 to 95; all patients satisfied |
| **Open Treatment of External Snapping Hip** | | | | |
| Brignall and Stainsby, 1991 | 6 (8) | Open Z-plasty lengthening of ITB | 3 years (1 to 8 years) | Relief of snapping and pain in all hips; 1 revision required |
| Larsen and Johansen, 1986 | 24 (31) | 27: resection of the posterior half of the ITB; 4: suturing of a posterior flap of the ITB to the anterolateral fascia | 4 years | 71% symptom free; 19% snapping, no pain; 10% residual snapping or pain; 2 revisions required |
| Provencher et al., 2004 | 8 (9) | Open Z-plasty lengthening of ITB | 23 months (7 to 38 months) | All patients had relief of snapping; 8 of 9 returned to full, unrestricted activity level |
| White et al., 2004 | 15 (16) | Open longitudinal incision of ITB with alternating step cuts for lengthening | 32.5 months (9 to 74 months) | 88% had complete relief of snapping and pain; 2 revisions required; all patients contacted were satisfied |
| Zoltan et al., 1986 | 7 (7) | Open ellipsoid resection of ITB and bursectomy | 55 months (12 to 76 months) | All athletes returned to sports participation; 1 revision required |
| **Arthroscopic Treatment of External Snapping Hip** | | | | |
| Ilizaliturri et al., 2006 | 10 (11) | Arthroscopic bursectomy and diamond-shaped resection of ITB | 2 years (1 to 3 years) | 100% resolution of pain; 91% resolution of snapping; mean WOMAC score improved from 81 to 94 |

*ITB*, Iliotibial band; *VAS*, visual analog scale; *WOMAC*, Western Ontario and McMaster Universities osteoarthritis index.

candid discussion with the patient regarding realistic expectations. The majority of patients have preexisting altered lower limb biomechanics and comorbidities that may preclude complete relief. In the patient with external coxa saltans, pain and snapping are typically relieved with lengthening of the ITB and bursectomy. Residual painless snapping is not uncommon and requires no further operative treatment.

## ANNOTATED REFERENCES

**Baker CL Jr, Massie RV, Hurt WG, et al. Arthroscopic bursectomy for recalcitrant trochanteric bursitis. *Arthroscopy*. 2007;23:827–832.**

Twenty-five patients were reviewed at a mean of 26 months after undergoing arthroscopic bursectomy. There were significant improvements in mean Harris Hip Scores (51 to 77), mean Visual Analog Scale (VAS) scores for pain (7.2 to 3.1), mean physical function scores on the Short Form 36 (SF-36) (33.6 to 54), and mean pain scores on the SF-36 (28.7 to 51.5). One patient developed a seroma that required repeat surgery, and another patient required open revision bursectomy for relief.

**Bradley DM, Dillingham MF. Bursoscopy of the trochanteric bursa. *Arthroscopy*. 1998;14:884–887.**

This article is a case report of a Division I male basketball player with bilateral trochanteric bursitis who was treated successfully with bursoscopy and bursectomy.

**Brignall CG, Stainsby GD. The snapping hip: treatment by Z-plasty. *J Bone Joint Surg Br*. 1991;73:253–254.**

Six patients (8 hips) with external coxa saltans were treated with an open Z-plasty lengthening of the ITB. One hip required revision lengthening, and snapping was relieved in all patients at a mean length of follow-up of 3 years.

**Brooker AF Jr. The surgical approach to refractory trochanteric bursitis. *Johns Hopkins Med J*. 1979;145:98–100.**

Five patients underwent open excision of the bursa, debridement of the greater trochanteric prominence, and ITB release. A circular defect was created for 1 patient's release, and a cruciate incision in the ITB was performed for the remaining 4 patients. All of the patients had satisfactory pain relief at a minimum follow-up of 1 year.

**Farr D, Selesnick H, Janecki C, et al. Arthroscopic bursectomy with concomitant iliotibial band release for the treatment of recalcitrant trochanteric bursitis. *Arthroscopy*. 2007;23:905 e1–5. Epub 2007 Jan 25.**

Two patients were treated with arthroscopic resection of the trochanteric bursa in combination with a longitudinal release of the ITB with the use of an electrocautery probe. At an average of 41 months of follow-up, there were no recurrences with the resumption of the full activity level.

**Fox JL. The role of arthroscopic bursectomy in the treatment of trochanteric bursitis. *Arthroscopy*. 2002;18:E34.**

Twenty-seven patients underwent arthroscopic bursectomy, with good to excellent results obtained in 23 of the patients. At 5 years of follow-up, there were three recurrences. No treatment was directed at the ITB.

**Gordon EJ. Trochanteric bursitis and tendinitis. *Clin Orthop*. 1961;20:193–202.**

The signs and symptoms of a group of 61 patients with trochanteric bursitis are presented. The author details the method and success of conservative treatment. The diagnosis and correction of associated disorders are emphasized.

**Govaert LH, van der Vis HM, Marti RK, et al. Trochanteric reduction osteotomy as a treatment for refractory trochanteric bursitis. *J Bone Joint Surg Br*. 2003;85:199–203.**

Ten patients (12 hips) with refractory trochanteric bursitis had a 5-mm to 10-mm-thick slice of the greater trochanter removed, with the remaining trochanter advanced and fixed distally and medially. The authors concluded that the procedure is safe and effective with good pain relief at a mean of 23.5 months after surgery.

**Ilizaliturri VM Jr, Martinez-Escalante FA, Chaidez PA, et al. Endoscopic iliotibial band release for external snapping hip syndrome. *Arthroscopy*. 2006;22:505–510.**

Ten patients (11 hips) with external coxa saltans underwent endoscopic trochanteric bursectomy and resection of a diamond-shaped portion of the ITB, and they were evaluated at an average follow-up of 2 years. Pain was relieved in 100% of hips, and snapping was relieved in 91% of hips.

**Kagan A II. Rotator cuff tears of the hip. *Clin Orthop Relat Res*. 1999;368:135–140.**

The author reports about seven patients who were found during surgery for trochanteric bursitis to have partial tears of the gluteus medius tendon attachment to the trochanter. All of these tears were repaired with heavy nonabsorbable suture. At a mean follow-up of 45 months, all patients were free of pain.

**Larsen E, Johansen J. Snapping hip. *Acta Orthop Scand*. 1986;57:168–170.**

In 31 patients (31 hips) with external snapping hip, 27 underwent the resection of the posterior half of the ITB and 4 underwent the suturing of a posterior flap of the iliotibial tract to the anterolateral fascia. At an average follow-up time of 4 years, 71% of patients (22 hips) were symptom free. The femoral neck angle was significantly decreased in affected patients as compared with healthy controls (128 degrees versus 134 degrees).

**Provencher MT, Hofmeister MP, Muldoon MP. The surgical treatment of external coxa saltans (the snapping hip) by Z-plasty of the iliotibial band. *Am J Sports Med*. 2004;32:470–476.**

Nine patients with symptomatic hips with external coxa saltans were treated with an open Z-plasty lengthening of the ITB. At an average follow-up of 23 months, all patients had complete resolution of snapping symptoms, and all but 1 patient returned to a full activity level. The authors felt that this technique provided predictable, excellent results.

**Slawski DP, Howard RF. Surgical management of refractory trochanteric bursitis. *Am J Sports Med*. 1997;25:86–89.**

Five patients (7 hips) underwent open trochanteric bursectomy via a longitudinal incision in the ITB. All patients reported marked improvement postoperatively with a return to all activities. Occasional discomfort was noted after athletic activity in the majority of hips.

**White RA, Hughes MS, Burd T, et al. A new operative approach in the correction of external coxa saltans: the snapping hip. *Am J Sports Med*. 2004;32:1504–1508.**

Sixteen patients (17 hips) with external snapping hip underwent open ITB release with a longitudinal incision and alternating transverse step cuts. Fourteen of the 16 hips (88%) evaluated during follow-up had resolution of pain and snapping. Two patients required revision release at 3 and 6 months after the initial surgery.

**Zoltan DJ, Clancy Jr WG, Keene JS. A new operative approach to snapping hip and refractory trochanteric bursitis in athletes. *Am J Sports Med*. 1986;14:201–204.**

Seven athletes with external coxa saltans and associated greater trochanteric bursitis were treated with an open ellipsoidal excision of the ITB and the removal of the trochanteric bursa. The procedure was performed under local anesthesia to allow for the dynamic assessment of elimination of snapping. At a mean follow-up of 55 months, all patients had returned to sports activities, although one had required a more extensive revision resection for relief.

# CHAPTER 17

# Arthroscopic Hip "Rotator Cuff Repair" of Gluteus Medius Tendon Avulsions

*James E. Voos, Travis Maak, and Bryan T. Kelly*

## INTRODUCTION

Advances in hip arthroscopy have increased the understanding of both intra-articular and extra-articular hip pathology. The anatomic and surgical techniques involved in hip arthroscopy have been described. Increasing enthusiasm for hip arthroscopy and minimally invasive surgery in addition to advances in magnetic resonance imaging of the hip have broadened arthroscopic application. Intra-articular pathologies—including loose bodies, labral tears, ligamentum teres tears, chondral lesions, synovial chondromatosis and femoroacetabular impingement—have now been arthroscopically treated.

Hip arthroscopy has recently been expanded to allow for the visualization and treatment of extra-articular pathology, specifically in the peritrochanteric compartment. Disorders in this compartment include external coxa saltans or snapping hip, trochanteric bursitis, and gluteus medius and gluteus minimus tears (Tables 17-1, 17-2, and 17-3). These pathologies, which were underappreciated before hip arthroscopy, have now been identified as significant causes of lateral hip pain. The previous treatment of these disorders with conservative modalities or open surgery has had varied efficacy, and it has been associated with significant postoperative morbidity. Conservative treatment is often the preferred treatment modality and includes corticosteroid and anesthetic injections in combination with a structured physical therapy regimen. Patients for whom conservative treatment is ineffective have previously required open surgery.

## INDICATIONS

- External coxa saltans
  - Generally asymptomatic or can be treated conservatively with rest, activity modification, stretching, corticosteroid injections, and physical therapy
  - Recalcitrant cases as defined by unabated symptoms may be addressed with either open or arthroscopic treatment
- Trochanteric bursitis
  - Conservative treatment with local corticosteroid and anesthetic preparation injections in combination with physical therapy as the mainstay of diagnosis and treatment
  - Refractory cases treated with open and arthroscopic trochanteric bursectomy
- Gluteus medius and minimus tears

  - Present as refractory trochanteric bursitis or iliotibial band syndrome with lateral hip pain and an ambulatory limp likely related to hip abductor weakness
  - Treatment described in an open and arthroscopic fashion when conservative treatment has failed

## BRIEF HISTORY AND PHYSICAL EXAMINATION

An in-depth patient history is one of the most effective tools for evaluating a complaint of hip pain. A historic description of hip pain can differentiate intra-articular versus extra-articular pathology. Extra-articular complaints can then be localized to lateral hip pain in the peritrochanteric compartment. When a description of extra-articular lateral hip pain is achieved, the diagnostic differential can be narrowed with descriptive characteristics specific to each peritrochanteric space disorder. External coxa saltans, or "snapping hip," is characterized by a palpable or audible snapping as the hip moves from flexion to extension; this is often seen during athletic activity. Trochanteric bursitis and greater trochanteric pain syndrome are characterized by chronic intermittent aching pain over the lateral aspect of the hip; these conditions are prevalent among older females. Gluteus medius and gluteus minimus tears often produce symptoms that are similar to those of trochanteric bursitis but on a shorter time line.

Lateral hip pain can arise from direct pain from the peritrochanteric space or from referred pain from intra-articular pathology. Palpation of the lateral hip aids in the differential diagnosis, because referred pain may be reproduced with passive and active joint motion but should not produce tenderness with direct palpation. In this vein, palpation should begin with the origin of the gluteus maximus at the inferoposterior aspect of the ileum and sacrum. The insertion can then be examined in two locations: the lateral base of the linea aspera on the proximal femur and the tensor fascia latae. Next, the gluteus medius should be palpated from its origin on the anterior and middle aspect of the ileum to its two insertions on the middle and superoposterior facets of the greater trochanter. The gluteus minimus can be examined from its origin deep to the gluteus medius to its insertion at the greater trochanter anterior facet. The greater trochanteric bursa should also be appreciated overlying the greater trochanter at the mid-posterior proximal aspect of the femur. The physical examination of muscle strength can be used to evaluate abductor strength in the presence or absence of pain. This examination should be conducted with the hip in flexion to assess the tensor fascia latae, in neutral to evaluate the gluteus medius, and

### Table 17-1 EXTERNAL COXA SALTANS

|  | Treatment | Response |
|---|---|---|
| Conservative | Rest, activity modification, stretching, corticosteroid injection, physical therapy | Varied |
| Open | Excision of ellipsoid portion of iliotibial band and trochanteric bursa | 80% improvement or full symptomatic relief |
| Arthroscopic | Transverse step cuts in the fascia and one longitudinal fascial incision | 88% with full symptomatic relief |
|  | Iliotibial band release (Z-plasty) | 95% full symptomatic relief |

### Table 17-2 TROCHANTERIC BURSITIS

|  | Treatment | Response |
|---|---|---|
| Conservative | Local corticosteroid and anesthetic injection with physical therapy | 66% excellent response and 33% improved symptoms |
| Open | Trochanteric reduction osteotomy | 50% excellent, 42% great, 8% fair improvement |
| Arthroscopic | Endoscopic bursectomy | Significant improvement in Harris Hip Score, visual analog scale results, and SF-36 score |

### Table 17-3 GLUTEUS MEDIUS AND MINIMUS TEARS

|  | Treatment | Response |
|---|---|---|
| Conservative | Local corticosteroid and anesthetic injection with physical therapy | Up to 90% pain relief |
| Open | Tendon repair | No clinical data |
| Arthroscopic | Debridement of calcification and degenerated tendon | 100% asymptomatic |
|  | Tendon repair | 100% asymptomatic; 9 out of 10, full strength recovery |

## IMAGING AND DIAGNOSTIC STUDIES

All patients who present with hip pain are evaluated with an anteroposterior radiograph of the pelvis as well as a Dunn lateral radiograph (90 degrees of hip flexion, 20 degrees of abduction, and the beam centered on and perpendicular to the hip) to assess for avulsions of the greater trochanter, cam and pincer lesions, loss of joint space, crossover sign, acetabular dysplasia, and sacroiliac joint pathology. Magnetic resonance imaging provides the most information about the soft tissues that surround the hip (Figure 17-1). Every magnetic resonance imaging study of the hip should include a screening examination of the whole pelvis that is acquired with use of coronal inversion recovery and axial proton-density sequences. Detailed hip imaging is obtained with use of a surface coil over the hip joint, with high-resolution, cartilage-sensitive images acquired in three planes (sagittal, coronal, and oblique axial) with use of a fast-spin-echo pulse sequence and an intermediate echo time. Other alternatives include the use of magnetic resonance arthrography of the hip for the evaluation of hip pathology. Ultrasound is used most commonly to confirm the placement of injections into the trochanteric space for diagnostic and therapeutic purposes. Dynamic ultrasound has also been described to evaluate external coxa saltans; it provides real-time images of the sudden abnormal displacement of the iliotibial band or the gluteus maximus muscle overlying the greater trochanter as a painful snap during hip motion. In addition, sonography can identify gluteus medius and gluteus minimus tendinopathy and provide information about the severity of the disease.

## SURGICAL TECHNIQUE

The importance of proper portal placement is critical during hip arthroscopy. For arthroscopy of the peritrochanteric space, a technique has been described that involves the use of both traditional and unique portals (Figure 17-2). The technique

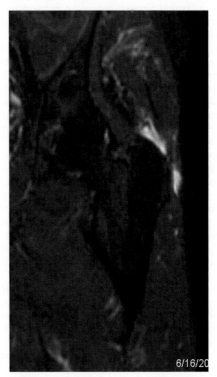

**Figure 17-1** Magnetic resonance image of the left hip that reveals increased signal at the greater trochanter; this is consistent with a tear of the gluteus medius tendon.

in extension for the gluteus maximus. This examination should be performed with the knee both flexed and extended to allow for the tension and relaxation of the iliotibial band, respectively. External coxa saltans can be replicated with audible or palpable snapping during physical examination. Gluteus medius and gluteus minimus tears often present with pain along the lateral aspect of the greater trochanter and may mimic trochanteric bursitis.

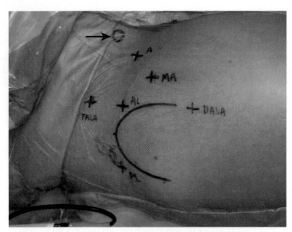

**Figure 17–2** Intraoperative photograph of the right hip anterolateral *(AL)*, mid-anterior *(MA)*, distal anterolateral accessory *(DALA)*, posterolateral *(PL)*, and proximal anterolateral accessory *(PALA)* portals for entry into the peritrochanteric space. The anterosuperior iliac spine is denoted by the arrow.

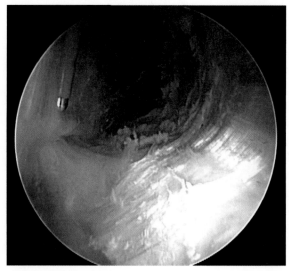

**Figure 17–3** Arthroscopic image of the attachment of the gluteus maximus tendon to the linea aspera. This is the starting point to gain orientation in the peritrochanteric space and to begin a systematic evaluation of the compartment. *(From Shindle MK, Voos JE, Heyworth BE, et al. Hip arthroscopy in the athletic patient: current techniques and spectrum of disease. J Bone Joint Surg Am. 2007;89 Suppl 3:29–43.)*

begins with the accurate identification of the trochanter and the marking of the arthroscopic portals. The procedure begins with routine central compartment hip arthroscopy to rule out associated intra-articular pathologies. Although intra-articular pathologies typically result in primary anterior or groin symptoms, it is also possible for these pathologies to result in primary lateral-sided hip pain. Central compartment arthroscopy is performed in all cases of peritrochanteric space endoscopy to document and treat any associated labral or chondral pathology that may coexist with the lateral-based pathology. The anterolateral portal is first established with the use of the standard Seldinger technique of a cannulated trochar over a guidewire, which is performed with the aid of fluoroscopy. To minimize trauma to the lateral femoral cutaneous nerve, a mid-anterior portal is then established. This portal is made slightly more lateral and distal than the traditional anterior portal. The portal is critical to get into the peritrochanteric space, because it is the initial primary viewing portal. Thus, fluoroscopy is used to assist with the optimal placement of the mid-anterior portal over the lateral prominence of the greater trochanter. Before entry into the peritrochanteric space and after the completion of the central compartment evaluation, the peripheral compartment should be entered if there is any concern about peripheral compartment pathology.

Diagnostic arthroscopy of the peritrochanteric space begins with a blunt trochar placed in the mid-anterior portal, which is then used to swipe between the iliotibial band and the vastus ridge in a controlled manner that is similar to that performed in the subacromial space in the shoulder. The trochar is aimed directly for the lateral prominence of the greater trochanter; this is the safest starting position for blunt trochar placement. If the trochar is placed too proximally initially, violation of the gluteus medius musculature may occur; if it is placed too distally, the trochar may disrupt the fibers of the vastus lateralis. The use of fluoroscopy helps to precisely identify the starting position to avoid iatrogenic injury to the surrounding soft tissue. Unlike the central compartment, in the peritrochanteric space, traction is not necessary. At times, however, minimal traction is used to maintain tension on the abductors.

After the space has been defined, a 70-degree scope is placed in the mid-anterior portal. The camera is oriented so that both the light source and the camera base are pointed distally. Such an orientation places both the tail of the 70-degree scope and the light source on the proximal portion of the patient, with visualization directed distally.

The first structure to be visualized is the gluteus maximus tendon inserting on the femur just below the vastus lateralis (Figure 17-3). This structure is a reproducible landmark that provides good orientation within the space. It is typically unnecessary to work distal to the gluteus maximus tendon, and one should avoid exploration posterior to the tendon, because the sciatic nerve lies within close proximity (i.e., 2 cm to 4 cm). The camera light source is then directed to the lateral aspect of the femur, where the longitudinal fibers of the vastus lateralis can be visualized and followed proximally to the vastus ridge. The insertion and muscle belly of the gluteus medius are located proximal to this, whereas the gluteus minimus is located more anteriorly and is mostly covered. Finally, the iliotibial band is identified with the camera looking proximally and laterally.

## Trochanteric Bursectomy

After a diagnostic arthroscopy is performed, a spinal needle is placed under direct arthroscopic visualization 4 cm to 5 cm distal to the anterolateral portal. This portal is the distal anterolateral accessory portal, which is roughly in line with the anterolateral portal.

An arthroscopic shaver is then placed in the distal anterolateral accessory portal, and a thorough trochanteric bursectomy is performed over the distal portion of the space. Initially, distended bursal tissue and fibrinous bands are cleared off of the gluteus maximus tendinous insertion distally. The bursectomy is then performed from distal to proximal. An additional portal can be made 2 cm to 3 cm proximal to the anterolateral portal (i.e., the proximal anterolateral accessory portal) to access the most proximal portions of the inflamed bursal tissue. This portal can also be used as a viewing portal to obtain a more complete perspective on the underlying pathology.

## Iliotibial Band Release and Lengthening

After a thorough bursectomy has been performed, attention is turned to the iliotibial band. The pathologic entity is the thickened posterior third of the iliotibial band, which, with flexion, snaps over the trochanter. A "kissing lesion" can often be seen on the lateral prominence of the trochanter, where a bruised or erythematous zone of injury corresponds with the site of impact. With the 70-degree scope in the mid-anterior portal, the proximal anterolateral accessory portal is made under direct visualization. A beaver blade is then placed in this portal, and a controlled transverse or cruciate-style lengthening is performed. When this is performed within the peritrochanteric space, it is fairly easy to confirm adequate release, because the direct visualization of the region of injury on the trochanter is possible.

### Gluteus Medius Repair

If there is evidence of significant gluteus medius pathology, an arthroscopic repair is performed (Figure 17-4). Occasionally, gentle distraction of the hip is needed to place the gluteus medius muscle fibers on tension to more clearly delineate proximal bursal tissue from gluteus medius muscle fibers. The 70-degree arthroscope is then placed in the proximal anterolateral accessory portal to get a more global view of the abductors, whereas the working instruments can be placed in the mid-anterior and distal anterolateral accessory portals.

Most commonly, the medius is degenerated and torn off of its distal insertion onto the lateral facet of the trochanter with proximal extension. Often the tear is predominantly an undersurface tear that is analogous to an articular-sided rotator cuff tear, which then extends posteriorly to become a full-thickness tear. Close scrutiny of the magnetic resonance images is critical to correlate intraoperative findings with the preoperative imaging. Sometimes the initial intraoperative finding is the significant thinning of the tendon insertion, which requires the completion of the tear with facet bone preparation and subsequent reattachment.

The technique for fixing these tears is quite similar to that of repairing rotator cuff tears. First, a probe or grasper is used to manually reduce the tear to its anatomic position in the footprint. With a burr, the lateral facet is burred to a bleeding edge of bone in a similar fashion as is done to the greater tuberosity during a rotator cuff repair. A spinal needle is placed to find the proper angle for anchor placement, and then two metallic anchors are usually placed as a result of the hard nature of the bone in the trochanter. These anchors can be placed percutaneously to achieve the optimal angle into the bone. Fluoroscopy is again useful at this stage of the procedure to confirm the proper

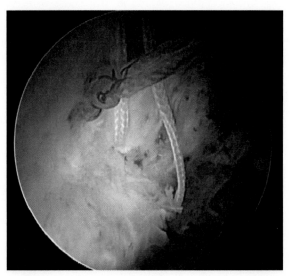

**Figure 17–5** Arthroscopic image of the hip after suture anchors have been placed in the greater trochanter. The sutures are passed through the tendon in preparation for repair.

positioning of the anchors. A suture-passing device is then used to pass the suture through the tendon from posterior to anterior in a sequential fashion (Figure 17-5). Proper suture management is critical. Extra-long cannulas are used to help manage the suture and to tie arthroscopic knots. Finally, after all of sutures are passed, arthroscopic sliding, locking knots are created, with a knot pusher securing the medius back to its native footprint on the trochanter (Figure 17-6).

### TECHNICAL PEARLS

- The placement of the initial mid-anterior portal should be performed under fluoroscopic guidance to confirm placement over the lateral prominence of the greater trochanter to avoid entry into the vastus lateralis distally and the gluteus medius muscle proximally.
- The initial view in the space should be directed toward identifying the gluteus maximus tendon insertion into the linea aspera. This allows the surgeon to gain proper orientation in the space, and it provides a boundary to protect the sciatic nerve, which is 4 cm posterior to the insertion point.
- A complete bursectomy should be performed before tendon evaluation.
- Slight axial traction on the limb will help to tension the gluteus medius fibers to allow for easy distinction between the inflamed bursa and the normal gluteus medius muscle tissue.
- Place anchors perpendicular to the trochanter with fluoroscopic assistance.
- A small stab incision at level of the posterolateral peritrochanteric portal is an ideal location for anchor placement.
- Extra-long plastic threaded cannulas should be used during suture passage to provide for optimal suture management.

### POSTOPERATIVE REHABILITATION

Rehabilitation for patients after bursectomy or iliotibial band release limits weight bearing to 20 lb with the foot flat as tolerated with crutches for the first 2 weeks postoperatively. Full weight bearing is advanced without crutches as the patient's pain tolerates. Range of motion and hip strengthening without restrictions begin as soon as the patient's pain allows. It is important to avoid aggravating the lateral hip with therapy that is too aggressive immediately after surgery.

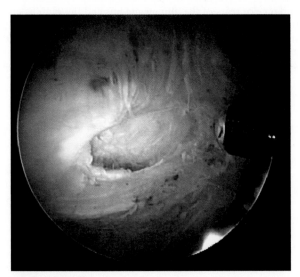

**Figure 17–4** Arthroscopic image that reveals a full-thickness tear of the gluteus medius tendon.

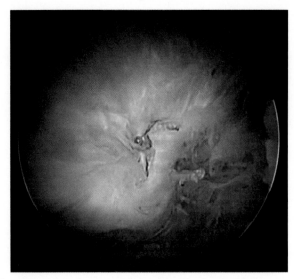

**Figure 17–6** Arthroscopic image of the hip after the final repair of the gluteus medius tendon edge to its footprint on the greater trochanter. The knots were secured with the use of arthroscopic knot-tying techniques.

For patients undergoing the repair of gluteus medius and gluteus minimus tears, physical therapy consists of 6 weeks of 20-lb flat-foot weight bearing with crutches. The patient is fitted with a hip abduction brace that blocks active abduction, and no limitation of hip flexion or extension is required. Isometric strengthening of the hip abductors should begin at 6 weeks. At 12 weeks, more aggressive strengthening and activity are introduced. Running is not allowed until the patient displays equal abductor strength bilaterally to support the pelvis.

## RESULTS AND OUTCOMES

In most cases, external coxa saltans is asymptomatic, or it can be treated conservatively with rest, activity modification, stretching, corticosteroid injections, and physical therapy (Table 17-4). Zoltan and colleagues described an open surgical technique for the treatment of recalcitrant external coxa saltans that involved the excision of an ellipsoid-shaped portion of the iliotibial band overlying the greater trochanter and the removal of the trochanteric bursa. Postoperative follow up demonstrated that 80% of patients (4 out of 5) had significant improvement or relief of their symptoms, whereas 20% (1 out of 5) had no improvement. A minimally invasive technique that makes use of transverse step cuts into the fascia along a longitudinal facial incision has

also been described. Fourteen of 16 hips remained asymptomatic postoperatively. The treatment of external coxa saltans with endoscopic iliotibial band release has been described by multiple authors with promising results. At an average follow up of 2 years, Ilizaliturri and colleagues reported 10 of 11 patients as having the complete resolution of pain and symptomatic snapping.

Conservative treatment in the form of one or two local corticosteroid and local anesthetic preparation injections in combination with physical therapy is the mainstay of diagnosis and treatment. This therapeutic regimen has resulted in excellent responses in 66% of cases and improvement in the remaining 33%. However, conservative therapy is not without its drawbacks. Multiple or inappropriately placed corticosteroid injections have been associated with gluteus medius injury, and open trochanteric bursectomy has been described for these refractory cases (Table 17-5). Trends toward arthroscopic treatment have also produced descriptions of endoscopic bursectomy. Baker and colleagues recently published a prospective follow up report of 25 patients treated with endoscopic bursectomy at a mean of 26.1 months postoperatively. Significant improvement was found in visual analog scale results, Harris Hip Scores, and Short Form 36 (SF-36) results. One postoperative complication occurred: a seroma that required repeat surgery. One patient had a failed arthroscopic bursectomy and subsequently underwent open bursectomy that resulted in the resolution of symptoms. Improvements in a patient's status that are likely to be lasting are usually evident by 1 to 3 months after surgery.

The insertions of the gluteus medius and the gluteus minimus at the greater trochanter and tears at this insertion have been described synonymously with tears of the rotator cuff tendons (Table 17-6). As a result of the similarities, injuries to the abductor tendons have been called *rotator cuff tears of the hip*. Tears were initially identified in the setting of open debridement for recalcitrant trochanteric bursitis, total hip arthroplasty, and the treatment of femoral neck fractures. Descriptions of calcific tendonitis of the hip have also included relationships with gluteus medius and gluteus minimus tears, thus further substantiating the rotator cuff similarity. Conservative treatment has included physical therapy and corticosteroid injection. Treatment has been described in an open fashion when encountered in the setting of refractory iliotibial band syndrome and total hip arthroplasty. The true incidence of gluteus medius and gluteus minimus tears is not known. A prospective study by Bunker and colleagues of 50 patients with fractures of the femoral neck revealed a 22% incidence of tears of the gluteus medius and the gluteus minimus. In addition, Howell and colleagues conducted another prospective study of 176 consecutive patients who underwent total hip arthroplasty for osteoarthritis, and they identified 20% of these patients as having degenerative pathology.

### Table 17–4 EXTERNAL COXA SALTANS

| Author | Title | No. of Hips | No. of Months of Follow Up | Results |
|---|---|---|---|---|
| Zoltan et al., 1986 | A new operative approach to snapping hip and refractory trochanteric bursitis in athletes | 5 | 55 | 4 out of 5, significant improvement; 1 out of 5, complete recurrence |
| White et al., 2004 | A new operative approach in the correction of external coxa saltans: the snapping hip | 16 | 32.5 | 16 out of 16, asymptomatic hips |
| Ilizaliturri et al., 2006 | Endoscopic iliotibial band release for external snapping hip syndrome | 11 | 24 | 10 out of 11, complete resolution; 1 out of 11, nonpainful snapping |

**Table 17–5** TROCHANTERIC BURSITIS

| Author | Title | No. of Hips | No. of Months of Follow Up | Results |
|---|---|---|---|---|
| Ege Rasmussen et al., 1985 | Trochanteric bursitis. Treatment by corticosteroid injection | 36 | 24 | 24 out of 36, excellent response; 12 out of 36, improvement; 9 out of 36, relapsed |
| Schipira et al., 1986 | Trochanteric bursitis—a common clinical problem | 72 | 24 | 65 out of 72, complete pain resolution |
| Govaert et al., 2003 | Trochanteric reduction osteotomy as a treatment for refractory trochanteric bursitis | 12 | 23.5 | 6 out of 12, excellent response; 5 out of 12, great improvement; 1 out of 12, fair improvement |
| Baker et al., 2007 | Arthroscopic bursectomy for recalcitrant trochanteric bursitis | 25 | 26.1 | Pain score decreased from 7.2 to 3.1; Harris Hip Score increased from 51 to 77; physical function increased from 33.6 to 54 on SF-36 |
| Fox et al., 2002 | The role of arthroscopic bursectomy in the treatment of trochanteric bursitis | 27 | 60 | 26 out of 27, outcome satisfaction; 2 out of 27, recurrence |
| Wiese et al., 2004 | Early results of endoscopic trochanter bursectomy | 45 | 25 | Japanese Orthopedic Association Hip Score improvement from 40.5 to 72.6 |

**Table 17–6** GLUTEUS MEDIUS AND MINIMUS TEARS

| Author | Title | No. of Hips | No. of Months of Follow Up | Results |
|---|---|---|---|---|
| Kandemir et al., 2003 | Endoscopic treatment of calcific tendinitis of gluteus medius and minimus | 1 | 3 | 1 out of 1, asymptomatic |
| Voos et al., 2009 | Arthroscopic repair of "rotator cuff tears of the hip" | 10 | 12 to 31 | 10 out of 10, asymptomatic; 9 out of 10, full strength recovery; Harris Hip Score, 91.7; Hip Outcomes Score, 92.4 |

Recently, the arthroscopic treatment of trochanteric bursitis and calcific tendonitis of the gluteus medius and the gluteus minimus has been reported by Kandemir and colleagues. Voos and colleagues reported about an arthroscopic approach that provides access for the repair of gluteus medius and gluteus minimus tendon tears. Results of this technique for 10 patients with 12 to 31 months of follow up demonstrated the full resolution of pain in 100% of patients, with 9 out of 10 patients recovering their full former strength. Moreover, an increasing understanding of the gluteus medius tendon attachment morphology may help in the development of future reparative techniques.

## COMPLICATIONS

There are few complications inherent to surgical procedures in the peritrochanteric space. The main complications include fluid extravasations into the soft tissues and hematomas. There have been no formal reports in the literature regarding the incidence of these complications.

The recurrence of trochanteric bursitis, painful external coxa saltans, and the retearing of gluteus medius tendon repairs can all occur, although the incidences of these complications

have not been reported. The senior author had one deep venous thrombosis occur postoperatively after addressing peritrochanteric space pathology.

## ANNOTATED REFERENCES AND SUGGESTED READINGS

**Allen WC, Cope R. Coxa saltans: the snapping hip revisited.** *J Am Acad Orthop Surg.* 1995;3:303–308.

Three causes of snapping hip are described in this report including external, internal, and intra-articular. The mechanism, diagnosis, radiographic imaging, and treatment algorithm are detailed.

**Baker Jr CL, Massie RV, Hurt WG, et al. Arthroscopic bursectomy for recalcitrant trochanteric bursitis.** *Arthroscopy.* 2007;23:827–832.

This study evaluated arthroscopic treatment of trochanteric bursitis in patients who had failed conservative therapy. Significant improvements in Harris Hip Scores, SF, 36, and visual analog scale were documented. They concluded that recalcitrant trochanteric bursitis may be effectively treated with this therapeutic modality.

**Bunker TD, Esler CN, Leach WJ. Rotator-cuff tear of the hip.** *J Bone Joint Surg Br.* 1997;79:618–620.

Tears at the insertion of the gluteus medius and minimus may be significantly under-reported in the literature. 22% of patients with femoral neck fractures have these tears and thus such pathology should be appreciated with this fracture pattern.

**Byrd JW. Hip arthroscopy. *J Am Acad Orthop Surg*. 2006;14:433–444.**

This article describes the indications, contraindications, surgical technique, and outcomes of hip arthroscopy. Pathology included in this report are loose bodies, labral lesions, degenerative disease, chondral injuries, femoroacetabular impingement, osteonecrosis, synovial disease, instability, adhesive capsulitis, joint sepsis, and snapping iliopsosas tendon.

**Byrd JW. Hip arthroscopy: surgical indications. *Arthroscopy*. 2006; 22:1260–1262.**

Outcomes of hip arthroscopy are significantly affected by patient selection. Indications for appropriate selection are identified in this article.

**Choi YS, Lee SM, Song BY, et al. Dynamic sonography of external snapping hip syndrome. *J Ultrasound Med*. 2002;21:753–758.**

Dynamic sonographic findings of external snapping hip syndrome was closely correlated with specific movements of the iliotibial band and the gluteus maximus muscle and replicated the painful snapping reported by the patient. This modality may be effectively used in the diagnosis of this syndrome.

**Connell DA, Bass C, Sykes CA, et al. Sonographic evaluation of gluteus medius and minimus tendinopathy. *Eur Radiol*. 2003;13:1339–1347.**

Ultrasonography was used to identify gluteus medius tendonopathy and tear in patients with point tenderness over the greater trochanter. Twenty-eight patients demonstrated tendonopathy, 16 patients had partial tear, and 9 had complete rupture of the gluteus medius. In addition, gluteus minimus tendonopathy was identified in 10 of 75 patients.

**Ege Rasmussen KJ, Fano N. Trochanteric bursitis. Treatment by corticosteroid injection. *Scand J Rheumatol*. 1985;14:417–420.**

Chronic trochanteric bursitis was identified to be a prevalent pathology in older females. Significant relief of symptoms can be achieved with corticosteroid injection. However, 25% of patients may have recurrent symptoms after 2 years.

**Fox JL. The role of arthroscopic bursectomy in the treatment of trochanteric bursitis. *Arthroscopy*. 2002;18:E34.**

Data from arthroscopic treatment of recalcitrant trochanteric bursitis are presented in this report. Excellent follow-up of 5 years demonstrated asymptomatic results in 25 of 27 patients.

**Govaert LH, van der Vis HM, Marti RK, et al. Trochanteric reduction osteotomy as a treatment for refractory trochanteric bursitis. *J Bone Joint Surg Br*. 2003;85:199–203.**

A new operative approach for the treatment of chronic trochanteric bursitis in the form of a trochanteric reduction osteotomy is described in ten patients who had failed conservative therapy. Good to excellent responses were demonstrated in all but one patient, who reported a fair result.

**Howell GE, Biggs RE, Bourne RB. Prevalence of abductor mechanism tears of the hips in patients with osteoarthritis. *J Arthroplasty*. 2001;16:121–123.**

Patients who have undergone total hip arthroplasty for osteoarthritis may have degenerative tears of the abductor mechanism. The gluteus medius and minimus tendons may be involved in this pathology.

**Ilizaliturri Jr VM, Martinez-Escalante FA, Chaidez PA, et al. Endoscopic iliotibial band release for external snapping hip syndrome. *Arthroscopy*. 2006;22:505–510.**

This article evaluated treatment of external snapping hip syndrome by endoscopic release of the iliotibial band. Eleven patients were treated with 10 of 11 asymptomatic and one patient with non-painful snapping.

**Kagan A 2nd. Rotator cuff tears of the hip. *Clin Orthop Relat Res*. 1999;135–140.**

Lateral hip pain commonly attributed to trochanteric bursitis in the setting of weak hip abduction may be related to partial gluteus medius tear. In this study, open reattachment or repair of this tendon significantly alleviated the preoperative pain.

**Kandemir U, Bharam S, Philippon MJ, et al. Endoscopic treatment of calcific tendinitis of gluteus medius and minimus. *Arthroscopy*. 2003;19:E4.**

This case report focuses on calcific tendonitis and the potential endoscopic treatment modalities including resection of these calcium deposits.

**Kelly BT, Williams RJ 3rd, Philippon MJ. Hip arthroscopy: current indications, treatment options, and management issues. *Am J Sports Med*. 2003;31:1020–1037.**

In this report, indications, surgical technique as well as specific radiographic analysis of hip pathology were described. Clinical criteria specific to arthroscopic hip pathology are also included.

**LaBan MM, Weir SK, Taylor RS. "Bald trochanter" spontaneous rupture of the conjoined tendons of the gluteus medius and minimus presenting as a trochanteric bursitis. *Am J Phys Med Rehabil*. 2004;83:806–809.**

This case report identifies a 66-year-old female who had continued lateral hip pain diagnosed by exam and MRI as consistent with trochanteric bursitis. Refractory symptoms prompted repeat MRI that diagnosed a full-thickness tear of the gluteus medius muscle and retraction of tendon.

**Robertson WJ, Gardner MJ, Barker JU, et al. Anatomy and dimensions of the gluteus medius tendon insertion. *Arthroscopy*. 2008;24:130–136.**

This cadaveric study described the anatomy of the gluteus medius footprint with specific focus on its area, dimensions, and orientation. Use of the described dimensions may aid in future arthroscopic and open repair of gluteus medius tears.

**Schapira D, Nahir M, Scharf Y. Trochanteric bursitis: a common clinical problem. *Arch Phys Med Rehabil*. 1986;67(11):815–817.**

**Shindle MK, Voos JE, Heyworth BE, et al. Hip arthroscopy in the athletic patient: current techniques and spectrum of disease. *J Bone Joint Surg Am*. 2007;89(suppl 3):29–43.**

Advances in hip arthroscopy have led to application of this surgical modality to athletes. Clinical exam and radiographic imaging of associated pathology are crucial to appropriate surgical indications. Arthroscopic treatment of pathologies including labral tears, loose bodies, femoroacetabular impingement, coxa saltans, ligamentum teres, and capsular laxity are all described.

**Tortolani PJ, Carbone JJ, Quartararo LG. Greater trochanteric pain syndrome in patients referred to orthopedic spine specialists. *Spine J*. 2002;2:251–254.**

The prevalence and patient characteristics of greater trochanteric pain syndrome were documented in this article. The prevalence was 20.2% with significantly more women than men. This entity may be far more prevalent in patients complaining of low back pain than previously appreciated.

**Voos JE, Rudzki JR, Shindle MK, et al. Arthroscopic anatomy and surgical techniques for peritrochanteric space disorders in the hip. *Arthroscopy*. 2007;1246;23:e1–e5.**

The arthroscopic anatomy of the peritrochanteric space has been only recently described. This study details the surgical technique, clinical findings, and associated pathology of this anatomic region.

**Voos JE, Shindle MK, Pruett A, Asnis P, Kelly BT. Endoscopic repair of gluteus medius tendon tears of the hip. *Am J Sports Med*. 2009;37(4):743–747.**

**White RA, Hughes MS, Burd T, et al. A new operative approach in the correction of external coxa saltans: the snapping hip. *Am J Sports Med*. 2004;32:1504–1508.**

External coxa saltans can be treated with a simple minimally invasive surgical procedure. Fourteen of sixteen hips remained asymptomatic after the final surgical release.

**Wiese M, Rubenthaler F, Willburger RE, et al. Early results of endoscopic trochanter bursectomy.** *Int Orthop.* **2004;28:218–221.**

This article describes 45 endoscopic bursectomies following 6 months of failed conservative treatment. Significant improvements in the Japanese Orthopaedic Association disability hip scores were identified.

**Zoltan DJ, Clancy Jr WG, Keene JS. A new operative approach to snapping hip and refractory trochanteric bursitis in athletes.** *Am J Sports Med.* **1986;14:201–204.**

This article describes an open excision of an ellipsoid-shaped portion of the iliotibial band over the greater trochanter coupled with a greater trochanteric bursectomy for treatment of snapping iliotibial band syndrome.

# CHAPTER 18

# Arthroscopic Iliopsoas Release and Lengthening

*Victor M. Ilizaliturri, Jr.*

## INTRODUCTION

Iliopsoas tendon lengthening has traditionally been a procedure that is performed with an open approach and that is used mainly for the treatment of coxa saltans interna or medial snapping hip syndrome. Other indications include iliopsoas irritation syndrome after hip arthroplasty and spastic hip subluxation. The evolution of surgical techniques and technology for hip arthroscopy has allowed for endoscopic techniques for the release or lengthening of the iliopsoas tendon.

## SNAPPING PHENOMENON OF THE ILIOPSOAS TENDON

The internal snapping hip syndrome is produced by the iliopsoas tendon passing over the iliopectineal eminence or the femoral head. The iliopsoas tendon is located lateral to the iliopectineal eminence when the hip is in full flexion; with hip extension, the tendon is displaced medially until it is positioned medial to the iliopectineal eminence when the hip is in a neutral position. The snapping phenomenon occurs without pain in up to 10% of the general population and should be considered a normal occurrence.

Iliopsoas impingement can be present in up to 4.3% of patients after total hip replacement. This phenomenon mainly occurs as a result of prominent anterior cup rims of reinforcement rings and extruded cement.

## INDICATIONS

- Internal snapping hip syndrome or coxa saltans interna
- Iliopsoas impingement after total hip replacement
- The treatment of soft-tissue contractures in spastic patients

## HISTORY AND PHYSICAL EXAMINATION

The symptomatic internal snapping hip syndrome always presents with pain in the groin associated with the snapping phenomenon. The snapping phenomenon is reproduced when bringing the hip to extension from a flexed position. Patients with this condition report snapping while climbing stairs or when standing up from sitting in a chair. The snapping phenomenon is always voluntary and reproducible. It commonly affects women, with the typical patient having a history of participating in sports. Ballet dancers have a high incidence

of snapping hip syndromes. The snapping phenomenon may occur initially without pain and become painful after a traumatic event or after prolonged participation in sports.

The physical examination of patients with the internal snapping phenomenon is performed with the patient supine; the affected hip is flexed to more than 90 degrees and extended to a neutral position. This may be accentuated with abduction and external rotation in flexion and by adducting and internally rotating the hip while extending it. The snapping phenomenon is not visible at the groin. It may be audible, or it may be palpated by placing the hand over the affected area of the groin. There is always an apprehension response from the patient when the snapping occurs.

## IMAGING STUDIES

The plain radiographs obtained for these patients are usually normal. In some cases, a femoroacetabular impingement deformity may be seen on a plain x-ray; this deformity may be related to the iliopsoas snapping phenomenon.

Psoas bursography may outline the tendon, and, in combination with fluoroscopy, it may document the snapping phenomenon dynamically. The main problem is that this type of imaging depends on the ability of the technician to reproduce the snapping while examining hip motion within the range of view of the C-arm, and it is an invasive study. Ultrasonography of the iliopsoas tendon is a dynamic, noninvasive study that may document both the snapping phenomenon and the pathologic changes of the iliopsoas tendon and its bursa. Psoas ultrasonography also depends on the ability and experience of the examiner. Because almost half of patients with internal snapping hip syndrome have associated intra-articular hip pathology, magnetic resonance arthrography is the diagnostic study that our practice prefers. It may demonstrate intra-articular pathology as well as changes related to the iliopsoas tendon and the bursa. The snapping phenomenon cannot be documented with the use of magnetic resonance arthrography.

Treatment is initially conservative with physical therapy, nonsteroidal anti-inflammatory drug therapy, and corticosteroid injections. If there is no positive response to conservative treatment, then surgical treatment is indicated.

## SURGICAL TECHNIQUE

The endoscopic release of the iliopsoas tendon can be performed with the use of one of two different techniques: release at the level of the insertion of the tendon on the lesser trochanter or release at the level of the hip joint by accessing the bursa through an anterior hip capsulectomy. With both techniques, hip arthroscopy is performed first. Intra-articular lesions are identified and treated before the hip periphery and the psoas bursa are accessed.

## Patient Positioning

The supine position and the lateral decubitus position have both been described for hip arthroscopy, and iliopsoas tendon release can be performed with the patient in either one.

We prefer to use the lateral decubitus technique. We position the patient lateral and resting on the nonoperative side on a fracture table with special accessories (Maquet, Rastatt, Germany). A horizontal perineal post with a diameter of 10 cm is positioned horizontally on the operating table; it is then positioned laterally on the patient's medial thigh and elevated to provide a lateralization vector to the traction force. The lateralization also distances the post from the pudendal nerve. The foot on the surgical side is fixed to the traction device of the fracture table, and the nonoperative side rests free on the table. Before traction is applied, the patient's genitalia should be inspected to verify that they are free from compression.

The hip is positioned in 20 degrees of flexion to relax the anterior hip capsule. Flexion of more than 20 degrees does not improve the distraction of the hip joint, and it in fact increases the possibility of injury to the sciatic nerve. Abduction is kept neutral to maximize the separation of the iliofemoral joint. Neutral rotation is preferred while establishing arthroscopic portals to maximize the distance between the posterior edge of the greater trochanter and the sciatic nerve.

The C-arm is positioned horizontally under the table to provide an anteroposterior view of the hip. A traction test is performed to confirm effective separation of a minimum of 10 mm between the femoral head and the acetabulum at the image intensifier. After a successful traction test is performed, the hip is flexed 35 degrees, abducted, and externally rotated to confirm the mobility of the setup; this mobility will provide adequate access to the hip periphery. The hip is brought back to a neutral position, and the surgical area is prepared for surgery in the standard fashion.

## Iliopsoas Release at the Lesser Trochanter

Arthroscopy of the central compartment is performed first with the use of traction. Three portals are usually established for arthroscopy of the central compartment: an anterolateral portal, a posterolateral portal, and a direct anterior portal. Traction is released to access the peripheral compartment, and accessory portals are usually required to access the hip periphery.

After hip arthroscopy of the central and peripheral compartments is complete, the instruments are taken out of the joint. The hip is positioned in 20 degrees of flexion and external rotation to expose the lesser trochanter at the image intensifier (Figure 18-1). A spinal needle is introduced through an accessory portal (i.e., the superior accessory portal) that is established about 2 cm distal to a horizontal line directed anteriorly from the tip of the greater trochanter and 2 cm anterior to the anterior femur (Figure 18-2). The needle is directed toward the lesser trochanter and navigated by the image intensifier (Figure 18-3). Orientation in the coronal plane is provided by the image intensifier. Orientation in the sagittal plane is provided by palpating the anterior aspect of the femur until the needle is positioned on the lesser trochanter; this will position the needle inside of the iliopsoas bursa. After the spinal needle has been successfully positioned in the iliopsoas bursa, the stylus is removed, and a flexible guidewire (Nitinol) is introduced. The needle is removed, and a cannulated switching stick

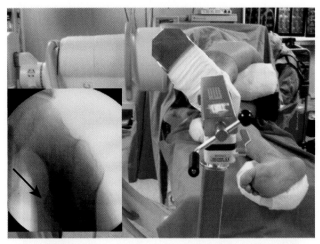

**Figure 18-1** This photograph demonstrates a patient positioned for hip arthroscopy on the left side. Only the left foot is fixed to the traction device. Note the extra-padded perineal post in a horizontal position and the image intensifier placed horizontally under the table. The hip is without traction and externally rotated to expose the lesser trochanter at the image intensifier. To the left, a photograph from the image intensifier demonstrates the exposure of the lesser trochanter with external rotation *(arrow)*. Note that the hip is without traction.

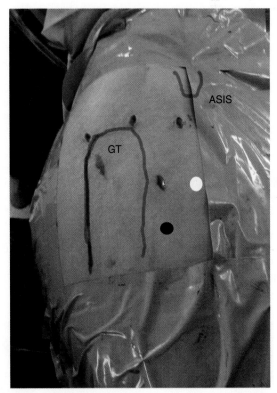

**Figure 18-2** This photograph demonstrates portal sites. The greater trochanter *(GT)* and the anterosuperior iliac spine *(ASIS)* have been outlined. The anterolateral portal and posterolateral portal are at the anterosuperior and posterosuperior corners of the greater trochanter. The direct anterior portal is 1 cm medial to the crossing of a horizontal line from the tip of the greater trochanter and a vertical line from the anterosuperior iliac spine. An anteroinferior accessory portal is located distal to the central compartment portals (i.e., the anterolateral, posterolateral, and direct anterior portals) 1 cm to 2 cm anterior of the anterior aspect of the proximal femur. The black circle indicates our preferred site for the working portal in the case of an iliopsoas tendon release at the lesser trochanter. The white circle indicates our preferred site for the working portal in the case of a transcapsular iliopsoas tendon release.

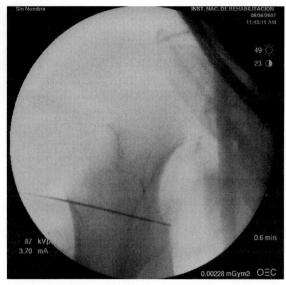

**Figure 18–3** Fluoroscopy photograph of a right hip. Note the lesser trochanter exposed by external rotation. A spinal needle has been introduced through an accessory portal into the iliopsoas bursa and on to the lesser trochanter. Note that the hip is without traction.

is passed into the iliopsoas bursa over the flexible guidewire. A 4.5-mm, double-valve, rotatable arthroscopic cannula is passed over the switching stick, which is then removed, and then a 4-mm, 30-degree arthroscope is introduced. The fluid pump is started, and the iliopsoas tendon is identified. A second accessory portal 3 cm to 4 cm distal to the first one is established (i.e., the inferior accessory portal). A spinal needle is triangulated toward the tip of the arthroscope inside of the iliopsoas bursa. The image intensifier can be used to assist with the navigation of the needle. The tip of the needle is identified endoscopically inside of the iliopsoas bursa, and a working portal is established with the use of a flexible guidewire, a cannulated switching stick with a dilator, and a slotted cannula (Hip Access System, Smith and Nephew, Andover, MA). A shaver is introduced through the slotted cannula, which is then removed. The shaver is used to resect synovial tissue from the iliopsoas bursa and to dissect the iliopsoas tendon. The slotted cannula is reinserted with the use of the shaver as a guide. The shaver is removed, and a radiofrequency hook probe is inserted; the slotted cannula is removed, and the radiofrequency probe is used to release the iliopsoas tendon close to its insertion on the lesser trochanter

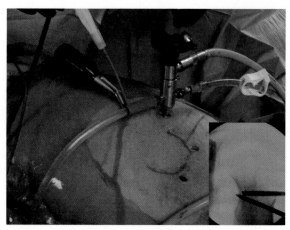

**Figure 18–4** This photograph demonstrates the arthroscope in position at an accessory portal. A slotted cannula is in position at the distal accessory portal, and a radiofrequency instrument is being introduced through the slotted cannula. The fluoroscopy image demonstrates the position of instruments above the lesser trochanter.

(Figures 18-4 and 18-5). The image intensifier can be used to verify the position of the radiofrequency hook probe before the release of the iliopsoas tendon.

### Transcapsular Iliopsoas Tendon Release

The iliopsoas tendon also can be released endoscopically at the level of the hip joint through an anterior hip capsulectomy. We perform this procedure with the patient in the lateral decubitus position, but it can also be performed with the patient in the supine position. After arthroscopy of the central compartment is complete, the instruments are taken out of the joint, and the traction is released. The hip is flexed 30 degrees and externally rotated, and the hip periphery is accessed through an accessory portal as described for the iliopsoas tendon release at the lesser trochanter. The spinal needle is directed to the hip capsule at the level of the anterior femoral neck in an angle that is almost perpendicular to the femoral neck, and cannulated instruments are used to establish a viewing portal. A second accessory portal (i.e., the working portal) is established with the use of a spinal-needle–guidewire technique and cannulated instruments by triangulating toward the tip of the arthroscope inside of the

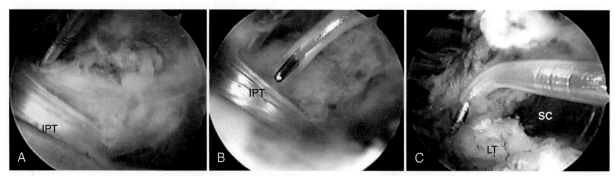

**Figure 18–5** Bursoscopic sequence of photographs of an iliopsoas tendon release at the lesser trochanter of the right hip. **A,** A slotted cannula *(SC)* is in position in the iliopsoas bursa. The iliopsoas tendon *(IPT)* is at the bottom of the photograph and surrounded by synovial tissue. **B,** The synovial tissue around the iliopsoas tendon *(IPT)* has been resected with a shaver. A radiofrequency hook probe is being introduced for the retrograde release of the iliopsoas tendon. **C,** The iliopsoas tendon has been released. The lesser trochanter *(LT)* is at the bottom of the photograph. A radiofrequency hook probe is being removed from the bursa through a slotted cannula *(SC)*. The muscle fibers of the iliacus are behind the hook probe.

hip periphery. The working portal is usually distal to the central compartment portals (i.e., the anterolateral, posterolateral, and direct anterior portals) and between the first accessory portal and a vertical line that descends from the anterosuperior iliac spine (Figure 18-6; see also Figure 18-2). The iliopsoas tendon is located immediately anterior to the hip capsule; it is always found in the space between the anterior zona orbicularis and the anterior labrum proximal and anterior to the medial synovial fold. A communication may exist at this level between the hip capsule and the iliopsoas

bursa. In most cases, the hip capsule is thinner at this region, and the iliopsoas tendon can be visualized through the thin portion of the hip capsule. A capsulectomy is performed at this level to gain access to the iliopsoas bursa and the tendon; we use a radiofrequency hook probe passed through a slotted cannula. After the capsulectomy is performed, synovial tissue from around the tendon is resected with the use of a shaver. The tendon is released with a radiofrequency hook probe (Figure 18-7). A slotted cannula is also used to introduce and interchange instruments in the iliopsoas bursa through the defect on the anterior hip capsule.

After the tendinous portion of the iliopsoas has been released, the iliacus muscle is visible behind the retracted tendon stumps. In our practice, we do not release the iliacus muscle (Figure 18-8). Partial release with both techniques is achieved by not releasing the fibers from the iliacus muscle.

**Figure 18–6** Fluoroscopy photograph that demonstrates the position of instruments introduced to the iliopsoas bursa through an anterior hip capsule window.

## TECHNICAL PEARLS

- Endoscopic techniques for iliopsoas tendon release must be combined with hip arthroscopy (at least 50% of patients present with intra-articular pathology).
- The patient can be positioned supine or lateral on a traction device (e.g., fracture table, dedicated hip arthroscopy distractor).
- Fluoroscopy is necessary to navigate instruments into the central compartment via the hip periphery of the iliopsoas bursa.
- The use of special hip arthroscopy cannulated instruments is mandatory.
- When releasing the iliopsoas tendon, we prefer to use a radiofrequency device:
  - Radiofrequency devices only cut when power is applied.
  - Cut in a retrograde motion to cut away from the branches of the femoral nerve.

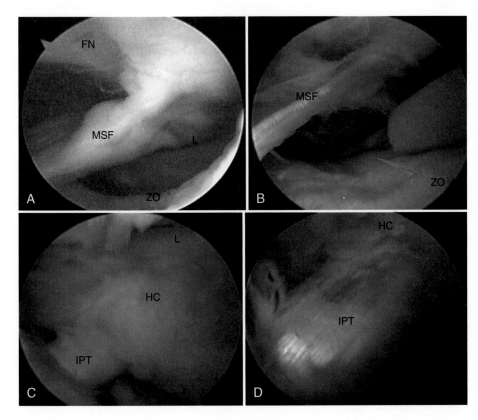

**Figure 18–7** Arthroscopic sequence that demonstrates the transcapsular release of the iliopsoas tendon in a right hip. **A,** Arthroscopy of the hip periphery. The inferior femoral neck *(FN)* is at the top of the photograph, with the medial synovial fold *(MSF)* below it. The anteroinferior labrum *(L)* is to the right of the photograph. The zona orbicularis *(ZO)* is at the bottom. **B,** The medial synovial fold *(MSF)* is at the top of the photograph, with the anterolateral labrum *(L)* to the left. A radiofrequency hook probe is being used to create a window at the anterior hip capsule between the labrum and the zona orbicularis *(ZO)*. The red line indicates the direction of the cut. **C,** The window on the anterior hip capsule *(HC)* has been completed. A shaver is being used to resect the synovial tissue around the iliopsoas tendon *(IPT)*. The labrum *(L)* is to the right of the photograph. **D,** The iliopsoas tendon *(IPT)* had been completely exposed. The inferior limit of the hip capsule *(HC)* window is at the top of the photograph.

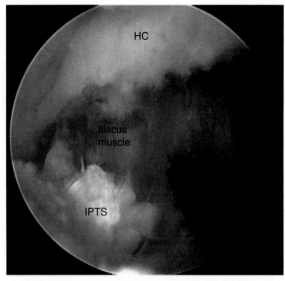

**Figure 18–8** Arthroscopic photograph after the release of the iliopsoas tendon. The iliopsoas tendon stump *(IPTS)* is at the bottom of the photograph. The iliacus muscle is behind the stump. Part of the hip capsule *(HC)* is visible at the top of the photograph.

## POSTOPERATIVE REHABILITATION

Successful iliopsoas tendon release or lengthening will always produce a loss of flexion strength that usually returns 6 to 8 weeks after surgery. Patients are advised about this situation before surgery, and no active hip flexor exercises are indicated during this period. Quadriceps and hip abductor strength exercises are indicated as soon as the first day after the procedure. There is no restriction of the range of motion with iliopsoas tendon release. Extension stretching exercises are indicated from the first postoperative week to prevent contractures, capsular scarring, and adhesions. Findings of hip arthroscopy should be considered during rehabilitation if microfractures were performed to treat cartilage lesions in load-bearing areas; partial weight bearing should be indicated for 6 weeks. If an osteochondroplasty was performed on the femoral neck for the cam type of femoroacetabular impingement, partial weight bearing should be indicated for 6 to 8 weeks. We do not restrict weight bearing in the case of isolated labral repairs of partial resections.

## RESULTS

The reported results of endoscopic iliopsoas release compare favorably with those of open procedures. Regarding the effective treatment of the snapping phenomenon, there are fewer cases of resnapping reported with endoscopic techniques than with open procedures. Hip arthroscopy is also an advantage of endoscopic techniques, which are always performed in conjunction with the arthroscopic examination of the central and peripheral compartments of the hip joint. This provides access for the diagnosis and treatment of intra-articular injuries and peripheral compartment pathologies (e.g., femoroacetabular impingement, loose bodies). The results of iliopsoas tendon release are reported in Table 18-1.

## COMPLICATIONS

The most significant complication is the failure of iliopsoas tendon release or lengthening, which results in the need for repeat surgical treatment. Massive heterotopic bone formation after the procedure is also an important complication that requires additional intervention (personal communication, J.W.T. Byrd, Nashville, TN, 2006); this complication can be treated with the resection of heterotopic bone (with either an open or an arthroscopic procedure) and with postoperative irradiation to prevent recurrence.

## ANNOTATED REFERENCES

**Allen WC, Cope R. Coxa saltans: the snapping hip revisited. *J Am Acad Orthop Surg*. 1995;3:303–308.**

Coxa saltans or snapping hip has several causes that can be divided into three types: external, internal, and intra-articular. Snapping of the external type occurs when a thickened area of the posterior iliotibial band or the leading anterior edge of the gluteus maximus snaps forward over the greater trochanter with flexion of the hip. The internal type has a similar mechanism except that it is the musculotendinous iliopsoas that snaps over structures that are deep to it (usually the femoral head and the anterior capsule of the hip). Intra-articular snapping is the result of lesions in the joint itself. The diagnosis of the external and internal types is usually made clinically. Most cases of snapping hip are asymptomatic and can be treated conservatively. However, if the snapping becomes symptomatic, surgery may be required.

**Byrd JWT. Evaluation and management of the snapping iliopsoas tendon. *Tech in Orth*. 2005;20:45–51.**

Surgical intervention is indicated after the failed conservative treatment of symptomatic internal snapping hip syndrome. Nine

### Table 18–1 RESULTS OF THE OPEN AND ENDOSCOPIC SURGICAL TREATMENT OF INTERNAL SNAPPING HIP SYNDROME

| Author | No. of Hips | Technique | Length of Follow Up | Pain | No. of Cases of Resnapping |
|---|---|---|---|---|---|
| Taylor et al. | 16 | Open release | 17 months | 0 | 5 occasional, 1 painful |
| Jacobson et al. | 20 | Open Z-plasty | 20 months | 2 (reoperated) | 6 |
| Dobbs et al. | 11 | Open Z-plasty | 4 years | 0 | 1 |
| Gruen et al. | 12 | Open Z-plasty | 3 years | 0 | 0 |
| Byrd et al. | 9 | Endoscopic release at lesser trochanter | 20 months | 0 | 0 |
| Ilizaliturri et al. | 7 | Endoscopic release at lesser trochanter | 21 months | 0 | 0 |
| Wettstein et al. | 9 | Endoscopic release (preserving iliacus muscle), transcapsular | 3 months (technique report) | 0 | 0 |
| Flanum et al. | 6 | Endoscopic release at the lesser trochanter | 12 months | 0 | 0 |

cases were treated with the endoscopic release of the iliopsoas tendon at its insertion on the lesser trochanter, which resulted in a 100% success rate for the relief of snapping. More than half of the patients in this study presented with intra-articular pathology.

**Cardinal E, Buckwalter KA, Capello WN, Duval N. US of the snapping iliopsoas tendon. *Radiology*. 1996;198:521–522.**

Dynamic ultrasound of the hip was performed for 3 patients with snapping hip syndrome. An abnormal jerk was documented in the affected hip as compared with the contralateral side, where a smooth movement of the iliopsoas tendon was observed at the front of the hip.

**Dienst M, Seil R, Godde S, et al. Effects of traction, distension and joint position on distraction of the hip joint: an experimental study in cadavers. *Arthroscopy*. 2002;18:865–871.**

This anatomic study analyzed the separation of the femoral head from the acetabulum with the hip in different positions, and it compared traction force and the distention of the hip capsule in the presence of introduced saline.

**Dobbs MB, Gordon JE, Luhmann SJ, Szymanzki DA, Schoenecker PL. Surgical correction of the snapping iliopsoas tendon in adolescents. *J Bone Joint Surg Am*. 2002;84(Am):420–424.**

This study addressed open lengthening in 9 adolescent patients (11 hips). At an average follow up of 4 years postoperatively, only 1 patient had mild recurrent snapping.

**Dora C, Houweling M, Koch P, Sierra RJ. Iliopsoas impingement after total hip replacement. *J Bone Joint Surg (Br)*. 2007;89(B):1031–1035.**

The reported incidence of iliopsoas impingement after total hip replacement is up to 4.3%. This phenomenon usually occurs in the presence of a prominent acetabular implant anterior rim or as a result of cement extrusion. The authors present a series of 30 hips with psoas impingement after hip replacement. The patients were divided into three groups: Group 1 was treated with conservative treatment, Group 2 underwent iliopsoas open release, and Group 3 experienced acetabular revision. The patients improved significantly more in Groups 2 and 3, with more complications seen in Group 3.

**Flanum ME, Keene JS, Blankenbaker DG, Desmet AA. Arthroscopic treatment of the painful "internal" snapping hip: results of a new endoscopic technique and imaging protocol. *Am J Sports Med*. 2007;35:770–779.**

This was a report of about 6 patients treated with endoscopic iliopsoas tendon release at the lesser trochanter. At 12 months of follow up, the authors reported a 100% success rate.

**Gruen GS, Scioscia TN, Lowenstein JE. The surgical treatment of internal snapping hip. *Am J Sports Med*. 2002;30:607–613.**

This report presents 11 patients (12 hips) treated with iliopsoas lengthening that involved the use of an ilioinguinal intrapelvic approach. At an average follow up of 3 years, 100% of the patients were asymptomatic.

**Harper MC, Schaberg JE, Allen WC. Primary iliopsoas bursography in the diagnosis of disorders of the hip. *Clin Orthop Relat Res*. 1987;221:238–241.**

A technique of primary psoas bursography under fluoroscopy is described. Filling the bursa with contrast material allowed for the observation of the movement of the iliopsoas musculotendinous unit across the front of the pelvis during motion of the hip.

**Ilizaliturri Jr VM, Mangino G, Valero FS, Camacho-Galindo J. Hip arthroscopy of the central and peripheral compartment by the lateral approach. *Tech Orthop*. 2005;20:32–36.**

A technique for positioning the patient in the lateral decubitus position for hip arthroscopy is presented. Avoiding compression injuries during traction and maintaining the mobility of the setup without traction for access to the peripheral compartment are emphasized. Accessory portals for accessing the hip periphery are described.

**Ilizaliturri Jr VM, Villalobos FE, Chaidez PA, Valero FS, Aguilera JM. External snapping hip syndrome: treatment by endoscopic release of the iliopsoas tendon. *Arthroscopy*. 2005;21:1375–1380.**

An endoscopic technique to release the iliopsoas tendon at the lesser trochanter to treat internal snapping hip syndrome is presented. Seven hips were treated successfully with the use of this technique. More than half of the patients presented with intra-articular pathology.

**Jacobson T, Allen WC. Surgical correction of the snapping iliopsoas tendon. *Am J Sports Med*. 1990;18:470–474.**

This report presents 18 patients with 20 symptomatic snapping hips who were treated with open lengthening with a step-cutting technique. At a mean postoperative follow up of 25 months, 6 patients had recurrence of mild snapping, and 2 hips required reintervention for painful snapping.

**McCulloch PC, Bush-Joseph CA. Massive heterotopic ossification complicating iliopsoas tendon lengthening. Case report. *Am J Sports Med*. 2006;34:2022–2025.**

A 25-year-old male elite college soccer player was treated with an open lengthening of the iliopsoas tendon after the failure of conservative treatment for internal snapping hip syndrome. Three months postoperatively, the patient complained of mild pain and a limited range of motion; massive heterotopic bone formation was diagnosed at the area of the lesser trochanter. Six months postoperatively, the ectopic bone formation was removed; it recurred 6 months later, another operation was performed to remove the heterotopic bone, and the patient was irradiated. No further recurrence was reported.

**Miller F, Cardoso Dias R, Dabney KW, Lipton GE, Triana M. Soft-tissue release for spastic hip subluxation in cerebral palsy. *J Pediatr Orthop*. 1997;17:571–584.**

Children with spastic hip subluxation as a result of cerebral palsy were treated with a standard protocol that focused on the early detection of the subluxation with the use of physical examination and anteroposterior pelvis radiographs. Using limited hip abduction of 30 degrees or less and subluxation of at least 25% migration percentage as indications, patients underwent open adductor and iliopsoas lengthenings with immediate postoperative mobilization and no abduction bracing. The protocol was applied to 74 children with a mean age of 4.5 years, and 147 hips were surgically addressed. Of these hips, initially, 20% were normal (migration percentage, <25%); 52% were mildly subluxated (migration percentage, 25% to 39%), 22% were moderately subluxated (migration percentage, 40% to 59%), and 6% were severely subluxated (migration percentage, ≥60%). At a final postoperative follow-up evaluation at 39 months, 54% of these hips were classified as good (migration percentage, <25%), 34% were considered fair (migration percentage, 25% to 39%), and 12% were thought to be poor (migration percentage, ≥40%). Of this patient population, 69% were nonambulators, and their outcomes were not statistically different from those of children who could walk. No child developed an abduction contracture or a wide-based gait that required treatment. With early detection and the application of this treatment algorithm, 80% of children with spastic hip disease should have good or fair outcomes. Longer follow-up times will be needed to determine how many children will require bony reconstruction to maintain stable and located hips when they have finished growing.

**Tannast M, Siebenrock KA, Anderson SE. Femoroacetabular impingement: radiographic diagnosis—what the radiologist should know. *AJR Am J Roentgen*. 2007;188:1540–1552.**

The purpose of this article is to describe the radiographic criteria that indicate the two types of femoroacetabular impingement. In addition, potential pitfalls in pelvic imaging that involve femoroacetabular impingement are shown.

**Taylor GR, Clarke NM. Surgical release of the "snapping iliopsoas tendon." *J Bone Joint Surg Br*. 1995;77(Br):881–883.**

This is a report about 16 open surgical releases that involved a medial approach. At a mean of 17 months of follow up, snapping was resolved in 10 hips, occasional painless snapping was present in 5 hips, and the condition was unchanged in 1 hip.

**Wettstein M, Jung J, Dienst M. Arthroscopic psoas tenotomy. *Arthroscopy*. 2006;22:907, e1–4.**

This article describes a surgical technique that involves access to the iliopsoas bursa from the hip periphery without traction via an anterior hip capsulectomy. The iliopsoas tendon is exposed through the anterior hip capsulectomy and then released, thus preserving the iliacus muscle. Nine patients were reported as having a 100% success rate at a minimum follow up of 3 months.

**Winston P, Awan R, Cassidy JD, Bleakney RK. Clinical examination and ultrasound of self-reported snapping hip syndrome in elite ballet dancers. *Am J Sports Med*. 2007;35:118–126.**

A snapping hip questionnaire was completed by 87 unselected elite ballet dancers. Twenty-six of these individuals (50 hips) were further examined by clinicians. Ninety-one percent reported snapping hip (80% bilateral), 58% had associated pain, and 7% had taken time off from dancing for this reason.

# CHAPTER 19

# Arthroscopic Femoral Osteoplasty

*Marc R. Safran*

## INTRODUCTION

In 1995, Ganz first described femoroacetabular impingement (FAI), and, in 1999, it was introduced into the English literature. Although the first case was pincer impingement as a result of acetabular overcoverage after a periacetabular osteotomy, further investigations by Professor Ganz and his group led to the recognition of a second type of impingement: cam impingement. This type of impingement is the result of loss of the femoral head–neck offset, which causes the joint to function like a mechanical cam device. The anatomy of cam impingement has been previously described as a pistol grip deformity or a tilt deformity (Figure 19-1). Many investigators have attributed this anatomy to subclinical slipped capital femoral epiphysis (SCFE), and certainly the residuals of an unreduced SCFE can result in cam impingement. Beaule and colleagues demonstrated in a computed-tomography–based study that cam impingement can occur without SCFE, which suggests that this condition is not the result of a subclinical SCFE. Wagner and colleagues demonstrated that the bone of the cam lesion is not reactive nor does it involve any inflammation; thus it is not likely the result of the impingement or arthritis. Because the deformity occurs at or near the femoral head physeal scar, it may be genetically predetermined or the result of stresses applied during development. Either way, this pistol grip deformity has been associated with premature osteoarthritis of the hip. It has also been suggested that cam impingement results in premature or idiopathic arthritis of the hip. However, Bardakos and Villar have shown that only two thirds of patients with cam impingement show radiographic progression of arthritis at 10-year follow up.

The anatomy of cam impingement can frequently be seen among those patients with idiopathic arthritis, although this is still a controversial subject. The suggestion that impingement results in hip arthritis is also likely when studying the pathologic findings of symptomatic impingement patients without arthritis, particularly of those with labral tears and chondral lesions that are thought to progress to arthritis when untreated. The majority of patients in Ganz's series had a combination of cam and pincer impingement, which has been confirmed in other published series as well as my own experience of several hundred patients with symptomatic FAI. Beck and colleagues found that the demographics and pathology do correlate with the different subtypes of impingements. Particularly, for those with isolated types of impingements, the cam type is the most common (17%). It tends to occur in 19-year-old males, whereas those with isolated pincer impingement are 40-year-old active females. For those with isolated cam impingement, the common pathologic findings initially are focal, deep chondral delamination lesions (anterolaterally and extending about 1 cm from the acetabular edge) (Figure 19-2). At first the labrum is intact, but it eventually separates from the acetabular articular cartilage edge before degenerating. The labrum often separates from the acetabulum and the articular cartilage, and the articular cartilage delaminates from the bony acetabulum (Figure 19-3). Alternatively, those with pincer impingement tend to have intrasubstance crushing of the labrum, and the articular cartilage damage extends only a couple of millimeters from the acetabular edge (Figure 19-4). Although the greatest depth of penetration of articular cartilage damage in pincer impingement is also anterolateral, the damage tends to be more global and to extend around the circumference of the acetabulum. In addition, there is often posterior acetabular (62%) and femoral head (31%) articular cartilage damage as a result of the contrecoup phenomenon of the femoral head levering against the anterior acetabulum as the patient tries to obtain hip motion, which results in shearing forces posteriorly (see Figure 19-4). It has been my experience that one type of impingement will predominate the intra-articular pathologic findings.

Although the overall goal of restoring the femoral head–neck offset to relieve the abutment is the same, there is controversy with regard to the approach to be taken to address the cam lesion. Beck and colleagues found that the restoration of the femoral head–neck complex can be most reliably performed through an open approach with a trochanteric osteotomy and surgical dislocation. Although the open approach to this problem is beyond the scope of this chapter, Ganz and colleagues stated that the hip arthroscopy "technique is difficult. Simultaneous assessment of movement of the hip and debridement is not possible." Furthermore, it has been suggested that the open approach, which is the gold standard, allows one to see the entire femoral head and the head–neck junction and thus allows for the use of templates to standardize the resection. This, in combination with the potential for complications of hip arthroscopy such as "nerve traction palsies, foot or perineal pressure sores, and iatrogenic damage to the articular cartilage of the joint," has led many to believe that arthroscopy is limited with regard to its usefulness. However, advances in hip arthroscopy and particularly in peripheral compartment arthroscopy without traction have enhanced the ability to arthroscopically observe impingement dynamically during arthroscopic osteoplasty of the femoral head–neck junction. It has also been suggested that the "constrained hip renders access to the underlying cause of impingement technically challenging, if not impossible." However, Sussman

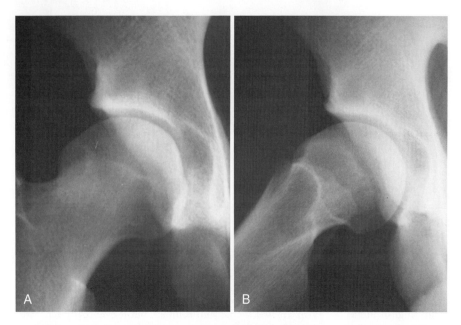

**Figure 19–1** Cam impingement. **A,** Anteroposterior hip radiograph (cropped from an anteroposterior pelvic view) and **B,** lateral radiograph of a 19-year-old collegiate basketball player with cam-type impingement with a mild crossing sign. Notice the loss of offset at the femoral head–neck junction and the convexity of the anterior femoral neck.

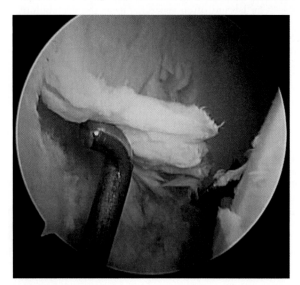

**Figure 19–2** Arthroscopic view of the chondral delamination of the acetabulum associated with cam impingement.

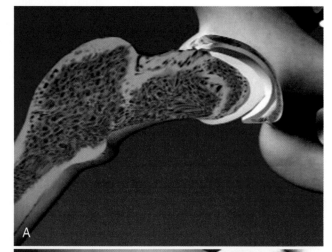

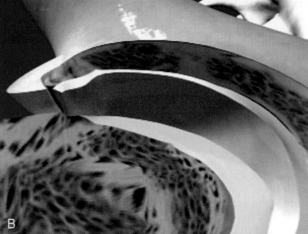

**Figure 19–3** **A,** Schematic representation of the pathophysiology of joint damage with cam impingement. The cam lesion slides underneath the labrum, thereby resulting in a labral chondral separation and the detachment of the labrum from the underlying acetabulum. This occurs anterolaterally. The articular cartilage is then abutted, which results in the delamination of the cartilage from the underlying bone. **B,** A close-up of the region of interest where the impringement occurs.

and colleagues performed a cadaveric comparison of open and arthroscopic techniques for cam impingement. With the use of subtraction computed tomography, those authors demonstrated that the accuracy and precision of arthroscopic osteoplasty approach that of open osteoplasty. They did report that the time for resection was faster with the open technique, although the time required to create the approach (e.g., trochanteric osteotomy, surgical dislocation) was not included. Those who perform the femoral osteoplasty or cheilectomy arthroscopically prefer this technique, because open surgical dislocation involves prolonged postoperative hospitalization (up to a week as compared with outpatient arthroscopic surgery), significant blood loss, a risk of trochanteric nonunion, and prolonged limited weight bearing (up to 12 weeks of crutch use as compared with 0 to 6 weeks). In addition, it is quite easy to see the entire central compartment arthroscopically as compared with the open surgical dislocation.

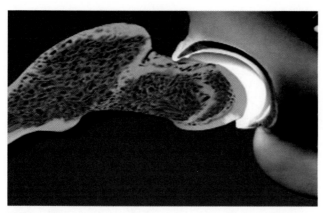

**Figure 19–4**  Schematic representation of the pathophysiology of joint damage as a result of pincer impingement. The overcoverage of the acetabulum results in the crushing of the labrum against the femoral neck. This may occasionally result in the notching of the femoral neck. There is some articular cartilage damage, although this is shallower than that seen with cam impingement. With continued motion, the femoral neck levers against the acetabulum. This results in posteroinferior subluxation of the femoral head and causes posterior femoral head and acetabular articular cartilage damage.

## INDICATIONS

Although some believe that FAI results in arthritis and thus that surgery should be performed to prevent the arthritis, that has not been the approach used in our practice, because there is no evidence at this point that arthritis can be prevented. I certainly believe that having the anatomy of impingement does put the patient at risk for chondral injury, labral injury, and, potentially, arthritis. However, on the basis of my experience with patients who are more than 60 to 70 years old with the anatomy of FAI but no evidence of arthritis or hip symptoms in combination with my extensive experience of cadaveric research involving specimens 80 to 90 years old with the anatomy of obvious cam and combined impingement without evidence of arthritis, I have concluded that not everyone with the anatomy of FAI will develop osteoarthritis (Figure 19-5). It is my belief that the anatomy of FAI does put patients at potential risk for joint damage. However, it likely requires the

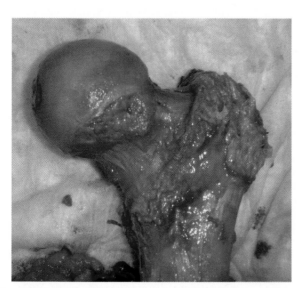

**Figure 19–5**  Photograph of a cadaveric specimen from an 85-year-old patient. Notice the obvious cam lesion and the lack of arthritic change.

individual to be involved in activities that require greater hip range of motion with or without pivoting (e.g., martial arts, soccer, running, golf) to result in impingement. After the tissues start breaking down, patients develop symptoms, because the labrum is a structure that is richly innervated. It is as soon as patients have confirmed intra-articular pain that surgery is indicated. Intra-articular anesthetic guided by fluoroscopy or ultrasound and that is given by itself or with contrast when performing magnetic resonance arthrography is a useful diagnostic test to confirm that the joint is the source of pain. Thus, the goal of surgery is to relieve intra-articular hip pain that is the result of impingement.

Jäger and colleagues demonstrated that there is no role for physical therapy in the treatment of FAI. Their finding is not unexpected, because the bony problem will not resolve with physical therapy. Furthermore, the structures that are injured have limited if any capacity to heal spontaneously. That being said, conservative management consists of activity modification (particularly the avoidance of extremes of motion and of flexion and internal rotation particularly) and nonsteroidal anti-inflammatory medications.

The pathologies that need to be addressed include labral pathology and chondral lesions in addition to the underlying bony cause. Nearly 90% of patients who undergo hip arthroscopy for labral tears have associated bony pathology. It has been shown that those undergoing hip arthroscopy for labral tears in which the FAI was not addressed had poorer results than those without FAI. Thus, addressing intra-articular pathology without addressing the underlying cause will be less likely to result in a good outcome. Although magnetic resonance imaging is not as good as one would hope for identifying chondral damage, Johnston and colleagues found that those patients with symptomatic cam impingement and an alpha angle of more than 62 degrees are at increased risk for chondral injury. As a result, all patients undergoing surgery for intra-articular damage (e.g., symptomatic labral tears, chondral lesions) who have the anatomy of FAI should have the bony impingement treated at the same time.

Thus, indications for surgery include the following:
- Hip pain with bony anatomy that is consistent with cam-type impingement
- Pain relief with intra-articular injection into the joint
- Concomitant labral surgery

## HISTORY AND PHYSICAL EXAMINATION

Those patients with FAI generally describe an insidious onset of groin aching or pain. Although the condition is frequently confused with hip tendonitis or other problems, patients will often note difficulty putting on or taking off their socks and shoes. The pain is usually described as being in the groin, the inguinal region, or deep inside the joint. The pain may be worsened with activities, particularly running and other impact types of activities. Sitting (especially in low seats or chairs) for prolonged periods of time may also result in pain, and there is frequently pain when arising from a seated position. Patients with cam impingement may also have pain when squatting, cutting, or pivoting or when making sudden stops and starts. Stair climbing may also be problematic for patients with impingement. Patients may note the limited hip range of motion, particularly during flexion, adduction, and internal rotation. If the patient has an associated labral tear or a chondral flap, there may be an acute onset of symptoms as well as mechanical symptoms (e.g., locking, catching). It is not uncommon for patients to complain of hip or groin pain for years.

It is also not uncommon for patients to have had other surgeries that may not have relieved their symptoms. This may be

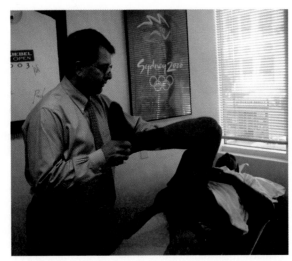

**Figure 19–6** Impingement test. The hip is flexed to 90 degrees, adducted, and internally rotated. The test is positive if pain is elicited. However, this test is not positive only in cases of femoroacetabular impingement.

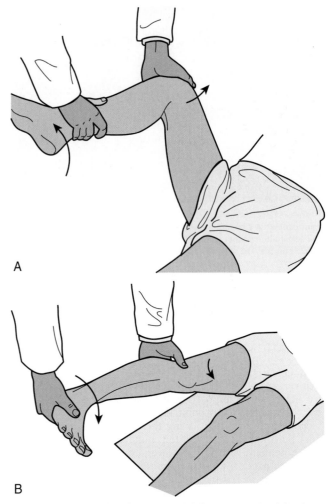

**Figure 19–7** The labral stress test: **A**, The supine patient's hip is brought to the position of flexion, abduction, and external rotation and **B**, then brought into extension, adduction, and internal rotation.

the result of radiating symptoms or the fact that cam impingement results in limited hip range of motion. The limited motion within the femoroacetabular joint may put stress on other structures, which may result in pain or injury in these remote locations as athletic patients try to get motion to perform their activities, such as the pubic symphysis (osteitis pubis), the sacroiliac joint (sacroiliac joint dysfunction), the lower back (strains, herniated disc), and the abdominal musculature (sports hernia/athletic pubalgia). As such, several patients have been successfully treated with arthroscopic FAI in my practice (and in other practices) who have had previous laparoscopy, laparotomy, inguinal hernia repair, athletic pubalgia surgery, osteitis pubis injections and surgery, orchiectomy, oophorectomy, lumbar spine injections, decompressions, diskectomies, and lumbar spine fusion.

Although a complete discussion of the evaluation of the hip is beyond the scope of this chapter, a brief discussion of the general concepts is appropriate. First, evaluation includes the inspection of the gait and of the skin around the hip. Patients are assessed for hip weakness and tightness with the use of the Trendelenburg and Ober tests. Hip range of motion is assessed while the patient is supine. Evaluation of hip adduction and abduction, as well as internal and external rotation, should be performed in hip flexion and extension. Also, hip motions evaluated include flexion, extension, and flexion contracture. There is usually limited hip internal rotation, particularly when the hip is in flexion, among patients with impingement. Furthermore, patients frequently have pain when the hip is flexed to 90 degrees, adducted, and internally rotated; this is known as the *impingement test* (Figure 19-6). The labral stress test and the resisted straight-leg raise are tests that commonly result in hip pain among patients with labral tears and symptomatic impingement (Figure 19-7). These tests are often positive among patients with both cam and pincer types of FAI, and they may also be positive among patients with other sources of intra-articular hip pain.

## IMAGING AND DIAGNOSTIC TESTS

Plain radiographs are extremely valuable for the assessment of patients with hip pain that is the result of hip impingement. The standard imaging series for patients with hip pain includes an anteroposterior pelvic view with the coccyx centered 1 cm to 3 cm above the pubic symphysis and a true

cross-table lateral radiograph (Figure 19-8). A frog-leg lateral view will demonstrate a lateral projection of the proximal femur and thus can be used for cam impingement assessment; however, this is not a lateral view of the acetabulum, so it has limited usefulness (see Figure 19-8, *B*). A cross-table lateral view, a Dunn view, and a modified Dunn view are true lateral views of the hip that can provide more information about the acetabulum (see Figure 19-8, *C*). The femoral head is generally symmetric, particularly the head–neck offset. A loss of the sphericity of the femoral head–neck region may be consistent with cam impingement (see Figure 19-8, *A* through *C*). This can be seen as a flattening of the concave surface of the lateral femoral neck and the appearance that the femoral head is not centered over the femoral neck. Leunig and colleagues demonstrated that, for patients with hip dysplasia, the apex of the femoral head is approximately 1 cm beyond the low point of the femoral neck, whereas in patients with impingement this distance was only 3 mm. In some situations, there may be a bump on the anterolateral surface of the femoral neck that may project beyond the femoral head or have a sharp transition or even a hook appearance at the head–neck junction. The alpha angle was originally described by Notzli and colleagues to quantify the head–neck offset on radially generated axial magnetic resonance imaging cuts of the femoral neck and head. These authors demonstrated that, in their normal population, the alpha angle averaged 42 degrees, whereas in those patients with impingement,

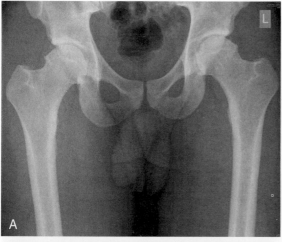

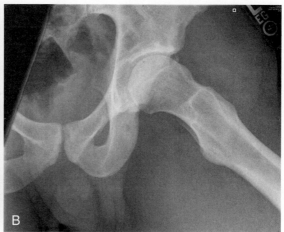

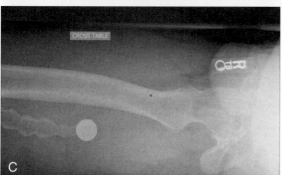

**Figure 19–8** Plain radiographs: anteroposterior pelvic and lateral views of a 22-year-old professional football player with cam impingement. **A,** Anteroposterior radiograph of the pelvis that demonstrates cam impingement. **B,** The frog-leg lateral view also shows the loss of the femoral head–neck offset. However, this view is not a lateral view of the acetabulum but only of the proximal femur. **C,** A true lateral view (this time of a collegiate lacrosse player). A Dunn view, or a modified Dunn lateral view may also be obtained.

this angle averaged 74 degrees. Most surgeons use 50 degrees or 55 degrees as their cutoff point for defining cam impingement. This angle has also been used when evaluating plain radiographs and computed tomography scans, although it has not been validated for these modalities. Additional plain radiographs may demonstrate a short femoral neck or a femoral neck–shaft angle that is varus, which may result in cam-type impingement. Untreated or residual deformity from SCFE or Legg-Calvé-Perthes disease may be seen on plain films, and this may result in cam impingement. Pincer impingement may also be seen on plain radiographs in association with coxa profunda, protrusio, retroversion, or

relative retroversion of the superior acetabulum and arthritic changes.

Computed tomography scans, particularly three-dimensional ones, are particularly useful for demonstrating the bony anatomy associated with cam impingement (Figure 19-9). Magnetic resonance imaging, particularly magnetic resonance arthrography, is beneficial for demonstrating the cam lesion by allowing for a way to measure the alpha angle and to demonstrate labral tears, edema, or cysts within the femoral neck (these are often seen with impingement); this type of imaging can occasionally demonstrate chondral lesions (Figure 19-10). Local anesthetic is usually introduced with the contrast used

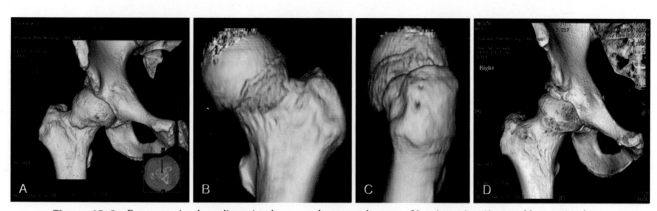

**Figure 19–9** Representative three-dimensional computed tomography scans of 3 patients: **A,** a 40-year-old recreational athlete; **B** and **C,** a 35-year-old world-class triathlete; and **D,** a 27-year-old recreational softball player. These images demonstrate the loss of the offset at the femoral head–neck junction, thus showing the usefulness of this type of scan for the identification of the extent of the cam lesion. Figure D also demonstrates an acetabular rim fracture seen with combined cam and pincer FAI.

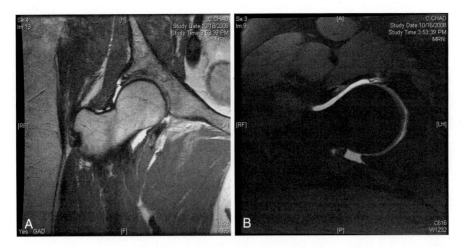

**Figure 19–10** **A,** Magnetic resonance arthrogram of a classic labrochondral separation in a patient with a cam lesion. **B,** Magnetic resonance arthrogram demonstrating an intrasubstance labral tear in a 32-year-old male laborer with combined FAI.

for magnetic resonance arthrography to determine whether the pain is temporarily relieved within the joint, which confirms the source of pain as being intra-articular.

## SURGICAL TECHNIQUE

The goals of surgery are to relieve the abutment between the femoral head–neck junction and the acetabular rim and to treat the associated pathology (i.e., labral tears and chondral lesions; Figure 19-11, *A* through *D*). Although this may be done with the patient in the supine or lateral position, my preference is the supine position, which is described in Chapter 9 of this book.

Surgery for cam impingement starts with the evaluation and treatment of pathology in the central compartment. With the patient lateralized relative to the perineal post and traction applied, the three standard central compartment portals—anterior, anterolateral, and posterolateral—are made. The anterolateral and posterolateral portals are the well-described portals that are made at the anterior and posterior margins just

proximal to the tip of the greater trochanter. The modified anterior portal that we have used for the past 3 years is 7 cm distal and anteromedial to the anterolateral portal at a 45-degree angle. This portal has been used for the following reasons: 1) it reduces the risk of injury to the lateral femoral cutaneous nerve; 2) it reduces the risk of postoperative rectus femoris tendonitis; and 3) it allows for a better approach to the joint if a labral repair becomes necessary. The entire joint is inspected with 70-degree and 30-degree lenses. All central compartment pathology is addressed before moving to the peripheral compartment to perform the cheilectomy or the femoral osteoplasty.

Chondral flaps are removed, and chondral defects and lesions are debrided to a stable edge. If the lesion is sufficiently large enough, a microfracture is performed (Figure 19-12, *A* through *C*). Our experience has been that femoral head chondral lesions do not do as well postoperatively as acetabular lesions do. However, when there are chondral lesions of the acetabular articular surface, the results of hip arthroscopy in general, including FAI surgery, are also less predictable as compared with patients in whom the articular cartilage is intact.

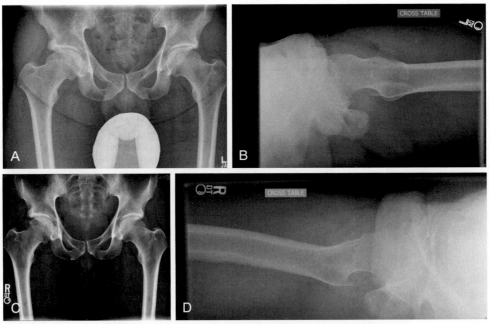

**Figure 19–11** **A,** Anteroposterior pelvic, and **B,** lateral hip radiograph of a 40-year-old engineer who had to give up martial arts as a result of hip pain. **C** and **D,** The same patient's postoperative radiographs 6 months after resection.

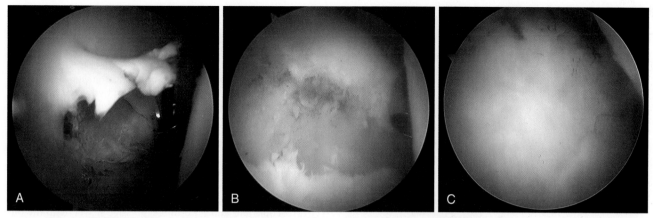

**Figure 19–12** The hip of a 32-year-old competitive triathlete. **A,** Chondral lesion at surgery with delamination of the articular cartilage. **B,** After microfracture. **C,** A second look 7 months after the initial surgery.

Labral tears are addressed next. If the labrum is intact and there is combined impingement, then an anterior portal at the junction of the anterosuperior iliac spine and the greater trochanter is made. An arthroscopic knife is then introduced to detach the labrum at the site of acetabular overcoverage or pincer impingement. A traction suture may be used to retract the detached labrum. The acetabuloplasty may then be performed with the use of a motorized burr. After other pathology has been addressed—including synovectomy, chondroplasty, and microfracture—the labrum is reattached with the use of suture anchors (Figure 19-13). If there is a labrochondral separation, which occurs more commonly with cam impingement, and if the labrum has minimal or no obvious intrasubstance damage, then this may be repaired with the use of suture anchors. Healing occurs from the acetabular bony blood supply and capsule. If there is significant intrasubstance damage and tearing of the labrum, then a partial labrectomy is carried out; there is limited blood supply within the labrum, and, as a result, the capacity to heal is limited. Partial labrectomy may be performed with the use of meniscal-type biters, shavers, or radiofrequency devices.

After the central compartment pathology has been addressed, attention is turned to the peripheral compartment and the cam lesion. This is performed with the traction taken off of the patient either by releasing the traction or taking the foot out of the traction boot altogether. The preferred technique on the fracture table is to keep the foot in the foot holder of the fracture table. The traction is removed to relax the capsuloligamentous structures, thus making the peripheral compartment more capacious and allowing for easier maneuverability.

Although many surgeons prefer to perform peripheral compartment arthroscopy with the hip flexed 20 degrees to 45 degrees to further relax the anterior capsule, I prefer to perform cam surgery decompression with the hip in neutral flexion and extension. When the extremity is in neutral flexion and extension, it is easier to get a truer fluoroscopic image, because the fluoroscope beam can be made perpendicular to the axis of the femur (Figure 19-14). Because fluoroscopy beams diverge, there is inherent distortion, which would be magnified if the central fluoroscopic beam is not perpendicular to the proximal femur; this may result in inadequate or excessive bony resection. While there are benefits to peripheral compartment arthroscopy in the neutral flexion-extension position, the trade-off, which the author accepts, is that it is necessary to perform a partial capsulectomy of the anterolateral capsule to allow for adequate visualization.

To perform peripheral compartment arthroscopy with the patient in the neutral flexion and extension position, the standard anterolateral portal is used along with a proximal antero-

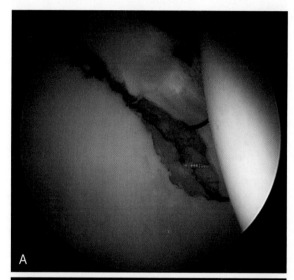

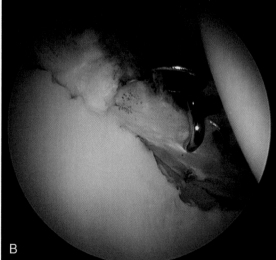

**Figure 19–13 A,** Labral tear and **B,** repair in a 29-year-old competitive marathon runner.

lateral portal that is 3 cm to 4 cm proximal to the standard anterolateral portal (Figure 19-15). The blunt trocar and the sheath for the arthroscopic camera are introduced via the anterolateral portal to the apex of the femoral head–neck deformity.

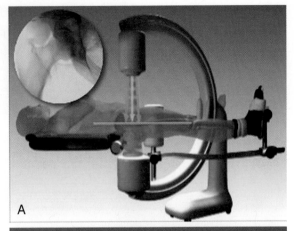

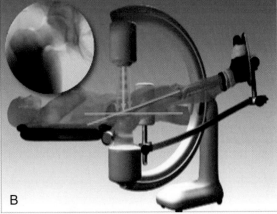

**Figure 19–14**  Comparison drawings of the fluoroscopic beam being perpendicular to the extremity versus the extremity being flexed. **A,** Because only the central beam in the fluoroscopic unit is truly perpendicular, maintaining the hip in neutral flexion and extension reduces the divergence and potential disorientation associated with **B,** performing the procedure with the hip in flexion with the fluoroscopic beam at an angular orientation.

The trochar is exchanged for the arthroscope within the cannula. The scope and cannula are maintained on the capsule and bone at the apex of the cam deformity. Next, the arthroscopic motorized shaver is introduced through the proximal anterolateral portal. With the use of triangulation, the shaver is brought to the tip of the camera in its sheath (Figure 19-16). At this point, the camera and the shaver are lying on the capsule directly over the apex of the bony deformity laterally; this is seen on the fluoroscopic monitor, which is projecting an anteroposterior view of the hip (see Figure 19-16). The shaver then is used to clear some of the soft tissue over the capsule. The shaver tip soon becomes visible, and the shaver is used to make a capsulotomy of the anterolateral capsule. This is enlarged as a partial capsulectomy to a size of 1 cm to 1.5 cm in diameter (Figure 19-17). This is generally performed with the use of a 30-degree arthroscopic lens and a 5.0-mm aggressive shaver, with the fluoroscopic monitor used for guidance. A radiofrequency device may also be used to perform the partial capsulectomy. Glick has shown that larger capsulectomies of the anterolateral capsule are safe and not associated with hip instability. Furthermore, he has shown that this capsule ultimately heals.

After the partial capsulectomy is completed, the shaver is introduced into the peripheral compartment. A partial synovectomy is performed to allow for the adequate visualization of the anterior, lateral, and posterior femoral head, with its cam deformity; the extra-articular acetabular rim; the labrum; and the capsular reflection on the acetabulum, in addition to many other peripheral compartment structures (see Figure 19-17). The lateral synovial fold with its retinacular vessels is also visualized, as is the medial synovial fold and the zona orbicularis. The hip can be flexed, adducted, and rotated to demonstrate the impingement arthroscopically, either with the traction boot attached to the fracture table or by removing it from the traction device.

With the use of a motorized burr, the femoral head–neck offset is restored when the surgeon removes the excessive bone. Not all cam impingement patients have the same anatomy, because the bumps differ: some may be lateral, some may be anterior, and most are anterolateral. Thus, the same operation (i.e., the location and amount of bone removed) is not performed on every patient. The surgery must be tailored to the

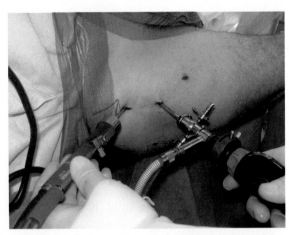

**Figure 19–15**  Patient supine with the head to the left and feet to the right. Notice the anterolateral portal (with the arthroscope in the cannula) and the proximal anterolateral portal with the arthroscopic shaver introduced into the portal. The modified anterior and posterolateral portal incisions can be seen without instrumentation placed in them.

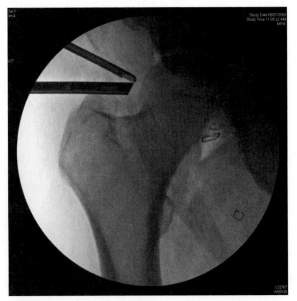

**Figure 19–16**  Fluoroscopic image of the trocar in the anterolateral portal and the shaver at the location of the maximal deformity.

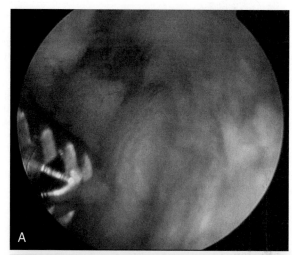

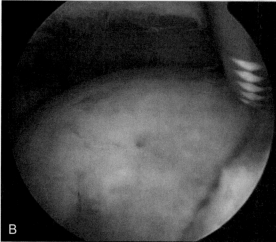

**Figure 19–17** Arthroscopic image **A,** of the shaver making the capsular window for cam decompression in a 20-year-old female collegiate soccer player. **B,** The view of the cam lesion after partial capsulectomy utilizing this approach.

patient's pathology. The goal is to restore the normal anatomy and offset for the patient (Figure 19-18). Bony resection and visualization may be enhanced by exchanging the scope with the shaver or burr so that the camera is introduced in the proximal anterolateral portal, whereas the burr is introduced from the standard anterolateral portal. The hip may be rotated, flexed, abducted, or adducted to help with bony resection.

The ideal amount of bone to resect has not been determined. Some clinicians start their resections 7 mm to 10 mm from the labral edge and work distally. However, to restore the alpha angle, one has to remove bone up to the labral edge. However, the removal of bone to the labral edge can result in the loss of the sealing function of the labrum. In addition, as is mentioned later in this chapter, the outcomes of decompression of the cam lesion do not correlate with the ability to restore the alpha angle to less than 50 degrees.

The amount of bone removed should be individualized on the basis of the patient's pathology. General guidelines suggest that the resection should be less than 1 cm deep, 8 mm from proximal to distal, and 15 mm from medial to lateral. Mardones and colleagues determined that the resection of more than 30% of the femoral neck width increases the risk of fracture of the femoral neck. Thus, resection is kept to less than 30% of the femoral neck width, and usually much less than that is necessary to eliminate the impingement. Sometimes the cam lesion is well circumscribed and demarcated, whereas other times it is not. Thus, fluoroscopy can help to identify the lesion and to assess how much bone is removed to avoid over-resection and increased risk of fracture. In addition, the hip may be dynamically assessed during the bony resection to ensure the adequacy of the bony resection.

Fortunately, cam lesions are almost exclusively anterior, anterolateral, or lateral. The blood supply to the femoral head, which is supplied by the posterior circumflex vessels, travels within the lateral synovial fold and the femoral neck posterolaterally, which is a safe distance from the resection (Figure 19-19). Injury to these vessels may result in avascular necrosis of the femoral head, although I am not aware of any reported cases of this condition after FAI surgery.

Occasionally cysts of the femoral head–neck junction are seen arthroscopically. These cysts, which were originally thought to be normal variants, are likely the result of the abutment of the femoral neck against the labrum; they are seen in a third of patients with FAI. Thus, the arthroscopic visualization and decompression of these femoral neck cysts help to confirm the location of the impingement and the adequacy of the bony resection (Figure 19-20).

Detailed descriptions of other techniques for cam resection are beyond the scope of this chapter. However, some considerations of other techniques will be discussed. Some clinicians prefer not to perform a partial capsulectomy. As a result, some surgeons position the hip in 20 degrees to 40 degrees of flexion. There are surgeons who perform the resection with the patient's hip in neutral rotation, and others prefer varying degrees of internal rotation with hip flexion. There are clinicians who perform a more extensive capsulotomy or capsulectomy that includes

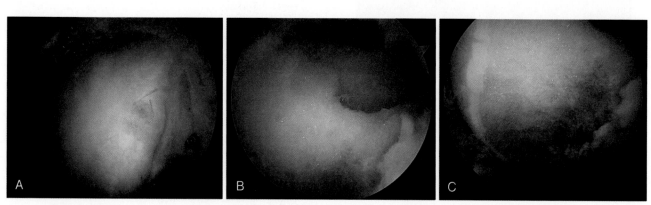

**Figure 19–18** Arthroscopic view **A,** before and **B** and **C,** after the resection of a cam lesion in a 21-year-old collegiate football player.

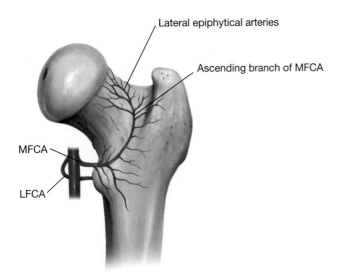

Lateral epiphytical arteries

Ascending branch of MFCA

MFCA

LFCA

**Figure 19–19** Drawing of the blood supply to the femoral head. Notice that the blood vessels from the lateral circumflex vessels enter the femoral head posterolaterally.

making an anterolateral longitudinal incision in the capsule initially and then making a transverse incision in the capsule at its acetabular insertion (i.e., essentially making a "T"). Some surgeons will start their hip arthroscopy in the peripheral compartment before entering the central compartment. By doing this, these surgeons may visualize the impingement first and address the cam lesion before entering the central compartment under arthroscopic visualization, which has the benefit of reducing the risk of iatrogenic labral damage. Other portals that can be used to address the peripheral compartment have also been described, including a distal anterolateral portal that is 7.5 cm distal to the anterolateral portal and an anterior portal that is one third of the distance from the anterosuperior iliac spine to the greater trochanter.

## TECHNICAL PEARLS

- The hip is the most difficult joint in which to perform arthroscopy, and there is a very steep learning curve.
- Femoral osteoplasty or cheilectomy should only be undertaken after the surgeon is comfortable performing central and peripheral compartment arthroscopy of the hip.
- In general, most of the complications of hip arthroscopy are related to patient positioning, traction, and fluid management.
- Be sure to adequately pad the compression points on the perineum and the feet.
- Compression of genitalia should always be avoided by careful positioning.
- Traction time should be limited to no more than 2 hours, although traction is not necessary when performing femoral neck osteoplasty or cheilectomy.
- Adequate traction is important to allow for appropriate maneuverability within the joint and to reduce the risk of iatrogenic damage to the articular cartilage and the labrum.
- Three-dimensional computed tomography scans can help to provide useful visualization of the three-dimensional relationships of the pathoanatomy of cam impingement.
- Adequate exposure of the deformity is mandatory.
- Partial capsulectomies and capsulotomies are necessary to expose deformities related to both cam and pincer FAI.
- The dynamic assessment of the peripheral compartment can help to confirm the diagnosis of cam impingement.
- The dynamic assessment of the peripheral compartment after resection, osteoplasty, or cheilectomy can help to confirm the adequacy of decompression.
- The judicious use of the fluoroscope, especially when learning this procedure, is helpful, because instrumentation movement in the peripheral compartment may be deceiving.
- Fluoroscopy is used to assist with navigating the depth of the resection and the extent of the lateral decompression on the femoral neck.
- A complete lateral decompression is important to avoid impingement in high degrees of motion.
- Although many surgeons perform peripheral compartment arthroscopy with the hip flexed to relax the anterior capsuloligamentous structures, this may distort the orientation of the structures of the hip. This is why I perform hip arthroscopy with the hip in neutral flexion and extension and why I make a 1-cm to 1.5-cm partial capsulectomy of the anterolateral capsule.
- Avoid femoral neck resection and dissection posterolaterally to reduce the risk of avascular necrosis.
- Resect only the deformity, and take care not to remove excessive bone. It is especially important not to remove more than 30% of the femoral neck, because doing so can increase the risk of femoral neck fracture.
- Individualize the resection to remove only the area of impingement; there are a variety of sizes and locations of cam lesions.

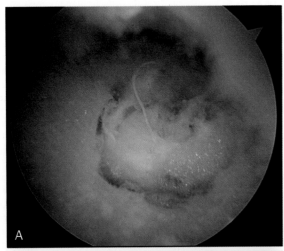

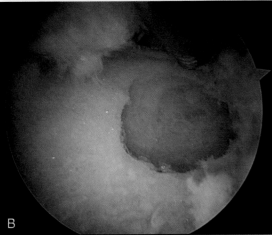

**Figure 19–20** Arthroscopic view of a cyst in the femoral neck **A,** before and **B,** after resection in a 30-year-old recreational athlete.

## POSTOPERATIVE REHABILITATION

There is very little science to guide postoperative rehabilitation after femoral osteoplasty or cheilectomy. Immediate full weight bearing after these arthroscopic procedures has been advocated by a minority of surgeons who also do not recommend physical therapy postoperatively. However, despite the work of Mardones, there have been isolated anecdotal reports of hip fracture after arthroscopic femoral osteoplasty or cheilectomy. It is my contention that postoperative stiffness and prolonged pain can be avoided by appropriate rehabilitation. As a result, I recommend a guided rehabilitation protocol that is advanced as patients reach particular milestones.

I recommend weight bearing to 20 lbs of force with crutches for 2 weeks after the procedure for most patients, provided that they have adequate bone quality and no concomitant microfracture. For women who are more than 39 years old and men who are more than 49 years old, I add an extra week of limited weight bearing per decade. We encourage early range-of-motion exercises, including the use of a continuous passive motion machine and passive circumduction exercises. Weight bearing occurs with the foot flat, because this reduces the amount of force across the hip and lessens the risk of hip flexor tendinitis. Rehabilitation includes range-of-motion exercises, stretching, and hip and core strengthening. Proprioception exercises are included early during the course of rehabilitation. The second phase of rehabilitation (usually the second month through the end of the third month) includes balance progression, stationary cycling with resistance, and increasing strength training, which includes double- and single-leg knee bends, side stepping, and elliptical training. During the fourth month, plyometrics are initiated and advanced, along with agility drills, running, and side-to-side movements. The goal is to return to sports participation between 4 and 6 months after surgery.

## RESULTS AND OUTCOMES

There have been only a few case series that have reported the results of hip arthroscopy for FAI, although the number of publications is growing rapidly. In fact, the number of patients and hips with FAI that have been treated arthroscopically is more than 800, which exceeds the number addressed in the literature regarding the open treatment of FAI. Although many of the early studies report the results of cam decompression, this is because arthroscopic acetabuloplasty techniques lagged behind. Unfortunately, most studies include patients with cam, pincer, or both types of impingements, and the outcomes and results are not differentiated. As noted previously, arthroscopic labral debridement in the setting of FAI in which the FAI is not treated does not have good results. The evaluation of the results of any procedure involving the nonarthritic hip suffers from the lack of an adequate, patient-generated, validated outcomes scale or score.

Philippon has shown that an alpha angle of more than 62 degrees correlates with chondral injury at the time of arthroscopy. However, Stähelin and colleagues and Brunner and colleagues have both reported that the outcomes of FAI surgery do not correlate with the clinical outcomes. This is not surprising, because the resection of the bone from the femoral head–neck region must be at the level of the labrum with the hip in neutral flexion and extension to restore the alpha angle for an anteriorly based loss of offset. By removing this much bone, the labrum loses its sealing effect. In addition, as noted previously, not all cam lesions are the same. The alpha angle measures the loss of anterior femoral head–neck offset, but, in reality, not all cam lesions are the same: some involve a loss of lateral offset, some are anterior, and some demonstrate both conditions; thus, the alpha angle measurement does not encompass the full extent of the pathology.

Table 19-1 reports the results of the arthroscopic treatment of FAI. A common theme that correlates with the results of the open surgical treatment studies is that concomitant chondral

---

**Table 19-1** ARTHROSCOPIC RESULTS

| Author | No. of Patients | Length of Follow Up | Results |
|---|---|---|---|
| Sampson, 2006 | 183 (194 hips) | Up to 29 months | 94% eliminated impingement sign; 3% THR; 1% fracture |
| Guanche and Bare, 2006 | 10 | 16 months | 80% good to excellent results |
| Philippon et al., 2007 | 45 athletes | 1.6 years | 93% returned to sports, with 78% still active at 20 months' follow up; 3 developed osteoarthritis |
| Philippon et al., 2009 | 112: 23 cam, 3 pincer, and 86 combined | 2.3 years | HHS improved from 58 to 84; 90% of patients satisfied with results; 10 patients progressed to THR at a mean of 16 months (range, 8 to 26 months); patients with better outcomes had higher preoperative HHS, joint space of 2 mm or more, and labral repair (versus debridement) |
| Larson and Giveans, 2008 | 96 (100 hips): 17 cam and 55 combined | 9.9 months | 75% of patients had good to excellent results; HHS improved from 61 to 83; SF-12 improved from 60 to 78; 3% of patients progressed to THR |
| Larson and Giveans, 2009 | 75 pincer and combined hips: 36 debrided and 39 refixated | 19 months: 21.4 months for debridement and 16.5 months for refixation | HHS with debridement, 88.9; HHS with refixation, 94.3; most recent follow up showed good to excellent results for 66.7% of debridement patients and 89.7% of refixation patients |
| Ilizaliturri et al., 2007 | 14 children | 30 months | WOMAC score improved from 78 to 87 |
| Ilizaliturri et al., 2008 | 19 | 24 months | 84% of patients improved; 100% had an alpha angle of less than 45 degrees after treatment |
| Stähelin et al., 2008 | 22 | 6 months | Pain score improved from 5.8 to 1.4; VAS improved from 49 to 74 |

*Continued*

**Table 19-1** ARTHROSCOPIC RESULTS—Cont'd

| Author | No. of Patients | Length of Follow Up | Results |
|---|---|---|---|
| Bardakos and Villar, 2008 | 71: 24 with cam treated plus debridement and 47 with cam not treated other than debridement | 1 year | HHS was 83 in cam-treated patients (versus 77; $P = .11$); good to excellent results were seen in 83% of treated versus 60% of debridement-only patients ($P = .043$) |
| Brunner et al. 2009 | 53 cam and combined hips | 2.4 years | Sports Frequency Score improved from 0.78 to 1.84; VAS improved from 5.7 to 1.5; NAHS improved from 54 to 86; patients were able to return to biking, hiking, and other fitness activities |
| Byrd and Jones, 2009 | 200 (207 hips): 163 cam and 44 combined | 16 months | HHS for cam patients improved 20 points (range –17 to 60); 83% of patients improved; in combination patients, there was a 19-point improvement (range, –15 to 49); MFx improved by 20 points (range, –17 to 58); there was 1 THR at 8 months and 3 reoperations for mech sx: 1 pudendal nn, 1 LFCN, and 1 HO |

*THR*, Total hip replacement; *HHS*, Harris Hip Score; *SF-12*, Short Form 12; *WOMAC*, Western Ontario McMasters Arthritis Scale; *VAS*, Visual Analogue Scale; *NAHS*, Non-arthritic Hip Score; *MFx*, microfracture; *mech sx*-mechanical symptoms; *nn*, nerve; *LFCN*, lateral femoral cutaneous nerve; *HO*, heterotopic ossification.

damage—and particularly arthritis—is a poor prognostic finding, with a larger proportion of failures occurring in this group of patients.

## COMPLICATIONS

In general, complications related to hip arthroscopy are related to traction: too much or too little, patient positioning, and fluid management. Complication rates are between 1.4% and 5.5%. Reported complications include the inability to perform the arthroscopy as a result of access issues in addition to neuropraxias of the sciatic, femoral perineal, pudendal, and lateral femoral cutaneous nerves that often resolve spontaneously. Also reported are infections, hematomas, portal bleeding, intra-articular instrument breakage, and vaginal tears and scrotal necrosis related to excessive lateral traction force. There have been several reported cases of intra-abdominal fluid extravasation, in addition to reports of avascular necrosis (not associated with FAI surgery). Heterotopic ossification has also been noted, including after FAI surgery. Labral repairs may not heal, and, in some cases, labral repairs have been associated with capsular adhesions postoperatively, which may limit motion and cause pain. Probably the most common complications that are under-reported are iatrogenic articular cartilage damage and labral injury. Although they have not been reported in the literature, deep venous thrombosis and pulmonary embolism related to hip arthroscopy have been anecdotally discussed among surgeons and at meetings and presentations where case series are presented along with their complications.

Complications related to the arthroscopic treatment of FAI include femoral neck fractures related to the over-resection of the femoral neck when treating cam impingement. Mardones and colleagues noted that the risk for femoral neck fracture is increased when the resection exceeds 30% of the femoral neck; thus, keeping the resection to less than that amount may reduce the associated risk. Another risk is the under-resection of the femoral neck, which results in the incomplete reshaping of the FAI deformity. This is also likely to be under-reported, although the exact amount and location from which to remove it still have not been defined. Although the main blood supply to the femoral head ascends on the posterolateral femoral neck, thus making it susceptible to injury during femoral osteoplasty, the cam lesion tends to occur anterolaterally and thus not in the region of the blood vessels. Nonetheless, avascular necrosis after the treatment of femoroacetabular impingement (FAI) is a potential concern, although no actual cases of the condition after FAI surgery have been reported. There is a concern that the anterior hip capsulotomy or capsulectomy may simulate injury to the iliofemoral ligament and result in hip instability; however, this phenomenon has not been reported in the literature.

## ANNOTATED REFERENCES AND SUGGESTED READINGS

**Bardakos NV, Vanconcelos JC, Villar RN. Early outcome of hip arthroscopy for femoroacetabular impingement: the role of femoral osteoplasty in symptomatic improvement.** *J Bone Joint Surg.* 2008;90(B):1570–1575.

This article compares the outcomes of 71 patients with cam-type FAI: 24 had arthroscopic resection of the cam lesion to restore the femoral headneck offset with debridement, whereas 47 age-matched patients only had arthroscopic debridement labral surgery. At 1 year of follow up, there was a trend toward better outcomes (as measured by the Harris Hip Score) in the osteoplasty group, and a higher proportion of those in the osteoplasty group had good to excellent results. Thus, at 1 year, patients with cam-type FAI tended to do better when the osteoplasty was performed in addition to arthroscopic debridement.

**Bardakos NV, Villar RN. Predictors of progression of osteoarthritis in femoroacetabular impingement. A radiological study with a minimum of ten years.** *J Bone Joint Surg.* 2009;91(B):162–169.

**Bartlett CS, DiFelice GS, Buly RL, Quinn TJ, Green DS, Helfet DL. Cardiac arrest as a result of intraabdominal extravasation of fluid during arthroscopic removal of a loose body from the hip joint of a patient with an acetabular fracture.** *J Orthop Trauma.* 1998;12:294–299.

**Beaule PE, Zaragoza E, Motamedi K, Copeland N, Dorey FJ. Three dimensional computed tomography of the hip in the assessment of femoroacetabular impingement.** *J Orthop Res.* 2006;23:1286–1292.

**Beck M, Kalhor M, Leunig M, Ganz R. Hip morphology influences the pattern of damage to the acetabular cartilage.** *J Bone Joint Surg.* 2005;87B:1012–1018.

**Beck M, Leunig M, Parvizi J, Boutier V, Wyss D, Ganz R. Anterior femoroacetabular impingement: Part II. Midterm results of surgical treatment.** *Clin Orthop Relat Res.* 2004;418:67–73.

**Brunner A, Horisberger M, Herzog RF. Evaluation of a computed tomography–based navigation system prototype for hip arthroscopy in the treatment of femoroacetabular cam impingement.** *Arthroscopy.* 2009;25:382–391.

**Byrd JW, Jones KS. Arthroscopic femoroplasty in the management of cam-type femoroacetabular impingement. *Clin Orthop Relat Res*. 2009;467:739–746.**

This article reports the outcomes of the arthroscopic treatment of cam-type FAI in 200 patients (207 hips) with a minimum 1 year of follow up (mean, 16 months). There was an average increase in the modified Harris Hip Score of 20 points, regardless of whether there was associated microfracture. There was a 1.5% complication rate, and 0.5% of patients underwent total hip replacements. This article confirms the efficacy of the arthroscopic restoration of the femoral head–neck offset.

**Byrd JW, Jones KS. Prospective analysis of hip arthroscopy with 2-year follow-up. *Arthroscopy*. 2000;16:578–587.**

**Clarke MT, Arora A, Villar RN. Hip arthroscopy: complications in 1054 cases. *Clin Orthop Relat Res*. 2003;406:84–88.**

**Funke EL, Munzinger U. Complications in hip arthroscopy. *Arthroscopy*. 1996;12:156–159.**

**Ganz R, Gill TJ, Gautier E, et al. Surgical dislocation of the adult hip: a technique with full access to femoral head and acetabulum without the risk of avascular necrosis. *J Bone Joint Surg*. 2001;83-B:1119–1124.**

**Ganz R, Parvizi J, Beck M, Leunig M, Notzli H, Siebenrock K. Femoroacetabular impingement: a cause for osteoarthritis of the hip. *Clin Orthop Relat Res*. 2003;417:112–120.**

**Glick JM. Complications of hip arthroscopy by the lateral approach. In: Sherman OH, Minkoff J, eds. *Current management of orthopaedics: arthroscopic surgery*. Baltimore: Williams & Wilkins; 1990:1–9.**

**Goodman DA, Feighan JE, Smith AD, Latimer B, et al. Subclinical slipped capital femoral epiphysis. *J Bone Joint Surg*. 1997;79A:1489–1497.**

**Guanche CA, Bare AA. Arthroscopic treatment of femoroacetabular impingement. *Arthroscopy*. 2006;22:95–106.**

This is one of the earliest articles about the arthroscopic management of cam impingement. These authors report about the technique and the results of treatment of 10 patients with 16 months of follow up. The 8 patients without degenerative joint disease had better outcomes than the 2 patients with arthritic changes.

**Haupt U, Volkle D, Waldherr C, Beck M. Intra- and retroperitoneal irrigation liquid after arthroscopy of the hip joint. *Arthroscopy*. 2008;24:966–968.**

**Ilizaliturri Jr VM, Nossa-Barrera JM, Acosta-Rodriguez E, Camacho-Galindo J. Arthroscopic treatment of femoroacetabular impingement secondary to paediatric hip disorders. *J Bone Joint Surg Br*. 2007;89(B):1025–1030.**

This article reviews the results of 13 patients (14 hips) who underwent the arthroscopic treatment of FAI as a result of residual deformity after pediatric hip disease. These 7 women and 6 men with a mean age of 30.6 years improved clinically (WOMAC) and radiographically after a mean follow-up time of 2.5 years. Thirteen hips experienced the successful restoration of the normal geometry radiographically, whereas only one had a residual deformity. The mean increase in the Western Ontario McMasters Osteoarthritis Index for the series at the last follow up was 9.6 points (range, 4 to 14). No patient developed avascular necrosis, sustained a fracture of the femoral neck, or had any other complication.

**Ilizaliturri Jr VM, Orozco-Rodriguez L, Acosta-Rodríguez E, Camacho-Galindo J. Arthroscopic treatment of cam-type femoroacetabular impingement: preliminary report at 2 years minimum follow-up. *J Arthroplasty*. 2008;23:226–234.**

This article describes the results of the arthroscopic treatment of cam impingement in 19 patients. Sixteen patients had improved symptoms after the procedure, whereas 3 patients deteriorated, with 1 requiring total hip arthroplasty at 2 years' follow up. There were no complications.

**Ito K, Minka MA II, Leunig M, Werlen S, Ganz R. Femoroacetabular impingement and the cam-effect. An MRI-based quantitative anatomical study of the femoral head-neck offset. *J Bone Joint Surg*. 2001;83B:171–176.**

**Jäger M, Wild A, Westhoff B, Krauspe R: Femoroacetabular impingement caused by a femoral osseous head–neck bump deformity: clinical, radiological, and experimental results. *J Orthop Sci*. 2004;9:256–263.**

**Johnston TL, Schenker ML, Briggs KK, Philippon MJ. Relationship between offset angle alpha and hip chondral injury in femoroacetabular impingement. *Arthroscopy*. 2008;24:669–675.**

**Kim KC, Hwang DS, Lee CH, Kwon ST. Influence of femoroacetabular impingement on results of hip arthroscopy in patients with early osteoarthritis. *Clin Orthop Relat Res*. 2006;456:128–132.**

**Kim YT, Azuma H. The nerve endings of the acetabular labrum. *Clin Orthop Relat Res*. 1995;320:176–181.**

**Larson CM, Giveans MR. Arthroscopic debridement versus refixation of the acetabular labrum associated with femoroacetabular impingement. *Arthroscopy*. 2009;25:369–376.**

This article describes a sequential series of patients who underwent arthroscopic treatment for pincer and combined cam and pincer types of FAI with 1 year of follow up. Thirty-six of the hips underwent labral debridement and were followed for an average 21 months, whereas 39 had labral refixation and were followed for an average of 16.5 months. The modified Harris Hip Score was higher in the labral refixation group at 1 year, and, at the most recent follow up, a greater proportion of patients with labral fixation reported good to excellent results as compared with the labral debridement group.

**Larson CM, Giveans MR. Arthroscopic management of femoroacetabular impingement: early outcomes measures. *Arthroscopy*. 2008;24:540–546.**

These authors report their early results of arthroscopic management of FAI in 100 hips (96 patients), with an average follow up of 9.9 months. Isolated cam impingement was identified in 17 hips, pincer impingement was found in 28 hips, and both types were noted in 55 hips. Thirty hips underwent labral repair and refixation. There was significant improvement seen with all outcome measures that were used: the Harris Hip Score, the Short Form 12, a visual analog score for pain, and the impingement test. Good to excellent results were observed in 75% of hips at a minimum of 1 year of follow up. The alpha angle was also significantly improved after resection osteoplasty. Complications included heterotopic bone formation (6 hips) and a 24-hour partial sciatic nerve neurapraxia (1 hip).

**Lavigne M, Parvizi J, Beck M, Siebenrock KA, Ganz R, Leunig M. Anterior femoroacetabular impingement. Part I. techniques of joint preserving surgery. *Clin Orthop Relat Res*. 2004;418:61–66.**

**Leunig M, Beck M, Kalhor M, Kim Y, Werlen S, Ganz R. Fibrocystic changes at anterosuperior femoral neck: prevalence in hips with femoroacetabular impingement. *Radiology*. 2005;236:237–246.**

**Leunig M, Podeszwa D, Beck M, Werlen S, Ganz R. Magnetic resonance arthrography of labral disorders in hips with dysplasia and impingement. *Clin Orthop Relat Res*. 2004;418:74–80.**

**Mardones RM, Gonzalez C, Chen Q, Zobitz M, Kaufman KR, Trousdale RT. Surgical treatment of femoroacetabular impingement: evaluation of the effect of the size of the resection. *J Bone Joint Surg*. 2005;87(A):273–279.**

**Murray RO. The aetiology of primary osteoarthritis of the hip. *Br J Radiol*. 1965;38:810–824.**

Myers SR, Eijer H, Ganz R. Anterior femoroacetabular impingement after periacetabular osteotomy. *Clin Orthop Relat Res.* 1999;363:81–92.

Nötzli HP, Wyss TF, Stoecklin CH, Schmid MR, Treiber K, Hodler J. The contour of the femoral head–neck junction as a predictor for the risk of anterior impingement. *J Bone Joint Surg.* 2002;84B:556–560.

Philippon MJ, Briggs KK, Yen YM, Kuppersmith DA. Outcomes following hip arthroscopy for femoroacetabular impingement with associated chondrolabral dysfunction: minimum two-year follow-up. *J Bone Joint Surg.* 2009;91(B):16–23.

These authors prospectively studied 112 patients who underwent arthroscopic surgery of the hip for FAI. Twenty-three patients underwent osteoplasty only for cam impingement, 3 underwent rim trimming only for pincer impingement, and 86 underwent both procedures for mixed-type impingement. The mean length of follow up was 2.3 years (range, 2.0 to 2.9 years). The mean modified Harris Hip Score improved 26 points, although 10 patients underwent total hip replacement at a mean of 16 months (range, 8 to 26 months) after arthroscopy. Predictors of a better outcome were the preoperative modified Harris Hip Score, joint space of 2 mm or more, and repair of labral pathology rather than debridement.

Philippon MJ, Maxwell RB, Johnston TL, Schenker M, Briggs KK. Clinical presentation of femoroacetabular impingement. *Knee Surg Sports Traumatol Arthrosc.* 2007;15:1041–1047.

Philippon M, Schenker M, Briggs K, Kuppersmith D. Femoroacetabular impingement in 45 professional athletes: associated pathologies and return to sport following arthroscopic decompression. *Knee Surg Sports Traumatol Arthrosc.* 2007;15:908–914.

Safran MR. Evaluation of the hip: history, physical examination and imaging. *Op Tech Orthop Sports Med.* 2005;13:2–12.

Sampson TG. Arthroscopic treatment of femoroacetabular impingement: a proposed technique with clinical experience. *Instr Course Lect.* 2006;55:337–346.

Sampson TG. Complications of hip arthroscopy. *Clin Sports Med.* 2001;20:831–835.

Sharma A, Sachdev H, Gomillion M. Abdominal compartment syndrome during hip arthroscopy. *Anesthesia.* 2009;64:567–569.

Stähelin L, Stähelin T, Jolles BM, Herzog RF. Arthroscopic offset restoration in femoroacetabular cam impingement: accuracy and early clinical outcome. *Arthroscopy.* 2008;24:51–57.

This article reports the results of 22 patients treated with the arthroscopic decompression of their symptomatic cam lesions. The authors noted that the alpha angle improved from a mean of 75 degrees to 54 degrees, although resection to "normal" alpha angles did not correlate with outcome. Hip range of motion increased in both internal rotation and flexion by 17 degrees. The pain score decreased, whereas the Non-arthritic Hip Score increased. Patients with early osteoarthritis did substantially worse than those without it.

Stulberg SD, Cordell LD, Harris WH, Ramsey PL, MacEwen GD. Unrecognized childhood hip disease: a major cause of idiopathic osteoarthritis of the hip. In: *The Hip: Proceedings of the Third Open Scientific Meeting of the Hip Society.* St. Louis, MO: CV Mosby; 1975:212–228.

Sussmann PS, Ranawat AS, Lipman J, Lorich DG, Padgett DE, Kelly BT. Arthroscopic versus open osteoplasty of the head-neck junction: a cadaveric investigation. *Arthroscopy.* 2007;23:1257–1264.

Tanzer M, Noiseux N. Osseous abnormalities and early osteoarthritis. The role of hip impingement. *Clin Orthop Relat Res.* 2004;29:170–177.

Wagner S, Hofstetter W, Chiquet M, et al. Early osteoarthritic changes of human femoral head cartilage subsequent to femoro-acetabular impingement. *Osteoarthritis Cartilage.* 2003;11:508–518.

Wenger DE, Kendell KR, Miner MR, Trousdale RT. Acetabular labral tears rarely occur in the absence of bony abnormalities. *Clin Orthop Relat Res.* 2004;426:145–150.

Wyss TF, Clark JM, Weishaupt D, Nötzli HP. Correlation between internal rotation and bony anatomy in the hip. *Clin Orthop Relat Res.* 2007;460:152–158.

# CHAPTER 20

# Arthroscopic Rim Resection and Labral Repair

*Marc J. Philippon, Chad T. Zehms, Karen K. Briggs, and David A. Kuppersmith*

## INTRODUCTION

Advances in arthroscopic techniques and the tools available have made hip arthroscopy an increasingly attractive alternative to longer, more invasive open approaches to address pathology within the hip joint. In particular, the challenges of femoroacetabular impingement have brought hip arthroscopy to the forefront of the current orthopedic literature in an attempt to address both the soft tissue and the bony pathology involved with this difficult diagnosis. Several authors have published their techniques, and their short-term results have demonstrated the efficacy of this approach. However, further efforts need to be made to make arthroscopic labral repair and femoroacetabular impingement surgery a further refined and more reproducible procedure.

The main controversy regarding the treatment of femoroacetabular impingement is whether it can be addressed more effectively with an open dislocation of the hip joint or with less invasive arthroscopic techniques. The work of Ganz and others has demonstrated excellent results with open dislocation. However, the morbidity associated with this procedure—in addition to the possible risks associated with the tenuous blood supply to the femoral head—in our opinion makes an open dislocation unnecessarily risky when considering recent improvements in arthroscopic techniques.

The purpose of this chapter is to discuss in detail the technique of labral repair and rim trimming in the setting of femoroacetabular impingement. Our goals are to describe our unique approach to this challenging diagnosis and to offer the orthopedic surgeon new tools with which to return patients and athletes to their daily lives and to their respective sports.

## INDICATIONS

Proper patient selection is the key to excellent outcomes. There are no absolute indications for rim resection and labral repair. However, it is important that any pathologic findings on plain radiographs or magnetic resonance images be correlated with the findings of the physical examination to determine the true cause of the patient's pain and dysfunction. The typical patients who undergo rim resection are those with coxa profunda or a relative retroversion to the acetabulum. These patients have either an acetabulum that is too deep and thus restrictive to motion or an abnormal amount of bone at the anterior lip of the acetabulum. The radiographic findings that demonstrate these two distinct pathologies will be discussed later in this chapter. These two patient populations have pincer-type impingement, and it can only be addressed by the resection of bone from the acetabular rim.

For labral repair, the indications are more varied. Labral tears can be caused by relatively minor to very extreme trauma. In the setting of pincer impingement, it is common to find a labral tear at the site of the excessive bone on the acetabulum. After this bone has been removed, it will be necessary to reattach the labrum to the acetabular rim. However, there are those cases in which a full-thickness tear of the labrum has not yet occurred; it is still possible to see dysfunction of the chondrolabral junction in these patients. In this setting, it is necessary to create a separation at the chondrolabral junction to remove the excessive acetabular bone.

The final indication would be the presence of an os acetabuli or a rim fracture at the acetabular rim. This piece of bone can either become painful itself as it moves with hip motion, or it can become fixed in place and create an external impingement source to the hip joint. There is debate among experts in the field regarding whether resection or fixation is the adequate approach in this patient population. The decision about which approach to use is typically made at the time of surgery, when the fragment of bone can be probed and evaluated in the natural environment of the hip joint.

## BRIEF HISTORY AND PHYSICAL EXAMINATION

The patient with pincer impingement or a labral tear may have had a multitude of varying diagnoses before the current evaluation. Typical patients will have prior diagnoses of sciatica, sports hernia, piriformis syndrome, coxa saltans, or various lumbar spine pathologies. It is important to elucidate from the patient the nature and quality of the pain when he or she first noticed his or her symptoms, any exacerbating conditions or positions, and his or her response to previous treatments. Each of these questions will help the surgeon to zero in on the cause of the patient's pain and dysfunction.

The physical examination is very important and very effective for determining the source of the patient's symptoms. First, an evaluation of the patient's lumbar spine and a focused neurologic evaluation should be performed; this allows the surgeon to rule out any non-hip pathologies that could be causing the patient's pain. In our practice, we then perform a series of tests that address the range of motion and strength of the musculature around the hip. It is common to see a reduction of internal rotation and pain during testing among patients with impingement. In addition, we will perform anterior and posterior impingement tests to further stress the labrum and to determine if there is a tear present. Finally, we will perform a hip dial test to determine the integrity of the anterior capsule and the iliofemoral ligament. With the patient in a supine position, we will evaluate the position of the lower extremity with respect to the long axis of the body. By pressing on the inside of the patient's foot and watching for rebound, we can determine how tight or lax this capsular tissue has become.

It is very important with any of these provocative tests to determine whether the pain that the patient is experiencing is the same pain that has brought that patient to your clinic. One effective way that this can be accomplished is to perform a lidocaine and Kenalog injection in the office. After sterile preparation, an 18-gauge spinal needle is placed within the hip capsule, and the steroid and lidocaine mixture is administered. After approximately 5 minutes, we repeat the physical examination tests and quantify the improvement in the patients' symptoms. This is typically diagnostic, and it can also be therapeutic during the time that the patient is awaiting surgical intervention.

## TECHNIQUE

All of our arthroscopic hip techniques are performed with the patient in the supine position. After a lumbar plexus block and a general anesthetic are administered to the patient, we are very meticulous with our setup. The patients' feet are wrapped in protective boots and placed in leather foot holders at the foot of the bed. Each lower extremity is attached to a bar that is freely mobile for abduction, adduction, flexion, and extension. The nonoperative extremity is placed in approximately 60 degrees of abduction, whereas the operative extremity will eventually be placed in neutral abduction. Before the feet are wrapped, electromyography monitors are placed near the tibial nerve for continuous monitoring during the procedure. After baseline signals are achieved, we are ready to begin the distraction of the operative extremity for optimal portal site placement. A C-arm fluoroscopy device is used to verify the amount of joint distraction that is achieved. The foot is internally rotated 90 degrees and then locked in place; this allows us to place the proximal femur nearly parallel with the floor. After the radiographic verification of adequate distraction is attained, we remove the C-arm and prepare the patient in a standardized fashion. A picture of our standard setup is shown in Figure 20-1.

Our portal placement has evolved after extensive experience with hip arthroscopy and the complications that can be related to portal placement. Although our lateral portal has remained mostly unchanged, we have changed the position of the standard anterior portal in an attempt to reduce the morbidity associated with the rectus muscles and the nearby nerves. In particular, the

lateral femoral cutaneous nerve and the smaller branches of the femoral nerve can potentially be irritated by the close proximity of the anterior portal.

We draw out specific landmarks on the patient's leg to properly identify the ideal location for our portals. The anterosuperior iliac spine and the outline of the greater trochanter are the most important of these landmarks. From the tip of the greater trochanter, we measure proximally 1 cm and anteriorly 1 cm; this is the ideal location for our lateral portal. From that site, we measure a distance between 5 cm and 6 cm distal and anterior on a 60-degree plane from horizontal for the placement of our unique mid-anterior portal (Figure 20-2). In our experience, these two portals are all that are necessary to achieve the adequate visualization of the most important aspects of both the central and peripheral compartments of the hip joint. We have also substantially reduced the morbidity associated with portal placement over the past year with the new position of our mid-anterior portal.

After our surgical team performs our standardized timeout for proper extremity identification, a No. 11 blade is used to incise the previously marked incision sites for our two portals. We place a standard hip arthroscopy needle into the hip joint through our lateral incision first. The needle is directed 20 degrees inferior and 20 degrees caudal for optimal placement within the central compartment. We no longer use C-arm fluoroscopy for this portion of the procedure; however, during the learning curve portion of hip arthroscopy, it may be useful to verify the position of the needle before entry into the hip joint while you are becoming comfortable with the procedure to lessen the chance that the femoral head or the labrum will be violated during needle placement. After the needle is placed within the hip joint, we insufflate the joint with approximately 30 ml

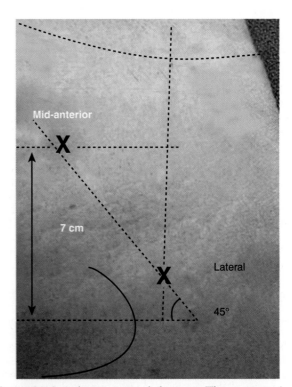

**Figure 20-2** Arthroscopic portal placement. The anterosuperior iliac spine and the outline of the greater trochanter are shown at the top and bottom of the image. A line is drawn through the tip of the greater trochanter. The lateral portal is placed 1 cm proximal from the greater trochanter and 1 cm superior. The mid-anterior portal is placed 5 cm to 7 cm distal to the lateral portal and at an angle of 45 degrees to 60 degrees from the longitudinal axis of the leg.

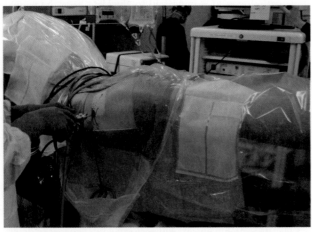

**Figure 20-1** Operative setup and patient positioning.

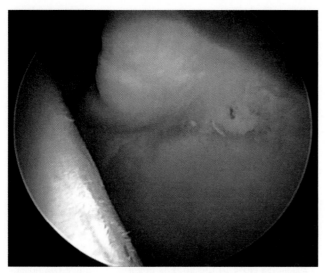

**Figure 20–3** Chondrolabral dysfunction "wave sign."

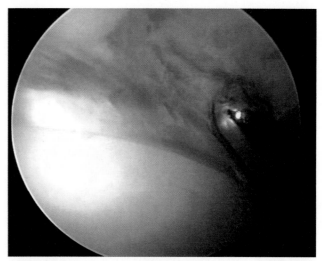

**Figure 20–4** Bruised acetabular labrum with associated pincer impingement.

of sterile fluid. We can positively identify the position within the hip joint by the presence of a sudden increase in pressure after an adequate amount of fluid is placed. The brisk outflow of fluid from the needle verifies needle placement. A guidewire is placed through the needle, and a 5-mm cannula is passed over the Nitinol wire. After the arthroscope is introduced into the hip joint through the lateral cannula, we place the mid-anterior portal with the use of direct visualization to lessen the risk of the cartilage of the femoral head and the labrum being violated. In our experience, C-arm fluoroscopy is not helpful during the placement of the mid-anterior portal.

Now that we have established a portal for the arthroscope and a working portal, we can begin the diagnostic portion of the arthroscopy to visualize all aspects of both the central and peripheral compartments. Our attention is first directed to the chondrolabral junction. We use a probe to determine if there are any areas in which the labrum has been separated from the acetabular rim. It is typical with cam-type impingement to see delamination of the acetabular cartilage at the site of the labral detachment. With the use of the blunt end of a shaver or with a probe, it is possible to see a "wave sign": the cartilage will buckle at sites where the labrum is damaged but not yet detached from the acetabular rim (Figure 20-3). It is very important to inspect these areas carefully. If they are not addressed at the time of the initial surgery, they can be the source of recurrent pain and disability as the junction between the labrum and the delaminated cartilage degenerates.

Before we perform our rim trimming and any necessary labral work, we measure the distance from the cotyloid fossa to the acetabular rim at the 3, 6, and 9 o'clock positions. We also measure the labral width at these three positions. This information, in combination with our preoperative x-rays and the measurement of the center-edge angle, provide us with a roadmap for our rim resection and the subsequent labral repair. Attention to detail during this portion of the procedure is essential to avoid the over- or under-resection of bone during the preparation of the acetabular rim.

## RIM TRIMMING

The typical pincer lesion is produced as a result of an abnormal growth of bone at the anterosuperior portion of the acetabulum (Figure 20-4). The pincer can be either primary or secondary to the chronic abutment of the femoral neck on the acetabular rim.

With respect to the normal anatomy and position of the acetabulum, this area creates a relative retroversion to the acetabulum. The x-rays in Figure 20-5 show this crossover sign. This is an area in which the anterior wall is farther lateral than the posterior acetabular rim. The goals of the rim resection should be to remove this area of bone and to restore the normal anatomy and relative position of the acetabulum with respect to the pelvis and the femoral neck. If this area is not addressed, subsequent labral damage and delamination of the cartilage will continue. Typically, this anterosuperior region of the acetabular rim also corresponds with the area of labral pathology. If the tear does not extend to this region, it is necessary to detach the labrum at this site for the proper resection of bone. After this has been completed, the labrum can then be reattached with the use of suture anchors.

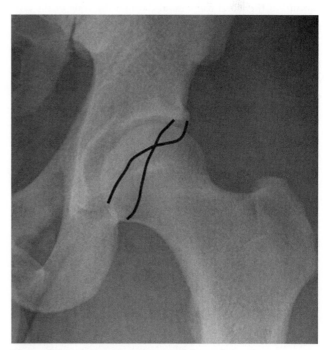

**Figure 20–5** Anteroposterior pelvic radiograph that shows a retroverted acetabulum and a crossover sign.

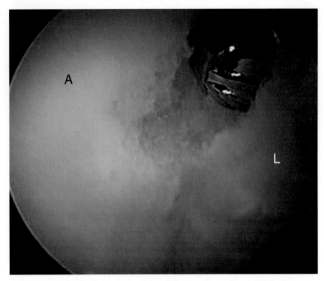

**Figure 20–6** Arthroscopic view of the burring of a pincer lesion. *A*, Acetabulum; *L*, labrum.

Before any bone removal occurs, the junction between the capsule and the labral tissue must be developed. This will allow for the removal of an adequate amount of bone without causing further damage to the labrum or disturbing the capsular integrity at this site. It is also important to maintain a meticulous dissection at the anterosuperior aspect of the rim as a result of the close proximity of the reflected head of the rectus. If this area is damaged, postoperative adhesions can cause significant dysfunction.

We perform the rim trimming with the use of a 5.5-mm motorized burr. With the labrum detached and safely out of the way, we slowly begin to remove bone from the anterosuperior margin of the rim. We continually stop and get a profile view of the acetabular rim with the arthroscope to determine the extent of our resection. This process is repeated until we have a normal acetabular profile and a healthy bed of tissue for reattaching the labrum. If the labral tear extends beyond the zone of the pincer lesion, we will also trim a small portion of the bone in that region as well to provide a good surface for our labral repair. An example of a typical rim resection is shown in Figure 20-6. It is not uncommon to encounter subchondral cysts during the rim resection; these cysts are evidence of chronic impingement and should be completely resected. If they are not addressed, it is possible to drill into them during suture anchor placement and thus achieve substandard fixation.

## LABRAL REPAIR

One of the most important aspects of this procedure—and also the most challenging arthroscopically—is the labral repair. The proper reattachment of the labrum to the acetabular rim provides the appropriate seal for the hip joint, the proper tracking of the labrum on the femoral head cartilage, and the surface area for pressure distribution within the hip joint. Failure in any one these three areas will cause subsequent pain, potential instability, and further degeneration of the cartilage.

Our technique requires the use of a very-small-diameter suture anchor. Because the acetabular rim can be both shallow and narrow, larger anchor devices are not as efficacious with this application. We use the 2.3-mm PEEK BioRaptor (Smith & Nephew, Andover, MA) for our fixation. We use a specially designed trocar with very sharp wings at the distal tip that help with the proper placement of the anchor; this allows us to get as

close to the acetabular rim as possible without penetrating the joint (Figure 20-7).

Depending on the size of the tear, we will typically use two to three anchors to adequately fix the labrum down to the rim. We usually start at the most anterior aspect of the tear and work posteriorly. The anchor placement is the only time during the procedure that we will use a plastic cannula. A 10-mm cannula is placed through the mid-anterior portal, and the trocar is subsequently passed and placed in an optimal position on the rim. After the drilling and seating of the anchor, we test its integrity by pulling on the free limbs of the suture. We use an arthroscopic suture passer to pass the suture closest to the rim around the intra-articular portion of the labrum and to retrieve both limbs through the cannula. It is possible to tie the labrum with too much force and to strangulate the tissue; it is also possible to have the suture too loose and to have it become a secondary source of impingement during the procedure. An example of the appearance of an appropriately tensioned knot is shown in Figure 20-8. A standard arthroscopic suture cutter is placed as close to the knot as possible to reduce the potential size of any foreign material within the hip joint. We will repeat these steps with subsequent anchors until the labrum is well fixed.

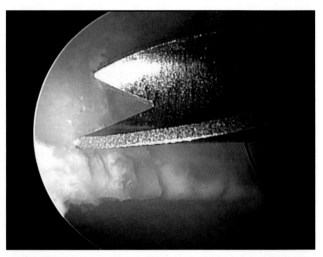

**Figure 20–7** Suture anchor guide device in place on the acetabular rim.

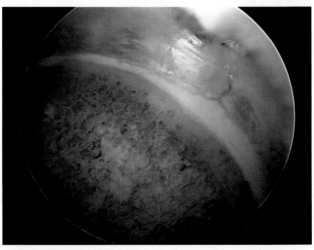

**Figure 20–8** Dynamic evaluation after labral repair, rim trimming, and osteochondroplasty that shows normal tracking of the labrum with the femoral head.

After we have completed the labral repair, we test its integrity and its ability to seal the hip joint. By releasing the traction and moving the arthroscope into the peripheral compartment, we can evaluate the labral repair. From the peripheral compartment, it is possible to see the entire labrum and its interaction with the femoral head and neck as it moves through a full range of motion (see Figure 20-8). We also perform a dynamic examination by testing the hip joint in full flexion and abduction to ensure that the labrum does not demonstrate excessive motion and that there is no evidence of impingement present.

If there is any component of cam impingement present, this must be addressed at the time of the initial arthroscopic intervention. We use the same 5.5-mm motorized burr to remove the excess bone from the femoral head–neck junction. After an adequate osteoplasty has been performed, we will again perform a dynamic examination to ensure that the labral tissue is not impinged during full flexion and abduction.

### TECHNICAL PEARLS

- The patient selection criteria are important. The joint space should be a minimum of 2 mm, and the patient should agree to following the postoperative protocol.
- The preoperative center-edge angle should be measured; this will allow the surgeon to plan the rim resection to avoid causing a dysplastic-like rim.
- Keep track of the amount of rim resected by measuring the distance from the cotyloid fossa to the acetabular rim both before and after rim resection.
- When placing suture anchors, keep the drill perpendicular to the acetabular rim.
- After the sutures have been placed, check the stability of the labrum. Additional sutures may be necessary if the labrum is not completely stable.
- After the repair of the labrum, always perform a dynamic examination to ensure that the labral repair is not moving or being impinged on by a lack of space as a result of pincer or cam impingement.

## POSTOPERATIVE REHABILITATION

Postoperatively, early emphasis is placed on preventing the formation of adhesions and regaining internal rotation. The prevention of adhesion formation consists of passive range-of-motion exercises and the use of a continuous passive motion machine for 2 weeks. Patients may also begin stationary biking as soon as it is tolerable to them. External rotation is restricted during the first 18 days in most cases, with this restriction being extended if more capsular work was performed. To protect the repaired labrum, a brace is worn while ambulating for the first 10 postoperative days to limit flexion to 90 degrees and to pre-

vent abduction. Passive external rotation exercises are begun 21 days postoperatively. Pneumatic foot pumps are worn while at rest for the first 2 weeks to prevent deep venous thrombosis.

## OUTCOMES

There are few reports that discuss the long-term outcomes of hip arthroscopy for labral dysfunction and associated femoroacetabular impingement (Table 20-1). We have recently reported about the outcomes of 45 professional athletes after arthroscopic intervention for femoroacetabular impingement and labral pathology. We used return to sport as an indicator for function, because these 45 professional athletes were unable to participate at the professional level before intervention. After arthroscopy, 93% of these patients returned to full competitive professional competition, and 78% remained active at the professional level an average of 1.6 years later.

We also looked at the early outcomes after arthroscopic acetabular labral repair. In this study, 52 patients underwent arthroscopic acetabular labral repair by a single surgeon. At an average follow-up length of 9 months (range, 6 to 15 months), patients showed significant improvement as measured by three clinical outcomes measures: the Modified Harris Hip Score, the Non-Arthritic Hip Score, and the Hip Outcome Score activities of daily living and sports subscales. The average patient satisfaction rate was 8.5 out of 10. This study showed that, during early follow up, patients exhibited significant improvement and high rates of satisfaction after arthroscopic acetabular labral repair.

In another study, early outcomes were documented after microfracture procedures in the hip. Nineteen patients underwent microfracture procedure for the treatment of grade 4 chondral defects on either the femoral head, the acetabulum, or both. At 1 year of follow up, patients showed significant improvements in all four of the previously mentioned clinical outcome measures, and the average patient satisfaction rate was 8.6 out of 10. Younger patients also experienced better outcomes. This study showed that patients who undergo microfracture for the treatment of grade 4 chondral defects in the hip can have good function, significant improvement, and high levels of patient satisfaction.

A continuation of the previous study looked at the ability of the microfracture clot to produce repair tissue. Nine patients underwent a microfracture procedure of acetabular chondral defects and had a subsequent hip arthroscopy in which the chondral defect fill could be quantified. The average time from the primary arthroscopy to the second look was 20 months. The average percentage of fill that was noted was 91% (range, 25% to 100%). Eight patients had a grade 1 or 2 repair product during the second look. The one patient who had 25% fill had diffuse osteoarthritis on both surfaces at the time of arthroscopy. This study showed that microfracture for the treatment of grade 4 acetabular chondral lesions shows an excellent ability to produce repair tissue as demonstrated during a second look at the area.

**Table 20–1** CLINICAL OUTCOMES

| Article | Arthroscopic or Open Procedure | No. of Patients | Modified Harris Hip Score | Patient Satisfaction Rate |
|---|---|---|---|---|
| Espinosa et al., 2006 | Open | 35 | 80% excellent | |
| Philippon et al., 2009 | Arthroscopic | 112 | 84 | 90% |
| Larson and Giveans, 2008 | Arthroscopic | 37 | 94 | |

The reason that a patient requires revision surgery is important for delineating the proper indications for hip arthroscopy. The purpose of this study was to report the major reasons that patients present for revision hip arthroscopy. Thirty-seven revision hip arthroscopies were performed by the senior surgeon. The most common reason that patients underwent revision hip surgery was for unaddressed or inadequately addressed impingement at the time of index arthroscopy, persistent labral pathology, chondral defects, and capsulolabral adhesions. The outcomes of this study showed that patients regained some of their lost function within the first year after revision hip arthroscopy and that the major reason that patients underwent revision hip arthroscopy was for persistent impingement.

## COMPLICATIONS

Unfortunately, there are no surgical interventions that are complication free, including hip arthroscopy. The keys to having successful outcomes are to recognize the potential complications and to take extraordinary steps to avoid them if at all possible.

In our practice, the most common complication after surgery has been postoperative tendonitis of the hip flexor. This will typically start to cause anterior groin pain with hip flexion approximately 6 weeks after surgery. Two interventions have been made to decrease the frequency of this complication. First, we changed the position of our anterior portal in an effort to move farther away from the hip flexor musculature. The mid-anterior portal allows for excellent visualization, and it is farther lateral than the anterior portal and thus farther from the hip flexors. Since the use of this portal, we have seen a dramatic improvement in hip flexor tendonitis. Second, we made multiple adjustments to the postoperative rehabilitation process with respect to the hip flexors. By limiting active flexion for the first 2 to 3 weeks after the procedure, patients have noted less pinching in the anterior groin.

Capsulolabral adhesions are also more frequent complications among our postoperative hip scope patients than we would prefer. Clinically, we will see a reduction in the previously attained range of motion. This reduction in motion then creates a vicious cycle of reduced motion, pain, deconditioning of the hip musculature, and then a further reduction of motion. The use of circumduction exercises postoperatively has limited the occurrence of postoperative adhesions. The addition of platelet-rich plasma (PRP) as part of our surgical intervention has been very beneficial with respect to this complication. The hemostatic properties of this injection directly at the site of the head–neck resection has reduced the frequency of capsulolabral adhesions among our patients.

There have been other complications described in the literature, including perineal numbness, transient neurologic symptoms (both motor and sensory), impotence, and bruising of the genitalia. Proper attention to detail during the setup of the operative theater is very important for avoiding these complications, and paying close attention to the amount of traction time is very effective for reducing them. Furthermore, the use of continuous nerve monitoring during the procedure is a good indicator of the amount of stress that is being placed on the nerves and on all of the associated structures within the lower extremities.

## CONCLUSIONS

Hip arthroscopy has provided the orthopedic surgeon with the ability to address pathologies related to the acetabular rim and the labral tissue with great effectiveness. The relatively low complication rates and the very high success rates are the driving forces behind the recent focus on this approach that have been seen in the orthopedic literature and at national meetings across the globe. Continuing innovations developed by pioneering orthopedic surgeons will further advance the successes that have been seen during the past 5 to 7 years.

## ANNOTATED REFERENCES

**Beck M, Leunig M, Parvizi J, Boutier V, Wyss D, Ganz R. Anterior femoroacetabular impingement: Part II. Midterm results of surgical treatment.** *Clin Orthop Relat Res.* 2004;418:67–73.

Beck and colleagues investigated 14 men and five women with a mean age of 36 years who were treated for femoroacetabular impingement using surgical dislocation and offset creation of the hip. Using the Merle d'Aubigné hip score, 13 hips were rated excellent to good, with the pain score improving from 2.9 points to 5.1 points at the latest follow-up. The authors found that surgical dislocation with correction of femoroacetabular impingement yields good results in patients with early degenerative changes not exceeding grade 1 osteoarthritis.

**Byrd JW, Jones KS. Prospective analysis of hip arthroscopy with 2-year follow-up.** *Arthroscopy.* 2000;16:578–587.

This prospective study investigated the 2-year outcomes on 38 procedures performed for various hip disorders. Modified Harris hip score improved from 57 to 85 points with the most statistically significant finding being that older men with longer duration of symptoms did worse. This was the first report to quantify the results to hip arthroscopy for a heterogeneous population.

**Byrd JW, Pappas JN, Pedley MJ. Hip arthroscopy: an anatomic study of portal placement and relationship to the extra-articular structures.** *Arthroscopy.* 1995;11:418–423.

Proper access to the hip joint depends on precise patient positioning with particular attention paid to critical anatomic landmarks. Byrd and colleagues aimed to describe the relationship between neurovascular structures and standard portals used during hip arthroscopy. Three standard arthroscopic portals were simulated in eight cadaveric hip specimens and the portals were determined to be safe distances from vital aspects of neurovascular anatomy.

**Espinosa N, Rothenflug DA, Beck M, Ganz R, Leunig M. Treatment of femoroacetabular impingement: preliminary results of labral refixation.** *J Bone Joint Surg Am.* 2006;88:925–935.

The authors of this study retrospectively reviewed the clinical and radiographic results of 52 patients (60 hips) with femoroacetabular impingement who underwent arthrotomy and surgical dislocation of the hip to allow trimming of the acetabular rim and femoral osteochondroplasty. In the first 25 hips (Group 1), the labrum was resected; in the next 35 hips (Group 2), the labrum was reattached to the acetabular rim. Comparison of the clinical scores between the two groups revealed significantly better outcomes for Group 2 at 1 year and at 2 years.

**Ganz R, Gill TJ, Gautier E, Ganz K, Krugel N, Berlemann U. Surgical dislocation of the adult hip: a technique with full access to the femoral head and acetabulum without the risk of avascular necrosis.** *J Bone Joint Surg Br.* 2001;83:1119–1124.

The authors of this study reported their experience using an anterior dislocation approach to the hip. They report on 213 hips over a 7-year period. They found that there is little morbidity associated with this technique and that it allows the treatment of a variety of conditions that may not respond well to other methods including arthroscopy.

**Lage LA, Patel JV, Villar RN. The acetabular labral tear: an arthroscopic classification.** *Arthroscopy.* 1996;12:269–272.

This study focused on the patterns of acetabular labral tears in 37 patients undergoing hip arthroscopy. Distinct categories of labral tears were observed and the authors worked to classify the tears with reference to etiology and morphology. The authors found 49% of the cohort had degenerative labral tears and 57% had radial flap tears.

**Larson CM, Giveans MR. Arthroscopic management of femoroacetabular impingement. Early outcomes measures.** *Arthroscopy.* 2008;24(5):540–546.

This study focused on 96 consecutive patients (100 hips) undergoing hip arthroscopy for radiographically documented FAI. A comparison of preoperative scores with those obtained at most recent follow-up revealed a significant improvement for all outcomes measured. No hip went on to undergo repeat arthroscopy and three hips subsequently underwent total hip arthroplasty. Good to excellent results were observed in 75% of the hips at a minimum 1-year follow-up.

**McCarthy JC, Lee JA. Hip arthroscopy: indications, outcomes, and complications. *Instr Course Lect*. 2006;55:301–308.**

McCarthy and colleagues aimed to describe the elements included in hip arthroscopy. Due to the nature of the procedure and its technically demanding requirements, the authors provided an educational description of its methods. These methods included the indications for surgery and the appropriate instrumentation involved with the operation. Additionally, they document outcomes and list complications involved with hip arthroscopy.

**Murphy KP, Ross AE, Javernick MA, Lehman Jr RA. Repair of the adult acetabular labrum. *Arthroscopy*. 2006;22:567.e1–567.e3.**

Murphy et al. worked to explain a method for repair of the acetabular labrum. The authors advocate labral repair to restore anatomic function rather than surgical debridement, which may lead to degenerative changes associated with osteoarthritis. The short-term results of labral repair are positive; however, long-term follow-up is still needed.

**Murphy S, Tannast M, Kim YJ, Buly R, Millis MB. Debridement of the adult hip for femoroacetabular impingement: indications and preliminary clinical results. *Clin Orthop Relat Res*. 2004;429:178–181.**

Murphy's study assessed 23 hips in 23 patients treated by surgical debridement for impingement. They found that at the most recent evaluation, 7 patients had been converted to total hip arthroplasty, 1 had arthroscopic debridement of a recurrent labral tear, and 15 patients have had no further surgery. Furthermore, the authors concluded that hips at greatest risk of failure have advanced arthrosis or a combination of impingement and instability preoperatively.

**Parvizi J, Leunig M, Ganz R. Femoroacetabular impingement. *J Am Acad Orthop Surg*. 2007;15:561–570.**

Parvizi outlines an anatomic description of femoroacetabular impingement as well as the consequences involved with the disorder. The authors describe the dislocation approach and osteoplasty technique as surgical management options. They report encouraging outcomes following femoroacetabular osteoplasty and arthroscopic treatment of femoroacetabular impingement.

**Peters CL, Erickson JA. Treatment of femoroacetabular impingement with surgical dislocation and debridement in young adults. *J Bone Joint Surg Am*. 2006;88:1735–1741.**

This study examined 30 hips with femoroacetabular impingement who underwent treatment utilizing debridement through a greater trochanteric flip osteotomy and anterior dislocation of the femoral head. The mean Harris Hip Score improved from 70 points preoperatively to 87 points at the time of final follow-up. The authors concluded that surgical dislocation and debridement of the hip for the treatment of FAI in hips without substantial damage to the articular cartilage can reduce pain and improve function.

**Philippon M, Schenker M, Briggs K, Kuppersmith D. Femoroacetabular impingement in 45 professional athletes: associated pathologies and return to sport following arthroscopic decompression. *Knee Surg Sports Traumatol Arthroc*. 2007;15:908–914.**

Philippon and colleagues examined 45 professional athletes who underwent arthroscopic treatment for femoroacetabular impingement. They found that 42 (93%) of these athletes returned to professional competition following arthroscopic decompression of FAI and the three who did not return had diffuse osteoarthritis at the time of arthroscopy. Thirty-five athletes (78%) remained active in professional sport at an average follow-up of 1.6 years.

**Philippon MJ, Briggs KK, Kuppersmith DA, Hines SL, Maxwell RB. Outcomes following hip arthroscopy with microfracture. *Arthroscopy* 2007;23(6):e11.**

Between March 2005 and June 2005, 19 hips underwent arthroscopy with microfracture. The authors of this study aimed to report 1-year outcomes in patients who underwent hip arthroscopy with microfracture treatment for full-thickness chondral defects. Modified Harris Hip Score improved from 58 preoperatively to 74 postoperatively and average patient satisfaction was 8.6 out of 10.

**Philippon MJ, Briggs KK, Yen YM. Outcomes following hip arthroscopy for FAI and associated chondrolabral dysfunction. *JBJS BR*. 2009;91:16–23.**

The purpose of this study was to report early results of function and patient satisfaction in 52 labral repair patients. Patients experienced improvement in function at least 6 months postoperatively, demonstrating that arthroscopic labral repair for the treatment of labral tears lead to improved level of function and high patient satisfaction.

**Philippon MJ, Maxwell RB, Johnston TL, Schenker M, Briggs KK. Clinical presentation of femoroacetabular impingement. *Knee Surg Sports Traumatol Arthrosc*. 2007;15:1041–1047.**

Philippon and colleagues prepared this study in order to identify subjective complaints and objective findings in patients treated for femoroacetabular impingement. Three hundred one arthroscopic hip surgeries were studied and the authors found that the most common subjective complaint was groin pain. There was a significant decrease in range of motion observed in operative hips compared to nonoperative hips.

**Philippon MJ, Schenker ML, Briggs KK, Kuppersmith DA, Maxwell RB, Stubbs AJ. Revision hip arthroscopy. *Am J Sports Med*. 2007;35:1918–1921.**

The purpose of this study was to describe reasons for revision hip arthroscopy. Between March 2005 and March 2006, 37 revision hip arthroscopies were performed by the senior author. Common findings among patients needing revision were hip pain, decreased range of motion, and functional disability. Revision procedures included 34 (95%) for femoroacetabular impingement, 32 (87%) for labral lesions, 26 (70%) for chondral defects, 23 (62%) for lysis of adhesions, and 13 (35%) for previously unaddressed instability. Outcomes showed patients regained some of their lost function within the first year following revision hip arthroscopy.

**Philippon MJ, Schenker L, Briggs KK, Maxwell RB. Can microfracture produce repair tissue in acetabular chondral defects? *Arthroscopy*. 2008;24.:46–50.**

Nine patients underwent revision hip arthroscopy after undergoing microfracture for the treatment of full-thickness chondral defects of the acetabulum. The authors of this study investigated the percent fill and repair grade of microfractured lesions from the primary arthroscopic procedure. They found that eight of the nine patients had 95% to 100% coverage of isolated acetabular chondral lesions. The remaining patient had diffuse osteoarthritis, with only 25% coverage with a grade IV appearance of the repair product 10 months after index arthroscopy.

**Philippon MJ, Stubbs AJ, Schenker ML, Maxwell RB, Ganz R, Leunig M. Arthroscopic management of femoroacetabular impingement: osteoplasty technique and literature review. *Am J Sports Med*. 2007;35:1571–1580.**

While published outcomes report successful mid-term results with the open surgical dislocation approach to treat femoroacetabular impingement, Philippon and colleagues set out to explain an arthroscopic technique and discuss the relevant literature on this topic.

**Seldes RM, Tan V, Hunt J, Katz M, Winiarsky R, Fitzgerald Jr RH. Anatomy, histologic features, and vascularity of the adult acetabular labrum. *Clin Orthop Realt Res* 2001;382:232–240.**

The authors studied 55 embalmed and 12 fresh-frozen adult hips in order to examine the anatomy, histologic features, and microvasculature of the acetabular labrum. Of these, 96% of the hips had labral tears, with 74% of the tears located in the anterosuperior quadrant.

The authors concluded that labral tears occur early in the arthritic process of the hip and may be one of the causes of degenerative hip disease.

**Sussmann PS, Ranawat AS, Shehaan M, Lorich D, Padgett DE, Kelly BT. Vascular preservation during arthroscopic osteoplasty of the femoral head-neck junction: a cadaveric investigation.** *Arthroscopy* **2007;23:738–743.**

The authors of this study evaluated the risk of vascular injury with arthroscopic osteoplasty of the femoral head-neck junction in a cadaveric model. Following arthroscopic osteoplasty, 7 of the 8 experimental specimens exhibited near-to-complete filling of the superior and inferior retinacula branches with no signs of latex extravasation. These findings show that arthroscopic osteoplasty can be performed without disrupting the vascular supply to the femoral head.

**Wahoff M, Briggs KK, Philippon MJ. Hip arthroscopy rehabilitation.** *Orthopaedic Knowledge Update.* **Chicago, IL: AAOS; 2009.**

This article describes the appropriate rehabilitation protocol in which one institution recommends for successful outcomes and functional return following hip arthroscopy. They focus on rehabilitative exercises as well as proper bracing and activity limitations that should follow surgical intervention of the hip.

# CHAPTER 21

# Arthroscopic Synovectomy and Treatment of Synovial Disorders

*Christopher M. Larson and Mehul M. Taylor*

## INTRODUCTION

The hip is a synovial joint that bears significant loads over a lifetime. There are various conditions that can lead to hip joint dysfunction and result in significant disability. Synovial hip disorders are less common hip conditions and include synovial chondromatosis, pigmented villonodular synovitis (PVNS), septic arthritis, and inflammatory arthropathies.

Much of the literature that addresses the management of hip synovial disorders is based on reports that involve the treatment of other joints. However, these conditions do affect the hip joint proper, and a systematic approach can lead to acceptable outcomes in appropriately selected individuals. This chapter will describe synovial disorders and their typical presentation, physical examination findings, appropriate imaging studies, and hip arthroscopy indications for the management of these less commonly encountered disorders. In addition, a detailed surgical technique for central and peripheral compartment synovectomy is described.

## BASIC SCIENCE

Synovial chondromatosis and synovial osteochondromatosis are the result of intrasynovial cartilage metaplasia, and it can cause the formation of multiple intra- and extra-articular loose bodies. These loose bodies may be primarily cartilaginous and associated with very little articular cartilage damage. With time, these loose bodies can ossify to variable degrees and result in progressive erosive changes near the hip joint proper. The cause and pathogenesis of PVNS remain unclear. The condition appears to be the result of a fibrohistiocytic chronic inflammatory or neoplastic response. It is associated with synovial proliferation (either diffuse or focal), joint effusion, and bony erosion with characteristic hemosiderin deposition within the synovial mass. Multiple loose bodies and PVNS of the hip are associated with more erosive and degenerative changes than those seen in the knee as a result of the more constrained nature of the hip joint proper. Rheumatoid arthritis is the most common inflammatory arthropathy that affects the hip joint. The initial pathology involves the inflammation of the synovium, which leads to the eventual destruction of the joint if left untreated. A septic hip results in microorganisms activating an inflammatory response that recruits polymorphonuclear cells. Bacteria, synovial cells, and polymorphonuclear cells release enzymes that facilitate the degradation of glycosaminoglycans and the subsequent loss of collagen; this ultimately results in the gross destruction of articular cartilage and the development of arthritis if untreated early during the course of its development.

## HISTORY

The typical history is quite variable for patients who present with synovial disorders. Patients with synovial chondromatosis are more commonly males in the third to fifth decade of life. They will typically present with deep groin and deep lateral hip pain that is often mechanical in nature as a result of loose bodies. These patients will frequently report catching and locking that may be quite unpredictable and that can have variable asymptomatic periods. Over time, the symptoms may become more frequent, with associated rest pain that is not related to activity; this may be the result of progressive articular cartilage destruction caused by the mechanical effects of the loose bodies. Pigmented villonodular synovitis typically presents during the third and fourth decades of life, with no gender predilection. It is typically monoarticular with associated aching and rest pain and variable mechanical symptoms. A longer duration of symptoms is associated with progressive degenerative and erosive changes and with a presentation that is similar to that of degenerative arthritis at a relatively young age. Patients will note progressive stiffness and range-of-motion limitations. Septic arthritis of the hip has a similar presentation to septic arthritis elsewhere. There is usually no history of trauma, and there may be a preceding illness. Septic arthritis of the hip is more prevalent among immunocompromised hosts and patients with frequent bacteremic episodes. Patients will often present with fever, chills, rapidly progressive groin pain, and irritability with range of motion. Joint aspiration is usually diagnostic. Inflammatory arthropathies that affect the hip joint can lead to end-stage arthritis. Earlier during the course of the disease, however, patients will occasionally present with hip joint irritability as a result of synovitis that is unresponsive to oral or injectable medication. Occasionally, this may be the first presentation of a patient with an undiagnosed inflammatory arthritis.

## PHYSICAL EXAMINATION

The physical examination findings of patients with synovial disorders can be variable. If intermittent mechanical symptoms are the primary complaint, the physical examination can be normal.

When synovitis is present, pain is typically experienced with range of motion of the hip, primarily at the end of the range. These patients may have secondary labral tears and chondral pathology. The anterior impingement test (i.e., hip flexion, adduction, internal rotation) is indicative of anterolateral rim pathology, and the posterior impingement test (i.e., hip extension, external rotation) indicates posterolateral rim pathology. A septic hip will often present with a severely antalgic gait and extreme pain with any attempts at range of motion, whereas an active synovitis caused by an inflammatory arthropathy will present with pain at the end of the range of motion with variable, less dramatic pain during early and mid–range-of-motion testing. Global restrictions of range of motion are usually indicative of advanced disease and end-stage hip joint destruction. A complete examination of the lower back, the pelvis, extra-articular hip structures, and, occasionally, the gastrointestinal and genitourinary systems is critical to rule out other causes of pain that can be referred to the hip region.

## IMAGING AND DIAGNOSTIC STUDIES

When evaluating a patient with symptoms that are consistent with hip joint pathology, plain radiographs should be obtained first. We typically obtain an anteroposterior radiograph of both hips with 2 cm to 4 cm between the pubic symphysis and the sacrococcygeal junction. A frog-leg lateral radiograph and a cross-table lateral radiograph with 15 degrees of internal rotation complete the initial series. Radiographic abnormalities may include arthritis, arthrosis, dysplasia, femoroacetabular impingement, and loose bodies. It has been reported that radiographs fail to diagnose loose bodies up to 50% of the time; this may be a result of the inconsistent calcification of these loose bodies and because they may be obscured by overlying structures. Large and multiple lucencies on plain radiographs are consistent with PVNS (Figure 21-1, *A*). Magnetic resonance arthrography (MRA) is the gold standard imaging technique for evaluating the hip joint proper. MRA has been shown to be very sensitive for labral tears and less accurate for chondral pathology. Filling defects can indicate loose bodies, as has been seen with synovial chondromatosis. As a result of hemosiderin deposition, pigmented villonodular synovitis is seen as a spotty or extensive low-signal area within proliferative synovial masses on T1 and T2 images; this condition is best seen on fast-field echo-sequence MRA images (see Figure 21-1, *B*). MRA imaging will typically reveal an effusion and variable degrees of synovitis in the setting of an acute septic hip; an aspiration can also be performed as part of this imaging. Chronic infection with associated osteomyelitis and adjacent abscesses should be ruled out in this setting before arthroscopic hip irrigation and synovial debridement are performed. MRA has important applications for imaging the rheumatoid joint. Bony erosions are visualized with MRA during the early stages of rheumatoid arthritis, and they are frequently detected before they appear on plain radiographs. MRA also detects bone marrow edema, which is another important feature that is associated with inflammatory joint disease and that may be a forerunner of erosion. Synovial membrane inflammation and hypertrophy are detected after contrast enhancement and also with the use of dynamic MRA techniques, which provide a noninvasive method for accurately measuring the inflammatory process.

## INDICATIONS

- Arthroscopic synovectomy of the hip is infrequently performed in isolation, and it is often performed along with the management of associated labral tears, chondral pathology, and loose bodies. The removal of loose bodies from patients with mechanical symptoms is one of the clearest indications for hip arthroscopy. These loose bodies may be the result of synovial chondromatosis, and, in this situation, a synovectomy is performed in addition to the removal of the loose bodies (Figure 21-2).
- Pigmented villonodular synovitis is best managed in its focal form. However, in diffuse PVNS it may not be possible to perform a complete synovectomy as the posterior and posterior inferior portions of the hip are difficult to access arthroscopically. In this situation we have performed a central compartment synovectomy (lunate fossa), followed by peripheral compartment (anteroinferior to posterosuperior) synovectomy (Figure 21-3). A T-capsulotomy and the addition of a postero-peritrochanteric portal allows for access to posterior capsular areas in some cases. A follow up MRI is obtained at 2 to 3 months and if residual disease is seen posteriorly, a limited open posterior approach to the hip can be performed to remove residual disease. Some nonarthroscopists would argue for open treatment primarily for diffuse PVNS.
- An arthroscopic irrigation, debridement, and synovectomy are effective for treating an acutely septic hip; these treatments result in less postoperative morbidity than an open arthrotomy. MRA images should be obtained before the performance of arthroscopy for a septic hip, because chronic infection, osteomyelitis, and the local extension of a periarticular abscess are contraindications to arthroscopic treatment.
- Arthroscopic synovectomy for inflammatory arthritis is less well defined, and the indications should be limited. Treatment of rheumatoid arthritis consists of immunosuppressive

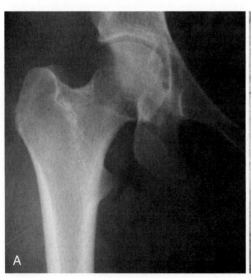
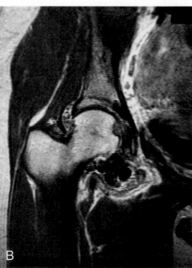

**Figure 21–1 A,** Plain anteroposterior radiograph of a 20-year-old female with progressive hip pain reveals lucencies around the hip joint that are consistent with pigmented villonodular synovitis. **B,** Magnetic resonance imaging reveals a massive hip joint effusion with multiple foci of low signal intensity and erosive changes that are consistent with pigmented villonodular synovitis.

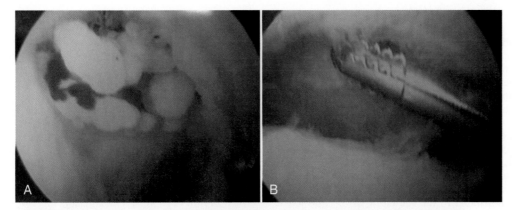

**Figure 21–2 A,** Arthroscopic view of the right hip of a 22-year-old male with increasing groin pain and mechanical symptoms. The peripheral compartment of the right hip reveals multiple chondral loose bodies that were not visualized during central compartment arthroscopy. **B,** Synovectomy has been performed in the peripheral compartment, and the loose bodies have been removed.

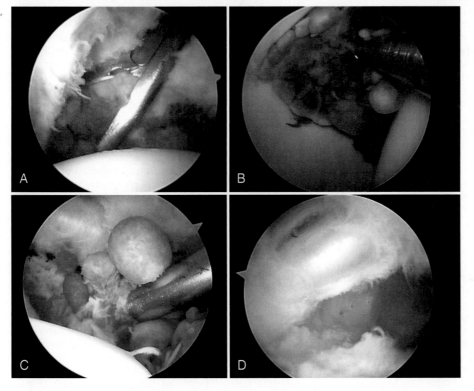

**Figure 21–3 A,** Arthroscopic view of the right hip of a 20-year-old female with pigmented villonodular synovitis (PVNS) of the hip. Disease is noted in the anterocentral compartment region. **B,** Arthroscopic view of the right hip foveal region reveals PVNS. **C,** Arthroscopic view of the peripheral compartment of the right hip reveals diffuse PVNS. **D,** Synovectomy of the peripheral compartment reveals the removal of the PVNS.

medication, disease-modifying agents, and anti-inflammatory medications. For patients with early rheumatoid arthritis with minimal degenerative disease and symptoms that are consistent with synovitis and unresponsive to oral and intra-articular medications, a synovectomy can be offered as an alternative treatment. There is no conclusive evidence that demonstrates that synovectomy slows the disease process and the eventual bony destruction. Again, it is difficult to access the posterior and posteroinferior hip joint arthroscopically, making a complete synovectomy very difficult if not impossible in many cases, which is a clear limitation to arthroscopic management.

- Moderate to advanced degenerative changes without primary mechanical symptoms as a result of loose bodies should be considered a relative contraindication to hip arthroscopy. Occasionally arthroscopy will reveal significantly more advanced degenerative changes than appreciated on plain radiographs or MRA, and this can help to expedite more definitive management (e.g., hip arthroplasty).
- In all of these situations, chondral and labral pathology may be encountered, and these can be treated during the same procedure.

## SURGICAL TECHNIQUE

Hip arthroscopic synovectomy can be performed with the patient in the supine or lateral position; the senior author (CML) prefers the supine position. The central compartment and the peripheral compartment need to be addressed for the full visualization of all of the pertinent structures and for the performance of a near-complete synovectomy, when indicated. The central compartment is visualized with traction on, and the peripheral compartment is best evaluated with hip flexion and variable degrees of abduction, adduction, and rotation. The structures visualized in the central compartment include the medial femoral head; the acetabular fossa (i.e., the ligamentum teres and the pulvinar); the anterior, superior, and posterior lunate articular cartilages and labrums; and the medioanterior, superior, and posterior capsule. The peripheral compartment arthroscopy allows for the visualization of the inferior, anterior, superior, and posterior femoral neck; the capsule, including the zona orbicularis; the peripheral capsular attachments; and the lateral femoral head–neck junction. The Weitbrecht fibers are visualized in the peripheral compartment as well and include the medial, anterior, and lateral (i.e., the retinacular vessel site) synovial folds.

The patient is initially placed in the supine position on a fracture table or a standard table with the addition of one of various available distractors. Intraoperatively, a preprocedure fluoroscopic "around the world" evaluation of the hip in extension is performed, with internal, neutral, and external rotation; a frog-leg lateral view with the trochanter superimposed on the femoral neck is obtained; and a cross-table lateral view with the hip in 15 degrees of internal rotation is also obtained to evaluate for bony abnormalities (e.g., femoroacetabular impingement), when indicated. Next, the leg is initially placed in slight hip flexion, neutral to slight hip abduction, and internal rotation. The minimum amount of traction that appropriately distracts the hip is then applied.

A spinal needle is placed at the level of the anterior paratrochanteric portal (i.e., just anterior to the proximal aspect of the greater trochanter), roughly parallel to the sourcil or the acetabular roof. Care is taken to not damage the femoral head articular cartilage and to place the needle between the labrum and the femoral head. The inner stylet is then removed, which releases the intra-articular negative pressure and allows for easier distractibility, if needed. A cannulated system is then used to introduce a blunt obturator into the joint over a guidewire, and this is followed by a 70-degree arthroscope. At this point, the anterior femoral head, the acetabulum, the acetabular labrum, and the anterior capsule are identified (Figure 21-4, *A*). An anterior portal 2 cm distal to the junction of the anterosuperior iliac spine and the proximal greater trochanter is made with the use of direct visualization. We make this portal farther distal than what is typically described, which allows for the better placement of anchors and for chondral work on the acetabulum without accessory portals when labral repair and/or chondroplasty procedures are indicated. A limited capsulotomy is then performed with a beaver blade to allow for improved maneuverability. At this point, the arthroscope is placed into the anterior portal looking back at the initial anterior paratrochanteric portal. If this portal has penetrated a portion of the labrum, then it is repositioned outside of the labrum and followed by a limited capsulotomy. The arthroscope is then placed back into the anterior paratrochanteric portal, and the superior and posterior portions of the femoral head, the labrum, and the acetabulum are visualized (see Figure 21-4, *B*). A spinal needle is placed in the posterior paratrochanteric portal initially for outflow; this portal can later be established as a working or arthroscopic portal if one is required for the procedure that is to be performed.

Next, a systematic evaluation of the central compartment is performed with the arthroscope initially in the anterior paratrochanteric portal. The anterior labrum, the medial femoral head, and the acetabular fossa with the associated ligamentum teres and pulvinar are evaluated (see Figure 21-4, *C*). External rotation of the hip should reveal a tightening of the ligamentum teres, if

it is intact. Loose bodies, synovitis, and PVNS will frequently be found in the acetabular fossa when managing these synovial disorders. Occasionally a 30-degree arthroscope will allow for the better evaluation of the acetabular fossa. Loose bodies are then removed with various available graspers, and the pulvinar can be debrided with a shaver if it is pathologic. PVNS can be resistant to standard shaving, and a more aggressive grasper can be used to remove this tissue and to send the tissue for confirmatory biopsy. Switching the working and arthroscopic portals allows for complete access to this region for the removal of loose bodies and pathologic pulvinar or synovium.

A 70-degree arthroscope is then used to evaluate the chondral surfaces of the femoral head, the acetabulum, and the acetabular labrum. The management of any pathology is then performed as described in other chapters. The anterior, superior, and posterior capsule is then evaluated, and a shaver can be used to perform a synovectomy in this region. Any bleeding can be controlled with various available ablation devices.

The hip is flexed to approximately 30 to 45 degrees initially, with a spinal needle placed through the incision for the anterior paratrochanteric portal to be created over the anterior femoral neck. Either a 30- or 70-degree arthroscope can be used to visualize the peripheral compartment. Secondary portals can then be established through the anterior portal and the posterior paratrochanteric portal, and an accessory (mid-lateral) portal can be made 2 cm to 4 cm distal to the previous portals and midway between the anterior portal and the anterior paratrochanteric portal. Limited capsulotomies can then be performed with a beaver blade to improve maneuverability. The peripheral compartment is visualized in a systematic fashion as previously described.

The peripheral compartment can be divided into seven distinct regions (Figure 21-5). We have modified this description on the basis of the evaluation of the anterior, posterior, inferior, superior, medial, and lateral anatomic regions as recently described by Ilizaliturri and colleagues. The anterior neck region is identified first with its associated anterior (adherent to the femoral neck) and medial synovial folds, zona orbicularis, and iliofemoral ligament (Figure 21-6). Looking further inferolaterally (caudally) reveals the inferior reflection of the capsule at the intertrochanteric crest (Figure 21-7). Moving the arthroscope farther inferior over the medial synovial fold reveals the inferior neck, the inferolateral femoral head, the anteroinferior labrum, and the transverse acetabular ligament (Figure 21-8). The arthroscope is then brought back superiorly to reveal the anterolateral femoral head and the anterior labrum (Figure 21-9). Looking farther superior will then bring the superolateral femoral head and superior labrum into view (Figure 21-10). The arthroscope is then brought down over the superior femoral neck, which brings the lateral synovial fold into view

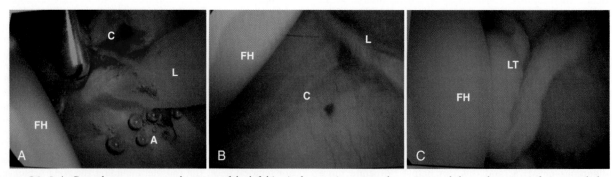

**Figure 21–4 A,** Central compartment arthroscopy of the left hip via the anterior paratrochanteric portal shows the anteroinferior acetabulum *(A)*, the labrum *(L)*, the capsule *(C)*, and the femoral head *(FH)*. A shaver has been introduced via the anterior portal. **B,** Central compartment arthroscopy of the left hip via the anterior paratrochanteric portal shows the posterosuperior femoral head *(FH)*, the labrum *(L)*, and the capsule *(C)*. **C,** Central compartment arthroscopy of the left hip reveals the acetabular fossa with the associated ligamentum teres *(LT)* and the medial femoral head *(FH)*.

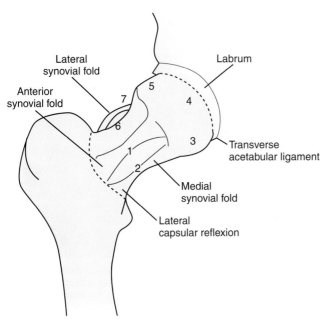

Figure 21-5  A systematic approach to peripheral compartment arthroscopy and to identifying the peripheral compartment anatomy is described with the use of the modification of a prior description by Dienst and colleagues. *1*, Anterior neck area; *2*, inferior neck area; *3*, inferolateral head area; *4*, anterolateral head area; *5*, superolateral head area; *6*, superior neck area; *7*, posterior area.

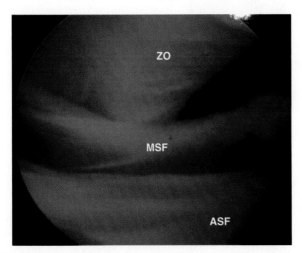

Figure 21-6  Peripheral compartment arthroscopy that reveals the anterior neck area (area 1) of the left hip. The anterior synovial fold *(ASF)*, the medial synovial fold *(MSF)*, and the zona orbicularis *(ZO)* are readily identified.

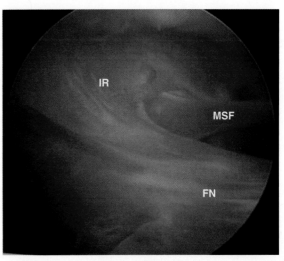

Figure 21-7  Further caudally in the peripheral compartment, the inferior capsular reflection *(IR)* at the intertrochanteric crest is visible, along with the anterior femoral neck *(FN)* and the medial synovial fold *(MSF)*.

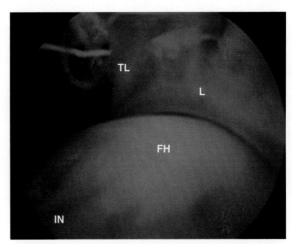

Figure 21-8  The anteroinferior region of the peripheral compartment (areas 2 and 3) reveals the inferior femoral neck *(IN)*, the inferolateral femoral head *(FH)*, the anteroinferior labrum *(L)*, and the transverse acetabular ligament *(TL)*.

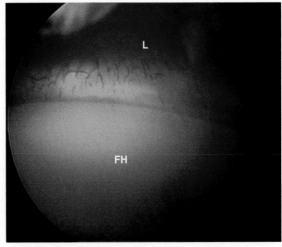

Figure 21-9  The anterior region (area 4) of the peripheral compartment reveals the anterolateral femoral head *(FH)* and the anterior labrum *(L)*.

(Figure 21-11, *A* and *B*). The arthroscope is then brought between the zona orbicularis and the lateral synovial fold to view the posterior femoral neck, the posterolateral femoral head, and the posterior capsule (Figure 21-12). This completes the systematic evaluation of the peripheral compartment. Exchanging the 30- and 70-degree arthroscopes will allow for the visualization of all of these areas in most patients. The shaver and the arthroscope can be exchanged among the anterolateral, anterior, posterolateral, and mid-lateral portals to perform a near-complete peripheral compartment synovectomy. Varying degrees of flexion, abduction, and rotation and the occasional removal of the perineal post will assist with the visualization of the previously named regions.

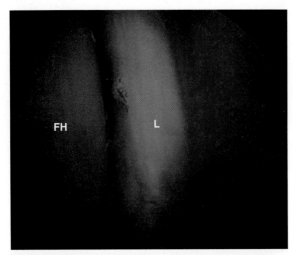

**Figure 21–10** The superior region (area 5) of the peripheral compartment reveals the superolateral femoral head *(FH)* and the superior labrum *(L)*.

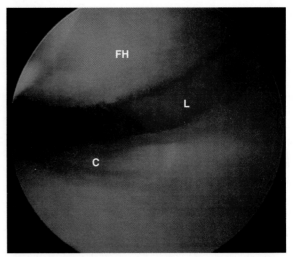

**Figure 21–12** By passing the arthroscope between the zona orbicularis and the lateral synovial fold, the posterior area (area 7) is visualized, with the posterior femoral head *(FH)*, the labrum *(L)*, and the posterior capsule *(C)*.

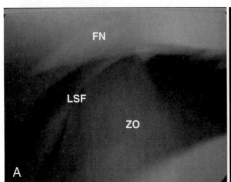
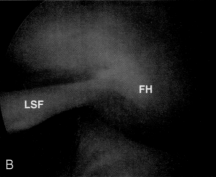

**Figure 21–11 A,** The superior region of the femoral neck *(FN)* is brought into view (area 6) with the associated lateral synovial fold *(LSF)* and the zona orbicularis *(ZO)*. **B,** The lateral synovial fold *(LSF)* is then followed to its insertion onto the lateral femoral head neck junction *(FH)*.

## OUTCOMES

Outcomes are limited with respect to arthroscopic management of synovial disorders. Much of the arthroscopic literature focuses on septic arthritis. There have been case reports and several series that report excellent results after arthroscopic treatment of septic hip arthritis. One series reported 10 patients treated arthroscopically for septic hip arthritis with no recurrences at a mean 5-year follow up. These results have shown that this approach is safe with less morbidity than an open approach. When a surgeon with hip arthroscopic skills is treating this condition, arthroscopy may be the preferred approach.

There are fewer reports on arthroscopic management of synovial chondromatosis or ostechondromatosis of the hip. One large series reported on 120 patients who underwent hip arthroscopy for synovial chondromatosis of the hip with mean follow up of 78.6 months. More than one arthroscopy was required in 20.7%, and 37.8% went on to open surgery. Arthroscopy was beneficial with good to excellent results reported in greater than 50% of the cases. When discussing treatment options with these individuals, the potential for future surgeries open and arthroscopic should be stressed. A large number of loose bodies seen on MRI and plain radiographs in the posterior capsular region may be an indication for an open approach or result in a greater chance of requiring an open approach after arthroscopic treatment.

There is very little outcomes data with respect to arthroscopic management of PVNS. The majority of the literature discussed the utility of hip arthroscopy for treatment of focal disease and for tissue biopsy. Based on the limited literature, one should be cautious when managing this disorder and stress the potential need for future surgery if there is persistent or recurrent disease. Although a combined arthroscopic and limited posterior open approach may allow for management of diffuse PVNS with less morbidity than a combined anterior and posterior or open surgical dislocation approach, there are no reports in the literature on this technique.

## CONCLUSION

Arthroscopic synovectomy is indicated for select hip joint disorders. A detailed history, a physical examination, and imaging studies will help to identify those patients who may benefit from arthroscopic synovectomy. A systematic evaluation of the central and peripheral compartments allows for a predictable evaluation of much of the hip joint proper. Focal and near-complete synovectomies are possible when treating patients with synovial hip disorders. The decision to perform the open management (as compared with arthroscopic management) of synovial hip disorders should be individualized on a case-by-case basis and determined on the basis of surgeon experience, technical feasibility, and location and extent of pathology.

# ANNOTATED REFERENCES

**Blitzer CM. Arthroscopic management of septic arthritis of the hip.** *Arthroscopy.* **1993;9(4):414–416.**

This is a report of 4 patients with septic hip arthritis treated successfully arthroscopically with mean 20.4-month follow-up.

**Boyer T, Dorfmann H. Arthroscopy in primary synovial chondromatosis of the hip: description and outcome of treatment.** *J Bone Joint Surg Br Mar.* **2008;90(3):314–318.**

This study reports the results of 120 patients who underwent hip arthroscopy for synovial chondromatosis of the hip with mean follow-up of 78.6 months. More than one arthroscopy was required in 20.7%, and 37.8% went on to open surgery. Arthroscopy was beneficial with good to excellent results reported in greater than 50% of the cases.

**Cheng XG, You YH, Liu W, Zhao T, Qu H. MRI features of pigmented villonodular synovitis (PVNS).** *Clin Rheumatol.* **2004;23(1):31–34, Epub 2004 Jan 9.**

This article reviews the typical magnetic resonance imaging features of 23 patients with documented pigmented villonodular synovitis of various joints. Nine patients in particular had hip joint involvement.

**Chung WK, Slater GL, Bates EH. Treatment of septic arthritis of the hip by arthroscopic lavage.** *J Pediatr Orthop.* **Jul-Aug 1993;13(4):444–446.**

This study reports 9 cases of septic arthritis of the hip treated arthroscopically with successful results in every case.

**Cotton A, Flipo RM, Chastaner P, et al. Pigmented villonodular synovitis of the hip: review of radiographic features in 59 patients.** *Skeletal Radiol.* **1995;24(1):1–6.**

This article describes the typical locations, histories, physical examinations, and radiographic findings of 58 patients with documented pigmented villonodular synovitis of the hip joint. The majority of patients had large and multiple lucencies that were seen on plain radiographs.

**Dienst M, Godde S, Seil R, Hammer D, Kohn D. Hip arthroscopy without traction: in vivo anatomy of the peripheral hip joint cavity.** *Arthroscopy.* **2001;17(9):924–931.**

This is a classic article that describes the surgical technique for peripheral compartment hip arthroscopy. A systematic surgical approach and detailed peripheral compartment anatomy are described.

**Doward DA, Troxell ML, Fredericson M. Synovial chondromatosis in an elite cyclist; a case report.** *Arch Phys Med Rehabil.* **Jun 2006;87(6):860–865.**

This article reports a case of an Olympic cyclist with synovial chondromatosis treated arthroscopically. The patient returned to full athletic activity without symptoms at 17 months' follow-up.

**Godde S, Kusma M, Dienst M. Synovial disorders and loose bodies in the hip joint. Arthroscopic diagnostics and treatment.** *Orthopade.* **2006;35(1):67–76.**

This is an excellent review of the role for hip arthroscopy in the treatment of synovial disorders. The advantages and disadvantages of arthroscopy compared to arthrotomy are described. A focus on patient selection and technique are described in order to maximize results in this patient population.

**Ilizaliturri V, Byrd JW, Sampson T, Larson CM, et al. A geographic zone method to describe intra-articular pathology in hip arthroscopy: cadaveric study and preliminary report.** *Arthroscopy.* **May 2008;24(5):534–539.**

This article compares the traditional "clock-face" description of the hip joint with a new proposed zone system for describing the arthroscopic hip joint anatomy. The accuracy of each method is tested by several hip arthroscopy master instructors and the identification of lesions in a cadaveric model.

**Kelly BT, Williams RJ 3rd, Philippon MJ. Hip arthroscopy: current indications, treatment options, and management issues.** *Am J Sports Med.* **2003;31(6):1020–1037.**

This is an excellent review of current diagnostic methods and indications for hip arthroscopy, including labral tears, capsular laxity and instability, chondral lesions, ligamentum teres lesions, snapping hip, iliopsoas bursitis, and synovial chondromatosis.

**Kim SJ, Choi NH, Ko SH, Linton JA, Park HW. Arthroscopic treatment of septic arthritis of the hip.** *Clin Orthop Relat Res.* **2003;(407):211–214.**

This article describes the arthroscopic technique and treatment of 10 patients with septic arthritis of the hip. All patients had an excellent result without complications at a mean follow up of almost 5 years.

**Krebs VE. The role of hip arthroscopy in the treatment of synovial disorders and loose bodies.** *Clin Orthop Relat Res.* **2003;(406):48–59.**

This is a detailed review of the current indications and outcomes for the arthroscopic management of various synovial disorders. This article includes a review of synovial chondromatosis, rheumatoid arthritis, pigmented villonodular synovitis, and septic arthritis of the hip.

**McQueen MF. MRI imaging in early inflammatory arthritis: what is its role.** *Rheumatology.* **2000;39:700–706.**

This review article describes the use of magnetic resonance imaging as a diagnostic tool for inflammatory arthritis. The strengths and weaknesses of this imaging modality are discussed as they apply clinically to inflammatory disorders.

**Nusem I, Jabut MK, Playford EG. Arthroscopic treatment of septic arthritis of the hip.** *Arthroscopy.* **2006;22(8):902, e1–e3.**

This article describes the arthroscopic management of septic arthritis of the hip in 6 patients. Arthroscopic irrigation, debridement, and postoperative antibiotics led to excellent outcomes in all patients at 6 to 42 months of follow up.

**Shabat S, Kollender Y, Merimsky O, et al. The use of surgery and yttrium 90 in the management of extensive and diffuse pigmented villonodular synovitis of large joints.** *Rheumatology (Oxford).* **2002;41(10):1113–1118.**

This article reports good results of the treatment of 10 patients with documented diffuse pigmented villonodular synovitis of large joints, including the hip. Patients were treated with a debulking surgery that was followed by the postoperative intra-articular injection of yttrium 90, and they were followed for a mean 6 years.

**Yamamoto Y, Ide Y, Hachisuka N, Maekawa S, Akamatsu N. Arthroscopic surgery for septic arthritis of the hip joint in 4 adults.** *Arthroscopy.* **Mar 2001;17(3):290–297.**

This study reports successful treatment of septic hip arthritis in 4 patients with hip arthroscopy. There were no recurrences at latest follow-up of 1 to 6 years.

# CHAPTER 22

# Arthroscopic Microfracture and Chondroplasty

*Jason Koh*

## INTRODUCTION

Articular cartilage defects are one of the pathologies that are most commonly encountered during hip arthroscopy. Limited information is available regarding the best treatment of these lesions; however, microfracture has been demonstrated to be effective for the treatment of articular cartilage defects of the knee and other weight-bearing joints, and several small series and case reports have been published that have described the use of microfracture for the treatment of articular cartilage defects in the hip. Several investigators are conducting ongoing outcome studies with regard to this treatment.

There are many conditions that can cause chondral defects that necessitate microfracture and chondroplasty, and these conditions can be acute, chronic, traumatic, or atraumatic. Defects can be full or partial thickness. Acute causes include hip dislocation, hip subluxation, and direct blows to the hip. Chronic causes include labral pathology, femoral acetabular impingement, loose bodies, dysplasia of the hip, a history of slipped capital femoral epiphysis, avascular necrosis, and degenerative joint disease.

It is critical to note that the diagnosis of these lesions is often only established intraoperatively, and patients should be aware that labral pathology is often associated with articular cartilage damage. The postoperative rehabilitation process and the patient's prognosis can be significantly different if such a lesion is discovered, and the patient and surgeon should be prepared for this possibility. A working knowledge of chondroplasty and microfracture will be helpful for any orthopedic surgeon who attempts to treat these diseases.

## BASIC SCIENCE

Microfracture is a type of a marrow-stimulating technique. After the removal of the avascular calcified cartilage layer, perforations are made through the subchondral plate to allow blood and marrow elements to enter the area of the articular cartilage defect. These marrow elements include stem cells as well as clotting and growth factors. The factors are crucial to the formation of a fibrin clot, which ultimately serves as an environment for nourishing pluripotent and mesenchymal stem cells. Initially, the regenerated tissue is fibrous tissue; however, with the use of appropriate biomechanical stimuli, a durable fibrocartilage repair tissue can be formed that will fill the defect.

## INDICATIONS

Indications for microfracture of the hip are largely derived from the knee literature and the author's experience. Factors that have been associated with good outcomes are listed here, although the particular indications for any procedure should be based on the physician's best judgment.

- Absence of generalized arthritis or articular cartilage loss
- Well-circumscribed Outerbridge grade IV full-thickness defect
- Intact subchondral bone
- Healthy surrounding cartilage
- The ability of the patient to comply with the postoperative protocol of decreased weight bearing
- Patient age of less than 40 years
- Symptom duration of less than 12 months
- Defect size of less than 200 mm$^2$ (Mithoefer 2006)

## BRIEF HISTORY AND PHYSICAL EXAMINATION

As with other musculoskeletal conditions, a careful history and physical examination are warranted. An understanding of the acuity and cause of the injury has important prognostic indications. Acute injuries (e.g., hip dislocations, subluxation events) are often associated with significant articular cartilage lesions that are sometimes asymptomatic. A direct lateral blow to the greater trochanter (e.g., a fall) can cause a medial impaction injury to the femoral head. A more gradual onset of pain or discomfort suggests a degenerative or impingement cause of the articular cartilage injury.

The location, frequency, and radiation of pain should be determined. Furthermore, alleviating or worsening symptoms or activities should be noted. Attention should be paid to any presence of mechanical symptoms (e.g., clicking, snapping, popping), because chondral defects can be associated with labral injuries. Defects associated with impingement may result in a history of pain with daily activities that involve hip flexion (e.g., prolonged sitting).

Physical examination features will be similar to those of other intra-articular pathologies, with pain usually experienced deep in the groin rather than posteriorly or laterally. The passive and active range of motion should be assessed. Specific testing for impingement symptoms should be performed, which includes the assessment of pain with combined hip flexion, internal rotation, and adduction. A loss of internal rotation with the hip flexed suggests a potential cam- or pincer-type deformity. Limited range of motion during the logrolling of the supine patient's leg suggests either synovitis or another, more diffuse pathology (e.g., arthritis, synovial chondromatosis). Unfortunately, there is no single clinical examination that reveals the presence or absence of a chondral defect. If a specific area of the joint is suspected of being damaged, weight-bearing activity that loads the area of the defect may elicit symptoms.

## IMAGING AND DIAGNOSTIC STUDIES

Plain radiographs may initially provide the most information. Degenerative joint disease, dysplasia, loose bodies, avascular necrosis (AVN), cam- or pincer-type impingement, and a history of slipped capital femoral epiphysis (SCFE) may be apparent on plain films. We recommend the use of a weight-bearing anteroposterior pelvic film and a frog-leg lateral view to evaluate bony morphology around the hip joint, with attention paid to the femoral head–neck offset and crossover lesions of the acetabulum in addition to the standard evaluation of loose bodies. A joint space narrowing of more than 2 mm to 3 mm is indicative of arthritis, and we would not recommend microfracture for this patient population. A pure cross-table lateral view has also been advocated by some authors to obtain additional information about the femoral head–neck offset.

Magnetic resonance imaging may be helpful to obtain a cause of the pain; however, many authors have noted that articular cartilage defects are frequently not clearly identified by the imaging sequences and resolutions that are often used (Keeney CORR 2004). Secondary signs of articular cartilage damage may be identified, such as subchondral bony cysts, bone edema (Figure 22-1), and joint effusions. High-resolution images may demonstrate distinct defects (Figure 22-2), articular cartilage thinning, or heterogeneity of the articular cartilage signal (Figure 22-3). The use of a surface coil with high-resolution, cartilage-sensitive images in the axial, coronal, and sagittal planes may provide a higher spatial resolution that could be helpful for diagnosis. Magnetic resonance arthrography improves the ability to evaluate the articular surface, but current techniques lack reliable sensitivity. In the future, the use of delayed gadolinium-enhanced MRI of cartilage (dGEMRIC) may provide additional information about the proteoglycan content of the articular cartilage.

## SURGICAL TECHNIQUE

The patient should be positioned on a fracture table or with a hip distraction system and in either a supine or lateral position, depending on surgeon preference. In most cases, the

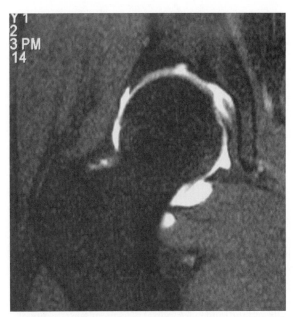

**Figure 22–2** Magnetic resonance image of a 16-year-old football player with a focal chondral defect in the acetabulum.

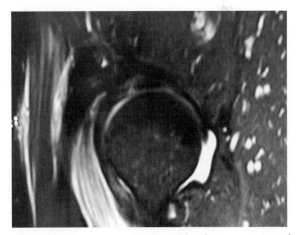

**Figure 22–3** Magnetic resonance image that demonstrates irregular articular cartilage with thinning subchondral edema.

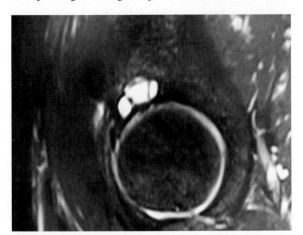

**Figure 22–1** Magnetic resonance image of the hip of a 41-year-old woman with associated subchondral cysts and irregular heterogeneous articular cartilage.

author prefers to have the patient in the supine position, with a commercially available hip distraction system placed on the leg that allows for the free movement of the limb. The hip is generally slightly internally rotated, flexed, and in neutral coronal alignment. The affected extremity is placed in 25 lb to 50 lb of longitudinal traction to distract the joint. A well-padded perineal post should be used to decrease the risk of pudendal nerve injury. The joint can then be distracted 7 mm to 15 mm under fluoroscopic guidance. The patient should be prepared and draped in the usual sterile fashion. Typically, after the surgical preparation solution has been applied and has dried, a large, clear drape with an adhesive central section (i.e., a "shower curtain" drape) is applied to the lateral aspect of the hip, and the top of the drape is allowed to cover the contralateral limb.

A spinal needle is then placed into the hip joint, and the stylet is removed; this breaks the vacuum seal and decreases the force needed to distract the joint. If necessary, the needle should be repositioned to avoid the labrum. This initial portal should be placed so that the tip of the needle enters the fovea of the acetabulum; this helps to ensure the good visualization of

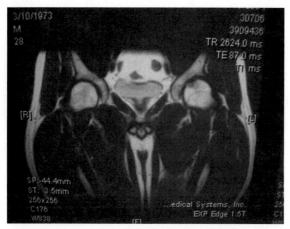

**Figure 22–4** Magnetic resonance image of the pelvis that demonstrates irregular articular cartilage at the medial femoral head lesion.

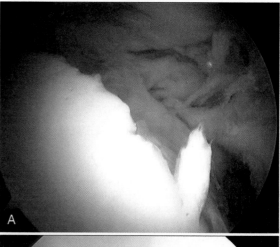

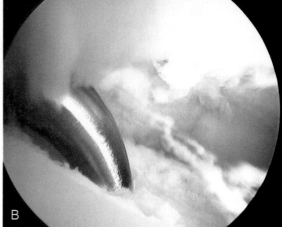

**Figure 22–6** Intraoperative arthroscopy image that demonstrates **A,** the medial articular cartilage flap on the femoral head and **B,** the use of the microfracture awl.

the joint. After the appropriate placement of the initial spinal needle and the guidewire, portal placement with the use of cannulated trocars can be performed to allow for access to the joint for visualization and instrumentation. A thorough diagnostic examination of the hip should occur, and this should involve the use of multiple portals. In some cases, defects on the femoral head are relatively medial (Figure 22-4), and careful instrument placement (Figure 22-5) is necessary to identify and treat defects (Figure 22-6, *A* and *B*).

After a defect is identified, the area should be debrided thoroughly with a motorized shaver, curette, or arthroscopic knife. All unstable cartilage should be debrided down to exposed bone until smooth vertical walls of healthy cartilage remain (Figure 22-7). Delaminated articular cartilage flaps are common adjacent to cam-type labral detachment lesions and should be removed (Figure 22-8). Thorough chondroplasty helps to ensure that the fibrin clot that forms after the microfracture stays within the defect.

Arthroscopic awls should be placed through portals that allow for access to the defect. The insertion and positioning of these instruments are significantly aided by the use of a slotted cannula (Figure 22-9). The semicylindric shape of this cannula allows irregularly shaped tools to enter into the joint.

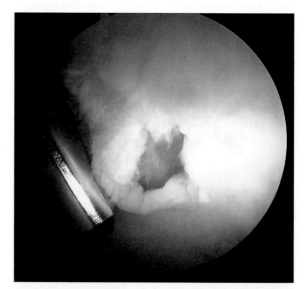

**Figure 22–7** Delamination of an articular cartilage defect.

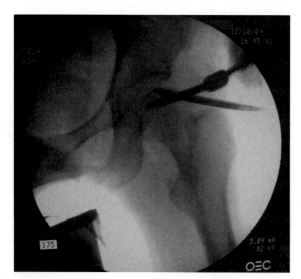

**Figure 22–5** Intraoperative fluoroscopy that shows the microfracture awl at the medial femoral head.

Subsequently, the slotted cannula can be removed to allow for the freer movement of the awl. As a result of the direction of instrument insertion into the joint, higher-degree angle-tipped awls (i.e., up to 90 degrees) are often used (Figure 22-10). Gentle punctures through the subchondral bone are created and spaced 3 mm to 4 mm apart to cover the area of the defect. If they are

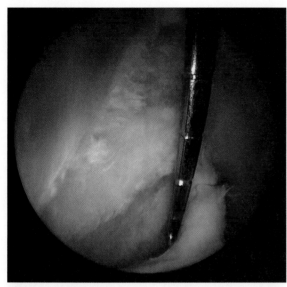

**Figure 22–8** Chondral flap.

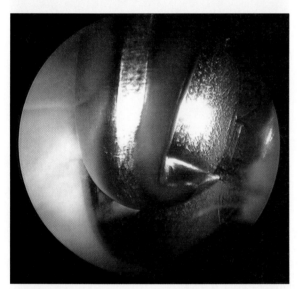

**Figure 22–9** Insertion of a 90-degree awl using a slotted cannula.

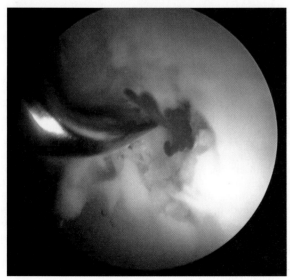

**Figure 22–10** Demonstration of the use of a 90-degree awl.

placed closer to one another, a bone fragment may break off, and the clot may not be retained. In addition, excessive force can cause the fracture holes to spread. Special attention should be paid to the depth of the awl puncture. A puncture depth of 2 mm to 4 mm will ensure that blood and fat droplets are discharged from the holes. The verification of an adequate depth of penetration can be performed by the application of suction to the area to see if blood or fat emerges (Figure 22-11). When the surgeon is satisfied with the microfracture, the instruments and the arthroscopic fluid should be removed from the joint. The incisions should be closed in the surgeon's preferred manner, and a sterile dressing is then applied.

### TECHNICAL PEARLS

- Many defects are not identified until surgery; the patient and the surgeon should both be aware of the potential for microfracture preoperatively.
- Access to the joint is significantly improved with the use of a slotted cannula to introduce instruments.
- Debride until perpendicular walls of healthy cartilage remain.
- Holes should be 2 mm to 4 mm deep to penetrate the subchondral plate.
- Holes should be spaced 3 mm to 5 mm apart to minimize bone fragmentation.
- Apply suction at the conclusion of the procedure to verify that blood and fat droplets emerge from the perforations.
- Continuous passive motion postoperatively substantially improves patient function.
- Patient compliance is critical.

## POSTOPERATIVE REHABILITATION

Before proceeding to the operating department for any hip arthroscopy, it is vital to have a well-informed discussion with the patient regarding his or her ability to comply with weight-bearing restrictions. This is a mandatory conversation as a result of the limitations of current radiologic techniques to discover cartilage defects that may only be found incidentally during hip arthroscopy. Microfracture may not have a successful result if patients do not understand and consent to weight-bearing limitations before they proceed into the operating department. In addition, range-of-motion limitations are indicated if concomitant labral repair is performed.

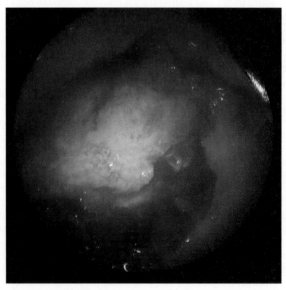

**Figure 22–11** Bleeding into a prepared defect.

Rehabilitation is similar to that of knee microfracture methods. A period of 6 to 8 weeks of toe-touch weight bearing with crutches is implemented. Passive range-of-motion exercises begin immediately postoperatively, and a continuous passive motion machine is extremely valuable for improving the quality of the repair and for significantly decreasing postoperative hip stiffness and hip flexor tendinitis. Physical therapy may also begin during this period, with a focus on range-of-motion exercises and an avoidance of extreme hip flexion, adduction, and internal rotation. Nonresistive stationary bicycling as tolerated may also begin, although patients will typically be more comfortable if the seat is raised to avoid hip flexion of more than 90 degrees. After 8 weeks, weight bearing may be advanced to full capacity, and physical therapy sessions can begin to focus on strengthening exercises. Athletes can typically return to sports 4 to 6 months postoperatively.

## RESULTS

In our experience, extensive areas of delamination or articular cartilage lesions are indicative of degenerative disease and are typically not successfully treated with microfracture. In addition, we have observed that hip arthritis can progress extremely rapidly over a period of several months and that it is unlikely in these cases that the treatment of focal defects will alter the course of the disease. The most successful results are found among young patients with acute pathology without any degenerative condition. Articular cartilage lesions associated with labral pathology and femoroacetabular impingement have had less satisfactory results if the underlying impingement pathology is untreated. At times, this requires labral detachment, the debridement of a pincer lesion that typically encompasses part of the cartilage defect, and labral refixation (Figure 22-12).

Results of the treatment of chondral defects with microfracture are somewhat difficult to interpret, because concomitant procedures are performed in the vast majority of cases, and it is difficult to identify the specific benefit that can be attributed to the microfracture procedure itself. However, subjective patient outcome data and second-look arthroscopies have demonstrated the efficacy of microfracture for the treatment of these defects.

Multiple authors have noted that the incidence of chondral defects is high when a labral injury is present, most likely as a result of femoroacetabular impingement. McCarthy noted that, in a series of 436 hip arthroscopies, 54% of defects occurred in the anterior acetabular quadrant.

There are only a limited number of studies that have evaluated the efficacy of microfracture (Table 22-1). Byrd and Jones looked at 21 cases of microfracture (19 acetabular cases, 1 femoral head case, and 1 case that involved both of these areas) and found an improvement in the mean Harris Hip Score from 51.4 to 75.2. Magnetic resonance imaging and arthrography revealed the pathology in only 19% of cases, and the average defect size was 12.2 mm$^2$ (range, 6 mm$^2$ to 17.5 mm$^2$). Labral tears were found in 17 of these cases, and degenerative ligamentum teres tears were found in 3 cases. The mean age of the patients was 35 years. At a minimum of 2 years of follow up, the authors found that 86% of patients had improved from the time of surgery. These authors also reported about 9 patients who were treated for inverted articular labrums. Three patients had chondral defects that were treated with microfracture, and these patients subsequently had the best outcomes of the group: they returned to their original baseline of activity and increased their Harris Hip Scores by an average of 36 points. In another study of arthroscopy and dysplasia, the investigators performed 8 microfracture procedures, with similar improvements seen in

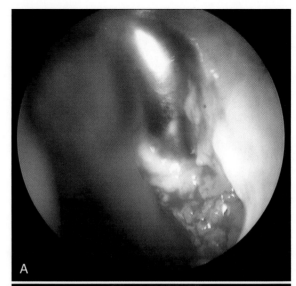

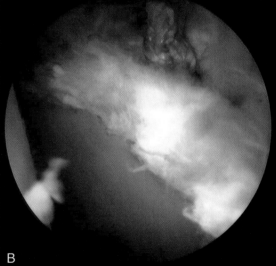

**Figure 22–12 A,** Anchor insertion into the debrided acetabular rim, as seen in Figure 22–7. **B,** The same area after repair with the arthroscopic mattress stitch.

the Harris Hip Scores. Again, almost all of these patients had concomitant labral debridement.

McCarthy noted that, in a series of 10 elite athletes (including 4 who had chondral defects), all patients returned to compete in their sports. Similarly, Bharam noted that, in a series of 28 professional athletes, 19 had chondral defects in addition to other pathology; these patients were also able to return to full sports activity.

Kocher and colleagues reported about chondroplasty of the acetabulum and the femoral head in 10 pediatric cases. These authors noted that there was an overall increase in the Harris Hip Scores from 53.1 to 82.1. However, the series did not isolate the improvement in hip scores for the chondroplasty group, because the chondroplasties were likely performed with other procedures.

Our experience with microfracture has been good for patients with small acute defects, who have returned to full athletic function. Patients with avascular necrosis have been treated with chondroplasty and microfracture of the femoral head in areas of articular cartilage loss and the retrograde injection of demineralized bone matrix into a cleared area of necrotic bone. These patients have done well clinically without subsequent collapse.

**Table 22-1** RESULTS SUMMARY

| Author | Title | No. of Patients | Length of Follow Up | Results |
|---|---|---|---|---|
| Byrd and Jones, 2003 | Hip arthroscopy in the presence of dysplasia | 48 | Minimum of 1 year | Improvement of HHS from 53 to 75; 8 patients treated with microfracture, 25 treated with chondroplasty |
| Byrd and Jones, 2004 | Microfracture for grade IV chondral lesions of the hip | 21 | 2 years | 86% had quantitative improvement |
| Byrd and Jones, 2002 | Osteoarthritis causes by an inverted acetabular labrum: radiographic diagnosis and arthroscopic treatment | 9 | 2 years | Increase in HHS by an average of 36 points in a subpopulation of 3 patients who underwent microfracture |
| Byrd and Jones, 2000 | Prospective analysis of hip arthroscopy with 2-year follow up | 15 | 2 years | Increase in HHS of 18 points |
| Kocher et al., 2005 | Hip arthroscopy in children and adolescents | 42 (54 hips) | Minimum of 1 year | 10 of 54 hips were treated with chondroplasty; all patients showed a significant improvement in HHS |
| Philippon et al., 2008 | Can microfracture produce repair tissue in acetabular chondral defects? | 9 | Average of 20 months | 91% fill of defect; 8 of 9 patients improved to modified Outerbridge grade 1 or 2 |
| Philippon et al., 2007 | Revision hip arthroscopy | 37 (23 hips) | Average of 12.7 months | HHS improved to an average of 77 points for all patients |

*HHS*, Harris Hip Score.

Philippon and colleagues recently reported about a series of 9 patients who underwent second-look procedures for acetabular defects who had been treated with microfracture. All of these patients had labral pathology. The average defect size was 163 mm$^2$ (range, 40 mm$^2$ to 240 mm$^2$). These patients had an average fill of 91%. The single patient in the study who did poorly had advanced osteoarthritis, which was noted as a contraindication for the procedure. One of the patients went on to total hip arthroplasty at 5.5 years postoperatively, despite 95% fill being found during a second-look arthroscopy 3 years after the procedure. Furthermore, Philippon and colleagues reported that microfracture or chondroplasty occurred in 70% of the revision cases.

Evidence exists to support these promising techniques, which have been well described for other joints. Improved data collection and analysis will help to further refine indications for this procedure. In addition, improved imaging of the articular cartilage will be helpful for the preoperative and postoperative evaluation of defects and their healing. Finally, a randomized controlled study that demonstrates the effectiveness of these techniques would also be welcome.

## COMPLICATIONS

There have been no studies that have reported the complication rates of microfracture with hip arthroscopy. It is important to pay attention to the articular surface while the arthroscopic awl is intra-articular. Any iatrogenic injury to healthy cartilage must be avoided. This type of injury can occur during the performance of a diagnostic procedure as well, and careful technique must be used to limit any unnecessary defects. In addition, as with other arthroscopic hip operations, traction neuropraxia, fluid extravasation, and neurovascular injury may occur.

## ANNOTATED REFERENCES AND SUGGESTED READINGS

**Bharam S, Draovitch P, Fu FH, Philippon MJ.** Return to competition in pro athletes with traumatic labral tears in the hip. Abstract, American Orthopaedic Society for Sports Medicine (AOSSM), Orlando, FL, June 2002.

**Byrd JWT, Jones KS.** Hip arthroscopy in the presence of dysplasia. *Arthroscopy.* 2003;19:1055–1060.

Byrd and Jones looked at 48 patients with either dysplasia or borderline dysplasia. From this population, they reported the results of various procedures that were performed, including chondroplasty and microfracture. The Harris Hip Score improved from 53 to 75 in the chondral damage group.

**Byrd JWT, Jones KS.** Microfracture for grade IV chondral lesions of the hip. *Arthroscopy.* 2004;20:e41.

This abstract provides 2 years of follow up for 21 patients who received microfracture for their grade IV lesions. Overall, 86% of patients improved. Interestingly, the abstract also comments on the ineffectiveness of magnetic resonance imaging and arthrography to diagnose the articular pathology that was discovered intraoperatively.

**Byrd JWT, Jones KS.** Osteoarthritis caused by an inverted acetabular labrum: radiographic diagnosis and arthroscopic treatment. *Arthroscopy.* 2002;18:741–747.

This study found that 9 out of 220 arthroscopic hip patients developed osteoarthritis as a result of an inverted acetabular labrum. The authors discovered that a subset of 3 patients who were treated with microfracture did the best out of the group: their Harris Hip Scores increased the most, and they returned to normal activity.

**Byrd JWT, Jones KS.** Prospective analysis of hip arthroscopy. *Arthroscopy.* 2000;16:578–587.

This article is a case series report about 38 procedures that were performed in 35 patients. Chondral injury was treated and resulted in an overall improvement in the Harris Hip Score of 18 points. Specific treatments were not listed.

Crawford K, Philippon MJ, Sekiya JK, Rodkey WG, Steadman JR. Microfracture of the hip in athletes. *Clin Sports Med.* 2006;25:327–335.

The authors provide an excellent review of the current literature that supports microfracture. In addition, this article supplies information about the workup and treatment of microfracture.

Frisbie DD, Oxford JT, Southwood L, et al. Early events in cartilage repair after subchondral bone microfracture. *Clin Orthop.* 2003;407:215–227.

This excellent basic science article describes and demonstrates changes in subchondral bone after microfracture.

Keeney JA, Peelle MW, Jackson J, Rubin D, Maloney WJ, Clohisy JC. Magnetic resonance arthrography versus arthroscopy in the evaluation of articular hip pathology. *Clin Orthop Relat Res.* 2004;249:163–169.

Kocher MS, Kim YJ, Millis MB, et al. Hip arthroscopy in children and adolescents. *J Pediatr Orthop.* 2005;25:680–686.

This study looked at 54 arthroscopies in 42 pediatric patients. Included in the cumulative data are 10 cases of chondroplasty. Significant improvement in the Harris Hip Score occurred with a minimum of 1 year of follow up.

McCarthy J, Barsoum W, Puri L, Lee JA, Murphy S, Cooke P. The role of hip arthroscopy in the elite athlete. *Clin Orthop Relat Res.* 2003;406:71–74.

McCarthy JC, Noble PC, Schuck MR, Wright J, Lee J. The Otto E. Aufranc Award: the role of labral lesions to development of early degenerative hip disease. *Clin Orthop Relat Res.* 2001;393:25–37.

Mithoefer K, Williams RJ 3rd, Warren RF, Wickiewicz TL, Marx RG. High-impact athletics after knee articular cartilage repair: a prospective evaluation of the microfracture technique. *Am J Sports Med.* 2006;34(9):1413–1418.

Philippon MJ, Schenker ML, Briggs KK, Kuppersmith DA, Maxwell RB, Stubbs AJ. Revision hip arthroscopy. *Am J Sports Med.* 2007;35:1918–1921.

Philippon and colleagues provide a look at 37 patients who required revision hip arthroscopy. In the study, impingement accounted for most revisions, with chondral defects being a close second. Outcomes demonstrated that patients regain some function within the first year.

Philippon MJ, Schenker ML, Biggs KK, Maxwell RB. Can microfracture produce repair tissue in acetabular chondral defects? *Arthroscopy.* 2008;24:46–50.

The authors provide a case series regarding second looks at acetabular defects that underwent microfracture. Eight of 9 patients had 95% to 100% coverage with grade 1 or 2 appearance of cartilage at an average follow up of 20 months.

Shindle MK, Voos JE, Heyworth BE, et al. Hip arthroscopy in the athletic patient: current techniques and spectrum of disease. *J Bone Joint Surg Am.* 2007;89:29–43.

This article provides a good review of the history and diagnostic features of hip disease. It also provides pearls to consider with regard to the radiologic workup.

# CHAPTER 23

# Arthroscopy for Symptomatic Hip Arthroplasty

*Vikas Khanduja and Richard N. Villar*

## INTRODUCTION

Arthroscopic surgery of the hip has gained immense popularity during recent years as a minimally invasive and low-risk surgical procedure for the treatment of many intra- and extra-articular conditions in the hip. A resurgence of interest in sports medicine and a proficiency in arthroscopic techniques has led to an expansion of the indications for—and, in some cases, perhaps a stretching the limits of—this procedure. The latest trends seem to be accessing the peripheral compartment on a regular basis; arthroscopic excision of the cam femoroacetabular impingement lesion; labral detachment; rim trimming and labral refixation for pincer impingement; and the treatment of several extra-articular conditions, such as snapping hip and iliopsoas tendonitis.

Alternatively, resurfacing arthroplasty of the hip is also increasingly being performed worldwide, and the early to mid-term results warrant optimism. Early complication rates have decreased, and this seems to have become the procedure of choice for the younger patient with end-stage arthritis and good bone stock. However, problems do occur, and assessing the radiologically well-fixed but symptomatic resurfacing arthroplasty can be a difficult task. Soft-tissue problems such as adhesions, iliopsoas tendonitis, trochanteric bursitis, synovitis, sports hernia, and metallosis can occur around the resurfacing; these are extremely difficult to diagnose initially. Secondary bony or soft-tissue impingement can also be fairly symptomatic, and these conditions do not always show up on the radiographs. Finally, septic or aseptic loosening can also result in a painful resurfacing with minimal or no radiologic changes.

Therefore, despite thoroughly investigating the patient, a definitive diagnosis is not always possible. Undertaking a revision of the resurfacing is perhaps the only solution, even when it is not warranted. However, an arthroscopy of the symptomatic joint could be useful in this scenario. Arthroscopy has already been reported to provide a diagnosis and possible treatment of symptomatic joint replacements of the knee, the elbow, the shoulder, and, in some cases, the hip. Larger series are available that have described the results of knee arthroscopy after total knee arthroplasty, with varying results. Although treatment options are often limited, obtaining a definite diagnosis with the use of a minimally invasive approach is undeniably advantageous, precluding further major surgery. On the basis of these reports and the large arthroscopic experience of our unit, we performed arthroscopies for patients with these symptomatic resurfacings, and we found that the procedures can be of great diagnostic and therapeutic value. This chapter outlines our experiences with these challenging but interesting patients.

## INDICATION

The sole indication for this procedure is a patient with a painful hip resurfacing in the presence of normal or indeterminate investigations.

## HISTORY AND PHYSICAL EXAMINATION

The assessment of a patient with a symptomatic resurfacing is quite challenging and should begin with a thorough history and physical examination. The patient typically presents with a history of pain in the buttock, groin, or thigh after the resurfacing. The character of the pain can provide some indication of the possible cause: a throbbing ache signifies underlying infection, whereas a sharp ache during weight bearing or start-up pain suggests possible implant loosening. The site of pain is also very helpful for determining the anatomic area of the possible pathology: pain in the buttock suggests problems with the acetabular component, whereas pain in the groin and the thigh suggests the femoral component. Patients who engage in strenuous physical or sports activity should be questioned about pain in and around the hernial orifices, because small sports hernias that are often missed can present with groin ache after a resurfacing. Patients with groin pain should also be questioned about the position or activity during which the pain is aggravated to elicit iliopsoas, adductor, or abductor tendonitis. Finally, referred pain from the lower back can also be a cause of pain in the buttock; a specific history that pertains to this pain should be elicited.

After a detailed history has been obtained, a physical examination that concentrates on the gait, the lower back, and the hip should be conducted. A limitation of the range of movement of the hip could be a result of soft-tissue or bony impingement lesions. The hernial orifices and the attachments of the iliopsoas, the adductors, the hamstrings, and the abductors should be palpated to ensure that pathology in these regions is not missed. Patients in whom there are clinical findings that are suggestive of sports hernias or muscle strains should be referred to a sports physician with an interest in groin pathology.

## INVESTIGATIONS

The patient should be thoroughly investigated before this procedure is performed. Initial investigations should include a full blood count, an erythrocyte sedimentation rate, a C-reactive protein test to rule out infection, and a biochemical screen. For a patient with reported hypersensitivity, a full immunologic screen and a referral to an immunologist or a physician with experience in this arena is warranted. Radiologic investigations should include plain anteroposterior and lateral radiographs of the affected hip and an isotope bone scan, which is helpful for identifying the early loosening of the components. For a patient with a suspected sports hernia or groin strain, an ultrasound scan of the groin and occasionally a magnetic resonance scan with metal-suppression sequences is beneficial. The magnetic resonance scan can also be helpful for identifying edema around the trochanteric bursa, the iliopsoas tendon, and the adductor tendons, if there is pathology in these areas. Finally, a diagnostic local anesthetic block can help to elucidate whether the pain is intra- or extra-articular in origin.

## SURGICAL TECHNIQUE

The operation is performed as a day-care procedure with the patient under general anesthesia or with the use of a combination of a general anesthetic and a lumbar plexus block. We prefer to have the patient in the lateral position, but the supine position can also be used. The patient is placed in the lateral decubitus position, and appropriate abduction, flexion, and longitudinal traction are obtained with a distractor that can be attached to a standard Maquet table. The image intensifier is placed obliquely across the patient, and images of the resurfacing arthroplasty are obtained. It should be kept in mind that a large amount of longitudinal traction is not necessary for this procedure. Therefore, the hip is distracted to about 1 cm under fluoroscopic control, and a 17-gauge spinal needle is inserted into the joint. This allows for the negative intra-articular pressure to be equalized with the atmospheric pressure, and it also allows for the mandatory aspiration of the synovial fluid for culture before saline is instilled in the joint.

Standard lateral paratrochanteric and anterior paratrochanteric portals are made to access the central compartment; this allows for the visualization of the edge of the acetabular component, the bone–component interface (Figure 23-1), and the synovial membrane, and the surgeon is also able to look for any possible metallosis. If debridement is required, it is performed with an arthroscopic shaver or a radiofrequency probe. Synovial biopsy and further aspirates from the bone implant interface may also be obtained at this time.

Releasing the traction completely and flexing the hip to relax the anterior capsule allows for easy access to the peripheral compartment of the arthroplasty. The main portal for the peripheral compartment is made approximately 4 cm anterior

and superior to the direct lateral paratrochanteric portal. Entry into the peripheral compartment allows for the visualization of the base of the femoral component (Figure 23-2) for assessing component stability. It also provides an opportunity to diagnose and treat capsular pathology, fibrosis, adhesions (Figure 23-3), iliopsoas tendonitis (Figure 23-4), and soft-tissue and bony impingement lesions (Figure 23-5).

However, the greatest advantage of arthroscopy for resurfacing lies in its dynamic component. The dynamic component involves the internal and external rotation of the hip during flexion, which leads to the micromovement of the acetabular component or the femoral component if either one is loose. A ring-handle spike or the arthroscopy hook can also be used at this stage to assess the stability of the components.

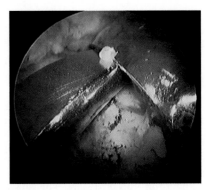

**Figure 23–2** Arthroscopic view of bone resorption at the base of the femoral component, with a bone spike in the resorbed area.

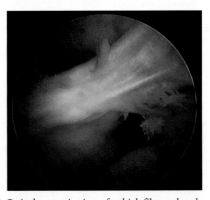

**Figure 23–3** Arthroscopic view of a thick fibrous band seen in the peripheral compartment. This band causes pain and restriction of the range of motion.

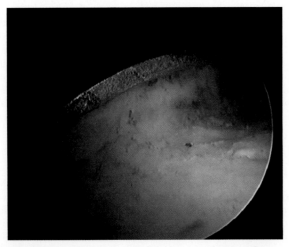

**Figure 23–1** Arthroscopic view of the bone–implant interface.

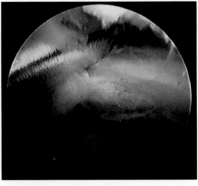

**Figure 23–4** Arthroscopic view of iliopsoas tendonitis in the peripheral compartment.

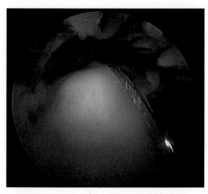

**Figure 23–5** Arthroscopic view of a bony impingement lesion in the peripheral compartment.

## TECHNICAL PEARLS

- Patients should be thoroughly investigated before the procedure begins.
- All of the investigations should be normal or indeterminate.
- Accurate patient positioning and portal placement are essential.
- Only a minimal amount of traction is required.
- One has to be extremely careful while inserting instruments to avoid scratching the surface of the components.

## POSTOPERATIVE REHABILITATION

As mentioned previously, the operation is carried out as a day-care procedure. If there is no obvious sign of infection during arthroscopy, we inject the joint and the portal sites with 20 mL of 0.5% Chirocaine for postoperative analgesia. Oral analgesia is also prescribed on a regular basis for the first week after surgery. The patient is mobilized with the use of partial weight bearing with crutches 3 to 4 hours after the operation. When the patient is mobilizing safely, he or she can be discharged from the ward.

When the patient is out of the hospital, our rehabilitation protocol includes a program of exercises to reestablish a full and pain-free range of motion. This involves progressing from partial weight bearing to full weight bearing after the prescribed period of crutch use within the limits of pain; the process usually lasts for approximately 4 weeks. Gait reeducation is essential for all patients, because surgery almost always follows prolonged pain and dysfunction. This can lead to altered biomechanics of the lower limb and abnormal movement patterns, which need to be assessed and corrected after surgery.

Gym-based rehabilitation is arranged at this stage and commonly involves a static cycle, an elliptical trainer, and a treadmill. Further progressions and resistance are added at the therapist's discretion. Hydrotherapy and swimming are begun after the wound has healed. The patient is reassessed at 2 weeks by his or her personal physician and then at 6 weeks at our clinic, where further management is discussed.

## RESULTS

Twelve consecutive patients with painful resurfacing and normal or indeterminate investigations underwent arthroscopy of the hip in our unit. There were 8 female patients in the series, and the mean age of the patients was 53.7 years (range, 38 to 70 years). Seven patients had a fully uncemented hydroxyapatite-coated resurfacing arthroplasty (Cormet 2000, Corin Medical Ltd., Cirencester, UK), and 5 patients had a hybrid BIRMINGHAM HIP Resurfacing procedure (Midland Medical Technologies Ltd., Birmingham, UK). The mean period from the index operation to the arthroscopy was 25 months (range, 6 to 48 months). More complete details about all of the patients and their intraoperative diagnoses and treatments are shown in Table 23-1.

Two of the 12 patients were suspected of having an aseptic loosening of the acetabular component, but there was no obvious osteolysis apparent on the plain radiographs to confirm this (Figure 23-6). One of these patients was found to have that condition during arthroscopy, but both of the patients were revised to an uncemented total hip replacement; the femoral component, although well fixed, showed osteolysis at the base. None of the cultures of the aspirates sent at arthroscopy came back as being positive.

## Table 23–1 RESULTS

| Patient No. | Age | Sex | Type of Implant | Time Since Implantation | Arthroscopic Diagnosis | Procedure |
|---|---|---|---|---|---|---|
| 1 | 55 | F | Cormet | 24 months | Bony FAI | Synovectomy and excision of the impingement lesion |
| 2 | 57 | F | Cormet | 36 months | Loosening of the acetabular component | Assessment and biopsy |
| 3 | 64 | M | Cormet | 36 months | Normal | Assessment and aspiration |
| 4 | 43 | F | Birmingham | 24 months | ALVAL | Assessment, synovectomy, and biopsy |
| 5 | 63 | M | Cormet | 24 months | Fibrous adhesions | Synovectomy and capsular release |
| 6 | 55 | F | Cormet | 12 months | Bony FAI with psoas tendonitis | Excision of the impingement lesion and iliopsoas tenotomy |
| 7 | 38 | F | Cormet | 6 months | Psoas tendonitis | Iliopsoas tenotomy |
| 8 | 70 | F | Birmingham | 12 months | Trochanteric bursitis | Excision of the trochanteric bursa |
| 9 | 53 | F | Cormet | 12 months | Psoas tendonitis | Synovectomy and iliopsoas tenotomy |
| 10 | 44 | M | Birmingham | 40 months | Soft-tissue impingement with psoas tendonitis | Excision of the impingement lesion and iliopsoas tenotomy |
| 11 | 65 | M | Birmingham | 48 months | Bony FAI with psoas tendonitis | Excision of the impingement lesion and iliopsoas tenotomy |
| 12 | 38 | F | Birmingham | 26 months | Loose cement particles with synovitis (see Figure 23-7) | Removal of loose cement and synovectomy |

*ALVAL*, acute lymphocytic vascular associated lesions; *F*, female; *M*, male; *FAI*, femoroacetabular impingement.

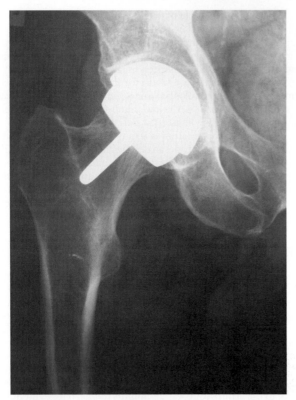

**Figure 23–6** Radiograph of a patient 3 months after a resurfacing arthroplasty. The patient is symptomatic, but there is no apparent osteolysis.

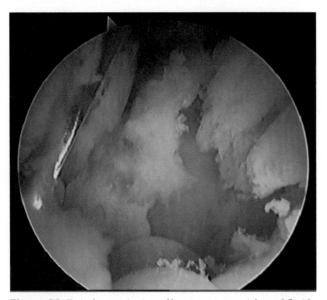

**Figure 23–7** Arthroscopic view of loose cement particles and florid synovitis.

## COMPLICATIONS

The procedure is relatively safe, and we did not have any complications in our series. However, apart from the general complications of hip arthroscopy related to traction, one has to be extremely vigilant during the insertion of instruments into the joint to avoid the iatrogenic scratching of the surfaces of the femoral and acetabular components. In addition, it should be kept in mind that a large amount of traction is not required for this procedure, thus circumventing the complications that could arise as a result of traction. Finally, one has to be vigilant while inserting wires into the resurfaced joint, because there is a high possibility of breaking them, and removing them is certainly not a task for the amateur.

## CONCLUSION

The assessment of a symptomatic resurfacing is usually difficult, and it becomes more challenging in the setting of normal or indeterminate investigations. However, we found that, in experienced hands, hip arthroscopy can be used as an effective tool for both diagnosis and therapeutic intervention for these patients.

Further possibilities of an arthroplasty include assessing polyethylene wear; replacing misplaced liners of the acetabular components; performing arthroscopically assisted revision hip replacements by allowing for easy access to the femoral canal for the retrieval of cement; performing sequestrectomy for infection; and excising recurrent synovial osteochondromatosis that may occur despite an arthroplasty.

It is important to note that resurfacing remains a highly specialized procedure that should not be undertaken without appropriate training.

## ANNOTATED REFERENCES

Fontana A, Zecca M, Sala C. Arthroscopic assessment of total hip replacement and polyethylene wear: a case report. *Knee Surg Sports Traumatol Arthrosc.* 2000;8:244–245.

The authors' report the case of a patient who showed clinical and radiological signs of massive polyethylene wear 3 years after total hip replacement. Arthroscopy was performed to assess the loosening of the acetabular cup. The procedure showed the polyethylene element to be broken into three pieces in the area corresponding to the upper border.

Hersch JC, Dines DM. Arthroscopy for failed shoulder arthroplasty. *Arthroscopy.* 2000;16:606–612.

The purpose of this study was to describe the specifics of technique and results of arthroscopic evaluation and treatment of failed shoulder arthroplasties in 10 patients with early and late complications of shoulder arthroplasty.

Hyman JL, Salvati EA, Laurencin CT, et al. The arthroscopic drainage, irrigation, and debridement of late, acute total hip arthroplasty infections: average 6-year follow-up. *J Arthroplasty.* 1999;14:903–910.

The authors present their experience with arthroscopy for the treatment of late, acute periprosthetic hip infections in 8 consecutive patients. After a hip aspiration confirmed the presence of bacterial infection, all patients underwent prompt arthroscopic drainage, lavage, and debridement. At a mean follow-up of 70 months (range, 29–104 months), no recurrence of infection occurred.

Khanduja V, Villar RN. The role of arthroscopy in resurfacing arthroplasty of the hip. *Arthroscopy.* 2008;24(122):e1–e3.

The authors report on the successful use of hip arthroscopy in a patient with persistent pain following a resurfacing arthroplasty, identifying loosening of the acetabular component. It was perhaps the only way to identify component micromovement in the background of all other investigations' being normal or indeterminate.

Klinger HM, Baums MH, Spahn G, et al. A study of effectiveness of knee arthroscopy after knee arthroplasty. *Arthroscopy.* 2005;21:731–738.

The purpose of this study was to investigate the outcome of arthroscopy in painful knee arthroplasty without evidence of infection, fracture, wear, and component loosening or malposition that had been refractory to conservative treatment. In addition, a literature review of 498 cases was performed. The authors concluded that arthroscopic treatment of painful knee arthroplasty provides reliable expectations for improvement in function, decrease in pain, and improvement in knee scores for most patients.

Mastrokalos DS, Zahos KA, Korres D, et al. Arthroscopic debridement and irrigation of periprosthetic total elbow infection. *Arthroscopy.* 2006;22(1140):e1–e3.

The authors report on the successful arthroscopic treatment of a patient with septic arthritis of a total elbow replacement.

# CHAPTER 24

# Arthroscopic Management of the Trauma Patient

*Aaron Perdue and James A. Goulet*

## INTRODUCTION

Hip arthroscopy has been described as part of treatment regimens for hip trauma and related sequelae for decades, but the role of hip arthroscopy for this application has expanded rapidly during recent years. As early as 1931, Burman noted a role for a form of hip arthroscopy for loose body or fragment removal. The role for surgical debridement of the hip expanded substantially with the observation that loose bodies were ubiquitous with hip fracture dislocations. Epstein advised that all hip fracture–dislocations should be treated with debridement in an attempt to delay the appearance of traumatic arthritis and to minimize its severity. He advocated open debridement rather than arthroscopic debridement. The prevalence of loose bodies after injury to the hip and their impact on the development of hip joint arthrosis certainly contributed to the imperfect long-term results of dislocations and fractures around the hip joint (Figures 24-1 and 24-2). Until recently, loose bone and cartilage fragments were almost always retrieved with open arthrotomy. Advances in arthroscopic tools and techniques have made arthroscopic loose-body removal highly efficient. Arthroscopy advantages include diminished blood loss, smaller incisions, decreased recovery time, reduced potential for neurovascular damage, and decreased disruption of capsuloligamentous structures. Indications for arthroscopic debridement after trauma have been extended to include the extraction of bullets, the removal of broken hardware from the joint, and joint lavage for the treatment of infection or contamination in association with bullet fragments passing through the bowel and communicating with the hip joint.

The arthroscopic treatment of acetabular labral pathology most typically involves atraumatic tears or labral disease associated with impingement or hip dysplasia. Isolated cases of traumatic labral pathology have been reported since 1959, when Dameron described a bucket-handle tear of the acetabular labrum that prohibited the reduction of a posterior dislocation of the hip that subsequently required open repair. Labral injury has more recently been described as a relatively common but previously poorly recognized phenomenon in association with acetabular fractures. Ganz described reproducible labral pathology in 14 patients with displaced transverse acetabular fractures

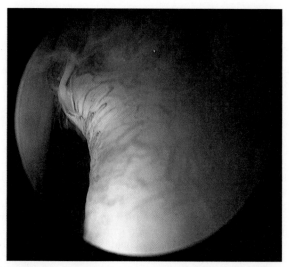

**Figure 24–1** A 31-year-old male who sustained a femoral head fracture and hip dislocation that were treated with open reduction and internal fixation 6 months earlier. Persistent groin pain was relieved with intra-articular anesthetic. A hypertrophied and inflamed labrum is evident.

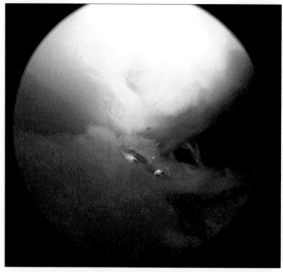

**Figure 24–2** Another view of the same patient shown in Figure 24-1. Femoral head chondrolysis is evident. Intervention was limited to labral debridement, chondroplasty of the femoral head, and lavage.

who had been treated with open reduction and internal fixation. The labrum was partially or completely detached from the superior acetabular rim in all cases. In this series, an avulsed portion of the labrum was left if it was stable and undamaged, resected if it was unstable and damaged, and repaired if it was unstable but intact or attached to a bony fragment. Ganz proposed arthrotomy at the time of acetabular fracture fixation to search for associated intracapsular injuries in displaced transverse acetabular fractures and to treat injuries accordingly. In the case of acetabular fractures, multiple authors have identified reduction as the most important factor for avoiding the development of arthrosis and for obtaining a good clinical outcome, but they have noted that even anatomic fracture reduction fails to guarantee excellent outcomes. It is likely that additional factors such as chondral damage at the time of injury, loose fragments, and labral injuries all contribute to the patient's final long-term outcome (Figures 24-3 and 24-4).

## INDICATIONS

- Foreign bodies (e.g., bullets, osteochondral and chondral fragments, broken fracture implants)
- Contaminated or septic joints
- Labral tears
- Chondral injuries
- Ligamentum teres ruptures
- Femoral head fractures (limited indication)

## BRIEF HISTORY AND PHYSICAL EXAMINATION

Patients with high-energy trauma require more urgent and comprehensive treatment than patients who have experienced lower-energy or focal trauma to the hip. The initial evaluation of a patient with high-energy trauma is based on the Advanced Trauma Life Support protocol and includes the "ABCs"—airway, breathing, and circulation—of the primary survey. The treatment of high-energy trauma patients is directed by general surgical colleagues with prompt cooperation from orthopedic surgeons. Standard radiographic trauma

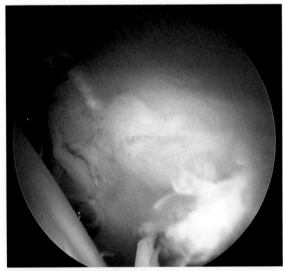

**Figure 24-3** A 28-year-old female who sustained a displaced both-column acetabular fracture at the age of 19 years. She had a gradual onset of groin pain over the previous year, with nonspecific findings of magnetic resonance imaging and pain relief with intra-articular anesthetic injection. Extensive fibrillation and cartilage loss on the femoral head are seen.

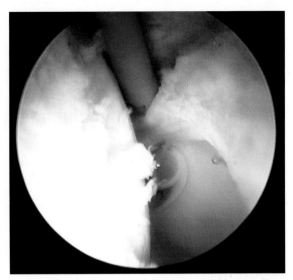

**Figure 24-4** Another view of the same patient shown in Figure 24-3. There is a small anterior labral tear. The labral tear and the femoral head were debrided.

series include an anteroposterior pelvic radiograph, an anteroposterior chest radiograph, and a lateral cervical spine radiograph. The orthopedic examination includes the palpation of the spine and all extremities to look for crepitance, deformity, open injuries, and dislocation. A high index of suspicion for a posterior hip dislocation is maintained when a patient presents with a shortened extremity with the affected hip held in flexion, abduction, and internal rotation. Alternatively, an anterior dislocation leaves the hip in extension and neutral or slight abduction. The examiner must complete a thorough trauma evaluation, because 95% of patients with a hip dislocation have at least one other organ-system injury. Of the patients who have high-energy hip dislocations, 15% have abdominal injuries, 21% have thoracic injuries, 21% have craniofacial injuries, 24% have closed head injuries, and 33% have other orthopedic injuries.

## IMAGING AND DIAGNOSTIC STUDIES

An anteroposterior pelvic radiograph is a routine part of the evaluation of a traumatically injured patient. If there is a disruption of the anterior or posterior pelvic ring, then the evaluation routinely includes pelvic inlet and outlet views. Similarly, if an associated acetabular fracture is present or suspected, radiographic evaluation should include the 45-degree oblique views described by Judet and Letournel. The closed reduction of a dislocated hip must be confirmed by a repeat anteroposterior pelvic radiograph. Follow up studies should also include pelvic computed tomography (CT) scans with 1.5-mm cuts through the acetabulum to search for loose bodies, to assess acetabular fractures, and to evaluate the reduction status of associated femoral head fractures. Final complete radiographs should include a dedicated hip series as well as full-length views of the ipsilateral femur to evaluate for associated fractures. In the case of gunshot wounds, metallic markers should be placed at all identifiable entrance and exit wounds to facilitate an understanding of the bullet's trajectory. Radiographs and CT scans may not reliably demonstrate loose bodies within the hip joint. In a series of 36 patients who were treated with arthroscopy, Mullis and Dahners found loose bodies in 33 patients, including 7 out of 9 patients who had no loose bodies seen on preoperative radiographs or CT scans with 3-mm cuts.

Labral tears are best evaluated with magnetic resonance arthrography. Typically, labral tears associated with high-energy trauma have not been routinely addressed or even recognized acutely unless they are specifically sought intraoperatively during open fracture fixation. Thus, magnetic resonance arthrograms may be most frequently indicated for traumatically injured patients who continue to have unexplained pain during convalescence. Labral injuries have been demonstrated in association with acetabular fractures, and traumatic labral pathologies should be addressed. The extent to which minor labral injuries associated with high-energy trauma will become symptomatic or contribute to arthrosis remains unknown.

## SURGICAL TECHNIQUE

The patient can be placed supine or in a lateral position, depending on surgeon preference. Because one must take into consideration other injuries of the traumatized patient (e.g., spine injury) when positioning him or her, a supine position is often required. By contrast, an obese patient's pannus may interfere with the maneuverability of arthroscopic equipment if he or she is in the supine position, so a lateral position should be considered for these individuals. A standard fracture table or a custom distraction device is necessary to distract the joint space. In our practice, we prefer to use a commercially available distraction device system that accommodates hip arthroscopy. Distractor systems must possess a stable distraction mechanism and a well-padded perineal post; most described complications encountered with hip arthroscopy are neuropraxias caused by compression against an underpadded post or by distraction, especially if it is prolonged. In addition, the perineal post must be offset laterally against the medial thigh of the operative leg to achieve a sufficient vector to distract the hip joint. The hip is slightly abducted and flexed to relax the anterior hip capsule. Both feet are generously padded and securely placed into the foot holders. Fluoroscopy is introduced from the nonoperative side of the patient before the sterile preparation of the injured extremity to confirm the ability to distract the joint. Approximately 50 lb of traction is needed to distract the hip joint; however, less force may be needed for the distraction of recently injured hips with traumatic capsular disruptions.

Three standard portals have been described for hip arthroscopy: anterior, anterolateral, and posterolateral. All of these may be necessary for the retrieval of intra-articular fragments, particularly if the fragments have been impacted and are relatively immobile. The anterolateral portal lies most centrally in the safe zone for arthroscopy and therefore should be established first for the introduction of the arthroscope and direct visualization while introducing the remaining portals. The anterolateral portal is placed 1 cm proximally and 1 cm anterior to the tip of the greater trochanter. The posterolateral portal is made at the superoposterior margin of the greater trochanter. The anterior portal is placed at the intersection of a line drawn distally from the anterosuperior iliac spine and a transverse line from the tip of the greater trochanter. Alternative arthroscopic portals have been described, including an inferomedial approach to remove an intra-articular bullet. With this approach, the hip is placed in extension and in approximately 30 degrees of abduction. A 3-cm incision is made posterior to the adductor longus tendon to allow for the blunt dissection and identification of the psoas tendon. The capsule is then penetrated medial to the tendon and distended with saline.

The hip is distracted a minimum of 8 mm to avoid chondral and labral injuries during the insertion of instruments. Portals are made with the use of specially designed extra-long

arthroscopic instruments, including a long spinal needle and a flexible guidewire. A long 18-gauge spinal needle is placed first under fluoroscopic imaging at the anterolateral portal. Special attention must be paid to avoid the penetration of the labrum. If the labrum is penetrated with the spinal needle, it will be subsequently damaged with the passage of the trocar. As the needle penetrates the capsule, a decrease in resistance is noted, whereas if the needle contacts the labrum, the resistance increases. The joint is then distended with saline, and intracapsular positioning is confirmed by the backflow of fluid. The guidewire is passed, and the spinal needle is removed. A sharp cannulated trocar is then introduced over the guidewire that is penetrating the joint capsule, and this is followed by a blunt cannulated trocar to avoid damage to the articular cartilage. The anterior portal can then be made by direct intra-articular visualization of the anterior triangle, which is comprised of the capsule, the labrum, and the femoral head. A long 18-gauge spinal needle is inserted within this triangle under direct visualization, and the steps are then repeated to introduce a trocar.

The inspection of the hip joint is accomplished systematically. One may switch among the three established portals with the use of a combination of 70- and 30-degree arthroscopic cameras. The 70-degree arthroscope is most commonly used, and it affords the best view of the labrum, the femoral head, and the acetabulum, including the most inferior portion of the acetabular fossa, which contains the ligamentum teres. The 30-degree arthroscope provides the best view of the central portion of the acetabulum, the femoral head, and the superior part of the fossa. Joint hematoma is addressed first to increase visualization. Subsequently, peripheral pathology is inspected and dealt with accordingly, with labral repair or excision, loose-body removal, or chondroplasty. Debridement within the acetabular fossa is performed last, because bleeding will obscure visualization. Electrocautery, epinephrine added to the pump fluid, and hypotensive anesthesia may be employed to optimize visualization. In addition, a high-flow pump may be used to allow for sufficient flow without requiring increased fluid pressure, which may be maintained at 60 mm Hg. Loose bodies can often be flushed from the joint with simple fluid lavage, whereas larger bodies require removal with a grasper.

Labral tears associated with hip trauma can be repaired with suture anchors if detached from the bone or with suture lassos if an intrasubstance tear is present. The suture anchor is positioned on the acetabular rim away from the articular surface. The anchor may be inserted with fluoroscopic assistance, but typically this is not necessary. The anchor is gently tapped into place while aiming away from the articular surface and simultaneously visualizing the joint surface to identify improper placement into the articular cartilage. With the anchor solidly in position, a curved spectrum is used to capture capsular tissue, and a suture passer is delivered through the spectrum. The passing suture and one limb of the anchor suture are retrieved with a grasping instrument through the anterior portal, and these are tied tightly together. The other end of the passing suture is then pulled out through the anterior portal, carrying with it the anchor suture limb through the capsular tissue and back out through the anterior portal. The passing suture is then untied from the suture anchor limb. The second suture anchor limb is retrieved from the joint through the anterior portal with a grasping instrument. The authors prefer a Weston knot, which results in a vertical mattress and the maintenance of the knot on the capsular side of the labrum. The suture is cut with a boxed suture cutter, and the technique is repeated as needed to reattach the labrum to the acetabular rim. Alternatively, intrasubstance tears may be repairable if a stable outer rim is present. The cleavage plane is initially debrided of nonviable tissue to healthy bleeding edges to facilitate healing. A curved spectrum is passed through the portion of the labrum that is attached to the acetabular rim. A passing suture is passed through the spectrum, delivered through the portal, and tied to a suture, which is pulled through the joint back out through the working cannula. A bird's beak is then used to pierce the labrum peripheral to the tear. The suture is grasped, and the free end is brought out through the working cannula. A Weston knot is placed on the capsular side, and the free sutures are cut with a boxed suture cutter. Additional sutures are placed as needed to stabilize the tear.

To address a ligamentum teres tear, the arthroscope is first placed in the anterolateral portal. The ligament is most readily accessed from the anterior portal. External rotation of the hip will help to deliver a portion of the ligament anteriorly to allow for debridement with an arthroscopic shaver. To completely debride the ligament, one must address the acetabular attachment via the posterolateral portal. The released ligament is then drawn to the mechanical debrider with suction.

Bullet extraction is accomplished with an appropriate portal that depends on the location of the missile. Cory and Ruch described removing a bullet from the femoral head with a pituitary rongeur through the anterior portal. Goldman used a mini open posterior approach and freed the missile with osteotomes to lever the bullet from the femoral head. In that particular case, the bullet fragmented on the first attempt to remove it, and a second hip arthroscopy was undertaken to remove all fragments. Singleton described the removal of a bullet from the acetabulum via the anterior portal by seating a pin with a threaded tip into the bullet and then extracting the bullet with the pin.

Broken fracture implants may rarely be considered for arthroscopic removal. A case study by Lu described the use of an arthroscope after the removal of a dynamic hip screw to examine the hip joint cavity. Hip arthroscopy in this case revealed synovitis, which was debrided, and an osteochondral defect that was caused by lag screw penetration. The new screw length was measured with the assistance of the arthroscopic camera.

A traumatically contaminated hip joint can be irrigated with arthroscopy. Irrigation is generally accomplished with an arthroscopic camera with associated inflow in the anterolateral portal, whereas the outflow trocar is placed in the anterior portal position. Synovial or hematoma debridement can be accomplished with a standard arthroscopic shaver in the anterior portal and with a high-flow pump that delivers at least 9 L of saline. Antibiotics can be added to the saline bags at the surgeon's discretion. The joint should be inspected for loose bodies as well, especially when hip contamination is associated with a gunshot to the hip.

Hip arthroscopy has reportedly been used to visualize the reduction of femoral head fractures. We have no experience with this technique, and we do not anticipate using the technique for significantly displaced or highly comminuted fractures. However, the technique may be useful to verify the minimal displacement of femoral head fractures and to confirm that fracture debris is absent from the joint.

## TECHNICAL PEARLS

- Plan portal sites depending on the need for access, especially for foreign bodies such as bullets.
- Attempt hip arthroscopy in acute fractures cautiously, and consider avoiding it completely. Fluid extravasation can have devastating consequences and may be avoided by using low pump pressures and strict fluid management. Signs of fluid extravasation include the inability to distend the joint, increased fluid requirements to maintain distention, the frequent cutoff of pump irrigation systems, and abdominal distention or thigh swelling.

## POSTOPERATIVE REHABILITATION

The postoperative rehabilitation period is significantly affected by the nature of the trauma to the hip and the associated injuries. Hip arthroscopy performed for the retrieval of loose bodies or foreign bodies or after simple dislocations without concomitant fractures is treated with partial weight bearing for 3 weeks followed by full weight bearing as tolerated. Alternatively, fractures of the femoral head or the acetabulum or other ipsilateral injuries are not compatible with early weight bearing; progress to full weight bearing occurs only as the healing of the fracture allows, which is typically 3 months after the injury. Patients who do not progress as expected during the first month postoperatively undergo formal physical therapy with strengthening and range-of-motion exercises.

## RESULTS AND OUTCOMES

The majority of results for hip arthroscopy performed for traumatic injuries are extracted from case reports, which typically have minimal follow up (Table 24-1). Keene and Villar described two cases of posterior hip dislocation with the successful removal of retained loose bodies with hip arthroscopy. Byrd described three cases of hip arthroscopy for the management of posttraumatic loose fragments. At 14 to 33 months of follow up, each case had a reportedly successful outcome with no mechanical symptoms. Svoboda discussed a case of loose-body removal from a posterior hip dislocation in a 23-year-old military recruit that was confirmed with a postoperative CT scan. Mullis reported about 36 patients with either a simple dislocation, a fracture dislocation, or a wall fracture. When arthroscopy was performed, 92% of these patients were found to have loose bodies. Interestingly, loose bodies were found even in 7 of the 9 patients in which standard radiographic studies (anteroposterior pelvic imaging and CT scanning) failed to demonstrate them.

The use of hip arthroscopy for bullet extraction has been documented mostly with case reports that have minimal follow up times. Goldman described a mini open posterior arthroscopic approach for bullet extraction from the hip, whereas Meyer described an intra-articular bullet removal via a lateral approach. Their case reports did not include patient follow up or outcome. In 1998, Ruch removed a .44-caliber bullet and associated loose fragments from the femoral head of a 45-year-old male. Clinical examination at 1 year of follow up revealed a full range of motion, negative heel impaction, and no mechanical symptoms. Radiographic evaluation revealed joint space narrowing with subchondral sclerosis and no evidence of avascular necrosis. Teloken described an inferomedial approach for bullet removal. In this case report, the bullet was removed, and this resulted in a full range of motion without crepitus or pain at 18 months of follow up. Singleton detailed a case of a bullet lodged in a patient's acetabulum after traversing through the rectum. The patient underwent hip arthroscopy, irrigation, debridement, and missile removal, with no evidence of subsequent hip infection.

Violent trauma to the hip, including dislocations, is frequently associated with injury or rupture of the ligamentum teres (Figure 24-5). Isolated injuries may present a diagnostic challenge. In 2001, Kashiwagi published a case report of a 10-year-old girl who fell awkwardly from a swing onto her leg, which resulted in an avulsion of the ligamentum teres from its acetabular attachment. The patient presented with pain and the inability to bear weight on the affected leg. On physical examination, her hip lay in an abducted position, with limited range of motion. Radiographs demonstrated a slightly widened joint space, and a CT scan confirmed a bone fragment that was associated with the avulsed ligamentum teres. The patient was treated with hip arthroscopy, and the osteochondral fragment

**Table 24–1** RESULTS SUMMARY

| Author | Title | No. of Patients | Length of Follow Up | Results |
|---|---|---|---|---|
| Byrd, 1996 | Hip arthroscopy for posttraumatic loose fragments in the young active adult: three case reports | 3 | 14 to 33 months | No mechanical symptoms |
| Cory, 1998 | Arthroscopic removal of a .44 caliber bullet from the hip | 1 | 12 months | Final range of motion: hip flexion, 120 degrees; abduction, 65 degrees; external rotation, 60 degrees; internal rotation, 50 degrees No mechanical symptoms, but radiograph demonstrated joint space narrowing with subchondral sclerosis |
| Teloken et al, 2002 | Hip arthroscopy: a unique inferomedial approach to bullet removal | 1 | 18 months | No mechanical symptoms or evidence of avascular necrosis |
| Meyers et al, 2002 | Retrieval of an intact, intra-articular bullet by hip arthroscopy using the lateral approach | 1 | 12 months | Normal lead levels; returned to previous level of activity |
| Ilizaliturri et al, 2007 | Arthroscopic retrieval of a broken guidewire fragment from the hip joint after cannulated screw fixation of slipped capital femoral epiphysis | 1 | 6 months | No clinical or radiographic evidence of chondrolysis or avascular necrosis |
| Kashiwagi et al, 2001 | Arthroscopic treatment for traumatic hip dislocation with avulsion fracture of the ligamentum teres | 1 | 12 months | Asymptomatic with normal hip range of motion and normal radiographs |
| Byrd et al, 2003 | Traumatic rupture of the ligamentum teres as a source of hip pain | 23 | Mean of 29.2 months | Average of 90 points on a 100-point Modified Harris Hip Scale at final follow up |

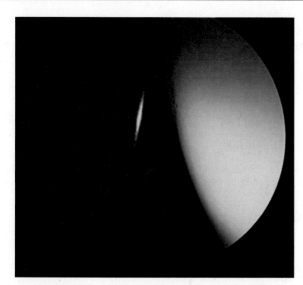

**Figure 24–5** A 29-year-old male who sustained a minimally displaced anterior column acetabular fracture from a fall that was associated with an anterior hip dislocation. Pain persisted after reduction. The image demonstrates a small bone fragment attached to ligamentum teres. The bone fragment was debrided, which resulted in pain relief and the return of function 1 year later.

was removed from the anterior portal using forceps. The girl was asymptomatic with a full range of hip motion and no abnormal radiographic findings at 1 year postoperatively. Byrd treated 23 patients with traumatic injuries to the ligamentum teres (15 violent injuries, including 6 dislocations and 8 twisting injuries). The duration of symptoms averaged 28.5 months and included deep anterior groin pain in all patients; 19 patients had mechanical symptoms, and 4 patients had pain during activity. On examination, 15 patients had pain during logrolling of the hip, whereas 23 had pain with maximal flexion and internal rotation.

Upon intervention, it was found that 12 patients had complete ruptures and that 11 had partial tears. Most commonly, there was associated pathology (9 labral tears, 5 loose bodies, 5 chondral injuries). The average preoperative Modified Harris Hip Score of 47 improved to 90 postoperatively.

## COMPLICATIONS

Complication rates associated with hip arthroscopy range from 0.5% to 6.4%. The majority of complications encountered during hip arthroscopy are neuropraxias. Funke performed hip arthroscopy with the patient in the lateral decubitus position on 19 patients and noted three complications: neuropraxia of the pudendal nerve, hematoma of the labia majora, and a postoperative acute onset of abdominal pain that was surmised to result from fluid extravasation into the retroperitoneum that caused peritoneal irritation. Griffin reported an overall complication rate of 1.6% in 640 patients. Complications in this series included neuropraxias of the sciatic and femoral nerves, a small vaginal tear, a portal hematoma, and the breakage of two arthroscopic instruments in the joint. Sampson reported 34 complications in 530 cases performed since 1977. Complications included 20 transient nerve injuries (10 peroneal, 4 pudendal, 4 sciatic, 1 that was both femoral and sciatic); 9 cases of fluid extravasation, which was felt to be related to prolonged surgery with a pump; and 1 case of avascular necrosis of the femoral head. Clarke reported about 1054 consecutive hip arthroscopies with an overall complication rate of 1.4%. The complications included neuropraxia, portal wound bleeding, portal hematoma, trochanteric bursitis, and instrument breakage.

The prospect of using hip arthroscopy for acute traumatic injuries of the hip or the acetabulum can be complicated by fluid extravasation. Bartlett and colleagues reported about a patient who underwent open reduction and internal fixation for a 3-week-old acetabular fracture. Hip arthroscopy was performed 12 days after the open reduction and internal fixation of the acetabular fracture for persistent intra-articular fragments and slight hip subluxation. In this report, an abdominal compartment syndrome developed as a result of intra-abdominal extravasated arthroscopy fluid that occurred during the procedure, which led to cardiopulmonary arrest, presumably as a result of paradoxic bradycardia from compression of the inferior vena cava. This report highlights the importance of strict fluid management and the maintenance of low intra-articular pressure to safely perform hip arthroscopy in the presence of acute acetabular trauma. This is especially important for intra-articular fractures or those that involve the tectal region, which can allow for extravasation into the retroperitoneum. Signs of fluid extravasation include the inability to distend the joint, increased fluid requirements to maintain distention, the frequent cutoff of pump irrigation systems, and abdominal distention or thigh swelling.

## ANNOTATED REFERENCES AND SUGGESTED READINGS

Bartlett CS, DiFelice GS, Buly RL, Quinn TJ, Green DS, Helfet DL. Cardiac arrest as a result of intraabdominal extravasation of fluid during arthroscopic removal of a loose body from the hip joint of a patient with an acetabular fracture. *J Orthop Trauma.* 1998;12(4):294–299.

Burman MS. Arthroscopy or the direct visualization of joints: an experimental cadaver study. *J Bone Joint Surg.* 1931;13:669–695.

Byrd JW. Hip arthroscopy for post-traumatic loose fragments in the young adult: three case reports. *Clin J Sport Med.* 1996;6:129–134.

Byrd JW, Jones KS. Traumatic rupture of the ligamentum teres as a source of hip pain. *Arthroscopy.* 2003;20(4):385–391.

Clarke MT, Arora A, Villar RN. Hip arthroscopy: complications in 1054 cases. *Clin Orthop Relat Res.* 2003;(406):84–88.

Cory JW, Ruch DS. Arthroscopic removal of a .44 caliber bullet from the hip. *Arthroscopy.* 1998;14(6):624–626.

Dameron TB Jr. Bucket-handle tear of acetabular labrum accompanying posterior dislocation of the hip. *J Bone Joint Surg.* 1959;41-A:131–134.

Epstein HC. Posterior fracture-dislocations of the hip; long-term follow-up. *J Bone Joint Surg Am.* 1974;56:1103–1127.

Funke EL, Munzinger U. Complications in hip arthroscopy. *Arthroscopy.* 1996;12(2):156–159.

Griffin DR, Villar RN. Complications of arthroscopy of the hip. *J Bone Joint Surg Br.* 1999;81(4):604–606.

Goldman A, Minkoff J, Price A, Krinick R. A posterior arthroscopic approach to bullet extraction from the hip. *J Trauma.* 1987;27(11):1294–1300.

Ilizaliturri VM Jr, Zarate-Kalfopulos B, Martinez-Escalante FA, Cuevas-Olivo R, Camacho-Galindo J. Arthroscopic retrieval of a broken guidewire fragment from the hip joint after cannulated screw fixation of slipped capital femoral epiphysis. *Arthroscopy.* 2007;23(2):227.e1–227.e4. Epub 2006 Sep 11.

Judet R, Judet J, Letournel E. Fractures of the acetabulum: classification and surgical approaches for open reduction—preliminary report. *J Bone Joint Surg Am.* 1964;46:1615–1646.

Kashiwagi N, Suzuki S, Seto Y. Arthroscopic treatment for traumatic hip dislocation with avulsion fracture of the ligamentum teres. *Arthroscopy.* 2001;17(1):67–69.

Keene GS, Villar RN. Arthroscopic loose body retrieval following traumatic hip dislocation. *Injury.* 1994;25:507–510.

Lee GH, Virkus WW, Kapotas JS. Arthroscopically assisted minimally invasive intraarticular bullet extraction: technique, indications, and results. *J Orthop Trauma.* 2008;56:513–516.

During a 5-year period, 3 out of 11 patients with retained intra-articular missiles in the hip underwent arthroscopically assisted minimally invasive bullet extraction. The four associated bullets were successfully extracted without complication.

Leunig M, Sledge JB, Gill TJ, Ganz R. Traumatic labral avulsion from the stable rim: a constant pathology in displaced transverse acetabular fractures. *Arch Orthop Trauma Surg.* 2003;123(8):392–395.

Lu KH. Arthroscopically assisted replacement of dynamic hip screw for unrecognized joint penetration of lag screw through a new portal. *Arthroscopy.* 2004;20(2):201–205.

Meyer NJ, Thiel B, Ninomiya JT. Retrieval of an intact, intraarticular bullet by hip arthroscopy using the lateral approach. *J Orthop Trauma.* 2002;16(1):51–53.

Mullis BH, Dahners LE. Hip arthroscopy to remove loose bodies after traumatic dislocation. *J Orthop Trauma.* 2006;20(1):22–26.

Philippon MJ, Schenker ML, Briggs KK, Maxwell RB. Can microfracture produce repair tissue in acetabular chondral defects? *Arthroscopy.* 2008;24:46–50.

The authors wrote a case series about second-look arthroscopy for acetabular defects that had been treated with microfracture. Eight out of 9 patients had 95% to 100% coverage with grade 1 or 2 appearance of the cartilage at an average follow up of 20 months.

Sampson TG. Complications of hip arthroscopy. *Clin Sports Med.* 2001;20(4):831–835.

Singleton SB, Joshi A, Schwartz MA, Collinge CA. Arthroscopic bullet removal from the acetabulum. *Arthroscopy.* 2005;21(3):360–364.

Svoboda SJ, Williams DM, Murphy KP. Hip arthroscopy for osteochondral loose body removal after a posterior hip dislocation. *Arthroscopy.* 2003;19:777–781.

Teloken MA, Schmietd I, Tomlinson DP. Hip arthroscopy: a unique inferomedial approach to bullet removal. *Arthroscopy.* 2002;18(4):E21.

Upadhyay SS, Moulton A. The long-term results of traumatic posterior dislocation of the hip. *J Bone Joint Surg Br.* 1981;63B:548–1541.

The authors reviewed 81 cases of patients with traumatic posterior dislocation of the hip who were treated between 1936 and 1974. The average follow-up period was 12.5 years. The overall results were surprisingly poor despite the early reduction of the dislocation in the majority of cases. The authors found that, at 15 years after simple dislocation, 24% of cases had a poor result by both clinical and radiologic criteria. The results deteriorated with more severe injuries, with 73.3% of the patients being graded as fair or poor.

Watson D, Walcott-Sapp S, Westrich G. Symptomatic labral tear post femoral shaft fracture: case report. *J Orthop Trauma.* 2007;21:731–733.

A 33-year-old male fell 4.5 m and sustained a Winquist type III left femoral shaft fracture, which was treated with a standard reamed statically locked antegrade femoral nail. The patient presented 22 months after his fall with significant groin pain that was worse with activity and an occasional sharp pain associated with a catching sensation in the hip. The patient underwent hip arthroscopy, with which a large labral tear was confirmed and treated with debridement back to a stable edge. At his 2-month postoperative visit, the patient had no complaints of groin pain, and he was walking better than he had for the previous 2 years. The incidence of hip pain with antegrade femoral nailing is reported to be as high as 26% with an incomplete resolution of symptoms after nail removal, whereas even those patients treated with retrograde femoral nails have a 4% reported incidence of residual hip pain. The authors propose that labral tears may be an underinvestigated and underestimated cause of hip pain after femoral shaft fracture that can be confirmed and treated safely with arthroscopy.

**Yamamoto Y, Ide T, Ono T, Hamada Y. Usefulness of arthroscopic surgery in hip trauma cases. *Arthroscopy*. 2003;19:269–273.**

Eleven joints from 10 hip trauma cases with hip fracture dislocations, including 5 femoral head fractures, were studied. All of the patients underwent successful hip arthroscopy with lavage, debridement, loose-body removal, and arthroscopically assisted fracture fixation in 2 patients. Their results at final follow up more than 5 years postoperatively showed that none of the arthroscopically treated hip joints with or without fractures had developed osteoarthritis.

# CHAPTER 25

# Arthroscopic Management of Pediatric Hip Disease

*Yi-Meng Yen and Mininder S. Kocher*

## INTRODUCTION

Injuries of the hip and pelvis in the pediatric population are increasing and receiving more attention. The majority of injuries are soft-tissue or apophyseal injuries that heal with nonoperative treatment. However, with the advent of hip arthroscopy and the development of more advanced imaging of the hip that involves magnetic resonance arthrography, internal derangements of the hip (e.g., labral tears, loose bodies, chondral injuries) are being diagnosed and treated with increased frequency. Hip arthroscopy has obvious advantages as compared with arthrotomy and surgical dislocation for the pediatric population. It is significantly less invasive than arthrotomy, and it allows for a quicker recovery and a sooner return to activities. Most of the experience in hip arthroscopy has been with hip disorders in adults; the role of hip arthroscopy for children and adolescents has been less well characterized.

Historically, arthroscopy of the hip in the pediatric population was used as a diagnostic and therapeutic tool for slipped capital femoral epiphysis, septic arthritis, and various arthropathies. The most common indication has been in cases of Legg-Calvé-Perthes disease, both for the diagnosis of severity and treatment, including the removal of loose bodies. In a review of 24 hip arthroscopies performed in 21 patients between the ages of 11 and 21 years old, Schindler and colleagues concluded that hip arthroscopy was effective for synovial biopsy and loose-body removal; however, as a diagnostic procedure, the arthroscopy failed to correlate with the presumptive cause of symptoms in 11 hips (46%). In many of the general series reported in the current literature, the role of hip arthroscopy for pediatric and adolescent athletes is rarely addressed. As our understanding of the mechanisms and anatomic abnormalities of hip pathology increases, the role of hip arthroscopy for the pediatric population will continue to expand.

## BRIEF HISTORY AND PHYSICAL EXAMINATION

Pediatric and adolescent patients are different from adults in that they frequently do not complain about hip pain. It is common for hip pathology to be discovered only after the examination of a young patient who complains of knee pain: up to a quarter of patients with stable slipped capital femoral epiphysis (SCFE) report knee pain. Another frequent presentation is in the limping child who has not experienced any known injury. As with any orthopedic patient, a detailed history is mandatory. On average, less than half of patients can recall a traumatic event that led to the injury. Running, jumping, and kicking activities are frequently involved in labral pathology, and patients often report an acute twisting injury. A gradual history of pain is frequently more common. Subjective complaints of catching, locking, and giving way point to mechanical symptoms that can benefit from surgical intervention. These symptoms should be carefully distinguished from popping or snapping sensations, which may indicate extra-articular pathology (e.g., psoas tendon bursitis, coxa saltans externa or interna).

The physical examination of the hip begins with the examination of the range of motion. A decreased range of motion as compared with the contralateral unaffected hip is a useful sign of hip pathology. Loss of flexion and internal rotation are usually the earliest signs in these patients. Hip contractures should be examined, and leg lengths and pelvic obliquity should be noted. An impingement test with flexion, adduction, and internal rotation appears to be predictive of intra-articular pathology. An examination of the low back, including straight-leg raising, should be conducted to rule out any contribution of the spine.

## IMAGING AND DIAGNOSTIC STUDIES

Plain-film radiography remains the primary screening tool, because it is widely available and relatively inexpensive; however, it must be performed properly. An anteroposterior radiograph with cross-table lateral views of the hips should be obtained. The anteroposterior radiograph is used to assess dysplasia and acetabular version. There should not be any excessive tilt of the pelvis, and, in general, the tip of the coccyx should be approximately 2 cm above the pubis. The cross-table lateral view with the hip in internal rotation is useful to determine the presence of a cam-type lesion in a patient with femoroacetabular impingement. To assess intra-articular pathology (e.g., labral or ligamentum teres tears, cartilage pathology), a unilateral magnetic resonance image with intra-articular gadolinium is used; in some centers, an "optimized nonarthrogram protocol" may be as accurate as a magnetic resonance image with gadolinium that includes the use of high resolution and a fast-spin-echo sequence. Occasionally a computed tomography scan can be used to further define the version of the femur and acetabulum and to visualize loose bony fragments and fracture. However, radiation doses to the pelvic organs can be substantial, and computed tomography should be used sparingly in the pediatric population.

## INDICATIONS

- Labral tears
- Loose bodies
- Osteoarthritis
- Osteonecrosis
- Osteochondral fractures
- Chondral injuries
- Hip dysplasia
- Septic arthritis
- Inflammatory arthritis
- Synovial chondromatosis
- Ligamentum teres tears
- Femoroacetabular impingement
- Legg-Calvé-Perthes disease
- Slipped capital femoral epiphysis

## SURGICAL TECHNIQUE

Hip arthroscopy can be performed with the patient in the supine or lateral decubitus position. Both positions allow for adequate visualization and positioning, and the one that is used is based on surgeon preference. We perform hip arthroscopy with the patient in the supine position, and it is generally performed as an outpatient procedure for the pediatric population. General anesthesia is used with muscle relaxation, although supplementation with regional anesthesia may be used, depending on the anesthesia available and patient preference. A standard fracture table or a specialized hip-scope table is used with a traction device and a large padded perineal post (Figure 25-1). The affected leg is prepped and draped along with a C-arm (Figure 25-2). The nonoperated side is placed in approximately 30 degrees of abduction, and firm traction is applied to that side so that the patient remains firmly against the perineal post. The operated leg is placed in neutral abduction to maintain a constant relationship between the topographic landmarks and the joint. A slight 10 degrees of flexion is used to relax the capsule; however, excessive flexion and traction can place tension on the sciatic nerve. Maximal internal rotation is used to make the femoral neck parallel with the floor. Traction is applied to achieve joint distraction between 5 mm and 10 mm, and this is confirmed by fluoroscopy; this will typically demonstrate the "vacuum sign" when viewed with the use of fluoroscopy. In general, approximately 50 lb to 75 lb of force is needed to distract a joint. The goals are to use the minimal force necessary to achieve distraction and to keep traction times as brief as possible (in general, less than 2 hours is considered optimal).

### Portals

Two to three operating portals are typically used. The anterolateral and posterolateral portals are placed at the superior margin

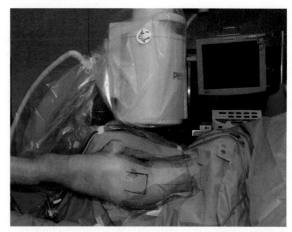

**Figure 25–2** A patient draped with a C-arm fluoroscope in position.

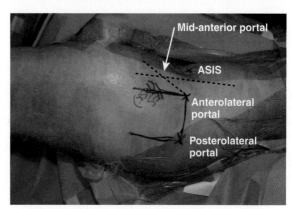

**Figure 25–3** The locations of the arthroscopy portals. The greater trochanter is outlined, and, with the foot internally rotated, the neck of the femur is parallel to the floor. The locations of the posterolateral and anterolateral portals are on the posterior and anterior borders of the greater trochanter. The mid-anterior portal is established by drawing a line parallel to the anterior border of the greater trochanter halfway between the border and the anterosuperior iliac spine *(ASIS)*. A line 45 degrees from the anterolateral portal is drawn, and the intersection of the two lines is the location of the mid-anterior portal.

of the greater trochanter at the anterior and posterior borders (Figure 25-3). The mid-anterior portal is made by first drawing a sagittal line from the anterosuperior iliac spine and another line at the anterolateral portal; a sagittal line is then drawn equidistant to these two lines. The entry point for the mid-anterior portal is approximately 45 degrees from the anterolateral portal on the middle sagittal line. With careful attention paid to these landmarks, the portals can be safely made away from neurovascular structures. The lateral femoral cutaneous nerve typically

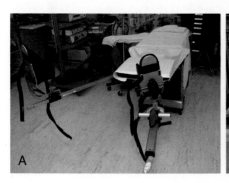

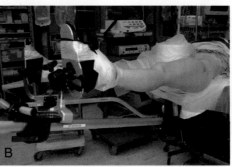

**Figure 25–1 A,** Standard table with special hip-scope extension. **B,** Large perineal post with the operative leg in a neutral position, slightly flexed, and internally rotated.

lies just medial to the anterosuperior iliac spine; the femoral nerve and artery are even more medial.

After traction is applied, a spinal needle is placed from the anterolateral position under fluoroscopic control, and the joint is distended with fluid. Care must be taken to ensure that the labrum is not perforated and that the femoral head articular surface is not disturbed. A Nitinol wire is inserted through the spinal needle, and the camera trochar is inserted with the use of a twisting motion (never a forceful push). With the use of a 70-degree arthroscope, the mid-anterior and posterolateral portals are then established under direct visualization. A fluoroscope can also be used to help with the establishment of the portals.

The peripheral compartment is entered by releasing traction with the arthroscopic instruments out of the joint but remaining intracapsular. The hip is flexed to approximately 30 degrees to 45 degrees to relax the capsule. The anterolateral portal and the mid-anterior portal can be used, or an ancillary portal approximately 5 cm distal to the anterolateral portal can be established under direct visualization.

### Diagnostic and Surgical Arthroscopy

A diagnostic arthroscopy can be performed with the use of a combination of 70-degree and 30-degree scopes. Alternatively, an arthroscopic blade can be used to perform an arthrotomy of the hip capsule from the mid-anterior portal to the anterolateral portal. This provides extensive maneuverability within the joint.

Loose bodies still represent the clearest indication for hip arthroscopy. Most of the problematic loose bodies are intra-articular and can be addressed with standard arthroscopic methods (Figure 25-4), and many can be debrided with shavers or flushed out through large-diameter cannulas. Both the intra-articular and peripheral compartments must be addressed, because loose bodies can easily hide within the peripheral joint. Large fragments frequently need to be morselized or removed freehand with sturdy graspers. If the surgeon is removing pieces in a freehand manner, the portal may need to be enlarged and the capsule further incised to prevent the loss of the fragment in the capsule or the subcutaneous tissue.

Labral pathology represents one of the most common reasons that athletes undergo hip arthroscopy. Labrum degeneration can occur as part of the aging process, and evidence of labral pathology exists in patients without symptoms. In general, pediatric patients experience more traumatic labral tears, but conditions such as femoroacetabular impingement have been recognized to predispose even young individuals to labral tearing. Labral tears can be addressed in a way that is similar to that of a meniscus in the knee. The goal is to remove diseased labrum to a stable rim of healthy tissue (Figure 25-5). Debridement can be performed with an arthroscopic shaver or thermal ablation with a flexible wand; however, care should be taken with thermal devices to avoid deep heat penetration. The evolution of debridement of the labrum has been to repair it.

Currently, labral repair of the hip resembles that of the shoulder. Occasionally the labral tissue must be partially detached from the chondrolabral junction that surrounds the original tear to obtain adequate exposure for the trimming of the acetabular rim. The center-edge angle should be known preoperatively, and the version of the acetabulum should be assessed. For cases in which there is normal anteversion of the acetabular cup, the bony area of labral detachment on the acetabular rim should be roughened with a rasp or an arthroscopic burr to ensure an adequate bony bed for the reattachment of the labrum. For cases in which there is protrusio or acetabular retroversion, the rim of the acetabulum should be trimmed with the arthroscopic burr. After the bony bed is prepared, suture anchors should be inserted into the rim, with care taken not to pierce the acetabular cartilage. The concavity of the acetabulum can make this difficult, and fluoroscopy can be used to help with anchor placement. The sutures can be looped around the labrum or placed through the labrum, and the knot should be placed on the capsular side. Depending on the size of the tear and if further detachment of the labrum is necessary, we use between one and three anchors.

Special attention should be paid to the articular cartilage around the chondrolabral junction. The extent of damage to this area may play a role in the eventual clinical response to debridement. If this area contains a chondral flap, the flap should be debrided to stable edges, and a microfracture should be performed for grade IV articular lesions. Chondroplasty can be performed with a curved arthroscopic shaver to negotiate the convex and concave surfaces of the hip joint. Radiofrequency devices with flexible wands can be useful as well, but, again, great care should be taken to avoid heat penetration of the surrounding viable chondrocytes.

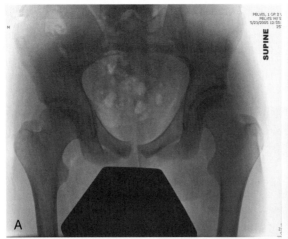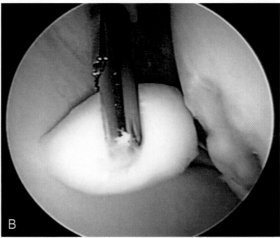

**Figure 25–4 A,** Radiograph of a patient with spondyloepiphyseal dysplasia and right hip pain. **B,** The removal of a loose body. Note the chondral damage to the femoral head.

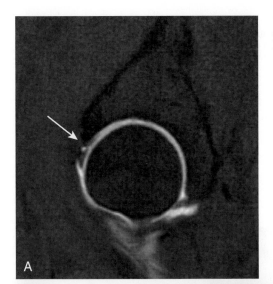

**Figure 25–5  A,** Magnetic resonance arthrogram of a labral tear. White arrow shows contrast behind the labrum indicative of a labral tear. **B1, B2,** Fraying of the labrum. **B3,** A thermal ablation device; **B4,** Debridement of the labrum with a shaver.

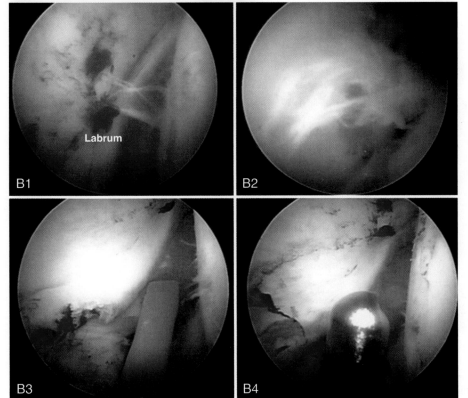

Ligamentum tears can also be debrided with an arthroscopic shaver or a radiofrequency thermal probe. Access to the ligamentum is typically easiest through the mid-anterior portal, and external rotation of the hip can also help to bring the ligamentum into view. Excessive debridement of the ligamentum should be avoided because of the potential to damage the blood supply to the femoral head in pediatric patients.

Synovitis frequently exists in the joint in response to other intra-articular pathology. A complete synovectomy cannot be performed, but the majority of inflamed synovial tissue can be removed with an arthroscopic shaver and radiofrequency ablation. For primary synovial disease, arthroscopy of both the intra-articular and peripheral compartments is necessary.

### Peripheral Compartment

After the work on the intra-articular side is completed, traction is released, and the hip is flexed to approximately 30 degrees to 45 degrees if surgery is to continue in the peripheral compartment. For synovial disease and loose-body removal, this compartment must be checked thoroughly. For patients with

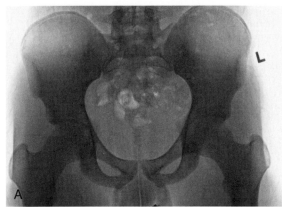

**Figure 25–6 A,** Radiograph of an adolescent patient with femoroacetabular impingement and left hip pain. **B1,** Entry into the peripheral compartment with the hip flexed at 30 degrees. Note the flattened head–neck offset. **B2, B3,** Recontouring of the femoral head–neck junction with a 5.5 mm arthroscopic burr.

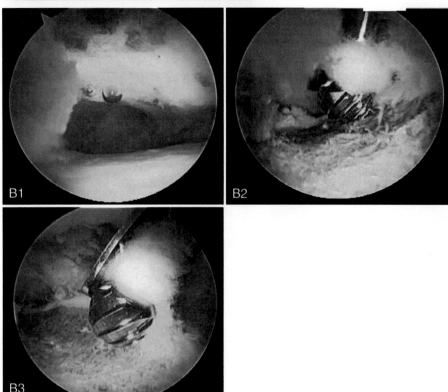

femoroacetabular impingement, the cam lesion can be addressed arthroscopically (Figure 25-6). Beginning with the arthroscope in the mid-anterior portal, the lateral edge of the cam lesion can be removed with an arthroscopic burr. Care must be taken not to remove too much bone and cartilage. The resection should begin above the lateral retinacular vessels and proceed medially across the neck; over-resection may predispose the patient to a femoral neck fracture. In the pediatric population, care should be taken not to disrupt the physis; localization with fluoroscopy may be necessary during the osteoplasty procedure.

### Closure

The wounds are closed with 2-0 Vicryl sutures subcutaneously and 3-0 nylon sutures in a mattress fashion for the skin. Alternatively, 3-0 Monocryl sutures in a buried subcuticular fashion can be used for the skin. Approximately 9 cc of 0.5% Marcaine and 40 mg of Depomedrol is injected into the hip joint before closure.

### TECHNICAL PEARLS

- *Traction:* Minimize traction time to less than 2 hours. Patients with an intact labrum may require more force to distract the joint. The use of muscle relaxation by anesthesiologists can help with the distraction of the joint.
- *Entry:* Fluoroscopy aids in the establishment of arthroscopic portals. Great care should be taken not to damage the articular cartilage during entry. The twisting of the cannula should be used instead of forceful pressure to prevent plunging into the joint. The direct visualization of other portals is useful to avoid iatrogenic injury.
- *Visualization:* Delay the inflow of saline until the outflow portal is established. A 70-degree scope provides the best visualization of the joint as a result of the concavity of the surfaces. A thorough hip capsulotomy allows for complete access to the joint.
- *Joint work:* The use of curved instruments, flexible tools, and slotted cannulas helps with joint entry and with the accessibility of different areas of the joint.

## POSTOPERATIVE REHABILITATION

The goal of rehabilitation is to return the patient to a preinjury level of activity. The first phase of rehabilitation involves protecting the repaired tissues while restoring hip motion and decreasing scarring. Patients are placed on crutches and allowed to be toe-touch weight bearing for approximately 2 weeks. If the patients had a microfracture procedure performed, they are made toe-touch weight bearing for 6 weeks. Gentle range-of-motion exercises are begun with a continuous passive motion machine, passive range-of-motion exercises, and stationary bicycling. If a labral repair is performed, we restrict external rotation and adduction for the first 2 weeks. Early passive range-of-motion exercises emphasize internal rotation and flexion, and isometric strengthening is begun for the gluteals, the quadriceps, the hamstrings, and the transverse abdominals. A continuous passive motion device (CPM) is used for 4 weeks. Approximately 6 weeks postoperatively, full range of motion should be achieved, and strengthening exercises can be started. Sport-specific training usually begins about 3 months postoperatively.

## RESULTS

There have been relatively few results published regarding the use of hip arthroscopy for pediatric hip disease. The studies are listed in Table 25-1, and, in general, they have had good results.

## COMPLICATIONS

The technique of hip arthroscopy is well described and considered to be safe for most patients. No cases of avascular necrosis after hip arthroscopy have been described to date. The most common complications involve nerve palsy injuries, with the sciatic and pudendal nerves being particularly at risk. Injuries to the lateral femoral cutaneous nerve, the extravasation of fluid into the abdominal cavity, equipment failure, and the inability to complete the procedure have all been reported, and recurrent labral tearing has been described as well. Attention to anatomic landmarks and minimizing traction times can decrease these complications.

### Table 25–1 OUTCOMES

| Authors | Title | No. of Patients | Length of Follow Up | Results |
|---|---|---|---|---|
| Kocher et al, 2005 | Hip arthroscopy in children and adolescents | 42 | Minimum of 1 year | Preoperative Modified Harris Hip Score of 53.1 versus a postoperative score of 82.9; $P < .001$ |
| Berend and Vail, 2001 | Hip arthroscopy in the pediatric adolescent and pediatric athlete | 8 | 33 months | Reportedly good |
| Bowen et al, 1986 | Osteochondritis dissecans following Perthes disease | 14 | Minimum of 2 years | Asymptomatic |
| Kim et al, 2003 | Arthroscopic treatment of septic arthritis of the hip | 10 | Minimum of 4 years | Excellent |

## ANNOTATED REFERENCES AND SUGGESTED READINGS

Berend KR, Vail TP. Hip arthroscopy in the adolescent and pediatric athlete. *Clin Sports Med.* 2001;20(4):763–778.

This is a review of hip problems in adolescent and pediatric athletes that details the authors' experiences with hip arthroscopy in 8 patients, with reportedly good results.

Bould M. Arthroscopic diagnosis and treatment of septic arthritis of the hip joint. *Arthroscopy.* 1993;9(6):707–708.

This is an early report about the use of arthroscope lavage for the treatment of septic arthritis of the hip as an alternative to formal arthrotomy.

Bowen JR, Kumar VP, Joyce JJ III, et al. Osteochondritis dessicans following Perthes disease. *Clin Orthop.* 1986;209:49–56.

This is a discussion of hip arthroscopy for the removal of osteocartilaginous fragments after Perthes disease. The joint is evaluated for degenerative joint disease as well.

Fischer SU, Beattie TF. The limping child: epidemiology, assessment, and outcome. *J Bone Joint Surg Br.* 1999;81B(6):1029–1034.

This article provides guidelines for the evaluation of the limping child in the emergency department. The epidemiology of limping is included, with the main diagnosis being transient synovitis (39.5%).

Futami T, Kasahara Y, Suzuki S, et al. Arthroscopy for slipped capital femoral epiphysis. *J Pediatr Orthop.* 1992;12:592–597.

In this study, hip arthroscopy was used to evaluate the hip after slipped capital femoral epiphysis that demonstrated the erosion of articular cartilage in the anterosuperior region and damage to the posterolateral aspect of the labrum. Findings were consistent with traumatic injury, and no arthroscopic treatment was performed.

Griffin DR, Villar RN. Complications in arthroscopy of the hip. *J Bone Joint Surg Br.* 1999;81B(4):604–606.

This article describes a complication rate of 1.6% among 640 hip arthroscopy patients. These complications included transient palsies of the sciatic and femoral nerves, perineal injuries, bleeding, bursitis, and instrument breakage.

Gross RH. Arthroscopy in hip disorders in children. *Orthop Rev.* 1977;6:43–49.

This article describes early experience with hip arthroscopy for patients with congenital dislocation of the hip, Perthes disease, slipped capital femoral epiphysis, and subluxation.

Holgersson S, Brattstrom H, Mogensen B, et al. Arthroscopy of the hip in juvenile chronic arthritis. *J Pediatr Orthop.* 1981;1(3):273–278.

Hip arthroscopy is described as a useful technique for the diagnosis of the hip among juvenile patients with arthritis because it provides better cartilage detail and useful synovial information.

Ikeda T, Awaya G, Suzuki S, et al. Torn acetabular labrum in young patients. *J Bone Joint Surg Br*. 1988;70B(1):13–16.

The authors describe diagnostic arthroscopy for a torn labrum in adolescent patients. Tears were located primarily on the postero-superior portion of the labrum. Repeat arthroscopy several months later did not demonstrate healing of the labrum, and one patient required open labral resection.

Kim SJ, Choi NH, Ko SH, et al. Arthroscopic treatment of septic arthritis of the hip. *Clin Orthop Relat Res*. 2003;407:211–214.

This article details a 4-year follow up of arthroscopic drainage of the septic hip in 10 patients, with good results.

Kocher MS, Bishop JA, Weed B, et al. Delay in diagnosis of slipped capital femoral epiphysis. *Pediatrics*. 2004;133(4):322–325.

In this study, up to 25% of patients with slipped capital femoral epiphysis presented with knee pain, which led to a delay in diagnosis. A delay in diagnosis correlates with the increased severity of the slip angle.

Kocher MS, Kim YJ, Millis MB, et al. Hip arthroscopy in children and adolescents. *J Pediatr Orthop*. 2005;25(5):680–686.

This is the largest published series of hip arthroscopies in pediatric patients. Labral debridement for isolated tears or as a result of hip dysplasia after periacetabular osteotomy and loose-body excision in patients with Perthes disease resulted in improvement.

Kuklo TR, Mackenzie WG, Keeler KA. Hip arthroscopy in Legg-Calve-Perthes disease. *Arthroscopy*. 1999;15(1):88–92.

This case report of debridement for an osteochondral lesion after Legg-Calve-Perthes disease demonstrated good results after 5 months.

Mintz DN, Hooper T, Connell D, Buly R, Padgett DE, Potter HG. Magnetic resonance imaging of the hip: detection of labral and chondral abnormalities using noncontrast imaging. *Arthroscopy*. 2005;21(4):385–393.

With the use of a noncontrast magnetic resonance imaging technique with a small pixel size and a fast-spin-echo sequence, the reliability of the detection of labral tears and cartilage defects was comparable to that of magnetic resonance arthrography and exceeded that of previous noncontrast magnetic resonance imaging techniques.

Schindler A, Lechevallier JJC, Rao NS, et al. Diagnostic and therapeutic arthroscopy of the hip in children and adolescents: evaluation of results. *J Pediatr Orthop*. 1995;15:317–321.

# Open Management

# CHAPTER 26

# The Bernese Periacetabular Osteotomy for Hip Dysplasia and Acetabular Retroversion

*Martin Beck and Reinhold Ganz*

## INTRODUCTION

Hip dysplasia in the adult can lead to pain and limping. Unfavorable leverages are responsible for the fatiguing of the abductors, whereas an insufficient coverage of the femoral head causes overload at the acetabular rim with shearing forces that result in lesions of the labrum and acetabular cartilage that eventually lead to osteoarthrosis (OA) of the hip.

The natural history of the dysplastic hip without subluxation is not well known, but it is estimated that 40% to 50% of patients with dysplasia develop OA before the age of 50 years and that approximately 50% have their first reconstructive surgeries before the age of 60 years. It appears that hips with a lateral center-edge angle (LCE angle) of less than 16 degrees or an acetabular index of more than 15 degrees will ultimately develop end-stage OA. Alternatively, it is well known that all dysplastic hips with subluxation evolve into OA during the second to third decade of life. Surgical interventions aim to alter the natural course of this degeneration.

Reorientation procedures include single, double, and triple osteotomies as well as spheric and periacetabular osteotomies. The inherent drawbacks of these osteotomies are a limited range of displacement; the potential narrowing of the pelvic cavity; and the need for a substantial internal fixation, because some techniques create a discontinuity of the pelvic ring. The medialization of the joint is difficult to achieve, and some osteotomies have an intra-articular course, because the radiologically visible teardrop remains in situ. To avoid these disadvantages, the Bernese periacetabular osteotomy (PAO) was developed in 1984. The polygonally shaped juxta-articular osteotomy respects the vascular blood supply to the acetabular fragment. It also facilitates extensive acetabular reorientation, including the correction of the version and mediolateral displacement. The posterior column remains intact, which protects the sciatic nerve and enables minimal internal fixation. The dimensions of the true pelvis remain unchanged, thus permitting unimpaired vaginal delivery. All steps of the acetabular osteotomy are performed with the use of the modified Smith-Petersen approach. During the early stages of this technique, some centers preferred the ilioinguinal approach; however, this was abandoned after several cases of thrombosis of the femoral artery, with serious consequences in some patients. In addition, the Smith-Petersen approach allows for an anterior capsulotomy for the inspection and correction of labral pathology and of potential femoroacetabular impingement. Initially, PAO was designed for the treatment of the dysplastic hip. With the recognition of orientation problems of the acetabulum—particularly retroversion—as a cause of impingement, the technique was also applied for the correction of acetabular pathologies other than dysplasia. It is currently used for the treatment of acetabular retroversion and for selected cases of protrusio.

## BASIC SCIENCE

The insufficient coverage of the femoral head by a too-small acetabulum leads to high loads at the acetabular roof. Most often, coverage is not only insufficient, but it is also maloriented with a steep acetabular roof. This results in a small inclined plane and leads to instability and the migration of the femoral head, thus further increasing load and shear stresses at the acetabular rim. The acetabular labrum initially hypertrophies to maintain the femoral head within the joint. If the chronic shear stresses persist, the labral soft-tissue compensation fails, and the labrum is torn off of the acetabular rim, sometimes with an osseous fragment. Acetabular rim fractures usually occur only in the presence of bone cysts, which have weakened the bony rim.

Histomorphologically, the labrum shows myxoid degeneration of its fibrocartilage structure and adjacent ganglion formation within the bone or soft tissues. In addition to increased femoral head instability, the joint-sealing function, which is required for cartilage lubrication and the distribution of joint pressures, is also lost. In this mechanically adverse situation, an increase of joint contact pressures at the acetabular rim is directly related to the onset of cartilage degeneration. As an adaptation to the increased load transmission, an increase in the subchondral bone density at the anterolateral acetabular rim can be observed.

### Principles of Pelvic Osteotomy

In the dysplastic hip, the goal of pelvic osteotomy is to change acetabular orientation to optimize the joint mechanics by increasing the weight-bearing area and by transforming shearing forces into compressive forces. The coverage of the femoral head can be increased by either an augmentation of the acetabular roof or by changing the spatial orientation of the acetabulum. Augmentation procedures such as the Chiari osteotomy and the shelf procedure reduce joint-loading forces by augmenting the weight-bearing area of the joint. With both methods, lateral osseous coverage can be reproducibly improved; however, the posterior aspect of the femoral head often remains uncovered. The interposed capsule undergoes metaplastic transformation to fibrocartilage, and the labrum remains within the main weight-bearing area. A high failure rate is reported after Chiari osteotomies when the labrum was torn. As compared with hyaline cartilage, fibrocartilage has inferior mechanical properties for withstanding axial loading. Although augmentation procedures can provide reliable pain relief for some years, they should be regarded as salvage procedures.

Reorienting procedures change the orientation of the acetabular articular surface, thereby correcting the area of deficiency. These procedures provide a greater surface area for load transmission while reestablishing or maintaining the stability of the joint. During reorientation procedures, coverage is achieved with hyaline cartilage supported by subchondral bone, which has optimal mechanical qualities for weight bearing. Reorientation procedures include single, double, and triple osteotomies as well as spheric and periacetabular osteotomies. The dysplastic acetabulum can be reoriented with the use of a single innominate osteotomy, such as that described by Salter. Although this may be beneficial for children, the degree of correction that is possible in adolescents and adults is limited by the age-related increase in the stiffness of the symphysis pubis. Moreover, this osteotomy retroverts and lateralizes the joint because of a hinged angulation of the acetabulum around a fixed axis. The dysplastic hip joint is usually relatively lateralized. Additional lateralization and distalization are undesirable, because they further increase adverse joint reactive forces. As a result, a variety of double and triple osteotomies and PAOs have been developed in an attempt to improve the degree and accuracy of correction. The double and triple osteotomies—as a result of their considerable distance from the acetabulum, the size of the fragment, and the tension of the sacropelvic ligaments—have a limited range of displacement. Triple osteotomies closer to the joint, as described by Le Coeur, Tönnis and colleagues and Carlioz and colleagues, permit a considerable correction, but they potentially narrow the pelvic cavity. In addition, they require a substantial internal fixation, because these techniques create a discontinuity of the pelvic ring. The spheric osteotomies allow for a good lateral and anterior correction, but the medialization of the joint can only be obtained with great difficulty. These osteotomies also run intra-articular, because the radiologically visible teardrop remains in situ. Finally, given the proximity of these procedures to the joint, the vascular supply depends on the vessels of the capsule and the acetabular branch of the obturator artery. After spheric osteotomies, the acetabular fragment relies on the blood supply provided through the acetabular artery and the capsule, so a simultaneous capsulotomy should not be performed. On the basis of both mechanical and biologic considerations and in the light of the limitations of previous techniques, the Bernese PAO was developed. The polygonally shaped juxta-articular osteotomy respects the vascular blood supply to the acetabular fragment. It facilitates extensive acetabular reorientation, including the correction of version and mediolateral displacement. The posterior column remains intact, which protects the sciatic nerve and enables minimal internal fixation. The dimensions of the true pelvis remain unchanged, thus permitting unimpaired vaginal delivery, even in cases with bilateral osteotomy. An anterior joint capsulotomy provides information about and treatment options for lesions of the acetabular rim, and it allows for the treatment of labral pathology and potential postcorrection femoroacetabular impingement. There are some concerns regarding the vascularity of the acetabular fragment with juxta-articular (spheric) osteotomies. The blood supply of the acetabular fragment is secured by the acetabular and supra-acetabular branches of the gluteal arteries.

## INDICATIONS

- Acetabular dysplasia around or after the closure of the physes
- Acetabular retroversion
- An anteroposterior pelvic radiograph that shows improved coverage of the femoral head and good congruence in 20 degrees to 30 degrees of abduction (abduction film)

In the presence of severe dysplasia or aspheric congruency, simultaneous femoral osteotomy for optimal positioning of the femoral head has to be evaluated.

## CONTRAINDICATIONS

- Marked cephalad dislocation
- Secondary acetabulum with fibrocartilage
- Deterioration of congruence on abduction films
- Osteoarthrosis with a Tönnis grade of more than 1

A definite upper age limit does not exist. However, patients who are more than 50 years old are rarely treated with an acetabular osteotomy. In contrast with distant pelvic osteotomies, the Bernese PAO crosses the posterior line of the triradiate cartilage. Therefore, this osteotomy is not indicated if substantial growth potential remains within this physis.

## BRIEF HISTORY AND PHYSICAL EXAMINATION

### History

The majority of patients treated with PAO are young adults with symptoms of labral pathology and pain related to the overload and fatigue of the abductor musculature. Labral pathology often presents as a sharp, knife-like groin pain that subsides as acutely as it presents. Occasionally, the hip appears to be mechanically blocked, but this can be relieved by shaking or twisting the leg. The groin pain may also have an aching, more chronic character, and prolonged sitting or walking can exacerbate the pain. The pain can be reproduced by activities that involve forced hip flexion, adduction, and internal rotation (e.g., breaststroke swimming, entering or exiting a motor vehicle, sport activities with cutting or twisting movements). As the symptoms increase in frequency, residual pain may result in a slight limp. Symptoms of muscular overload range from early fatigue to clear weakness of the abductors, with irritation at the tendinous insertion on the greater trochanter.

### Physical Examination

A complete physical examination includes the assessment of gait, limb length, muscle power, and range of motion as well as special tests. Abductor strength is assessed with the Trendelenburg test and with a leg raise against resistance in the lateral position. Range of motion, particularly for internal rotation, is often increased in a patient with hip dysplasia. With the onset of secondary osteoarthrosis, however, the range of motion may decrease again. A snapping psoas tendon is often present. A lesion of the acetabular rim (i.e., labral pathology) is suspected if the impingement test is positive. With the patient supine, the hip is flexed to 90 degrees. With additional internal rotation and adduction, the labrum will be squeezed between the femoral neck and the acetabular rim. In the presence of a damaged labrum, this will elicit the typical groin pain about which the patient is complaining. Occasionally a positive apprehension test may be possible, which is indicative of symptomatic anterior instability as a result of deficient anterior acetabular coverage. During this test, the patient lies supine, and the hip is extended, adducted, and externally rotated. Discomfort and a sense of instability are felt as the femoral head is subluxing anteriorly. In a very thin patient, this external rotation in extension can produce a mass in the inguinal region when the femoral head subluxes anteriorly; this is referred to as the *lump sign*.

Signs of trochanteric irritation indicate abductor muscle insufficiency. The bicycle test is performed by placing the patient in the lateral position with the affected hip up; a bicycle pedaling maneuver is then performed, and the lateral and posterior margins of the trochanter are palpated. Tenderness is most commonly palpated along the posterior border of the gluteus medius muscle.

## IMAGING AND DIAGNOSTIC STUDIES

### Conventional Radiography

An anteroposterior pelvic radiograph, a lateral cross-table view, and a false-profile view of the pelvis are required. The anteroposterior pelvic view allows for the visualization of the acetabular cover and version. The false-profile view permits the evaluation of the anterior acetabular coverage and the anterior migration or subluxation of the femoral head. The lateral cross-table view provides information about femoral torsion and the head–neck offset. Finally, anteroposterior abduction radiographs are used to assess the joint congruency that can be achieved with the reorientation of the acetabulum and the potential need for a concomitant femoral osteotomy.

### Magnetic Resonance Arthrography

Magnetic resonance arthrography (MRA) is currently the method of choice for the imaging of the hip joint. The application of intra-articular gadolinium-diethylenetriamine pentaacetic acid as a contrast agent allows for the improved visualization of intra-articular joint structures, particularly the acetabular labrum and the cartilage surface of the hip. The technique includes high-field-strength magnetic resonance imaging and the use of surface coils. In addition to standard T1- and T2-weighted sagittal oblique and coronal oblique images, MRA includes proton-weighted radial sequencing in the axis of the femoral neck. This has the advantage that the acetabular and femoral articular cartilage as well as the labrum are visualized orthogonally at any point around the circumference of the acetabular rim and the femoral head. MRA including radial sequences has been shown to be extremely helpful for detecting labral lesions, and it enables a better assessment of the cartilage damage, which is always more extensive than it appears on conventional radiographs.

## SURGICAL TECHNIQUE

The patient is in a supine position with the lower limb draped free. The iliac crest and the proximal half of the thigh should be accessible. Surgery is performed through a modified Smith-Petersen approach with osteotomy of the anterosuperior iliac spine (ASIS). The first part of the dissection is performed with the hip in extension. The incision starts at the gluteal tubercle of the iliac crest, curves just lateral to the ASIS, and continues in a curved way to the lateral aspect of the proximal thigh. The subcutaneous tissue is incised in line, and a lateral skin flap is developed until the fat layer between the fascia of the sartorius and the tensor fasciae latae becomes visible. The main branch of the lateral femoral cutaneous nerve lies in this fatty tissue.

The muscle belly of the tensor fasciae latae is identified, and its fascia is split lengthwise. The dissection follows the fascia medially into the interval between the tensor fasciae latae and the sartorius muscle. The tensor is pulled laterally with a narrow Langenbeck retractor. Slight abduction of the lower limb helps to relax this muscle. The floor of the muscle compartment is incised longitudinally, and the lateral border of the muscle belly and the tendon of the rectus femoris, including its reflected part, are visualized. The fascia between the rectus and the tensor can be of quite variable thickness, and, in the distal part of the incision, the ascending branch of the lateral femoral circumflex artery runs within this fascial layer between the rectus and the tensor fasciae latae. These blood vessels represent an important source of vascularization of the tensor fasciae latae and therefore have to be protected. The blood vessels are mobilized from the fasciae to allow for the spread of the deep layers of the approach.

The origin of the external oblique muscle that overhangs the iliac crest is lifted and detached subperiosteally from the iliac crest to about 1.5 cm from the ASIS. The ASIS is osteotomized about 1.5 cm to 2 cm proximal to the palpable tip of the ASIS. The osteotomized ASIS is mobilized medially together with the origin of the sartorius and the inguinal ligament. The dissection of the inner table of the iliac wing is continued strictly subperiosteally down to the pelvic brim. In approximately half of patients, the nutrient artery of the iliolumbar artery enters the iliac wing lateral to the pelvic brim. This blood vessel has to be visualized carefully and coagulated. There may be considerable backflow from the bone; if this happens, hemostasis can be performed with the use of bone wax to obstruct the blood vessel. In the other half of patients, the nutrient artery enters the bone medial to the pelvic brim and cannot be controlled. In these cases, blood loss through the supra-acetabular osteotomy can be substantial and can only be controlled by bone wax after the mobilization of the acetabular fragment. The periosteal and muscle connection with the osteotomized ASIS should be preserved, thus preventing a stretching of the femoral cutaneous nerve, even if the wound is considerably spread. The intact periosteum that covers the iliac muscle protects this muscle during the entire operation. The exposure of the inside of the pelvis is continued by detaching the origin of the iliac muscle along the interspinous crest until the origins of the direct and reflected heads of the rectus become visible. At this time, it is advantageous to hold the hip in 40 degrees of flexion with the leg holder to relax the medial soft tissues.

The direct head of the rectus is detached from the anteroinferior iliac spine (AIIS), and the indirect head is divided. The rectus femoris then is retracted medially with a Langenbeck retractor, and the lateral limit of iliocapsularis muscle becomes visible. Particularly among patients with dysplastic hips, the iliocapsular muscle (i.e., the capsular part of the iliac muscle) can be hypertrophic and well visible lying on the joint capsule. The main site of origin lies at the distal border of the AIIS.

The iliocapsular muscle is detached from the capsule by sharp dissection going from lateral to medial until the iliopectineal bursa is opened and the psoas tendon becomes visible. The psoas tendon is undermined and retracted medially with the use of a pointed Hohmann retractor driven into the pubic ramus 1 cm to 1.5 cm medial to the iliopectineal eminence. The psoas tendon protects not only the femoral nerve but also the femoral vessels from overstretching; therefore, it should never be divided. The iliocapsularis muscle is now completely detached from the capsule, thus exposing the anteroinferior part of the capsule around the calcar. Any accidental opening of the capsule should be closed, because a closed capsule being put under tension facilitates the dissection of the ischial ramus. During this stage, a large, curved pair of scissors with rounded ends is advanced along the anteroinferior capsule, and the space between the capsule and the obturator externus is enlarged by spreading the scissors (Figure 26-1). The transversely running muscle belly of the obturator externus can often be seen. Because the medial femoral circumflex artery that supplies the femoral head runs distal to the muscle belly, scissors and other instruments must stay strictly proximal to the muscle belly. If visualization is impossible, it is safe to keep the instruments in close contact with the capsule.

All osteotomies are performed with the patient's hip in 45 degrees of flexion. The first cut is the partial osteotomy of the ischium (Figure 26-2). The scissors follow the capsule in a posterior direction until the ischial ramus is reached in the area of the infracotyloid notch. With the tip of the scissors, one can palpate the posterior and inferior border of the facies lunata of the acetabulum. The width of the ischium is assessed by gliding the scissors medially into the obturator foramen and then laterally until a soft resistance prevents further dissection. The soft-tissue resistance is formed by the tendinous origins of the ischiocrural muscles, which exceed the lateral border of the ischium when the hip is flexed. Respecting this resistance helps to avoid the lateral slipping of an instrument and thus protects the sciatic nerve. A large periosteal elevator or a Cobb elevator can be used to assist with the introduction of a 15-mm curved pelvic osteotome. The infracotyloid notch is palpated with the osteotome. The osteotome should point in the direction of the contralateral shoulder to avoid exiting through the lateral cortex and putting the sciatic nerve in danger. The handle of the osteotome points in a posteroinferior direction. The entry point of the osteotome is carefully made, and it is then driven slowly to a depth of 20 mm to 25 mm while the direction of the handle is gradually changed so that, at the end of the insertion, the handle points posterosuperiorly. At this stage, it is important to remember that the posterior column is not osteotomized completely. With wiggling motions, the osteotome is pulled back to the entry point, but the blade remains in contact with the bone. By doing this, one can feel whether the medial and lateral cortical borders are still intact. At the level of the entry point, the osteotome is moved carefully onto the remaining medial

bone bridge and advanced with the same technique as used previously. The same technique is then applied to the lateral side. To relax and protect the sciatic nerve, the flexed hip has to be abducted and externally rotated. Of special importance is the fact that the medial cortex should be cut, whereas the lateral cortex should only be notched for the protection of the sciatic nerve. To determine whether the osteotomy is sufficiently deep and especially to be sure that the medial cortex is included in the osteotomy, the osteotomy is carefully repeated. The orientation as well as the depth of the partial osteotomy can be checked with the image intensifier. A sufficiently deep cut is the most important prerequisite for the problem-free displacement of the acetabulum at the end of all osteotomies.

The second cut is the osteotomy of the superior pubic ramus, which is made just medial to the iliopectineal eminence. To ease visualization, the flexed hip is slightly adducted. A 16-mm Hohmann retractor is placed 1 cm to 1.5 cm medial to the eminence. The periosteum of the superior pubic ramus is incised, and the base of the pubic ramus is exposed subperiosteally; two blunt retractors are inserted around it to protect the obturator nerve and vessel. With the use of a 15-mm Lexer osteotome, a complete osteotomy is made that starts medial to the iliopubic eminence and perpendicular to the long axis of the pubic ramus, with the osteotome pointed medially at a 45-degree angle. One of the blunt retractors is placed into the osteotomy of the superior pubic ramus.

For the remaining three osteotomy steps, the approach to the quadrilateral plate is completed, and the abductors have to be tunneled. For the approach to the quadrilateral plate, the periosteum along the anterior surface of the anterior wall of the acetabulum, starting at the iliopectineal eminence, is incised and stepwise detached medially and inferiorly. Beyond the pelvic brim, the use of a curved periosteal elevator is recommended. To improve the stability of the reversed blunt Hohmann retractor positioned on the ischial spine, the dissection should not be carried out into the greater sciatic foramen. Having cleared the entire surface of the medial acetabular wall, the reversed blunt Hohmann retractor is inserted and levered against the ischial

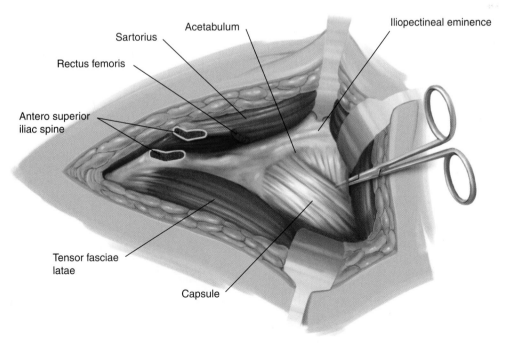

**Figure 26–1**   The completed approach. The osteotomy of the anterosuperior iliac spine allows for the preparation of the inner pelvis. A Hohmann retractor sits on the pubis. The iliocapsularis is detached from the capsule, and the scissors are placed arrownd it. With the tip of the scissors, the ischium is palpated.

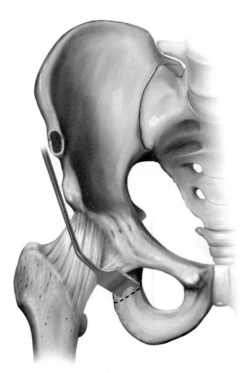

**Figure 26–2**  Osteotomy of the ischium.

spine. The entire space up to the sacroiliac ligaments can now be viewed. Adduction of the flexed leg allows for the reduction of the soft-tissue tension (Figure 26-3).

Only limited subperiosteal tunneling is necessary at the outer wall of the ilium; all that is needed is just enough to insert a reversed blunt Hohmann retractor down to the greater sciatic foramen to protect the muscles and the sciatic nerve during the supra-acetabular and retroacetabular osteotomies. Halfway

between the ASIS and AIIS and starting just distal to the osteotomy of the ASIS, the gluteus minimus is detached by sharp dissection over a distance of 3 cm and then freed with a curved periosteal elevator until the tip of a blunt reversed Hohmann retractor can reach the greater sciatic foramen. The tunneling proximally should not involve the remaining fibers of origin of the tensor fasciae latae; distally, an area approximately 3 cm wide should be left at the origin of the gluteus minimus. In this latter area, the supra-acetabular branch of superior gluteal artery is embedded to ensure the blood supply to the supra-acetabular region.

The supra-acetabular and retroacetabular osteotomies (i.e., the third and fourth steps) are performed in two parts. First, the planned line of osteotomy is marked on the inside of the ilium with a straight 10-mm Lexer osteotome. The marking starts on the lower border of the osteotomized ASIS and continues perpendicularly in a posterior direction, stopping short of the pelvic brim by 1.5 cm. The mark then continues, usually at an angle of 110 degrees to 120 degrees distally in the direction of the ischial spine. The determination of the apex and the degree of the angle can vary, depending on the patient's anatomy. It is important that the retroacetabular cut be made at a distance of at least 1 cm away from the greater sciatic notch. With an oscillating saw, the first step—the supra-acetabular osteotomy—is performed (Figure 26-4). Second, with a curved Simal osteotome, the remaining distance to the pelvic brim is osteotomized at an angle of 110 degrees to 120 degrees to the first cut. The purpose of this cut is to osteotomize the bone completely; therefore, it is important that the curved retractor introduced on the external side of the pelvis remains in situ to protect the abductors and the sciatic nerve (Figure 26-5). With a straight Simal osteotome, the cortical bone of the quadrilateral plate is cut at a distance of approximately 1.5 cm anterior to the greater sciatic notch (Figure 26-6). Only the first 20 mm to 30 mm must be osteotomized; the remaining bony bridge in the direction of the sciatic spine will be broken later on in a controlled fashion. Because the subchondral bone of the joint and the rim of the greater sciatic notch are very hard, this controlled fracture

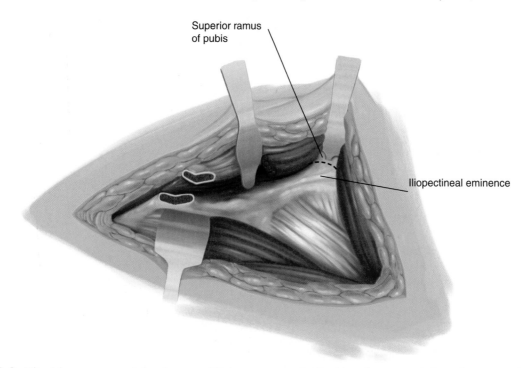

Superior ramus of pubis

Iliopectineal eminence

**Figure 26–3**  The abductors are tunneled, and a reversed Hohmann retractor is placed into the greater sciatic notch to protect the sciatic nerve. A second reversed Hohmann retractor is placed medially onto the sciatic spine to retract the intrapelvic musculature medially to allow for the wide exposure of the quadrilateral plate.

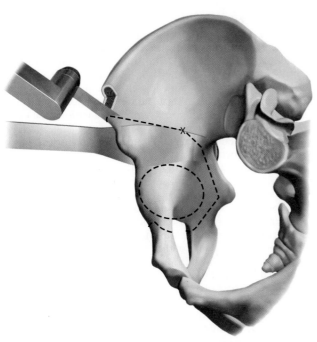

**Figure 26–4**  The supra-acetabular osteotomy starts at the distal end of the osteotomy of the anteroinferior iliac spine and runs in a perpendicular direction to a point approximately 1 cm lateral to the iliopectineal line.

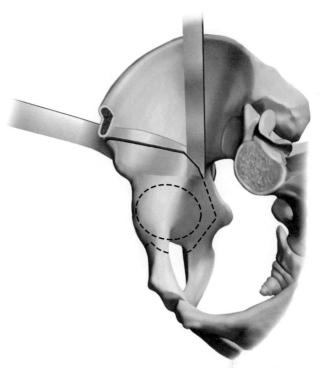

**Figure 26–6**  With a straight Simal osteotome, the cortical bone of the quadrilateral plate is cut at distance of approximately 1.5 cm anterior to the greater sciatic notch.

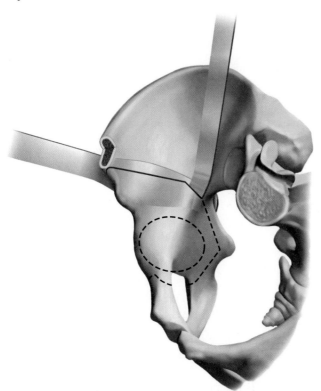

**Figure 26–5**  With a curved osteotome, the remaining distance to the pelvic brim is osteotomized. The osteotome is aimed at the lateral cortex. The soft tissues and the sciatic nerve are protected by the lateral retractor.

always succeeds without extending into the joint or the greater sciatic notch.

A 15-mm Lexer osteotome is introduced into the second posterior part of the osteotomy. By pulling the handle forward, a lever movement is exerted against the acetabulum until the

bridge toward the sciatic spine breaks. If this maneuver does not succeed with moderate force, then the posterior part of the osteotomy should be extended more distally. The acetabulum is still attached to the pelvis at the posterior and caudal corner through a bone bridge between the first ischial cut and the posterior part of the supra-acetabular osteotomy. A Schanz screw is inserted through the AIIS into the supra-acetabular bone and parallel to the inner wall. The remaining bone bridge is now put under tension. With a spreader inserted into the posterior part of the supra-acetabular osteotomy and pulled through at the Schanz screw in a distal and lateral direction, the acetabulum is tilted distally and laterally; this allows for a better view of the quadrilateral plate. A 20-mm-wide angled pelvic osteotome is advanced 4 cm below the pelvic brim at an angle of 50 degrees to the quadrilateral plate in the direction of the endpoint of the first ischial osteotomy (Figure 26-7). The osteotome is advanced with careful hammer blows until resistance ceases. This is repeated two to three more times with more distal positioning of the osteotome. A decrease in tension is felt by less resistance at the Schanz screw and by a loosening of the spreader. Under no conditions should the chisel be advanced beyond the point at which no more resistance is felt because of the risk of injury to the sciatic nerve. The complete mobilization of the acetabular fragment is done by opposing the forces of the Schanz screw and the spreader: the Schanz screw is rotated forcefully medially, whereas the spreader is rotated externally to the outside of the pelvis. By doing this, the last part of the posteroinferior bone bridge is fractured.

The acetabular fragment is now freely movable and thus can be reoriented. Because there is a tendency of the dysplastic joint to lateralize, the fragment must be correspondingly medialized. If the center of rotation is in a proper position, the correction is achieved by rotating the acetabular fragment around the femoral head. A supra-acetabular gap that appears during correction is always the result of hinging caused by incomplete posterocaudal

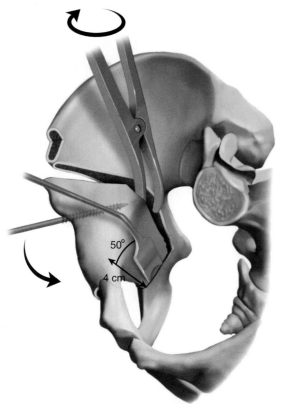

**Figure 26–7**   With a large spreader, the remaining bone bridge between the ischial osteotomy and the supra-acetabular osteotomy is put under tension. The osteotomy propagates more distally and is completed with the large special osteotome, and the fragment then is mobilized. The Schanz screw is rotated forcefully medially, whereas the spreader is rotated externally to the outside of the pelvis. By doing this, the last part of the posteroinferior bone bridge is fractured.

mobilization or a persisting bone bridge (Figure 26-8). The correction depends on the area of deficient cover. The pre-operative assessment of the anteroposterior pelvic radiograph includes an analysis of the lateral, anterior, and posterior coverage. Anterolateral deficiency is most commonly present, but one has to be aware that approximately 15% of these hips have a posterior deficiency (i.e., acetabular retroversion). For the most common type, the main correction is an anterior rotation in combination with some internal rotation. In general, this leads to sufficient lateral coverage. The correction is provisionally stabilized with two 2.5-mm threaded Kirschner wires advanced from the iliac crest into the fragment. The checking of the correction is performed with an anteroposterior radiograph of the entire pelvis that permits for a comparison with the opposite hip. The inclination of the weight-bearing area of the acetabulum should not go beyond the horizontal plane. The edges of the anterior and posterior wall should meet at the lateral edge of the sourcil. The center of the femoral head should lie neither too lateral nor too medial as measured by the distance between the medial border of the femoral head and the ilioischiatic line. Novices in particular run the risk of overcorrection, either by exaggerating the lateral coverage or by creating retroversion of the acetabulum. Overcorrection of the acetabulum may lead to a pincer type of femoroacetabular impingement. Even for the experienced surgeon, several adjustments and corresponding radiographs are necessary.

Occasionally, after preceding femoral osteotomies or in the presence of aspheric deformities of the femoral head, a simultaneous varus or extension osteotomy of the femur is necessary to stabilize the femoral head and to improve congruency. Intraoperative radiographs in abduction as well as abduction and flexion will supply the necessary information.

While waiting for the intraoperative radiographs, the joint is opened with a "T"-shaped incision, and the labrum is inspected. Only free-floating flaps or intralabral ganglia are removed. Should a large acetabular rim fragment be present, the pseudarthrosis is freshened, and the fragment is fixed with a mini screw. With the joint opened, the head–neck junction is evaluated for potential causes of impingement. If necessary, a bulge at the anterolateral transition between head and neck is shaped so that a normal neck diameter results and neither

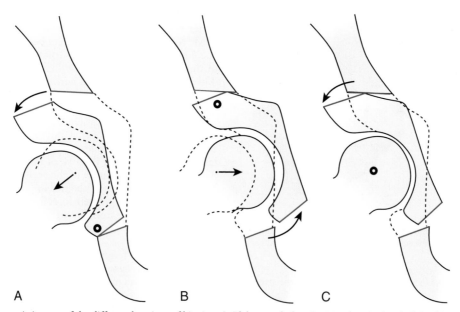

**Figure 26–8**   Schematic images of the different locations of hinging. **A,** If the acetabulum is rotated around an inferior hinge (i.e., an incomplete osteotomy of the ischium), the hip joint is lateralized. **B,** A completely free fragment allows for rotation around the center of the femoral head. **C,** Conversely, if the fragment is not mobilized completely cranially or in the area of the pubis, the correction will medialize the center of the rotation.

flexion nor flexion and internal rotation interfere with the acetabular rim. Flexion of up to 95 degrees and a balanced rotation to either side in 90 degrees of flexion is desirable.

The definite fixation is achieved with two 3.5-mm cortex screws of 60 mm to 80 mm in length that are introduced from the iliac crest into the acetabular fragment. An additional screw is inserted from the AIIS through the fragment and aimed at the sacroiliac joint. Occasionally a 3.5-mm reconstruction plate at the inner side of the pelvis is needed, particularly for patients with osteoporosis or after a substantial correction. The bone of the acetabular fragment that exceeds anteriorly is removed and inserted into the osteotomy cleft.

The capsule is closed loosely with resorbable sutures. The direct and reflected heads of the rectus are reinserted with the use of transosseous, nonresorbable sutures. The osteotomized ASIS is fixed with a 2.7-mm cortical screw. The abdominal muscles are reattached back to the iliac crest and the fascia of the proximal thigh is closed with absorbable sutures. Suction drains are placed subcutaneously (but not intrapelvicly), if necessary; because of the large cancellous osteotomy surfaces, the patient could be exsanguinated.

Figure 26-9 shows the preoperative and postoperative radiographs of a patient with bilateral dysplasia.

## TECHNICAL PEARLS

- The easiest way to find the interval between the tensor fasciae latae and the sartorius is to incise the fascia over the tensor and then dissect the fascia in a medial direction. By pulling the tensor laterally, the floor of the interval becomes visible and can then be incised.
- The detachment of the periosteum in the iliac fossa should only be extended to the superior pubic ramus after the osteotomy of the latter. If the periosteum is detached earlier, the superior curved retractor, which is used to protect the obturator nerve and vessel in the obturator foramen, is more difficult to keep in position and tends to slip away.
- The supra-acetabular osteotomy should start immediately at the distal end of the osteotomy of the ASIS to keep as much muscular attachment of the gluteus minimus to the external side of the acetabular fragment and thus preserve the blood supply. This also improves the stability of the Schanz screw.
- It is mandatory to perform an anterior arthrotomy for the inspection of the labrum and the assessment of the anatomy of the anterior head–neck junction. In a consecutive series of 100 patients, a resection osteochondroplasty of the head–neck junction was necessary in 34 hips that otherwise would have developed cam-type femoroacetabular impingement after acetabular correction. At least 90 degrees (and preferably more than 100 degrees) of passive unobstructed hip flexion and 30 degrees of internal rotation at 90 degrees of flexion are required.

## POSTOPERATIVE REHABILITATION

The leg is positioned in a foam splint with the hip in extension and the foot in a neutral position. After 1 to 2 days, the suction drains are removed, and the dressing is changed. Mobilization is started on the first or second postoperative day with two crutches. Touch-down weight bearing of approximately 15 kg is allowed for 8 weeks. At this time, physiotherapy is limited to instruction in and surveillance of proper gait and partial weight bearing. The lifting of the extended lower limb while in a supine position is not allowed for 6 weeks so as not to disturb the reattached hip flexors. After 8 weeks, the progression of the union is checked radiographically. If signs of bony union are present, progressive weight bearing and strengthening exercises of the hip abductors are started. Physiotherapy is now directed to gain back normal strength and coordination. Three months postoperatively, walking without a limp and a cane should be possible. Before allowing the patient to discontinue the use of crutches, the Trendelenburg sign should be negative and normal abductor strength should be present when the patient is tested in the lateral decubitus position.

## RESULTS AND OUTCOMES

Siebenrock and colleagues reported about 75 symptomatic dysplastic hip joints in 63 patients treated with the Bernese PAO. This group included the first series of PAOs performed between 1984 and 1987. The mean patient age was 29 years (range, 13 to 56 years), and the female-to-male ratio was 3.4 to 1. Fifty percent of the hips were Severin grade III, and 44% were Severin grade IV with signs of subluxation. Osteoarthrosis was present in 51% of the patients. Twenty-three patients (31%) had previous acetabular (14 hips) and femoral (9 hips) surgery for the treatment of the dysplastic hip. The average follow up time was 11.3 years (range, 10 to 13.8 years) in 71 hip joints (95%). In 58 patients (82%), the hip joint was preserved at the last follow up, with good to excellent results in 73% of these patients. Unfavorable outcomes were significantly associated with an older age of the patient, moderate to severe joint degeneration at the time of surgery, labral lesions, less anterior coverage correction, and a suboptimal acetabular index. The presence of joint degeneration was correlated with a significantly worse outcome. The analysis of the hip joints with only Tönnis grade 0 or 1 degeneration showed good to excellent outcomes in 88% of patients.

Major complications were encountered in the first 18 patients, including an intra-articular cut in 2 patients, excessive lateralization in 1 patient, a secondary loss of correction in 2 patients, and femoral head subluxation in 3 patients.

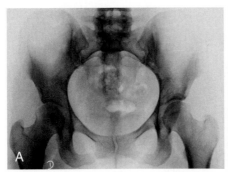
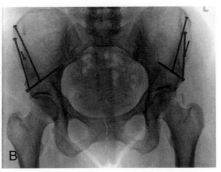

**Figure 26–9** **A,** Preoperative radiograph of a 35-year-old female patient with bilateral dysplasia. The left side shows already some mild joint space narrowing. **B,** The same patient 10 years (left side) and 9 years (right side) after periacetabular osteotomy. The joint spaces are stable without further signs of degeneration, and excellent results are seen on both sides.

Steppbacher and colleagues reevaluated the initial study group after 20 years. Four patients (5 hips) were lost to follow up, and 1 patient (2 hips) had died. The remaining 58 patients (68 hips) were followed for a minimum of 19 years (mean, 20.4 years; range, 19 to 23 years), and 41 hips (60%) were preserved at the final follow up. Forty-one hips (60%) had a preserved hip joint at 20 years, which corresponds with a cumulative Kaplan-Meier survivorship rate of 60.5% (range, 48.7% to 72.2%; 95% confidence interval). Twenty-six hip joints (38%) were converted to total hip arthroplasty, and one had a hip fusion at a mean time of 11.7 ± 5.9 years (range, 0.9 to 19.3 years). The 41 surviving hips (60%) had a mean Merle d'Aubigné score of 15.8 ± 2.1 at the final follow up. Of these, 81% (33 hips) were graded as good to excellent, 15% (6 hips) were graded as fair, and 5% (2 hips) were considered poor. No major changes in any of the radiographic parameters were observed during the 20-year postoperative period, except for the osteoarthrosis score. Six factors that are predictive of poor outcome were identified: 1) age at surgery; 2) preoperative Merle d'Aubigné score; 3) positive anterior impingement test; 4) limp; 5) osteoarthrosis grade; and 6) postoperative extrusion index.

In general, there is only very limited long-term experience with other reorienting acetabular osteotomies; in fact, there is only the study of Schramm and colleagues that involved 22 patients who underwent Wagner osteotomy for the treatment of the dysplastic hip. The mean age at surgery was 24.4 ± 9.7 years, and 19 women and 3 men were treated. Seventeen hips had no signs of osteoarthrosis. The authors reported a survivorship of 68% for the first 22 cases of spheric periacetabular osteotomy after a minimum follow up of 20 years. The remaining 15 hips had an average Harris Hip Score of 86 points (range, 50 to 100 points), and the clinical results were rated as good or excellent for 11 of the 15 patients. Risk factors for failure were the incongruency of the joint and a poor preoperative Harris Hip Score. The Kaplan-Meier survival rate estimate with conversion to total hip replacement as the endpoint was 86.4% at 20 years.

In a study that was specifically designed to assess the influence of osteoarthrosis on outcome, Trousdale and colleagues retrospectively reviewed 42 patients after PAO with and without intertrochanteric osteotomy performed between January 1984 and December 1990. There were 8 male and 34 female patients. The average age of the patients at the time of the operation was 47 years (range, 11 to 56 years). Ten patients had combined PAO and intertrochanteric osteotomies. Osteoarthrosis was graded according to the Tönnis classification: it was grade I in 15 patients, grade II in 18 patients, and grade III in 9 patients. Follow up averaged 4 years (range, 2 to 8 years). The Harris Hip Score improved significantly ($P < .0001$) from an average of 62 points preoperatively to an average of 86 points postoperatively. Results were excellent or good for 32 of the 33 patients with grade I or II osteoarthrosis. Eight of the 9 patients who had grade III osteoarthrosis had a Harris Hip Score of less than 70 points at the final follow up. Six patients subsequently underwent total hip arthroplasty, and 3 patients had an additional intertrochanteric osteotomy. Reported complications included heterotopic ossification in 14 patients (33%), nonunion of the pubic osteotomy in 2 patients (5%), and pain related to the hardware that led to its removal in 9 patients (21%). Overall, the study showed that the amount of preoperative arthrosis correlated with postoperative outcome.

There are several short-term outcomes reported from various centers. The results are remarkably consistent and can be summarized as follows: patients with minimal to moderate arthritic changes usually achieve pain relief and improved function after surgery. However, patients with advanced radiographic degenerative changes have less predictable success (Table 26-1).

## COMPLICATIONS

In addition to the usual surgical risks of bleeding, thrombophlebitis, embolism, and infection, there are some additional risks related to the surgical approach, the osteotomy, and the things that occur after treatment.

Risks associated with the approach include the avulsion of the reattached muscles (i.e., musculus sartorius, musculus rectus femoris); injury to vessels (i.e., obturator vessels, medial femoral circumflex artery) and nerves (i.e., lateral femoral cutaneous nerve, obturator nerve, femoral nerve, sciatic nerve); and heterotopic ossification. Most commonly, some damage to the lateral femoral cutaneous nerve is observed. The course of the nerve in the area of the ASIS is highly variable. To avoid damage to the main branch, the fascia over the tensor should be incised lateral to the fatty streak, including the nerve. The patient has to be advised that numbness of the proximal lateral thigh may occur. However, other nerve lesions are rare. In the series of the

| Author | Technique | No. of Patients | Length of Follow up | Results |
|---|---|---|---|---|
| **Table 26-1** SUMMARY OF RESULTS AFTER REORIENTING ACETABULAR OSTEOTOMIES | | | | |
| Siebenrock et al, 1999 | PAO | 63 (75 hips) | 11.3 years (range, 10 to 13.8 years) | Overall MdA score: good to excellent in 73%; MdA score for patients with OA grade 0 or 1, good to excellent in 88% |
| Steppbacher et al, 2008 | PAO | 63 (75 hips) | 20.4 years (range, 19 to 23 years) | 41 (60%) preserved hips with 81% good to excellent MdA scores; 28 patients converted to total hip replacement |
| Schramm et al, 2003 | Wagner | 22 | Minimum of 20 years | 15 hips preserved; average HHS of 86; 11 hips rated good to excellent |
| Trousdale et al, 1995 | PAO | 42 | Average of 4 years (range, 2 to 8 years) | Average HHS of 86 at follow up; 32 out of 33 hips with OA of less than 2 had good to excellent results; 8 out of 9 hips with OA of 3 had HHS of less than 70 |
| Clohisy et al, 2005 | PAO | 16 hips | Average of 4.2 years | Improvement in HHS from 73.4 to 91.3 points; all hips were rated Severin III or higher |
| Crockarell et al, 1999 | PAO | 19 hips | Average of 3.2 years (range, 2 to 4.3 years) | Improvement in HHS from 62 to 86 |

*PAO*, Periacetabular osteotomy; *MdA*, Merle d'Aubigné hip score; *OA*, osteoarthrosis Tönnis grade; *HHS*, Harris Hip Score.

senior author, 7 of more than 1000 PAOs result in the permanent loss of sciatic nerve function. Damage to the femoral nerve is very uncommon, but the nerve may become overstretched after a Sharrard procedure in which the iliopsoas muscle is transferred and thus no longer protecting the femoral nerve. The nerve may also incur damage during corrections that include substantial medial tilting of the acetabular fragment during the correction of acetabular retroversion. Heterotopic ossification is observed around the origin of the rectus femoris muscle; this ossification may cause extra-articular impingement with a painful limitation of flexion.

Complications associated with the osteotomy include intra-articular osteotomy, fracture of the posterior column, undercorrection, overcorrection, a loss of fixation, delayed union, and nonunion. Nonunion of the pubic ramus is rarely seen (it is more often seen with major corrections). In general, the condition is not painful, and it necessitated a revision in only one of our patients. A fracture through the posterior column may result in a nonunion of the ischium. In three of our patients, this was painful and required revision with bone grafting and plating.

Proud screw heads at the iliac crest may cause tenderness and may have to be removed. During the postoperative course, a loss of correction can result from weight bearing that occurs too early; surgical revision to realign the acetabular fragment should occur as soon as possible. Additional supra-acetabular fixation with a 3.5-mm reconstruction plate from the inside of the pelvis has to be considered. Avulsion of the reattached ASIS after a straight-leg raise has to be revised as well.

A consequence of the increased coverage of the femoral head—and not really a complication—is a slight decrease in the overall range of motion.

## ANNOTATED REFERENCES AND SUGGESTED READINGS

Beck M, Leunig M, Ellis T, Sledge JB, Ganz R. The acetabular blood supply: implications for periacetabular osteotomies. *Surg Radiol Anat.* 2003;25:361–367.

This injection study shows that blood supply to the acetabular fragment after a PAO is secured through the acetabular branches of the obturator and the superior and inferior gluteal arteries. The supra-acetabular branch of the superior gluteal artery is protected by its course within the gluteus minimus muscle. To further protect it, the osteotomy should be carried out as close as possible to the anterior superior iliac spine.

Carlioz H, Khouri N, Hulin P. Ostéotomie triple juxtacotyloidienne. *Rev Chir Orthop Reparatrice Appar Mot.* 1982;68:497–501.

Clohisy JC, Barrett SE, Gordon JE, Delgado ED, Schoenecker PL. Periacetabular osteotomy for the treatment of severe acetabular dysplasia. *J Bone Joint Surg Am.* 2005;87:254–259.

This article describes the short-term (mean, 4.2 years) follow up of 16 hips treated for severe acetabular dysplasia (i.e., group IV or V Severin classification). No hip had advanced degenerative changes, and 3 hips had undergone previous surgery. The average Harris Hip Score improved from 73.4 point preoperatively to 91.3 points at the final follow up. Two of the 13 patients were dissatisfied with the result; both had Severin V dysplasia with a false acetabulum. Overall, PAO was considered to be an effective technique for this particular subgroup of patients.

Crockarell J Jr, Trousdale RT, Cabanela ME, Berry DJ. Early experience and results with the periacetabular osteotomy. The Mayo Clinic experience. *Clin Orthop.* 1999;363:45–53.

This is a review of the early results of a small series of 19 patients. The Mayo Clinic hip scores improved from an average of 46 to 68 points, and the Harris Hip Score improved from 62 to 86 points.

Good correction was obtained uniformly. Complications included two transient peroneal nerve palsies, three ischial fractures, and three asymptomatic pubic nonunions. The authors also noted a slight decrease in hip motion.

Davey JP, Santore RF. Complications of periacetabular osteotomy. *Clin Orthop.* 1999;363:33–37.

This is a review of the learning curve for performing PAO and the complications associated with it. The authors found that the complication rate decreases significantly in proportion with increased experience.

Ganz R, Klaue K, Vinh TS, Mast JW. A new periacetabular osteotomy for the treatment of hip dysplasias. Technique and preliminary results. *Clin Orthop.* 1988;232:26–36.

This is the original description of the technique of periacetabular osteotomy.

Hempfing A, Leunig M, Nötzli HP, Beck M, Ganz R. Acetabular blood flow during Bernese periacetabular osteotomy: an intraoperative study using laser Doppler flowmetry. *J Orthop Res.* 2003;21:1145–1150.

This study addresses the laser Doppler flowmetry of acetabular perfusion during surgery. A drop in blood flow of 77% was measured; however, the pulsatility of the Doppler signal remained preserved, which indicated the viability of the acetabular fragment.

Hussel JG, Rodriguez JA, Ganz R. Technical complications of the Bernese periacetabular osteotomy. *Clin Orthop.* 1999;363:81–92.

This article is a discussion of potential complications that are related to the approach, to the osteotomy, to the positioning of the acetabular fragment, and to the morphologic particularities of the acetabulum and the proximal femur.

LeCoeur P. Corrections des défauts d'orientation de l'articulation coxofemorale par ostéotomie del'isthme iliaque. *Rev Chir Orthop.* 1965;51:211–212.

Leunig M, Siebenrock KA, Ganz R. Rationale of periacetabular osteotomy and background work. *J Bone Joint Surg Am.* 2001;83:438–448.

This is a review of the current knowledge of and rationale for the treatment of the dysplastic hip with the use of PAO.

Mast JW, Brunner RL, Zebrack J. Recognizing acetabular version in the radiographic presentation of hip dysplasia. *Clin Orthop.* 2004;418:48–53.

This review of 153 patients with dysplasia determined the frequency of acetabular retroversion. The frequency was found to be high, with retroversion being present in 1 out of 3 hips. Retroversion was commonly associated with lower values of the center-edge angle. This observation is important, because it must be taken into consideration when planning a corrective osteotomy to avoid overcorrection.

Murphy S, Deshmukh R. Periacetabular osteotomy: preoperative radiographic predictors of outcome. *Clin Orthop.* 2002;405:168–174.

This is a 2-year retrospective study of 52 hips after PAO. By Tönnis category, there were 0 failures among 21 grade I hips, 4 failures among 22 grade II hips, 1 failure among 8 grade III hips, and 1 failure in the 1 grade IV hip. Failures were attributed to a loss of correction during the early postoperative period, the remaining incongruency of the joint, a false acetabulum, or a lack of improvement of the joint space as compared with what was seen on the preoperative functional radiographs.

Myers SR, Eijer H, Ganz R. Anterior femoroacetabular impingement after periacetabular osteotomy. *Clin Orthop.* 1999; 363:93–99.

An increasing knowledge of hip mechanics (i.e., femoroacetabular impingement) enabled the authors to identify a cause of previously unrecognized secondary impingement after PAO with residual pain and limited range of motion. A lack of anterior or anterolateral femoral head–neck offset results in an abutment conflict between the femoral neck and the acetabular rim. Before correction, this is compensated for by the lack of anterior coverage; however, after correction, this mismatch becomes symptomatic. To avoid this complication, it is therefore mandatory to open the joint anteriorly, to assess for potential impingement, and, when necessary, to perform a resection osteoplasty to improve the femoral head–neck offset.

**Reynolds D, Lucas J, Klaue K. Retroversion of the acetabulum. A cause of hip pain. *J Bone Joint Surg Br*. 1999;81:281–288.**

This article describes and defines the features of acetabular retroversion and the problems related to it. As a treatment of symptomatic acetabular retroversion, a reversed PAO is proposed. With that technique, the anterior overcoverage is decreased, and the symptoms of impingement are alleviated.

**Salter RB. Innominate osteotomy in the treatment of congenital dislocation and subluxation of the hip. *J Bone Joint Surg Br*. 1961;43:518–539.**

**Schramm M, Hohmann D, Radespiel-Troger M, Pitto RP. Treatment of the dysplastic acetabulum with Wagner spherical osteotomy. A study of patients followed for a minimum of twenty years. *J Bone Joint Surg Am*. 2003;85:808–814.**

**Siebenrock KA, Schöll E, Lottenbach M, Ganz R. Bernese periacetabular osteotomy. *Clin Orthop*. 1999;363:9–20.**

**Steppbacher SD, Tannast M, Ganz R, Siebenrock KA. Mean 20-year followup of Bernese periacetabular osteotomy. *Clin Orthop*. 2008;466:1633–1644.**

**Tonnis D, Behrens K, Tscharani F. Eine neue Technik der Dreifachosteotomie zur Schwenkung dysplastischer Hüftpfannen bei Jugendlichen und Erwachsenen. *Z Orthop*. 1981;119:253–263.**

**Trousdale RT, Ekkernkamp A, Ganz R, Wallrichs SL. Periacetabular and intertrochanteric osteotomy for the treatment of osteoarthrosis in dysplastic hips. *J Bone Joint Surg Am*. 1995;77:73–85.**

# CHAPTER 27

# Trochanteric Distalization (Relative Femoral Neck Lengthening) for Legg-Calvé-Perthes Disease and Coxa Vara

*Karl F. Schultz*

## INTRODUCTION

Isolated distalization of the greater trochanter of the femur has been a relatively uncommonly used salvage procedure for various pediatric hip diseases. The procedure was first described in 1969 by Jani for the relative overgrowth of the greater trochanter, and since then there have been several publications that have discussed the functional results with the use of either a distalization technique, a lateralization technique, or combined techniques. Most commonly, the distalization is performed concomitantly with an intertrochanteric osteotomy and the functional lengthening of the femoral neck.

The relief of the Trendelenburg gait, a lessening of pain, and an improvement in the range of motion are common goals for all trochanteric distalization procedures. In the setting of total hip replacement, distalization procedures have been extensively studied. Although this technique falls outside of the scope of this chapter, some of the related conclusions can be helpful for surgical decision making for hip preservation.

## INDICATIONS

The distalization procedure is indicated for coxa brevis with minimal degeneration of the hip as a result of the following:
- Osteonecrosis as a complication of developmental dysplasia of the hip (DDH) treatment
- Legg-Calvé-Perthes disease
- Congenital coxa vara
- Bacterial coxitis

## BASIC SCIENCE

The purpose of the procedure is twofold: 1) to alleviate any bony impingement of the greater trochanter on the lateral ilium, thereby increasing the range of motion (particularly abduction in full extension); and 2) to increase the moment arm of the abductors as a result of the distal or lateral placement of the trochanter in addition to increasing the baseline tension.

In 1977, Gore and colleagues postulated that the distalization of the trochanter would be beneficial to hip biomechanics by increasing the abductor moment arm and by increasing the resting muscle tension. This was partially confirmed by Free and Delp in a computer model in the presence of a total hip replacement; the authors examined the effect of the distalization and lateralization of the greater trochanter on the moment arm of the abductors as well as the force-generating capacity of this procedure. The study showed a maximum increase of 11% for anterolateral transfer in a patient with normal anatomy. However, when the hip was shortened by the superior displacement of the hip center, which somewhat replicated the shortening of the abductors in the presence of coxa brevis, there was a 43% decrease in the force-generation capacity of the abductors. Although the moment arm of the abductors was not significantly changed with distalization in this setting, the force-generating capacity was restored via the restoration of the resting muscle length.

## HISTORY AND PHYSICAL EXAMINATION

The history is dependent on the presenting diagnosis, its severity, and how long the deformity has been present. Patients will usually present with a limp, varying degrees of pain with abduction, and substantially limited abduction of the hip. There is nearly always an accompanying diagnosis that has led to the coxa brevis, as mentioned previously. Presentation can be at any time during childhood or adulthood.

The physical examination will reveal a positive Trendelenburg sign. A positive "gear stick test" as described by MacNicol is a limitation of abduction in extension with an improvement of abduction in flexion, because the high-riding trochanter is allowed to slip posteriorly in flexion. A positive impingement sign may also be present. With the proximal femoral growth disturbance, there will usually be a limb-length discrepancy present.

## IMAGING AND DIAGNOSTIC STUDIES

An anteroposterior pelvic view and frog-leg lateral view of the affected hip are required. In addition, an abduction view may be obtained if there is a question of bony impingement after looking at the radiographs (Figure 27-1). For the purposes of isolated distalization or lateralization of the trochanter, these studies will usually suffice.

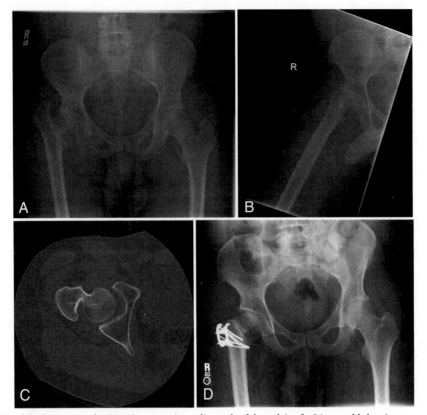

**Figure 27–1 A** and **B**, Case example: Anterior-posterior radiograph of the pelvis of a 24 year old showing a preserved hip joint, short femoral neck, trochanteric overgrowth and leg-length discrepancy. On physical exam, he has a vaulting gait due to leg length discrepancy and a positive Trendelenburg sign and positive trochanteric impingement sign on the right side with mild trochanteric tenderness and a positive gear stick test. **C**, An axial computed tomography image depicting the posterior position of the trochanter. **D**, Post-operative anterior-posterior radiograph after trochanteric distalization procedure with augmented fixation with claw plate due to the patients smoking history. At one year out, the osteotomy healed, Trendelenburg and gear stick sign were negative, and the patient was able to return to work with a shoe lift. R, Right.

## SURGICAL TECHNIQUE

The patient is placed in the lateral decubitus position. A bumper is placed between the patient's legs such that the leg is held in slight abduction. Great care should be taken to adequately pad all bony prominences, and an axillary roll should be placed. The surgical extremity is then prepped and draped free.

An 8-cm to 10-cm incision is made longitudinally over the lateral aspect of the trochanter and taken down to the fascia lata in line with the incision. Any bursal tissue is taken down to reveal the proximal border of the vastus lateralis at the vastus tubercle and the posterior border of the gluteus medius.

An osteotomy is performed with an oscillating saw from immediately proximal to the insertion of the vastus lateralis to just above the trochanteric (piriformis) fossa. The osteotomy is gently elevated with broad osteotomes superiorly. A bone hook can be used to retract the osteotomized fragment superiorly. Any remaining medial trochanter can be excised carefully and in a subperiosteal manner to protect the blood supply to the femoral head. After adequate mobilization of the fragment is achieved, a bone hook is used to distalize the fragment. During the distalization, some rotation of the trochanteric fragment can occur, which can be alleviated by releasing the tendinous insertion of the gluteus minimus on the anterior border of the trochanteric fragment. Additional bumps under the extremity are used to gain approximately 15 degrees of additional abduction.

The use of an image intensifier may help with the optimal final position of the fragment. The optimal placement of the

trochanter is achieved when the tip of the trochanter is level with the center of rotation of the femoral head.

After adequate distalization is achieved, the reduction is held with a bone hook (and, if necessary, a smooth Kirschner wire), and two 3.5-mm screws with or without washers are placed perpendicular to the osteotomy plane. The hip should be ranged to ensure a secure fixation.

The fascia is then closed, usually without great difficulty, with the hip in abduction. The subcutaneous tissue and skin are also closed, with or without a suction drain, as needed.

## POSTOPERATIVE TREATMENT

The patient is allowed to perform toe-touch weight bearing with a strict avoidance of active abduction or passive adduction. If necessary, a spica cast can be used for younger pediatric patients, or a hip abduction brace can be used for adults. In general, neither of these measures is necessary if the patient can be relied on to follow the weight-bearing precautions. These precautions can be eased at 8 weeks, at which point active abduction can be started.

## RESULTS AND OUTCOMES

The results of the related studies are summarized in Table 27-1.

**Table 27–1** RESULTS SUMMARY

| Study | Good Results | Fair Results | Poor Results | Complications | Technique |
|---|---|---|---|---|---|
| Lloyd-Roberts et al, 1985 | 9 out of 17 | | 8 out of 17 showed progressive degeneration | None | Distal |
| MacNicol, 1991 | 23 out of 27 | | 4 out of 27 | None | Distal |
| Takata et al, 1999 | 4 out of 4 | | | None | Distal |
| Pucher et al, 2000 | 33 out of 55 | 22 out of 55 | | None | Distal |
| Garrido et al, 2003 | 9 out of 11 | 1 out of 11 | 1 out of 11 | One fracture of a trochanteric fragment | Distal/lateral |
| Eilert et al, 2005 | 22 out of 28 | 4 out of 28 | 2 out of 28 | None | Based on a computer model |
| Schneidmueller et al, 2006 | 24 out of 24 | | | None | Distal/lateral |

## COMPLICATIONS

Complications are rare in the pediatric age group, but they include infection and deep venous thrombosis with the possibility of embolic events. As such, some form of anticoagulation should be used, particularly in the adult group.

Nonunion of the trochanter is also a possible complication, but it is very rare in the reported series. One trochanteric fragment fracture was reported.

In addition, it is possible to interrupt the vascular supply to the femoral head during the procedure (if osteonecrosis is not already present). Again, this was not reported as a complication in any of the case series in the literature.

## ANNOTATED REFERENCES AND SUGGESTED READINGS

Eilert RE, Hill K, Back J. Greater trochanteric transfer for the treatment of coxa brevis. *Clin Orthop Relat Res.* 2005;434:92–101.

Free SA, Delp SL. Trochanteric transfer in total hip replacement: effects on the moment arms and force-generating capacities of the hip abductors. *J Orthop Res.* 1996;14:245–250.

Garrido IM, Molto FJL, Lluch DB. Distal transfer of the greater trochanter in acquired coxa vara. Clinical and radiographic results. *J Pediatr Orthop B.* 2003;12:38–43.

Gore DR, Murray MP, Gardner GM, Sepic SB. Roentgenographic measurements after Muller total hip replacement: correlations among roentgenographic measurements and hip strength and mobility. *J Bone Joint Sur Am.* 1977;59:948–953.

Jani L. Die entwicklung des Schenkelhalses nach der trochanterversetsung. *Arch orthop Unfallchirurgie.* 1969;66:127–132.

Lloyd-Roberts GC, Wetherill MH, Fraser M. Trochanteric advancement for premature arrest of the femoral capital growth plate. *J Bone Joint Surg (B).* 1985;67–B:21–24.

MacNicol MF, Makris D. Distal transfer of the greater trochanter. *J Bone Joint Surg Br.* 1991;73–B:838–841.

Pucher A, Ruszkowski K, Nowicki J. et al. Distal greater trochanteric transfer in the treatment of deformity of the proximal femur caused by avascular necrosis. *Orthop Traumatol Rehabilitation.* 2006;8:41–47.

The authors reevaluated their distal greater trochanteric transfers at a mean of 15 years after the procedure. They found an increase of 22% in abductor torque as measured with strain gauges, and they concluded that transfer did improve hip function and delayed osteoarthritis of the hip.

Pucher A, Ruszkowski K, Bernardczyk K, Nowicki J. The value of distal greater trochanteric transfer in the treatment of deformity of the proximal femur owing to avascular necrosis. *J Pediatr Orthop.* 2000;20:311–316.

Schneidmueller D, Carstens C, Thomsen M. Surgical treatment of overgrowth of the greater trochanter in children and adolescents. *J Pediatr Orthop.* 2006;26:486–490.

Takata K, Maniwa S, Ochi M. Surgical treatment of highstanding greater trochanter. *Arch Orthop Trauma Surg.* 1999;119:461–463.

# CHAPTER 28

# Surgical Hip Dislocation for Femoroacetabular Impingement

*Michael Leunig, Anil S. Ranawat, and Reinhold Ganz*

## INTRODUCTION

The cause of hip osteoarthritis is a controversial topic. Historically, it was believed that arthritis was the result of intrinsic cartilage abnormalities and a biomechanical mismatch with axial loading that led to joint overload and subsequent cartilage wear. Recently, femoroacetabular impingement (FAI) has been shown to cause chondrolabral damage and leads to osteoarthritis. Although the pistol grip deformities have been described, the biomechanical concept of FAI as a unifying principle that explains how abnormal osseous parameters lead to arthritis is unique. FAI is a dynamic phenomenon that causes chondrolabral damage from repetitive hip motion, especially flexion and internal rotation. These "at-risk" hips have osseous structural abnormalities on either the femoral side, the acetabular side, or both. During the range of motion of the hip, particularly during flexion and internal rotation, these abnormalities produce the mechanical impingement of the femoral head against the acetabular cartilage or the femoral neck against the adjacent labrum. With time, repetitive impingement leads to acetabular cartilage damage, and this is followed by early osteoarthritis.

Two distinct mechanisms of FAI have been described; these are commonly referred to as *cam disease* and *pincer disease* (Figure 28-1, *A* through *D*). The descriptions of these conditions were based on the skeletal morphology and the pattern of chondrolabral damage observed during surgical hip dislocations. However, these morphologic patterns are not mutually exclusive; it is quite common for patients to have components of both cam and pincer types of impingements. With cam FAI, there is an abnormal bony prominence at the femoral head–neck junction that is often located anterosuperiorly. During hip flexion, the abnormal contoured femoral head engages the anterosuperior acetabulum and produces shear forces that lead to chondral abrasion, delamination, and, eventually, full-thickness cartilage loss. The natural history of this impingement process is initially acetabular cartilage injury, which is followed by labral injury and ultimately joint arthrosis. At first the labrum is uninvolved, but, with further impingement, labral injury results from the further loosening of the labrum at the transition zone between the peripheral cartilage and the labrum itself. With pincer FAI, there is increased acetabular coverage that leads to linear contact between the femoral head–neck junction and the acetabular rim. Acetabular overcoverage may be either generalized, as in coxa profunda and protrusio acetabuli, or localized, as in acetabular retroversion and anterior acetabular overhang. Unlike what occurs with cam FAI, the labrum is the first to get injured with intrasubstance degeneration, cyst formation, and bone apposition at the rim, which further deepens the socket and exacer-bates the problem. The prominent acetabular rim abuts with the femoral neck and causes the femoral head to lever in the acetabulum. This chronic levering of the head generates shear forces and injury to the posterior cartilage. Over time, this contrecoup mechanism leads to posteroinferior chondral damage and joint space narrowing.

## BASIC SCIENCE

The major breakthrough in impingement surgery was the safe surgical dislocation of the hip. The key to this procedure is an in-depth understanding of the blood supply to the femoral head. A recent latex injection study demonstrated that the medial femoral circumflex artery (MFCA) is the main blood supply to the femoral head. The vessel was surgically dissected and found to cross the obturator externus posteriorly and to then pass anteriorly to the short external rotators before perforating the joint capsule at the level of the superior gemellus. The study also demonstrated that the vessel remained undamaged during a controlled surgical hip dislocation, providing that the short external rotators and obturator externus remained intact. As a result of this study, an operative technique was developed that allowed for the safe surgical dislocation of the femoral head. Unlike the commonly used posterior approach, which requires the division of the short external rotators, a surgical dislocation protects these structures and, in doing so, preserves the blood supply to the femoral head.

Another critical basic science concept is that, in most cases, chondral injury usually leads to labral tears (and not vice versa). On the basis of our observations during several hundred surgical dislocations, the pattern of disease in cam FAI is that osseous abnormalities create mechanical "outside-in" shear forces and chondral damage, and, subsequently, the uninvolved labrum gets injured. This concept is supported by the fact that the majority of so-called labral tears occur at the anterosuperior portion of the acetabulum at the transition zone between the labrum and the articular cartilage and not the capsular margin. In addition, in early cam FAI, chondral damage is often observed without labral tears. Intrasubstance labral tears that are less frequently associated with chondral injuries have been observed in patients with early pincer FAI. Labral tears in the anterosuperior portion of the acetabulum are the result of FAI and not isolated traumatic injuries; this idea is supported by the observations that the majority of labral tears are also associated with chondral damage and radiographic evidence of abnormal skeletal morphology.

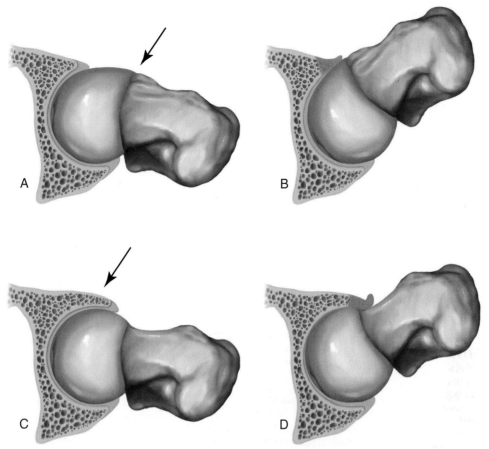

**Figure 28–1**   The two forms of femoroacetabular impingement (FAI) are shown. **A,** Cam FAI occurs when the lack of offset of the femoral neck *(arrow)* leads to mainly anterosuperior damage through repetitive inclusion of the femoral neck with subsequent shearing injury of the acetabular cartilage. **B,** During hip flexion, impingement causes chondral labral injury. **C,** Pincer FAI occurs as a result of acetabular overcoverage *(arrow)*. **D,** Pincer impingement causes anterosuperior impaction and subsequent leverage with contrecoup injury to the cartilage of the posteroinferior acetabulum during hip flexion. *Redrawn from Leunig, M., Robertson, W., and Ganz, R. Femoroacetabular impingement: diagnosis and management including open surgical technique.* Tech Sports Med *15:178-188, 2007.*

## TREATMENT, INDICATIONS, AND CONTRAINDICATIONS

Conservative treatment is usually attempted first, and this includes activity modification; rest; nonsteroidal antiinflammatory drugs; and a physical therapy regimen that focuses on core, lower back, and hip flexor strengthening. On occasion, one may use intra-articular injections for both diagnostic and therapeutic uses. We do not routinely perform intra-articular hip injections; however, for select cases in which the origin of a patient's symptoms remains unclear, we will perform a diagnostic intra-articular injection. In many cases, conservative management strategies may only partially relieve symptoms, and often they only mask symptoms. Attempts by physical therapists to improve the passive range of motion are often not beneficial and in fact may be counterproductive, because the limitation of internal rotation in patients with FAI is the result of abnormal osseous morphology. Although some patients receive temporary benefits from these conservative measures, young athletic patients often have difficulty complying with activity modifications.

The most important indications for FAI surgery are physical examination and radiographic findings that are consistent with FAI (Box 28-1). Proper imaging studies are critical to confirm and quantify the deformity and to assess the degree of arthritis. Unnecessary treatment delays also should be avoided.

The next critical issue is determining the surgical technique that should be used. Although this decision depends

> ### BOX 28-1   INDICATIONS
>
> - Failed nonoperative management
> - Groin pain and physical examination findings that are consistent with FAI
> - Osseous parameters that are consistent with FAI
> - Prearthritic hip (i.e., a Tönnis scale score of less than 2)
> - Large deformities that are not amenable to arthroscopic treatment

on numerous patient factors, the type, magnitude, and location of the underlying osseous abnormality are important. Although arthroscopy is an emerging technique for the treatment of FAI, it is technically challenging, and it has its limitations. Arthroscopy can easily handle the soft-tissue or secondary effects of FAI (e.g., the chondrolabral pathology), although how well it can handle the underlying osseous abnormalities remains debatable. Alternatively, a surgical dislocation of the hip provides a wide, safe exposure with the complete visualization of both the acetabular and femoral pathologies. In addition, the structural morphologic changes (e.g., the lack of an anterior femoral neck offset, acetabular overcoverage) can be addressed with relative ease. It has also been shown that the failure to address the underlying bony abnormality is likely to lead to continued symptoms, progressive joint degeneration, and poor outcomes. Another advantage of a surgical dislocation is that it is provides versatile exposure of the hip joint. It enables the surgeon to perform numerous impingement procedures as well as other procedures for soft-tissue injuries, osseous Bankart lesions, avascular necrosis, hip resurfacing, loose bodies, osteochondromatosis, and other non-FAI diagnoses. Contraindications for this technique are few, but the most obvious are extensive arthritic changes (e.g., a score of more than 2 on the Tönnis scale) and extensive destruction and deformity of the femoral head. Other contraindications include significant acetabular protrusio and dysplasia.

## HISTORY AND PHYSICAL EXAMINATION

FAI typically presents with an insidious onset of groin pain in young adults. Although patients often mistakenly associate the condition with a traumatic event, it is a more chronic process with intermittent pain and occasionally with acute exacerbations from activities that require forceful hip flexion and internal rotation. As a result of the often subtle findings on routine radiographs, these patients may experience a delay in diagnosis and be subjected to extensive nonorthopedic workups. Pincer-type FAI is more common among women, and it is often quite painful as a result of the crushing of the sensitive labrum between the acetabular rim and the femoral neck. This symptom often acts as a warning sign that causes patients with the condition to seek earlier orthopedic evaluation before significant chondral damage occurs. Alternatively, cam-type FAI is more common among young males. These patients have a pain pattern that involves more deep-seated groin symptoms, which are usually less severe than those experienced by patients with pincer-type FAI, because the labrum is commonly spared. These patients often do not seek evaluation until they have developed significant chondral injury.

It is crucial that all FAI patients receive a thorough physical examination, because there are many extra-articular diagnoses that can present with hip pain. The examination begins with detailed motor and sensory examinations. Next, the range of motion is assessed. Limited internal rotation of the flexed and adducted hip is seen in both cam and pincer FAI, but a greater loss of internal rotation is seen with cam FAI. This is followed by FAI-specific tests. An impingement test (Figure 28-2) is performed with the patient in the supine position; the affected hip is adducted and internally rotated as it is passively flexed. In patients with FAI, the femoral head–neck junction and the acetabulum abut, thus producing shear forces on the labrum and reproducing a sharp pain in the groin. A posteroinferior FAI test is performed with the patient supine on the edge of the examination table with the legs dangling free from the end. The examiner then extends and externally rotates the affected hip. Deep-seated groin pain during this maneuver is indicative of posteroinferior FAI, and it is frequently combined with limited external rotation. Finally, other critical examination maneuvers are performed to find associated pathology of the psoas, the iliotibial band, the lower back, and other related structures.

## IMAGING

A correctly performed anteroposterior pelvic radiograph is the most essential imaging study for the assessment of impingement. The radiograph should be standardized to ensure proper rotation (i.e., the sacrum bisects the pubis) and pelvic inclination (i.e., 2 cm to 5 cm of pubic–sacrococcygeal distance). Slight deviations in either of these parameters can lead to an inaccurate assessment of acetabular coverage, inclination, and anteversion.

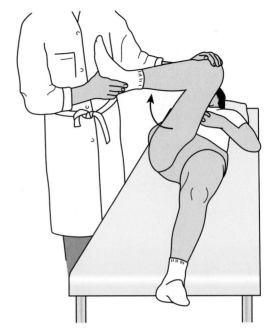

**Figure 28–2**   Clinical examination of the impingement test. *Redrawn from Leunig, M., Robertson, W., and Ganz, R. Femoroacetabular impingement: diagnosis and management including open surgical technique.* Tech Sports Med *15:178-188, 2007.*

After the adequacy of the radiograph has been verified, it should be reviewed in a systematic fashion. First, the radiograph should be assessed for the coverage of the femoral head (i.e., center edge angle and Tönnis angle) or for gross arthritic changes (i.e., Tönnis scale). Next, the acetabulum should be inspected for pincer-type FAI. Five radiographic structures must be identified: 1) the medial acetabular wall; 2) the ilioischial line; 3) the anterior wall of the acetabulum; 4) the posterior wall of the acetabulum; and 5) the femoral head. By understanding the relationship of these radiographic structures, all of the common causes of pincer FAI can be diagnosed. In a patient with coxa profunda, the medial acetabular wall approaches and overlaps (if it does not pass medial to) the ilioischial line, which causes a deep socket. In a patient with protrusio, the femoral head is medial to the ilioischial line. In a patient with true acetabular retroversion, the anterior and posterior acetabular walls overlap; they also have a positive crossover sign and a prominent ischial spine (Figure 28-3, *A*). In these cases, there may or may not be a sufficient posterior wall, but there is always a relative anterior overhang. Finally, one must assess for os acetabuli, which can represent either broken pincer lesions or unfused portions of the acetabulum (i.e., true os acetabuli).

On the femoral side, cam FAI is readily diagnosed with the proper radiographs. Given its mostly anterosuperior location, the cam lesion is often underappreciated on a standard anteroposterior radiograph, and it may be obstructed by the greater trochanter on a frog-leg lateral view. The aspheric head–neck junction is best visualized with either a 45-degree Dunn view or a cross-table lateral view with the leg in 15 degrees of internal rotation. The Dunn view, which is also known as an *extended neck lateral view*, is taken with the patient's hip in neutral rotation, flexed 45 degrees, and abducted 20 degrees. The internally rotated cross-table lateral view is often more practical for routine use, because positioning the patients for the Dunn view requires a leg holder or an assistant. Either image can be used to measure the head–neck offset and the alpha angle, both of which are abnormal parameters that can be used to assess cam FAI (see Figure 28-3, *B*). In addition, the femoral neck shaft angle should also be assessed for any significant varus deformities.

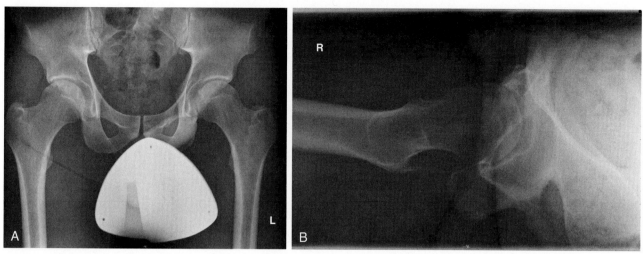

**Figure 28–3**   **A,** Anteroposterior radiograph that shows a crossover sign indicating acetabular retroversion. **B,** Cross-table lateral view that shows a lack of femoral offset. *L,* left; *R,* right.

In addition to radiographs, we routinely obtain a magnetic resonance arthrogram to accurately assess chondral delamination and full-thickness cartilage defects. In many cases of FAI, hips that produce normal radiographs (as defined by Tönnis grade) in fact have extensive chondral injury. Magnetic resonance imaging also assesses for labral pathology or subtle signs of FAI, such as fibrocystic changes at the head–neck junction; these changes are also known as *synovial herniation pits.* The magnetic resonance imaging should involve the use of cartilage-specific sequences, and it should be performed in radial-directed sections for the accurate measurement of angulation and the translation of the impingement lesions in the radiologic reference planes (Figure 28-4). Standard magnetic resonance imaging of the pelvis is often less sensitive, because it does not occur in the correct sequence plane with a resolution being far too low. In addition, although computed tomography scans provide a superior assessment of femoral anteversion, acetabular version, and femoral offset, they require radiation exposure during 20 radiologic pelvic overviews; thus, computed tomography should be used quite judiciously. Other advantages of obtaining a magnetic resonance image include the evaluation of stress

fractures and soft-tissue abnormalities as well as the measurement of the alpha angle and acetabular version.

## SURGICAL TECHNIQUE

The fundamental principle of the surgical treatment of impingement is an exposure that preserves the blood supply to the femoral head. The approach combined and made use of features from several previously described approaches, with the general principle being that of an anterior dislocation of the femoral head from a posterolateral approach. However, to protect the MFCA, the external rotators are left intact, and the joint capsule is exposed anteriorly with the use of a trochanteric osteotomy. The surgical technique is explained in detail later in this chapter.

General or spinal anesthesia is used. The patient is placed in the lateral decubitus position in well-padded bolsters, and care is taken to also protect the nonoperated limb. Correct orientation is important to allow for the accurate assessment of acetabular orientation during the procedure. The skin is cleansed with a standard preparation solution over the trochanteric region. The patient is prepared and draped in standard sterile fashion (Figure 28-5, *A*) with a free leg sterile bag drape placed on the opposite side of the operating table to receive the lower leg during hip dislocation (see Figure 28-5, *B*). A second-generation cephalosporin antibiotic is given for prophylaxis and continued for 24 hours. Image intensifying and laser Doppler flowmetry are not routinely used, but both can be helpful for either osteotomy fixation or to monitor the perfusion of the femoral head.

A straight lateral incision of approximately 20 cm to 25 cm in length is made along the anterior border of the greater trochanter. This incision has been more cosmetically favorable than a traditional Kocher-Langenbeck incision; in cases with excessive adipose tissue and the latter type of incision, unaesthetic bulges developed posteriorly toward the distal end of the incision. As a general rule, the more adipose tissue present, the longer the incision necessary for the adequate visualization for the trochanteric osteotomy and for the dislocation maneuver. The fascia lata is incised in line with the incision and extended proximally without any violation of the gluteus maximus fibers, as described by Gibson. The advantage of this approach is that it affords a wide exposure without any splitting of the gluteus maximus, thus avoiding damage to the muscle and its neurovascular supply. To locate the anterior margin of the gluteus maximus, the perforant vessels to the muscle are identified by

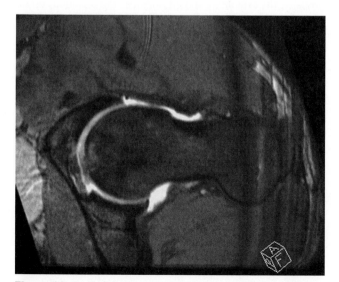

**Figure 28–4**   Radial sequence magnetic resonance image of the right hip showing cam-type FAI with a decreased head/neck offset.

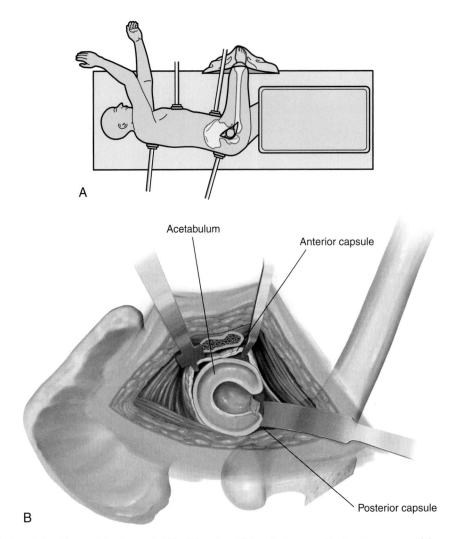

**Figure 28–5** **A,** The lateral decubitus position for surgical hip dislocation. This technique provides for the exposure of the entire femoral head and the acetabulum, which allows for the identification and treatment of femoroacetabular impingement. **B,** With the hip in flexion and external rotation, the femoral head can be dislocated to allow for an almost circumferential inspection of the entire acetabulum. *Redrawn from Leunig, M., Robertson, W., and Ganz, R. Femoroacetabular impingement: diagnosis and management including open surgical technique.* Tech Sports Med *15:178-188, 2007.*

undercutting the epifascial layer of the fatty tissue in an antero-cephalic direction. Care is taken to incise the intermediate fascia that rests on the gluteus medius and to retract it posteriorly with the mass of gluteus maximus muscle fibers, because this fascial plane retains the blood supply and innervation to the anterior part of the gluteus maximus. The intergluteal space is then developed with the hip in extension and internal rotation.

The next step is to make a gentle incision of the trochan-teric bursa close to its lateral edge and to then retract it in an anterior direction. The innominate tubercle and the border of the vastus lateralis origin are now visible. By careful, superficial exposure of the posterior margin of gluteus medius, the postero-cranial tip of the trochanter with the tendinous insertions of the gluteus medius can be seen and palpated. A small trochan-teric branch of the MFCA can be identified running anteriorly along the posterior border of the trochanteric crest and should be hemocauterized.

Before starting the osteotomy, one should inspect the tro-chanter. The osteotomy fragment should provide continuity between the gluteus medius and the gluteus minimus (specifi-cally the long tendon anteriorly) proximally and the vastus lat-eralis via the osteotomy fragment distally. Thus, the osteotomy is trigastric rather than digastric in nature. Conversely, the piri-formis and the short external rotators should remain attached to

the nonosteotomized femur (i.e., the stable trochanter). If done properly, the osteotomy should undercut the tendinous origin of the vastus lateralis distally and a few remaining incoming glu-teus medius fibers proximally at the tip of the trochanter. This will increase the certainty that the major part of the underlying piriformis muscle tendon will remain on the stable trochanter.

The trochanteric osteotomy begins with the internal rota-tion of the leg of about 20 degrees to 30 degrees on a Mayo stand to expose the posterior border of the gluteus medius. The osteotomy is generally performed with an oscillating saw at an angle that is roughly parallel to the rotation of the affected extremity. The osteotomy should run from the posterosuperior border of the greater trochanter distally toward the posterior border of the vastus lateralis muscle, and it should remain paral-lel with the long axis of the femoral shaft.

Although the osteotomy was originally described as a sin-gle plane cut, we now recommend using a triplanar osteotomy to increase the mechanical stability of the osteotomy fragment, especially among older patients, who may have compromised bone. The osteotomy should commence at the posterosuperior border of the greater trochanter with two broad chevron-type cuts, leaving a step of 5 mm between them. The distal cut should end more medial than the proximal one to offset the pull of the abductors. Moreover, it is recommended that the osteotomy not perforate the anterior cortex of the trochanteric crest but rather be left incomplete. An osteotome is used to lever the fragment forward with a controlled fracture of the anterior cortex. This creates a third plane to the osteotomy, because the anterior cortex typically detaches with an anterior lip of cortex attached. The advantages of this triplanar osteotomy are its increased stability and the ease of the anatomic refixation of the fragment.

The resulting mobile fragment should be approximately 10 mm to 15 mm in diameter. If the trochanteric osteotomy is too thick, the tendon of the piriformis muscle will adhere completely to the mobile trochanteric fragment. This may lead to insufficient mobilization of the trochanteric fragment and endanger the anastomosis with the inferior gluteal artery or the deep branch of the MFCA itself, with the consequent risk of femoral head necrosis. Alternatively, if the trochanteric osteotomy is too thin, fixation difficulties and the risk of fracture of the trochanteric fragment may arise.

The osteotomy fragment is then mobilized. Initially, an 8-mm Hohmann retractor is placed in the osteotomy site, and the fragment is retracted and mobilized anteriorly. The mobile osteotomy fragment is in continuity with the gluteus medius and the vastus lateralis. The fibers of the vastus lateralis originating at the posterior femur are gradually released to the middle of the height of the gluteus maximus tendon. The mobile fragment can now be tilted more anteriorly, especially after the anterolateral part of the vastus lateralis has been released subperiosteally from the femur with the hip in external rotation, flexion, and abduction. Proximally, the residual tendon insertions of the gluteus medius that are still attached to the stable part of the trochanter are cut. After releasing these fibers, the piriformis tendon becomes visible. Ideally, approximately 25% of the piriformis tendon should be attached to the mobile osteotomy fragment to ensure the appropriate thickness of the osteotomy. These residual piriformis fibers on the mobile fragment are then released to further mobilize the osteotomy fragment. Care must be taken during this portion of the procedure to avoid any damage to the short external rotators, because they protect the MFCA.

The next step is to develop and expose the hip capsule between the interval of the gluteus minimus and the piriformis. The limb is placed in extension and slight internal rotation. The interval between the gluteus minimus and the posterior capsule is carefully dissected posteriorly down to the acetabular rim; this interval offers the most certainty that the blood supply to the femoral head will be preserved. Furthermore, the constant anastomosis between the inferior gluteal artery and the deep branch of the MFCA is protected; this runs along the lower margin of the piriformis tendon, and it is of fundamental importance because it alone can guarantee the vascularization of the femoral head if there is injury to the deep branch. Finally, the limb is placed in abduction, flexion, and external rotation again. The anterosuperior capsular insertions of the gluteus minimus muscle are then released while preserving the long tendon insertion into the mobile fragment. After the gradual release of the posterior, superior, and anterior insertions of the gluteus minimus from the capsule, the hip capsule is completely exposed; however, the short external rotators have always remained protected and attached to the stable trochanter.

With the hip capsule completely exposed, a Z-shaped capsulotomy (for the right hip) or an inverse Z-shaped capsulotomy for the left hip is performed. It begins with a linear incision along the line of the femoral neck close to the superior border of the stable trochanter. The capsulotomy then runs posterosuperior along the acetabular rim from the inside out in a proximal direction to avoid injury to the retinaculum, the cartilage, and the labrum. Finally, an inferomedial extension of the capsulotomy is performed over the front of the anterior capsule and headed toward the lesser trochanter. It is important to avoid extending the capsulotomy cut past the lesser trochanter

to protect the MFCA, and the posterosuperior extension should not extend past the piriformis tendon, because the vessel may also be injured at this point. The labrum and the chondral surfaces are best preserved by an "inside-out" arthrotomy, which ensures the visualization of these structures at all times.

The next critical step is the careful dislocation of the femoral head and the appropriate positioning of the retractors to visualize the pathology. First, an 8-mm Hohmann hook is hammered into the bone below the capsular margin but above the labrum to hold the soft tissues back at the 12-o'clock position; a Langenbeck hook may also be adequate for this purpose. A bone hook is then placed around the femoral calcar, and the hip is gently subluxed with traction, flexion, and external rotation as the limb is prepared to be placed into the sterile leg bag. The ligamentum teres, which prevents complete dislocation, is then cut with parametrium scissors, with care taken not to damage the chondral surfaces of the acetabulum or the femoral head. On rare occasions, the hip is only subluxed, and all operative work is then performed with the limb in this position. The lower extremity is then dislocated anteriorly and placed in the sterile leg bag. Two additional retractors are placed: one at the anterior acetabular rim and the other inferiorly by the transverse acetabular ligament. There is now a 360-degree view of the entire acetabulum. Posterior retractors can also be placed, if necessary. Finally, a bump is placed on the femur to provide slight abduction, and a posterior force is placed on the femur by an assistant to assist with acetabular visualization.

The hip can now be inspected for evidence of injury as a result of FAI. Open inspection initially begins with a capsulotomy when the amount of synovial effusion and the degree of synovitis are documented. Next, attention turns to the acetabular chondrolabral surfaces. Note that, as soon as the cartilage is exposed, it should be protected from drying out with a constant trickle of physiologic salt solution. Damage to the acetabular cartilage and labrum is documented. A blunt probe can be used to examine the labrum for detachments or tears and to assess the cartilage for softening or delamination. By altering the position of the leg in flexion, all articular surfaces can be visualized, and any chondrolabral injuries in both the anterosuperior and posterosuperior regions are documented. If labral tears are unrepairable, then the labrum might be debrided or even replaced by graft tissue (round ligament, hamstrings, IT band, etc.). Likewise, grade IV contained chondral lesions are often microfractured. Larger lesions, particularly of the femoral head, might require cartilage repair techniques such as ACT, AMIC, or others.

If pincer FAI is noted preoperatively and confirmed intraoperatively, then an acetabular rim trimming is performed (Figure 28-6, *A* through *D*). First, the labrum must be detached from the acetabular rim with the use of sharp dissection. Because the typical location of acetabular rim lesions is the anterosuperior margin, the excessive rim segment can be removed with a curved osteotome. The amount of rim resected depends on the location of the crossover sign and the femoral head coverage (e.g., the value of the lateral center-edge angle, femoral head extrusion) seen on the preoperative plain radiograph. Ultimately, however, intraoperative tests are performed to assess the degree of overcoverage. These tests are performed after both the acetabular and femoral resections, if needed. Rim excision is performed until no impingement exists but not at the expense of creating instability or dysplasia. If there are full-thickness chondral lesions, then a microfracture is performed with angled awls. The labrum is then reattached with the use of two to four small bone anchors placed into the bed of bleeding cancellous bone approximately 10 mm to 15 mm apart. The nonabsorbable suture of the anchor should be passed through the base of the labrum and tied with the labrum firmly seated against the acetabular bone so that the knot lies on the nonarticular surface of the labrum.

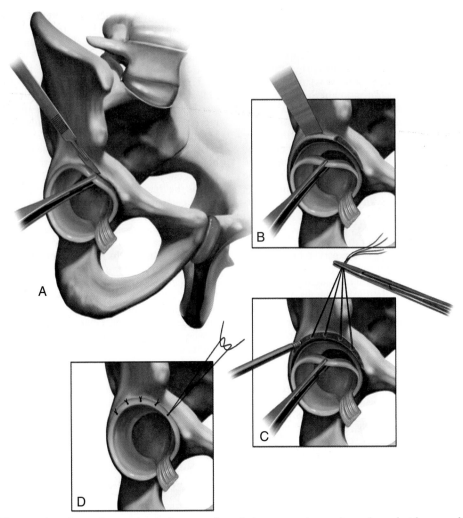

**Figure 28–6**  **A,** The resection of excessive anterior rim in a case of acetabular retroversion can be performed with a curved osteotome **B,** after labral detachment as part of the approach to the acetabular rim. **C,** After sufficient rim resection, **D,** labral refixation is performed with the use of bone anchors. *Redrawn from Leunig, M., Robertson, W., and Ganz, R. Femoroacetabular impingement: diagnosis and management including open surgical technique. Tech Sports Med 15:178-188, 2007.*

Attention now turns to the femoral side. The retractors are gently removed, the knee is lowered, and the femoral head can be elevated out of the wound so that, with rotation, about three fourths of the head circumference can be seen. First, the posterosuperior retinaculum and the vessels are identified and protected. Next, the sphericity of the femoral head can be assessed after two blunt retractors are placed under the femoral neck. Nonsphericity is tested with the use of appropriately sized transparent spheric templates. With these templates, a safe resection is predictable, and the risk of femoral neck fracture is minimized. A previous study has shown that up to 30% of the femoral neck can be resected.

The most common location for this pathology is the anterosuperior head–neck junction, with the abnormal cartilage having a slightly hypervascular, pink appearance. The presence of a cyst near the peripheral border of the nonspheric segment is sometimes noted, which indicates the point of maximum impingement. The abnormal bone can be removed carefully with the use of curved chisels until a normal head–neck offset is recreated, with great care taken not to laterally injure the terminal branches of the MFCA in the posterosuperior retinaculum (Figure 28-7, *A* and *B*). Unfortunately, this area may also be nonspheric, in which case the debridement should start proximally on the neck and reach the point at which the vessels enter

their intraosseous course. A periosteal elevator may also be used to strip a portion of the retinaculum off of the bone as well. Femoral resection should be performed cautiously with regular reassessment with the use of the spheric templates to avoid over-resection, which both increases the risk of femoral neck fracture (only with excessive resections) and endangers the loss of the labrum's suction seal effect with the femoral head.

Before relocation, the ligamentum teres is debrided. Perfusion should be assessed by observing bleeding from the fovea or from the raw cancellous surface that was created after the neck debridement. Bone wax (ideally resorbable) can be applied to the debrided surface before relocation. Hip relocation can be achieved with simple traction and controlled internal rotation, with care taken not to avulse the repaired labrum. Alternatively, although bone anchors have been placed during the acetabular preparation, the sutures can be tightened after the femoral head relocation, thus reducing the risk for avulsing labral refixation. After relocation, the range of motion can be assessed to look for any residual impingement before closure.

Capsular closure is performed without excessive tension to avoid the compression of the retinacular vessels. The trochanteric fragment is reduced anatomically according to the triplanar osteotomy step cuts, and it is reattached with the use of 3.5-mm or 4.5-mm screws. With the triplanar trochanteric osteotomy, 3.5-mm screws

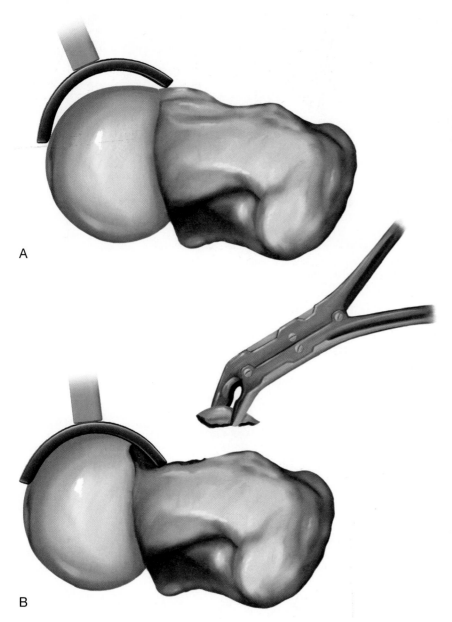

A

B

**Figure 28–7**  Resection osteoplasty from the femoral head–neck junction can be used to recreate the normal concave contour of the femoral neck. **A,** Transparent templates are used to determine the sphericity of the femoral head. **B,** Femoral osteochondroplasty is performed to restore the insufficient offset. *Redrawn from Leunig, M., Robertson, W., and Ganz, R. Femoroacetabular impingement: diagnosis and management including open surgical technique. Tech Sports Med 15:178-188, 2007.*

are sufficient for fixation, but if the patient develops any reactive bursitis, these screws are slightly more difficult to remove. Alternatively, 4.5-mm screws are much easier to remove if the patient becomes symptomatic. The fascia lata and the fat and cutaneous layers are then carefully closed in a layered fashion. Drains are rarely indicated. Box 28-2 reviews technical pearls for this procedure.

## REHABILITATION AND POSTOPERATIVE MANAGEMENT

A postoperative radiograph is obtained in the recovery department (Figure 28-8). The patient is usually immobilized postoperatively on crutches, with toe-touch weight bearing for 6 weeks for triplanar osteotomy or 8 weeks for classic slide osteotomy. The patient is prohibited from performing hip flexion of more than 70 degrees (or of more than 90 degrees after a triplanar procedure) and from actively abducting or adducting the hip to allow for the proper healing of the osteotomy site. Continuous passive motion with flexion limited to 70 degrees is started on postoperative day 1 and continued until discharge to prevent the formation of intra-articular adhesions between the femoral

---

### BOX 28-2 TECHNICAL PEARLS

- Create a straight lateral incision.
- Have an intimate understanding of the course of the MFCA.
- Use an angle of the oscillating saw that is parallel to the internal rotated lower limb.
- Use a triplane osteotomy to maximize the stability of the osteotomy.
- Keep the osteotomy fragment to 10 mm to 15 mm in thickness.
- Mobilize the fragment anteriorly.
- Approach the capsule between the piriformis and gluteus minimus muscles.
- Perform the acetabular procedures first, followed by the femoral procedures.
- Perform an intraoperative impingement test.

---

osteochondroplasty and the capsule. If a microfracture was performed, then the use of continuous passive motion is extended for up to 8 weeks. The patient is usually discharged after 5 days. All patients receive low-molecular-weight heparin until full mobilization occurs.

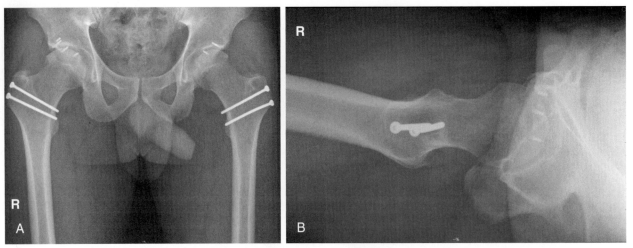

**Figure 28–8** Postoperative **A,** anteroposterior and **B,** lateral radiographs after bilateral surgical dislocations through a transtrochanteric approach with acetabular rim trimming, labral refixation, and femoral offset correction.

**Table 28–1** OPEN CLINICAL RESULTS OF SURGICAL DISLOCATION FOR FEMOROACETABULAR IMPINGEMENT

| Authors | No. of Hips | Length of Follow Up | Impingement Type | Other Information | Complications | Results |
|---|---|---|---|---|---|---|
| Beaule et al | 37 | 3.1 years | Cam | | No revisions or AVN; 9 ROH | Improvement in WOMAC, UCLA activity scale, and SF-12 scores; 6 out of 34 patients were dissatisfied |
| Bizzini et al | 5 | 2.7 years | Combined | Patients were professional hockey players | None | All patients returned to hockey participation |
| May et al | 5 | 16.3 months | Cam | Performed after arthroscopic labral debridement | None | Good |
| Peters et al | 30 | 2 years | Combined | Worse results with worse preoperative arthritis | None | 8 hips had progressive DJD, 4 had THA, and 2 had staged PAOs |
| Espinosa et al | 60 | 2 years | Combined | Labral refixation resulted in less arthrosis | None | 80% of patients with labral refixation as compared with 28% of patients with labral resection had good or excellent results |
| Beck et al | 19 | 4.7 years | Combined | Worse results with worse preoperative arthritis | No AVN | 5 patients had THA, whereas 13 hips were rated as good or excellent |
| Murphy et al | 23 | 2 to 12 years | Combined | Worse results with worse preoperative arthritis, combined impingement, and instability | None | 7 patients went on to THA, and 1 had arthroscopic labral debridement |

*AVN,* avascular necrosis; *ROH,* removal of hardware; *WOMAC,* Western Ontario and McMaster University Osteoarthritis Index; *UCLA,* University of Los Angeles; *SF-12,* short form 12; *DJD,* degenerative joint disease; *THA,* total hip arthroplasty; *PAO,* periacetabular osteotomy.

If after 6 to 8 weeks the radiograph shows evidence of healing at the osteotomy site, then weight-bearing and motion restrictions are advanced. If there is any concern, then therapy advancement is postponed for another 3 to 4 weeks. Full activities are allowed after the patient has regained full motion and strength, which usually takes about 3 months.

## RESULTS

A review of the literature and of the results of open impingement surgery is given in Table 28-1. To date, there have been seven series with approximately 199 patients. The patient's prognosis generally depends on the extent of articular damage. Stated another way, the extent of preoperative arthritis is an important predictor of outcome. In addition, it has been shown that labral refixation appears to yield better clinical and radiographic results, whereas cases that involve both impingement and instability have been shown to have worse results.

## COMPLICATIONS

General complications such as infection, blood loss, and venous thrombosis are quite rare. Specific complications of this procedure include iatrogenic head femoral necrosis, osteotomy nonunion, symptomatic hardware, undercorrection, overcorrection, and femoral neck fracture.

Although the risk of osteonecrosis is possible, in numerous series, the condition has not been reported. If one has a thorough understanding of the course of the MFCA, this potential complication is completely preventable. Similarly, these reports have all reported minimal trochanter fixation problems. If trochanter failure develops, then a repeat stable osteosynthesis is recommended. With the new triplane osteotomy, trochanter nonunions have been almost eliminated. Alternatively, symptomatic hardware is not infrequent. If indicated, this situation requires a small day procedure to remove the hardware, but minimal disability is associated with this condition and the procedure. Finally, undercorrection and overcorrection are also rare problems that can be eliminated with proper preoperative radiographic assessment in conjunction with carefully performed intraoperative impingement testing. Likewise, femoral neck fractures can be avoided with the use of templates to avoid excessive resection.

## CONCLUSION

The open treatment of FAI with a surgical dislocation has many potential advantages. It is a safe, reproducible, and versatile procedure. It also allows the surgeon to perform a real-time assessment of the impingement. The best mid-term results have been seen among patients with the least amount of osteoarthritis. As indications are better defined, clinical outcomes will continue to improve. By eliminating FAI, progressive osteoarthritic changes will hopefully be delayed or even prevented.

## ANNOTATED REFERENCES

Beaule PE, Le Duff MJ, Zaragoza E. Quality of life following femoral head-neck osteochondroplasty for femoroacetabular impingement. *J Bone Joint Surg Am.* 2007;89(4):773–779.

Level IV study using pre- and postoperative WOMAC, UCLA activity, and SF-12 scores on osteochondroplasty after open dislocation. The procedure was found to be safe and effective and improves quality of life in most patients.

Beck M, Kalhor M, Leunig M, Ganz R. Hip morphology influences the pattern of damage to the acetabular cartilage: femoroacetabular impingement as a cause of early osteoarthritis of the hip. *J Bone Joint Surg Br.* 2005;87(7):1012–1018.

Of the 302 hips analyzed, cam FAI caused damage to the anterosuperior acetabular cartilage, with separation between the labrum and cartilage. During flexion, the cartilage was sheared off the bone while the labrum remain untouched. In pincer FAI, articular damage was located circumferentially and included only a narrow strip. During movement, the labrum is crushed between the acetabular rim and the femoral neck, causing degeneration and ossification.

Beck M, Leunig M, Parvizi J, Boutier V, Wyss D, Ganz R. Anterior femoroacetabular impingement: part II. Midterm results of surgical treatment. *Clin Orthop Relat Res.* 2004;(418):67–73.

One of the first clinical papers following 19 hips after surgical dislocation and offset procedure. After 5 years, good results were found in patients with early degenerative changes not exceeding grade 1 OA.

Bizzini M, Notzli HP, Maffiuletti NA. Femoroacetabular impingement in professional ice hockey players: a case series of 5 athletes after open surgical decompression of the hip. *Am J Sports Med.* 2007;35(11):1955–1959.

Level IV study to describe the functional and sport-related outcomes 2 years after open surgical hip decompression in 5 young pro hockey players suffering from cam FAI.

Espinosa N, Beck M, Rothenfluh DA, Ganz R, Leunig M. Treatment of femoro-acetabular impingement: preliminary results of labral refixation. Surgical technique. *J Bone Joint Surg Am.* 2007;89(suppl 2) Pt.1:36–53.

A review of the open surgical technique for femoroacetabular impingement with labral refixation.

Espinosa N, Rothenfluh DA, Beck M, Ganz R, Leunig M. Treatment of femoro-acetabular impingement: preliminary results of labral refixation. *J Bone Joint Surg Am.* 2006;88(5):925–935.

Retrospective review of the clinical and radiographic results of 60 hips with FAI who underwent surgical dislocation. Twenty-five hips had labrum resection and 35 hips had labrum rerefixation. Patients treated with refixation recovered earlier and had superior clinical and radiographic results when compared with patients who had undergone resection of a torn labrum.

Ganz R, Gill TJ, Gautier E, Ganz K, Krugel N, Berlemann U. Surgical dislocation of the adult hip: a technique with full access to the femoral head and acetabulum without the risk of avascular necrosis. *J Bone Joint Surg.* 2001;83B(8):1119–1124.

A report of the technique to surgically dislocate the hip with minimal risk. Report describes experience in 213 hips, none of which developed avascular necrosis.

Ganz R, Leunig M, Leunig-Ganz K, Harris WH. The etiology of osteoarthritis of the hip: an integrated mechanical concept. *Clin Orthop Relat Res.* 2008;466(2):264–272.

Level V study discussing the theories of the etiology of OA, arguing that recent information supports so-called primary OA is related to subtle developmental abnormalities from FAI.

Ganz R, Parvizi J, Beck M, Leunig M, Notzli H, Siebenrock KA. Femoroacetabular impingement: a cause for osteoarthritis of the hip. *Clin Orthop Relat Res.* 2003;(417):112–120.

Detailed description of FAI including causes, clinical presentation, radiographic assessments, proposed mechanisms, different types, modes of surgical treatment, and surgical efficacy and importance.

Gautier E, Ganz K, Krugel N, Gill T, Ganz R. Anatomy of the medial femoral circumflex artery and its surgical implications. *J Bone Joint Surg Br.* 2000;82(5):679–683.

The classic description of the approach and technique commenting on the advantages of a posterior exposure of the hip joint.

Gibson A. Posterior exposure of the hip joint. *J Bone Joint Surg.* 1950;32B:183–186.

Description of the anatomy of the MFCA (primary blood supply of femoral head) and its branches based on 24 dissected hips after injection of neoprene-latex into the femoral or internal iliac arteries.

Guevara CJ, Pietrobon R, Carothers JT, Olson SA, Vail TP. Comprehensive morphologic evaluation of the hip in patients with symptomatic labral tear. *Clin Orthop Relat Res.* 2006;453:277–285.

A radiographic study correlating patients with symptomatic labral tear with radiographic osseous abnormalities.

Jamali AA, Mladenov K, Meyer DC, Martinez A, Beck M, Ganz R, Leunig M. Anteroposterior pelvic radiographs to assess acetabular retroversion: high validity of the "cross-over sign." *J Orthop Res.* 2007;25(6):758–765.

A study of 86 acetabuli in order to determine cranial, central, and caudal anatomic acetabular version (AV) from cadaveric specimens; establish the validity and reliability of the radiographic measurements of central acetabular anteversion; and determine the validity and reliability of the radiographic "cross-over sign" to detect acetabular retroversion.

Kalberer F, Sierra R, Madan S, Ganz R, Leunig M. Ischial spine projection into the pelvis. *Clin Orthop Relat Res.* 2008;466:677–683.

149 AP pelvic radiographs (298 hips) correlating the prominence of the ischial spine and the crossover sign as a sign of true retroversion.

Leunig M, Podeszwa D, Beck M, Werlen S, Ganz R. Magnetic resonance arthrography of labral disorders in hips with dysplasia and impingement. *Clin Orthop Relat Res.* 2004;(418):74–80.

Using MR arthrography, findings provide evidence that the anterosuperior acetabulum represents the initial fatiguing site of the hip in both FAI and dysplasia.

Locher S, Werlen S, Leunig M, Ganz R. [MR-Arthrography with radial sequences for visualization of early hip pathology not visible on plain radiographs]. *Z Orthop Ihre Grenzgeb.* 2002;140(1):52–57.

A description of a successful technique to improve MRI visualization of the hip.

Mardones RM, Gonzalez C, Chen Q, Zobitz M, Kaufman KR, Trousdale RT. Surgical treatment of femoroacetabular impingement: evaluation of the effect of the size of the resection. *J Bone Joint Surg Am.* 2005; 87(2):273–279.

A study to evaluate the amount of resection of the anterolateral aspect of the femoral head–neck junction that can be done safely. Resection of up to 30% of the anterolateral quadrant of the head–neck junction did not significantly alter the load-bearing capacity of the proximal part of the femur.

May O, Matar WY, Beaule PE. Treatment of failed arthroscopic acetabular labral debridement by femoral chondro-osteoplasty: a case series of five patients. *J Bone Joint Surg Br.* 2007;89(5):595–598.

A case series study in which 5 patients presented with persistent pain following arthroscopic labral treatment alone. All five had cam-type FAI that was treated by chondro-osteoplasty and had symptomatic improvement at mean follow-up of 16 months.

McCarthy JC, Noble PC, Schuck MR, Wright J, Lee J. The Otto E. Aufranc Award: the role of labral lesions to development of early degenerative hip disease. *Clin Orthop.* 2001;393:25–37.

Retrospective review of 436 hip arthroscopies and 54 cadavers to see whether labral lesions contribute to early degenerative hip disease. Arthroscopic and anatomic observations support the concept that labral disruption and degenerative joint disease are frequently part of a continuum of joint disease.

Mercati E, Guary A, Myquel C, Bourgeon A. [A postero-external approach to the hip joint. Value of the formation of a digastric muscle]. *J Chir (Paris).* 1972;103(5):499–504.

Classic description of the anatomic muscular insertions on the trochanter and the technique of how to perform a modified trochanteric osteotomy.

Meyer DC, Beck M, Ellis T, Ganz R, Leunig M. Comparison of six radiographic projections to assess femoral head/neck asphericity. *Clin Orthop Relat Res.* 2006;445:181–185.

A retrospective study of 21 desiccated femurs in order to determine which of six radiographic projections (anteroposterior, Dunn, Dunn/45° flexion, cross-table/15° internal rotation, cross-table/neutral rotation, and cross-table/15° external rotation) best identifies cam-type impingement. The Dunn view in 45-degree or 90-degree flexion or a cross-table projection in internal rotation best shows asphericity.

Murphy S, Tannast M, Kim Y-J, Buly R, Millis M. Debridement of the adult hip for femoroacetabular impingement. *Clin Orthop Relat Res.* 2004;429:178–181.

A follow-up study of 22 hips treated open for FAI. At most recent follow-up (range 2–12 years), 7 patients had THA, 1 had arthroscopic debridement of a recurrent labral tear, and 15 had no further surgery.

Murray RO. The aetiology of primary osteoarthritis of the hip. *Br J Radiol.* 1965;38(455):810–824.

Classical description of pistol grip deformity and early arthritis.

Notzli HP, Wyss TF, Stoecklin CH, Schmid MR, Treiber K, Hodler J. The contour of the femoral head-neck junction as a predictor for the risk of anterior impingement. *J Bone Joint Surg Br.* 2002;84(4):556–560.

A study to determine a simple method to describe concavity at the femoral head–neck junction performed by comparing MR scans of patients with groin pain, decreased internal rotation, and a positive impingement test with asymptomatic control subjects.

Parvizi J, Leunig M, Ganz R. Femoroacetabular impingement. *J Am Acad Orthop Surg.* 2007;15(9):561–570.

General review of FAI including its causes, consequences, and failed modes of treatment followed by a report of "encouraging results" of femoroacetabular osteoplasty and arthroscopic treatment of FAI.

Pauwels F. *Biomechanics of the Normal and Diseased Hip: Theoretical Foundation, Technique and Results of Treatment. An Atlas.* Edited. Berlin, Germany: Springer-Verlag; 1976.

Classic biomechanical description of hip biomechanics and osteotomies.

Peters CL, Erickson JA. Treatment of femoro-acetabular impingement with surgical dislocation and debridement in young adults. *J Bone Joint Surg Am.* 2006;88(8):1735–1741.

Clinical study of open surgical treatment of FAI at 2 years of follow up using HHS.

Reynolds D, Lucas J, Klaue K. Retroversion of the acetabulum. A cause of hip pain. *J Bone Joint Surg Br.* 1999;81(2):281–288.

A general overview of acetabular retroversion including a definition, possible causes, pathological changes that occur if untreated, clinical and radiographic parameters as well as proposed management techniques.

Robertson WJ, Kadrmas WR, Kelly BT. Arthroscopic management of labral tears in the hip: a systematic review of the literature. *Clin Orthop Relat Res.* 2007;455:88–92.

A lit review to determine the rate of patient satisfaction that can be expected following acetabular labral debridement. Patients can expect a patient satisfaction rate of approximately 67% at 3.5 years, good results by a modified HHS in patients and a complete resolution of mechanical symptoms in nearly 50% of patients.

Seldes RM, Tan V, Hunt J, Katz M, Winiarsky R, Fitzgerald RH Jr. Anatomy, histologic features, and vascularity of the adult acetabular labrum. *Clin Orthop.* 2001;(382):232–240.

Embalmed and frozen hips were studied to describe the anatomy, histologic features, and microvasculature of the acetabular labrum and labral tears. Description of study results indicates that labral tears occur early in the arthritic process of the hip.

Siebenrock KA, Kalbermatten DF, Ganz R. Effect of pelvic tilt on acetabular retroversion: a study of pelves from cadavers. *Clin Orthop Relat Res.* 2003;(407):241–248.

By defining the normal range of the distance between the symphysis and the sacrococcygeal joint on standard AP pelvic films, a technique was developed to evaluate pelvic inclination. Retroversion signs were significantly more pronounced and found at lower pelvic tilt angles in the pelves from males than from females.

Siebenrock KA, Schoeniger R, Ganz R. Anterior femoro-acetabular impingement due to acetabular retroversion. Treatment with periacetabular osteotomy. *J Bone Joint Surg Am.* 2003; 85-A(2):278–286.

Twenty-nine hips diagnosed with anterior FAI underwent a periacetabular osteotomy to evaluate the procedure's effectiveness. Procedure was deemed an effective way to reorient the acetabulum in young adults with symptomatic anterior femoro-acetabular impingement due to acetabular retroversion.

**Sussmann PS, Ranawat AS, Lipman J, Lorich DG, Padgett DE, Kelly BT. Arthroscopic versus open osteoplasty of the head-neck junction: a cadaveric investigation. *Arthroscopy.* 2007;23(12):1257–1264.**

A study to compare the precision and accuracy of arthroscopic versus open osteoplasty in treating FAI. Statistical analysis showed no differences between techniques regarding volume, depth, or overall arc of resection, confirming the ability to perform arthroscopic decompressions of the head–neck junction for isolated cam-type FAI.

**Tannast M, Siebenrock KA, Anderson SE. Femoroacetabular impingement: radiographic diagnosis—what the radiologist should know. *AJR Am J Roentgenol.* 2007;188(6):1540–1552.**

Describes important radiographic criteria that indicate the two types of FAIs. Also lists potential pitfalls in pelvic imaging.

**Tonnis D, Heinecke A. Acetabular and femoral anteversion: relationship with osteoarthritis of the hip. *J Bone Joint Surg Am.* 1999;81(12):1747–1770.**

A review of hip conditions including FAI, anteversion, and torsional deformities. It provides framework into understanding how hip pain is due to combined deformities on both the femur and acetabulum.

**Wenger DE, Kendell KR, Miner MR, Trousdale RT. Acetabular labral tears rarely occur in the absence of bony abnormalities. *Clin Orthop Relat Res.* 2004;(426):145–150.**

A retrospective review to evaluate the percentage of patients with acetabular tears who also have structural hip abnormality detectable by conventional radiography. Eighty-seven percent had at least one abnormal finding and 35% had more than one abnormality.

# CHAPTER 29

# Limited Open Osteochondroplasty for the Treatment of Anterior Femoroacetabular Impingement

*Murat Pekmezci and John C. Clohisy*

## INTRODUCTION

An abnormal relationship of the femur and the acetabulum that is characterized by repetitive abutment of the anterolateral femoral head–neck junction against the acetabular rim–labral complex is called the *femoroacetabular impingement syndrome* (FAI). Repetitive anterolateral impingement produces acetabular articular cartilage delamination, labral disease, and, eventually, osteoarthritis. To date, there is no prospective data that shows the natural history of untreated hip impingement. However, there are several retrospective case series that analyzed the structural anatomy associated with hip arthritis. These series demonstrated that deformity at the head–neck junction is commonly associated with osteoarthritis and that this may have a causative role in the disease pathogenesis. Currently, many investigators believe that untreated FAI has a poor prognosis and that the joint pathomechanics will lead to labral tears, articular cartilage injury, and progressive joint degeneration.

## PATHOPHYSIOLOGY

An appropriate relationship between the femoral head–neck junction and the acetabulum is a prerequisite for normal hip function. Normal hip range of motion requires a specific orientation of the acetabulum as well as of the proximal femur. The wide range of motion of normal hip function requires the appropriate orientation of the proximal femur and the acetabulum as well as normal femoral head–neck anatomy. Any deviation from this optimal orientation and alignment of the acetabulum and the femur may result in a decreased range of motion. For example, a decreased head–neck offset (i.e., the distance between the most prominent part of the anterior femoral neck and the articular surface of the anterior femoral head at the widest diameter of the head) results in less clearance between the neck and the bony acetabulum. As a result, the impingement of the femoral neck against the acetabulum and the labrum may occur within the normal range of hip motion. Activities that involve deep hip flexion (e.g., squatting, cycling) may aggravate the symptoms.

FAI has two types that depend on the anatomic location of the abnormality. The abnormality may be on the acetabular side (e.g., acetabular retroversion, coxa profunda) and result in abnormal coverage or overcoverage of the femoral head; this is called *pincer-type impingement*. If the abnormality is on the

femoral side in the form of an aspheric head–neck junction or an abnormal head–neck junction with a decreased head–neck offset (e.g., slipped capital femoral epiphysis, Perthes abnormalities, femoral neck malunions), it is called *cam-type impingement*. The third type of FAI is a combination of the cam and pincer types of impingements. In all scenarios, the impingement of either the femoral neck or the head–neck junction at the edge of the acetabulum results in repetitive trauma to the labrum. This leads to degenerative tears in the labrum and the disruption of the labrochondral junction, which leads to osteoarthritis of the hip. Although the degeneration starts in the anterolateral joint space, it may also affect the posteroinferior joint space as a result of the levering of the femoral head on the anterior edge of the acetabulum caused by anterior impingement.

## INDICATIONS

- The surgical strategy presented here has been primarily used for the treatment of cam-type deformities.
- Pincer abnormalities may be addressed with arthroscopic techniques or open procedures.
- Ideal surgical candidates have symptomatic anterior FAI, are well conditioned, are less than 50 years old, and have no or mild secondary osteoarthritis.

## HISTORY AND PHYSICAL EXAMINATION

The most common clinical presentation is activity-related groin pain in the young to middle-aged athletic individual. Associated lateral and posterior hip pain is also commonly observed. The symptoms are frequently intermittent, and the intensity ranges from mild to severe. High-demand sport activities that involve running, cutting, pivoting, and repetitive hip flexion (e.g., soccer) frequently exacerabate symptoms. Patients also complain of groin discomfort with prolonged sitting. Mechanical symptoms of locking and catching may also be problematic, and these presumably result from labral disease or unstable articular cartilage flaps. A history of hip trauma, childhood hip disease, and previous surgeries and treatments should be determined. These patients are commonly evaluated by multiple physicians and have been treated for tendonitis and synovitis. However, conservative treatment commonly fails as a result of the persistent structural abnormalities of the joint.

The physical examination starts with an observation of the patient's gait and sitting posture. Patients with FAI may avoid sitting erect in a chair. These patients may also have an antalgic gait, depending on the extent of the disease, and abductor weakness is common. Previous surgical scars are inspected to clarify the nature of previous procedures and to facilitate preoperative planning. A Trendelenburg test is used to assess abductor strength. During physical examination, the most common finding is the limited internal rotation of the hip, particularly with simultaneous hip flexion. The anterior impingement test is performed by passively flexing (90 degrees to 100 degrees), adducting (10 degrees to 20 degrees), and internally rotating (5 degrees to 20 degrees) the hip. This motion elicits the groin pain by moving the proximal anterolateral part of the femoral neck into contact with the rim of the acetabulum. A positive test can be indicative of anterior FAI. The Patrick test is performed by flexing, externally rotating, and abducting the hip by placing the ipsilateral foot on the contralateral knee. A positive test (i.e., the presence of groin pain) suggests the irritability of the hip joint and intra-articular hip disease. Finally, an examination of the lumbar spine and the entire limb is necessary to eliminate other sources of pain.

## IMAGING AND DIAGNOSTIC STUDIES

Plain radiographs are the traditional imaging modality for this condition. They can include a standing or supine anteroposterior pelvic view, a cross-table lateral view with 15 degrees of internal rotation, and a Dunn view or a frog-leg lateral view. The rotation and tilt of the pelvic x-ray should be assessed by observing the symmetry of the obturator foramens and the distance of the symphysis pubis to the sacrococcygeal joint, respectively. The normal value for the latter is 47 mm in females and 32 mm in males. Acetabular inclination and femoral head coverage should be evaluated to rule out associated hip dysplasia (i.e., structural instability). Acetabular version can also be assessed by looking for the presence of a crossover sign, which indicates acetabular retroversion. In addition, joint space narrowing, subchondral sclerosis, and periarticular cysts should be noted as indicators of secondary articular degeneration. The cross-table lateral view is helpful to evaluate the femoral head–neck junction. The femoral head–neck offset, the head–neck offset ratio, and alpha angle can be measured with the use of this view. These measurements have been shown to demonstrate abnormal femoral head morphology that is observed with cam-type impingement, and they can also be analyzed with the 45-degree and 90-degree Dunn views or the frog-leg lateral radiograph.

The next step in imaging should be magnetic resonance arthrography. This modality is sensitive for detecting intraarticular abnormalities (e.g., labral tears, chondral defects), and it is also helpful for excluding other diagnoses (e.g., osteonecrosis of the femoral head, stress fracture, neoplasm, infection). When evaluating patients with FAI, a computed tomography scan with three-dimensional reconstruction is informative with regard to the osseous deformity. The contour of the femoral head–neck junction and the extent of the femoral-sided disease can be appreciated in detail. The version of the acetabulum and associated osseous anomalies of the acetabular rim can also be defined.

Finally, diagnostic intra-articular hip injections provide valuable information about the presence or absence of intraarticular disease. Patients with intra-articular hip diseases (e.g., labral tears) usually report significant pain relief after injection. Alternatively, patients who do not have any pain relief should be re-evaluated for other causes of extra-articular hip disease (e.g., abdominal wall hernia, trochanteric bursitis, spinal stenosis).

## SURGICAL TREATMENT

The goal of the surgical treatment of FAI is to restore a more normal bony anatomy while addressing the associated soft-tissue problems (e.g., labral tears, acetabular cartilage lesions). The ideal surgical approach should possess the following properties:
- It should allow the surgeon to accurately visualize and evaluate disease characteristics.
- It should allow the surgeon to accurately reconstruct the structural hip anatomy.
- It should allow the surgeon to accurately treat the associated labral or acetabular cartilage disease.
- It should cause minimal morbidity while achieving these goals.

Different surgical approaches have been proposed to reach these goals. Ganz and colleagues popularized surgical dislocation and showed that this technique allowed for the 360-degree evaluation of the femoral head with complete access to the acetabulum. They did not observe any evidence of avascular necrosis after 2 to 7 years of follow up. Murphy and colleagues reported about 23 patients who were treated with open osteochondroplasty; 15 patients did not require further surgery, whereas 1 patient required hip arthroscopy to address a torn labrum. Seven patients were later converted to total hip arthroplasty. Spencer and colleagues reported about 19 patients who had osteochondroplasty or intertrochanteric osteotomy via surgical dislocation, and they concluded that this approach is safe and efficacious for treating FAI. Inferior clinical outcomes were observed among patients who had articular cartilage degeneration. Peters and Erickson reported about 20 patients with a minimum of 2 years of follow up. The authors noted severe acetabular cartilage lesions that were not appreciated on preoperative radiographs or magnetic resonance arthrography in 18 hips. Eight hips demonstrated a progression of arthritis, 3 hips were later converted to total hip arthroplasty, and 1 patient was considering total hip arthroplasty. The authors concluded that the prognosis of FAI largely depends on the status of the acetabular cartilage. Finally, Beck and colleagues reported excellent outcome among 13 out of 19 patients who had an open osteochondroplasty procedure after an average of 4.7 years. In summary, surgical dislocation of the hip seems to be an effective procedure for the treatment of FAI, and it is associated with clinical improvement for most patients.

To avoid the potential complications of surgical dislocation, Pierannunzii and d'Imporzano reported a modified anterior approach without surgical dislocation to address FAI. The authors proposed that this approach is advantageous because there is no risk of interference with the posterior blood supply. In addition, the approach provides direct exposure of the anterolateral head–neck junction. However, this approach relies on imaging for the evaluation of the acetabular cartilage, because it does not allow dislocation of the femoral head. The authors reported about 7 patients; all except 1, who had advanced arthritis, demonstrated significant clinical improvement.

An arthroscopic osteochondroplasty technique was proposed to avoid the potential complications involved with open surgical procedures and to expedite the recovery of the patients. Hip arthroscopy allows the surgeon to evaluate the labral and acetabular lesions with the use of a minimally invasive approach. The impingement can also be evaluated and addressed during the same procedure. However, the learning curve of the arthroscopic osteochondroplasty is steep, and the procedure usually takes longer than an open procedure. In addition, the evaluation of the adequacy of the resection is limited by the technique itself. Guanche and Bare reported about 10 patients who were treated with arthroscopic osteochondroplasty procedures with an average of 16 months of follow up. Eight patients without cartilage lesions did substantially better than the 2 patients who did have associated cartilage lesions.

## Preferred Surgical Technique

We prefer the surgical dislocation of the hip for cases that involve nonfocal impingement problems or severe deformities and for most cases that require acetabular rim trimming with labral repair. Specific examples include hips with nonfocal femoral head deformities or circumferential pincer impingement abnormalities. Alternatively, hip arthroscopy with limited open osteochondroplasty is an attractive treatment option for the management of cam-type impingement. Hip arthroscopy is performed first, and the surgeon evaluates and treats the intra-articular problems (e.g., labral tears, chondral flaps). If the surgeon chooses to proceed with osteochondroplasty, it is performed through a limited direct anterior approach. This approach eliminates the risk of interfering with the blood supply of the femoral head as well as the risk of trochanteric nonunion while allowing for the direct visualization of the anterolateral rim and the head–neck junction. The soft-tissue dissection is less than that required for a surgical dislocation, and the procedure does not require a trochanteric osteotomy.

## Anesthesia and Positioning of the Patient

We prefer general endotracheal anesthesia with muscle relaxation to help with the distraction of the joint. The patient is positioned supine on a fracture table with a hip arthroscopy traction attachment. The first stage of the operation is a hip arthroscopy to evaluate the severity of the disease and to address labral and articular cartilage lesions. The affected lower extremity and hip are maintained in a neutral position of flexion, extension, slight abduction (i.e., 5 degrees to 10 degrees), and neutral rotation. The contralateral extremity is placed in 40 degrees of abduction and 20 degrees of flexion. With the appropriate amount of countertraction on the contralateral extremity, the hip joint is distracted 8 mm to 10 mm with the use of the fracture table traction. The amount of distraction is monitored by fluoroscopy.

## Hip Arthroscopy

We make use of the anterior, anterolateral, and posterolateral portals for arthroscopic surveillance (Figure 29-1). These portals are established with fluoroscopic assistance by placing 4.0-mm, 4.5-mm, and 5.0-mm hip arthroscopy cannulas. The joint is systematically evaluated with 70-degree and 30-degree angled arthroscopes. The articular cartilage of the femoral head, the acetabulum, and the acetabular labrum are inspected. In patients with an anterior FAI complex, degenerative tears of the anterior and acetabular labrum are common. These lesions are frequently associated with the delamination of the adjacent articular cartilage at the transition zone, and they are addressed with the appropriate arthroscopic technique. After the joint is inspected, the final arthroscopic plan is developed.

## Limited Open Osteochondroplasty

During the second part of the procedure, the patient remains in the same position. After the traction is released, the central post is removed. An anterior longitudinal incision of 8 cm to 10 cm is made starting just distal and lateral (2 cm to 3 cm) to the anterosuperior iliac spine (see Figure 29-1). The dissection is extended laterally in the subcutaneous tissue to dissect directly onto the fascia of the tensor fascia lata muscle. The fascia is incised, the muscle belly is retracted laterally, and the fascia is retracted medially (Figure 29-2). This medial sleeve of tissue contains the lateral femoral cutaneous nerve, which should be protected by placing the fascial incision lateral to the tensor sartorius interval. The interval between the tensor and the sartorius is then developed, and the origin of the rectus femoris is identified (Figure 29-3). Next, the direct and reflected heads of the rectus femoris are released. The rectus is reflected distally, and the adipose tissue and the iliocapsularis muscle fibers are dissected off of the anterior hip capsule (Figure 29-4). Alternatively, the direct head of the rectus may remain intact and be retracted medially. An "I"-shaped capsulotomy is then performed to provide adequate exposure of the anterolateral head–neck junction (Figure 29-5). Most commonly, an outgrowth of osteochondral tissue is observed along the anterolateral head–neck junction (Figure 29-6). The offset from the femoral head to the neck in this region is deficient. The normal head–neck offset anteromedially serves as a reference point for the resection of the abnormal osteochondral lesion. In addition, we almost always observe a marked delineation between the normal articular cartilage

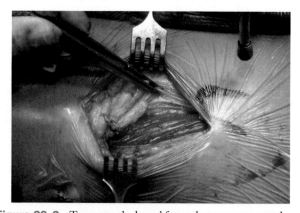

**Figure 29–2**  To protect the lateral femoral cutaneous nerve, the tensor fascia lata sheath is incised, and the muscle belly is retracted laterally. The soft-tissue sleeve with the lateral femoral cutaneous nerve is reflected medially.

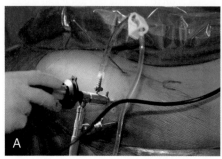

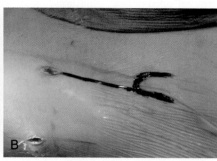

**Figure 29–1**  **A,** Hip arthroscopy is performed with the patient in the supine position through the anterior, anterolateral, and posterolateral portals. **B,** A 10-cm longitudinal incision is made just distal to the anterosuperior iliac spine. The anterior incision can also be made 2 cm to 3 cm farther lateral to minimize the risk to the lateral femoral cutaneous nerve.

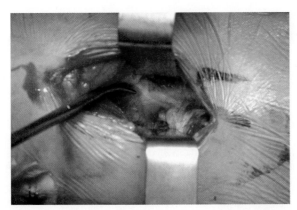

**Figure 29–3**    The rectus femoris tendon, which lies just above the anterior hip capsule, is exposed.

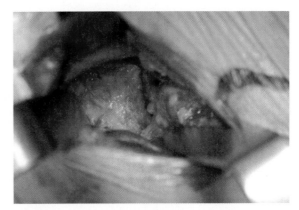

**Figure 29–4**    The rectus femoris tendon is released from its insertion into the anteroinferior iliac spine, which exposes the anterior hip capsule. Alternatively, the tendon can be reflected medially without release.

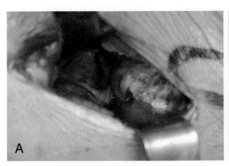

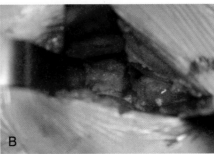

**Figure 29–5**    An "I"-shaped arthrotomy is performed, and the femoral head is exposed. **A,** Anterior hip capsule is shown before and **B,** after capsulotomy.

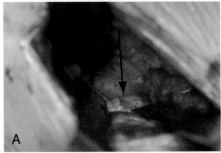

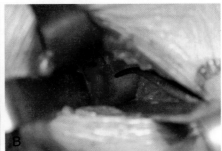

**Figure 29–6**    **A,** This limited anterior approach allows the surgeon to evaluate the deformity at the head–neck junction (*arrow*) and **B,** acetabulum.

of the femoral head and the impinging rim (see Figure 29-6). A ½-inch curved osteotome is used to perform an osteoplasty at the head–neck junction. The osteotome is directed distally and posteriorly to perform a beveled resection to prevent the delamination of the retained femoral head articular cartilage (Figure 29-7). After the osteoplasty is performed and the head–neck offset is re-established, the accuracy of the surgical resection is confirmed with intraoperative fluoroscopy. The Dunn view or the frog-leg lateral view is effective for visualizing the anterolateral head–neck junction and for assessing the reconstruction. The hip can also be examined at this time to assess impingement during hip flexion and during combined flexion and internal rotation; this is performed while palpating the anterior hip to test for residual impingement. If the anterior acetabular rim was overgrown as a result of labral calcification or osteophyte formation, this is carefully debrided until adequate clearance is achieved. Hip motion should improve at least 5 degrees to

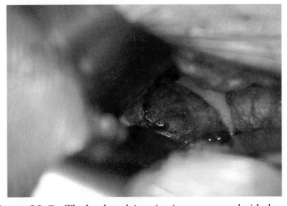

**Figure 29–7**    The head–neck junction is reconstructed with the use of direct visualization.

15 degrees in flexion and 5 degrees to 20 degrees in internal rotation. The goal of the osteoplasty is to remove all prominent anterolateral osteochondral tissue that contributes to an aspheric shape of the femoral head (Figure 29-8). Bleeding from the surface of the osteoplasty is controlled with bone wax. The joint is irrigated, and the longitudinal and superior transverse arms of the arthrotomy are closed with absorbable sutures. The direct and reflected heads of the rectus tendon, if released, are repaired with nonabsorbable suture, and the remainder of the wound is closed in a standard fashion.

### Labral Debridement or Repair

- Labral repair is considered when the tear is located at the capsular side, where there is increased vascularity and potential for healing.
- It is extremely important to be technically conservative with the partial labral resection.
- Unstable intra-articular flaps of the labrum should be removed.
- The stable capsular labral remnant should be preserved, when possible.
- Full-thickness resection of the labrum should be avoided.

### Articular Cartilage

- Articular cartilage delamination along the anterior and superolateral acetabular rim is common.
- Articular flaps should be debrided back to stable articular cartilage.
- Microfracture of acetabular rim disease can be performed for full-thickness defects.

### Limited Open Osteochondroplasty

- Wide exposure of the femoral head–neck junction should be obtained to safely and precisely perform the osteochondroplasty.
- Exposure can be enhanced with the release of the rectus tendon, if needed, and an "I"-shaped arthrotomy can be used to enable wide access to the anterolateral head–neck junction.
- A combination of ¼-inch and ½-inch angled and curved osteotomes facilitates the osteochondroplasty with the use of this surgical approach. A power burr may also be used.
- The dynamic examination of the hip and palpation through the arthrotomy ensures complete decompression of the impinging structures.
- Fluoroscopic examination of the hip after osteochondroplasty assists with the judging of the adequacy of the femoral head–neck junction recontouring.

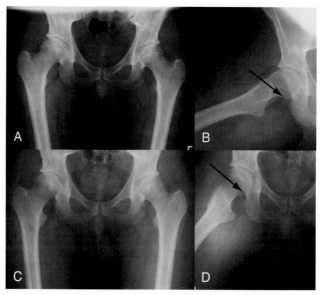

**Figure 29–8**  Preoperative AP pelvis **A,** and frog-leg lateral **B,** x-rays of a patient with cam-type impingement. The frog-leg lateral view demonstrates the deformity of the head–neck junction (*arrow*). The postoperative AP pelvis **C,** and frog-leg lateral **D,** x-rays demonstrate that all of the bony deformity was removed and that the head–neck offset was re-established (*arrow*).

## POSTOPERATIVE REHABILITATION

Patients are observed overnight in the hospital. A pillow is placed under the thigh to maintain hip flexion, thereby decreasing the stresses placed over the rectus repair. Active hip flexion exercises are also prohibited for the first 6 weeks. Abductor strengthening is instituted immediately and continued with a home exercise program. We currently have the patients bear 50% weight during the first 4 weeks, which is followed by gradual weight bearing as tolerated. Nevertheless, it is recommended that these patients avoid contact sports and impact activities (e.g., running) for at least 4 months to minimize the risk of pathologic femoral neck fracture. Enteric-coated aspirin (325 mg) is taken as thromboembolic prophylaxis, and sustained-release indomethacin (75 mg) is used for heterotrophic ossification prophylaxis. Both of these medications are taken for 6 weeks.

**Table 29–1**  RESULTS SUMMARY

| Author | Technique | No. of Patients | Mean Length of Follow Up (Range) | Results |
|---|---|---|---|---|
| Murphy et al., 2004 | Open osteochondroplasty | 23 | 62 months (24 to 144 months) | AVN rate, 0%; 15 patients improved, and 7 patients later required THA |
| Spencer et al., 2006 | Open osteochondroplasty with or without PFO | 19 | 12 months (4 to 25 months) | Osteochondroplasty: 7 patients improved, 4 were unchanged, and 2 worsened Osteochondroplasty with PFO: 5 out of 6 patients improved |
| Peters et al., 2006 | Open osteochondroplasty | 29 | 32 months | HHS improved from 70 to 87; 8 patients had progressive arthritis, and 3 patients later required THA |
| Beck et al., 2004 | Open osteochondroplasty | 19 | 56 months (48 to 62 months) | AVN rate, 0%; 13 patients improved, and 5 patients later required THA |
| Pierannunzii et al., 2007 | Open osteochondroplasty | 8 | 10 months (3 to 12 months) | HHS improved from 74.4 to 85.3 |
| Guanche et al., 2006 | Arthroscopic osteochondroplasty | 10 | 16 months (9 to 24 months) | McCarthy score improved from 75 to 95 |

*AVN,* Avascular necrosis; *THA,* total hip arthroplasty; *PFO,* proximal femoral osteotomy; *HHS,* Harris Hip Score.

## RESULTS AND OUTCOMES

The results of these procedures are summarized in Table 29-1, but highlights include the following:

- The documentation of clinical outcomes for the surgical treatment of hip impingement disease is limited.
- Early to mid-term results are now available for treament with surgical dislocation of the hip; these results are encouraging for most patients.
- Our experiences with hip arthroscopy and with combined limited open osteochondroplasty have been encouraging. An analysis of our first 36 consecutive cases demonstrated that 29 of the 36 hips had good or excellent clinical results at a mean of 24 months of follow up.

## COMPLICATIONS

- Neurovascular injury
- Deep venous thrombosis
- Heterotopic ossification
- Femoral neck fracture
- Infection
- Articular cartilage scuffing
- Arthroscopic instrument breakage

## ANNOTATED REFERENCES AND SUGGESTED READINGS

Beaule PE, Allen DJ, Clohisy JC, Schoenecker P, Leunig M. The young adult with hip impingement: deciding on the optimal intervention. *J Bone Joint Surg Am.* 2009;91(1):210–221.

Beck M, Leunig M, Parvizi J, Boutier V, Wyss D, Ganz R. Anterior femoroacetabular impingement: part II. Midterm results of surgical treatment. *Clin Orthop Relat Res.* 2004;(418):67–73.

Byrd JW. Hip arthroscopy. *J Am Acad Orthop Surg.* 2006; 14(7):433–444.

This article reviews the indications and the hip arthroscopy surgical technique used to treat various intra-articular hip pathologies.

Clohisy JC, McClure JT. Treatment of anterior femoroacetabular impingement with combined hip arthroscopy and limited anterior decompression. *Iowa Orthop J.* 2005;25:164–171.

This article reviews the general characteristics of FAI. In addition, it provides a detailed description of the limited open osteoplasty technique.

Ganz R, Parvizi J, Beck M, Leunig M, Nötzli H, Siebenrock KA. Femoroacetabular impingement: a cause for osteoarthritis of the hip. *Clin Orthop Relat Res.* 2003;(417):112–120.

This article reviews the pathomechanism of the development of osteoarthritis as a result of FAI. The authors propose that surgical treatment may decelerate the development of secondary arthritic changes by alleviating the femoral abutment against the acetabular rim.

Guanche CA, Bare AA. Arthroscopic treatment of femoroacetabular impingement. *Arthroscopy.* 2006;22(1):95–106.

Murphy S, Tannast M, Kim YJ, et al. Debridement of the adult hip for femoroacetabular impingement: indications and preliminary clinical results. *Clin Orthop.* 2004;429:178–181.

Peters CL, Erickson JA. Treatment of femoro-acetabular impingement with surgical dislocation and debridement in young adults. *J Bone Joint Surg Am.* 2006;88:1735–1741.

Philippon MJ, Maxwell RB, Johnston TL, Schenker M, Briggs KK. Clinical presentation of femoroacetabular impingement. *Knee Surg Sports Traumatol Arthrosc.* 2007;15(8):1041–1047.

The authors report the common symptoms and physical examination findings of 301 patients who had surgical treatment for the treatment of FAI.

Philippon MJ, Stubbs AJ, Schenker ML, Maxwell RB, Ganz R, Leunig M. Arthroscopic management of femoroacetabular impingement: osteoplasty technique and literature review. *Am J Sports Med.* 2007;35(9):1571–1580.

This article provides a review of certain aspects of FAI as well as arthroscopic osteoplasty and rim-trimming techniques that are used to address cam- and pincer-type impingement, respectively.

Pierannunzii L, d'Imporzano M. Treatment of femoroacetabular impingement: a modified resection osteoplasty technique through an anterior approach. *Orthopedics.* 2007;30(2): 96–102.

The authors describe a new approach to the treatment of FAI that involves an anterior approach without dislocation of the hip. They report favorable outcomes for 8 patients who had osteochondroplasty with the use of this technique.

Spencer S, Millis MB, Kim YJ. Early results of treatment of hip impingement syndrome in slipped capital femoral epiphysis and pistol grip deformity of the femoral head-neck junction using the surgical dislocation technique. *J Pediatr Orthop* 2006;26(3):281–285.

Tannast M, Siebenrock KA, Anderson SE. Femoroacetabular impingement: radiographic diagnosis—what the radiologist should know. *AJR Am J Roentgenol.* 2007;188(6):1540–1552.

This article reviews the radiographic criteria that are used to diagnose FAI as well as the potential pitfalls of pelvic imaging.

Tanzer M, Noiseux N. Osseous abnormalities and early osteoarthritis: the role of hip impingement. *Clin Orthop Relat Res.* 2004;(429):170–177.

This article combines the results of three different studies that demonstrated that the anterior femoral head offset deficiency is a common cause of various hip disorders, including labral tears, FAI, and idiopathic hip osteoarthritis.

# CHAPTER 30

# Nonvascularized Bone Grafting for the Treatment of Osteonecrosis of the Femoral Head

*Ronald E. Delanois, Mike S. McGrath, Lorenzo Childress,*
*Mario Quesada, David R. Marker, and Michael A. Mont*

## INTRODUCTION

Osteonecrosis of the femoral head, which is also known as *avascular necrosis*, describes the clinical picture that is observed after the death of bone marrow and osteocytes. Resorption of the dead bone marrow and subchondral tissue leads to the generation of weaker tissue. The newly formed bone is prone to both fracture and collapse, and this may cause pain and decreased function of the hip joint. Without intervention, the disease process usually leads to articular cartilage destruction and resulting osteoarthritis. Osteonecrosis is most often seen in individuals who are 40 years old or younger, with approximately 10,000 to 20,000 new cases identified in the United States each year.

Trauma is the most common cause of osteonecrosis, but it can also be classified as atraumatic, in which the cause is not well defined. Traumatic osteonecrosis is seen when the blood supply of the femoral head and neck is disrupted as a result of trauma to the joint. This may occur after femoral head and neck fracture, hip dislocation, or both. Some atraumatic conditions (e.g., Caisson disease, sickle cell disease, myeloproliferative diseases, coagulation disorders) may directly cause osteonecrosis via the impairment of blood supply to the bone. However, most cases of atraumatic osteonecrosis have unknown causes, although they have numerous associated risk factors, including corticosteroid use, alcohol abuse, smoking, systemic lupus erythematosus, chronic renal disease, inflammatory bowel disease, human immunodeficiency virus infection, and hypertension. Some individuals may also have a genetic predisposition for osteonecrosis.

Various treatment methods have been used in an attempt to alleviate the symptoms or to slow the progression of the disease, including nonoperative (e.g., limited weight bearing, medication) and operative modalities (e.g., core decompression, bone grafting, osteotomies, hip arthroplasty). Nonvascularized bone grafting is a surgical technique that attempts to remove necrotic bone, to increase the amount of viable bone present in the femoral head for remodeling, and to provide support to decrease damage to the articular cartilage. In this chapter, we will describe the basic science of osteonecrosis as well as the indications, diagnostic methods, surgical techniques, rehabilitation, results, and complications of nonvascularized bone grafting for the treatment of osteonecrosis of the femoral head.

## BASIC SCIENCE

In patients with traumatic osteonecrosis, the initial insult is a decrease in the blood supply that is caused by the disruption of the blood vessel. Bone marrow death follows within 12 hours of vascular compromise. The event that precipitates atraumatic osteonecrosis is less well defined, in part because of the lack of knowledge of the causes of this disease. Some causes are believed to incorporate the combined effects of metabolic factors, mechanical stresses, local factors that affect blood supply, and increased intraosseous pressure. Corticosteroid use and excessive alcohol intake are associated with the majority of cases.

The pathologic disease course that occurs after the initial insult is similar for both traumatic and atraumatic osteonecrosis. Reperfusion initiates a cascade of local metabolic factors that cause demineralization and trabecular thinning. Despite attempts to replace dead bone and repair weak bone, subchondral fractures occur. The resulting lack of mechanical support for the articular cartilage leads to altered joint mechanics and the degeneration of the hip joint.

## INDICATIONS

As with other treatment modalities, the successful employment of bone grafting is most dependent on the stage of the disease. Several classification systems, including the Ficat and Steinberg systems, have been used to define various stages of tissue involvement, as shown in Table 30-1. The goal of bone grafting is to preserve the structure of the bone and the articular cartilage, so the procedure is most useful during precollapse stages (Ficat and Steinberg stages I and II), especially when less than 30% of the femoral head is involved. Bone grafting may also be used for a limited number of patients who have smaller Ficat stage III lesions if the articular cartilage is mostly intact.

## HISTORY AND PHYSICAL EXAMINATION

Patients who have osteonecrosis of the femoral head often present in a similar manner to patients who have other hip diseases (e.g., osteoarthritis), except that patients with osteonecrosis are frequently 40 years old or younger. The most common symptom of osteonecrosis is groin pain, which often occurs

**Table 30–1** DESCRIPTIONS OF THE STAGES OF TWO WIDELY USED SYSTEMS FOR CLASSIFYING OSTEONECROSIS OF THE FEMORAL HEAD

| Stage | Ficat and Arlet | University of Pennsylvania* |
|---|---|---|
| 0 | No consistent findings on radiograph or bone scan. No symptoms. | No findings on radiographs, MRI, or bone scan. |
| I | No radiographic abnormality. Increased uptake on bone scan. | No radiographic abnormalities. Lesion present on MRI and/or bone scan. |
| II | Diffuse sclerosis and/or cystic lesions present on radiograph. | Diffuse sclerosis and/or lucent lesions present on radiograph. |
| III | Subchondral collapse (crescent sign present on radiograph, with or without femoral head flattening). | Subchondral collapse (crescent sign on radiograph without flattening of the femoral head). |
| IV | Femoral head flattening with acetabular involvement and joint destruction. | Flattening of the articular surface of the femoral head with a normal acetabulum. |
| V | N/A | Acetabular involvement (joint-line narrowing, sclerosis, lucencies, or osteophytes of the acetabulum). |
| VI | N/A | Advanced degeneration of the joint manifested by complete destruction of the joint line. |

*The University of Pennsylvania stages I–V are further subclassified into three grades: Grade A = mild, involving less than 15% of the femoral head. Grade B = moderate, involving 15 to 30% of the femoral head. Grade C = severe, involving greater than 30% of the femoral head. In Stage V, the grade is determined by averaging the extent of involvement of the femoral head and the acetabulum.

with weight bearing or other activity. Patients may describe the feeling of a groin pull (i.e., a sudden loss of hip stability) or groin fullness. Some patients who have an advanced stage of osteonecrosis may experience a sudden change in their ambulatory status. The physician should understand the risk factors for this disease. Patients may have a history of corticosteroid or alcohol use. Corticosteroid doses of more than 2 g of prednisone in 3 months or analogous doses of other steroids are generally associated with osteonecrosis. Alcohol exhibits a clear relationship with osteonecrosis, with higher doses of alcohol being associated with an increased risk of osteonecrosis. Other important risk factors include chronic conditions (e.g., systemic lupus erythematosus, renal disease) and immunocompromising conditions (e.g., human immunodeficiency virus, previous organ transplantation).

During the physical examination, pain is reproduced with passive as well as active internal rotation of the leg. The patient will point to the groin as the area of maximum pain, but he or she occasionally may point to the lateral trochanteric region, which may signify referred discomfort. Patients may be unable to fully bear weight on the affected extremity because of the pain. It is important to routinely perform a straight-leg raise and contralateral straight-leg raise to ensure that the cause of the pain is not the lumbar region.

## IMAGING AND DIAGNOSTIC STUDIES

When evaluating a patient who has hip pain, several imaging studies may facilitate the diagnosis of osteonecrosis, including plain radiographs, bone scans, and magnetic resonance imaging (MRI). Currently, the standard diagnostic studies include plain radiographs followed by MRI. Plain radiographs should include an anteroposterior pelvic view to include the contralateral hip as a comparison and a cross-table lateral view of the affected hip. The presence of sclerosis, cystic changes, a crescent sign, or collapse on the plain radiographs may indicate the presence of osteonecrosis. The MRI is the current gold standard for the diagnosis of osteonecrosis; it is considered to be 98% to 99% sensitive and specific for the condition, and it also allows for the quantification of the size of the necrotic segment on both the sagittal and coronal axes.

## SURGICAL TECHNIQUE

When performing a nonvascularized bone graft, the authors prefer to have the patient placed in the lateral decubitus position (Figures 30-1 through 30-6). The patient is secured to the operating table, pads and cushions are placed on the extremities, and the airway is controlled by the anesthesiologist. The direct lateral approach is the surgical approach of choice for the author, because the vasculature to the femoral head is more easily preserved. The posterior approach is also used, but greater care needs to be taken to avoid injury to the lateral epiphyseal vessel, which is the branch of the medial obturator vessel that supplies the femoral head. After the patient is appropriately positioned, prepared, and draped, an 8-cm to 14-cm incision is made overlying the center of the greater trochanter and brought proximally and distally. Sharp dissection is performed with the use of a No. 10 scalpel down to the level of the iliotibial band. The iliotibial band is then incised and retracted posteriorly and anteriorly. A blunt Hohmann retractor is placed posteriorly, again to avoid injury to the neurovascular structures located posterior to the greater trochanter. The bursa can be excised for the better

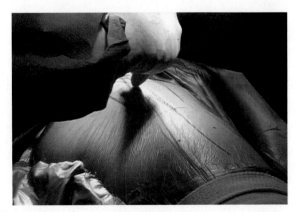

**Figure 30–1** The patient is in the direct lateral position, and the incision is centered over the trochanter.

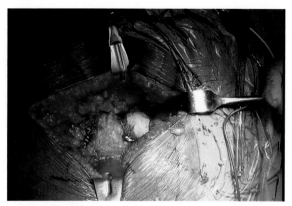

**Figure 30–2** At the completion of the bone grafting, the cortical window is replaced and fixed with the use of three bioabsorbable pins.

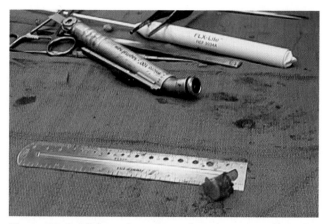

**Figure 30–5** A light can be used to evaluate the amount of bone that has been removed from the femoral head.

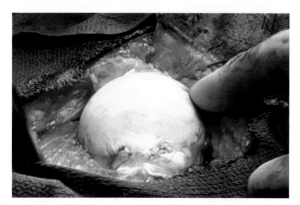

**Figure 30–3** With this approach, the femoral head does not need to be dislocated to allow for access to the anterior cortex or to preserve the posterior blood supply.

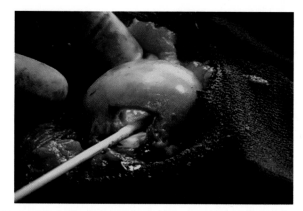

**Figure 30–6** Cortical cancellous chips are packed tightly into the femoral head.

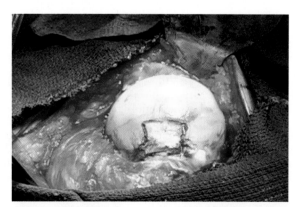

**Figure 30–4** The femoral head is delivered into the wound, thereby minimizing internal rotation and maximizing the protection of the posterior blood supply.

identification of the vastus ridge, the greater trochanter, and the insertion site of the gluteus medius muscle. With the use of an electrocautery device, the anterior 40% of the gluteus medius muscle is elevated from the anterior neck of the proximal femur in conjunction with the gluteus minimus muscle. The bursa between the iliopsoas muscle and the hip capsule is explored and retracted anteriorly with the use of a Cobb elevator; this allows for the preservation of the muscle and avoids injury to the neurovascular structures anteriorly. Care is taken to avoid the excessive stripping of the hip capsule. The gluteus medius and minimus tendons are taken proximally and held in place with the use of a Taylor retractor. Care is taken

to avoid injury to the neurovascular structures that innervate the gluteus medius and gluteus minimus tendons. Excessive dissection is not necessary posteriorly. If additional exposure is necessary, then a Cobb elevator is used to elevate some of the muscular attachments of the gluteus muscle onto the capsule. We prefer to place a Hohmann retractor anteriorly and a Taylor retractor superiorly, and this is followed by the use of a blunt Hohmann retractor posteriorly. These retractors allow for excellent exposure to the hip capsule. The hip capsule is incised from the femoral neck and extending to the acetabulum. It is important to avoid injury to the labrum of the acetabulum. The capsule incision is then extended from the base of the neck anteriorly and then posteriorly approximately 180 degrees around the circumference of the femoral neck. The posterior capsule is not violated. The capsule is also peeled off on the acetabular side approximately 180 degrees, thereby exposing the whole anterior lateral labrum. Next, the capsule incision is shaped like an "H," which allows for the visualization of the neck–cartilage junction. The anterior neck is outlined with the use of a surgical marker. A 1.5-cm by 1.5-cm square area of bone is identified. The surgeon should take great care to avoid extending this window too far medially and thus compromising the neurovascular structures or too far laterally and thus creating a potential stress riser for a femoral neck fracture. An oscillating saw is used to remove the area of bone. The authors prefer to bevel the bony cuts to allow for the replacement of the bony window after the bone grafting procedure is completed. A high-speed burr is used to remove all of the necrotic bone from the femoral head. This procedure can successfully be performed without dislocation, but if dislocation is necessary, then we recommend partial dislocation to obtain better visualization of the femoral head. A full dislocation increases the risk of complete femoral head death. After the necrotic segment within the femoral head is removed, a light is placed into the femoral head to ensure that the entire necrotic segment has been removed, and the remaining bone is observed to ensure that bleeding is still present. The authors prefer to use fresh-frozen bone graft that has been milled and then mixed with bone morphogenic protein to maintain the osteoinductive and conductive properties of the bone. Autograft is also used, when available. The autograft can be harvested from small cores within the greater trochanter or from a secondary incision along the iliac crest. The femoral head is packed tightly with the substrate. If a large volume of the head has been denuded of bone, then small cortical strips can be added to the substrate to provide structural integrity. The cortical window is then placed back onto the femoral neck and fixed with the use of three resorbable pins.

Closure is accomplished in the following manner. The capsule is reduced to its normal anatomic position and held in place with the use of bioabsorbable suture. The gluteus minimus tendon is separated from the gluteus medius tendon. The authors prefer to use No. 5 nonabsorbable polyester sutures to secure both the gluteus minimus and gluteus medius tendons back to bony tunnels onto the greater trochanter; this promotes tendon–bone healing, and the authors believe that this helps to reduce the incidence of postoperative limp. A drain is then placed deep into the wound, and closure is continued. The iliotibial band and the subcutaneous tissue are reapproximated, and the skin is often closed with staples. A sterile dressing is applied, and an abduction pillow is placed between the patient's legs.

## TECHNICAL PEARLS

- We recommend the anterolateral approach as compared with the posterior approach. Most osteonecrotic lesions are located in the anterosuperior region of the femoral head, and access is easiest from the anterolateral approach. This approach also increases the femoral head blood supply.
- When performing the trapdoor procedure, great care needs to be taken to avoid extension through the articular cartilage.
- The window should not exceed 2 cm in length or 2 cm in width.
- When creating the window, the cuts should be beveled inward so that, when the window is placed back in its normal position, it will not collapse into the femoral head.
- Postoperatively, patients should remain less than 20% weight bearing with two crutches or a walker for a minimum of 6 weeks. Patients are then advanced to 50% weight bearing with a cane at 6 weeks and to 100% weight bearing at 10 to 12 weeks.

## POSTOPERATIVE REHABILITATION

Patients who have undergone nonvascularized bone grafting procedures usually remain nonambulatory for 6 weeks. The authors recommend a maximum of 20% weight bearing with two crutches or a walker during this period. Patients are allowed to perform gentle range-of-motion exercises, but they are instructed to avoid excessive abduction in an attempt to protect the gluteus medius and gluteus minimus muscle repair. They are also encouraged to avoid hip flexion beyond 90 degrees, excessive hip rotation, and adduction to reduce the risk of dislocation. After 6 weeks, radiographs are obtained to confirm the lack of progression of osteonecrosis and the beginning of cortical remodeling. If adequate remodeling is present, then weight bearing is increased to 50% with a cane, abductor

strengthening exercises can begin, and gait training is encouraged. Radiographs are obtained 3 months, 6 months, and then yearly after the procedure. If adequate remodeling has occurred at 3 months, patients are advanced to full weight-bearing status. Strenuous activity is not allowed for a minimum of 6 months.

## RESULTS AND OUTCOMES

Multiple published studies have indicated the success of nonvascularized bone grafting procedures for the treatment of early-stage osteonecrosis. Ko and colleagues reported about the use of the "trapdoor" bone-grafting procedure in addition to a femoral or acetabular osteotomy to treat 9 teenagers (10 hips) who had severe osteonecrosis and articular surface collapse. Cancellous bone grafting was used to pack the femoral head. At an average follow up of 53 months (range, 2 to 9 years), 7 patients (8 hips) had good clinical results, and 2 patients (2 hips) had fair clinical results. Six hips were rated as good radiographically, 3 hips were rated as fair, and 1 hip was rated as poor.

Rosenwasser and colleagues examined the use of the "lightbulb" bone-grafting approach to treat 13 patients (15 hips) who had a mean age of 34 years and who had Ficat stage I, II, or III osteonecrosis of the femoral head. At a mean follow up of 12 years (range, 10 to 15 years), 11 patients (87%) remained pain free, with minimal progression of osteoarthritis. No fractures, infections, or thromboembolic events were reported.

Mont and colleagues reported about 30 trapdoor procedures that were performed on 23 patients who had Ficat stage III or early stage IV osteonecrosis of the femoral head. The mean Harris Hip Score improved from 41 points (range, 31 to 64 points) preoperatively to 92 points (range, 80 to 100 points) at the final follow up. In 2003, Mont and colleagues reported about the use of the lightbulb procedure to treat 19 patients (21 hips) who had Ficat and Arlet stage II or stage IIII osteonecrosis of the femoral head. The mean Harris Hip Score improved from 48 points (range, 25 to 62 points) preoperatively to 91 points (range, 80 to 100 points) at the final follow up.

Seyler and colleagues provided a retrospective study of 33 patients (39 hips) who had Ficat stage II or III lesions and who were treated with trapdoor procedures. At a mean follow up of 36 months (range, 24 to 50 months), 24 of the 30 hips (80%) that had small and medium-sized lesions did not require further surgery. Eighteen out of 22 hips that had stage II disease did not require further surgery. It was also noted that lateral lesions fared poorly as compared with centrally located lesions.

In summary, the lightbulb and trapdoor techniques have demonstrated excellent results in several studies of patients who have Ficat stages II and III osteonecrosis of the femoral head with small to medium-sized lesions.

## COMPLICATIONS

Complications associated with nonvascularized bone grafting are similar to those described for core decompression. These include infection, continued pain, progression of collapse, and femoral head or neck fractures. The most common complication that has been reported in the literature is the progression of the osteonecrosis that ultimately results in a hip replacement. In one study, 2 out of 15 hips (13%) that were treated with cancellous bone grafting required total hip arthroplasties for disease progression at a mean follow up of 12 years (range, 10 to 15 years). Mont and colleagues reported a 14% rate of conversion to total hip arthroplasty at a shorter follow up of 48 months. There were no reported cases of femoral neck fractures. In our experience, there were no femoral neck fractures after nonvascularized bone-grafting procedures. Seyler and colleagues reported that the size of the lesion plays a role in the need for a subsequent hip replacement. Their study revealed 9 large lesions that required conversion to total hip arthroplasties. There have been no reported cases of venous thromboembolism after this procedure.

## ANNOTATED REFERENCES

**Aldridge 3rd JM, Urbaniak JR. Avascular necrosis of the femoral head: etiology, pathophysiology, classification, and current treatment guidelines. *Am J Orthop*. 2004;33:327–332.**

This is a review of osteonecrosis of the femoral head, which discusses mechanisms of development of the disease, staging, and recommendations for treatment.

**Ficat RP. Idiopathic bone necrosis of the femoral head. Early diagnosis and treatment. *J Bone Joint Surg Br*. 1985;67:3–9.**

This report discusses the creation and validation of the Ficat-Arlet system of staging of osteonecrosis of the femoral head, with outcomes of treatment classified by various stages.

**Hungerford DS, Jones LC. Asymptomatic osteonecrosis: should it be treated? *Clin Orthop Relat Res*. 2004;429:124–130.**

This is a review of asymptomatic osteonecrosis, which states that the disease often progresses to a symptomatic stage. The authors recommend observation for small lesions (which typically do not progress) and large lesions (for which core decompression is often ineffective), while core decompression and/or bone grafting is the recommended treatment for moderate lesions.

**Ko JY, Meyers MH, Wenger DR. "Trapdoor" procedure for osteonecrosis with segmental collapse of the femoral head in teenagers. *J Pediatr Orthop*. 1995;15:7–15.**

This report examined the use of nonvascularized bone grafting via the trapdoor technique in conjunction with a femoral and/or acetabular osteotomy for 9 teenaged patients (10 hips) and found that 8 of 10 hips had a good clinical result and 2 had a fair result at a mean follow-up time of 53 months.

**Mont MA, Einhorn TA, Sponseller PD, Hungerford DS. The trapdoor procedure using autogenous cortical and cancellous bone grafts for osteonecrosis of the femoral head. *J Bone Joint Surg Br*. 1998;80:56–62.**

This report examined the use of the trapdoor technique of nonvascularized bone grafting to treat 23 patients who had late-stage osteonecrosis of the femoral head. At a mean follow-up time of 56 months (range, 30 to 60 months), the success rate was 83% for stage III hips and 33% for stage IV hips. Small and medium-sized lesions had greater success than larger lesions.

**Mont MA, Etienne G, Ragland PS. Outcome of nonvascularized bone grafting for osteonecrosis of the femoral head. *Clin Orthop Relat Res*. 2003;417:84–92.**

This report examined the use of the lightbulb technique of nonvascularized bone grafting with bone morphogenetic protein to treat 19 patients (21 hips) who had osteonecrosis of the hip. At a mean follow-up time of 48 months (range, 36 to 55 months), 86% of the hips had good outcomes and required no further treatment.

**Mont MA, Hungerford DS. Non-traumatic avascular necrosis of the femoral head. *J Bone Joint Surg Am*. 1995;77:459–474.**

This is a review of atraumatic osteonecrosis of the femoral head from 1995, including prevalence, risk factors, evaluation, diagnosis, prognosis, and treatment.

**Mont MA, Jones LC, Hungerford DS. Nontraumatic osteonecrosis of the femoral head: ten years later. *J Bone Joint Surg Am*. 2006;88:1117–1132.**

This is a complete review of osteonecrosis of the femoral head from 2006, including prevalence, pathogenesis, risk factors, radiographic factors, evaluation of patients, staging systems, prognoses, treatment methods, outcomes, and recommendation.

**Mont MA, Ulrich SD, Seyler TM, Smith JM, Marker DR, McGrath MS, Hungerford DS, Jones LC. Bone scanning of limited value for diagnosis of symptomatic oligofocal and multifocal osteonecrosis. *J Rheumatol*. 2008;35(8):1629–1634.**

This report assessed 48 patients who had osteonecrosis of at least one joint, and compared the sensitivity and specificity of bone scintigraphy with MRI. It found that bone scanning only identified 56% of the lesions that were found on MRI.

**Petrigliano FA, Lieberman JR. Osteonecrosis of the hip: novel approaches to evaluation and treatment. *Clin Orthop Relat Res*. 2007;465:53–62.**

This is an overview of treatments for osteonecrosis of the hip, including pharmacologic, biophysical, bone grafting, total hip arthroplasty, and surface replacement. The report also includes a discussion of staging and prognosis of atraumatic osteonecrosis.

**Rosenwasser MP, Garino JP, Kiernan HA, Michelsen CB. Long term followup of thorough debridement and cancellous bone grafting of the femoral head for avascular necrosis. *Clin Orthop Relat Res*. 1994;306:17–27.**

This report examined the use of the lightbulb technique of nonvascularized bone grafting to treat 13 patients who had osteonecrosis of the femoral head. The procedure had an 87% success rate, with little or no progression of the disease, at a mean follow-up time of 12 years (range, 10–15 years).

**Seyler TM, Marker DR, Ulrich SD, Fatscher T, Mont MA. Nonvascularized bone grafting defers joint arthroplasty in hip osteonecrosis. *Clin Orthop Relat Res*. 2008;466(5):1125–1132.**

This report examined the use of the lightbulb technique of nonvascularized bone grafting with bone morphogenetic protein-7 to treat 33 patients (39 hips) who had osteonecrosis of the femoral head. At a mean follow-up time of 36 months (range, 24 to 50 months), 80% of small and medium-sized lesions were successful, while 22% of large lesions were successful. The authors also reviewed numerous previously published reports of nonvascularized bone grafting.

**Steinberg ME, Hayken GD, Steinberg DR. A quantitative system for staging avascular necrosis. *J Bone Joint Surg Br*. 1995;77:34–41.**

This report discusses the creation and validation of the University of Pennsylvania system of staging of osteonecrosis of the femoral head, with outcomes of treatment classified by various stages and lesion sizes.

# CHAPTER 31

# Vascularized Fibular Grafting for Osteonecrosis of the Femoral Head

*J. Mack Aldridge, III, and James R. Urbaniak*

## INTRODUCTION

The first documented report of osteonecrosis of the femoral head (ONFH) appeared more than a century ago, yet, since then, few definitive conclusions have been reached regarding its causes or treatment. Approximately 20,000 new cases are diagnosed each year, and ONFH accounts for 5% to 12% of total hip replacements performed in the United States annually. The natural history of ONFH is subchondral collapse with a squaring of the femoral head that leads to hip degeneration. Because of this natural history and the fact that ONFH has a proclivity to manifest in younger patients, most surgeons have traditionally believed that procedures aimed at preserving the native hip are preferable to joint replacement.

Conceptually, the ideal procedure would remove the necrotic bone within the femoral head and replace this void with healthy bone that is replete with a nascent vascular source to improve the likelihood of restoring a vital subchondral plate. Such a procedure would relieve the patient's pain, preserve or restore the sphericity of the femoral head, and ultimately prevent the deterioration of the hip. Fulfilling these criteria would likely prevent the need for a second surgery (i.e., arthroplasty); this is an important objective, particularly for younger patients. We feel that the free vascularized fibular graft more closely addresses these objectives as compared with any other biologic-preserving procedure currently available; it is our preferred method for the treatment of ONFH. We have outlined our indications, contraindications, results, and surgical technique, and we have highlighted some of the critical steps that we feel are paramount to obtaining successful results with this procedure.

## BASIC SCIENCE

There are more than 100 conditions or factors that are known to activate intravascular coagulation and to potentially cause osteonecrosis. A growing body of evidence supports the theory that ONFH in adults and Legg-Calvé-Perthes disease in childhood is related to an underlying thrombophilia or hypofibrinolysis. A recent study reported that 136 of 206 patients (66%) with osteonecrosis revealed abnormal clotting values of the tested factors. In a follow up study of patients with ONFH, activated protein C resistance was the most frequent abnormality found, with a 50% prevalence. Lipoprotein A is also thought to play a role in the development of osteonecrosis, with a reported prevalence of 32% in one study of 124 subjects with ONFH.

Aberrant microvascular anatomy has also been implicated in the development of ONFH. With the use of digital subtraction angiography, one study showed that 94% of 99 hips with osteonecrosis demonstrated abnormal hip vasculature as compared with 31% (5 out of 16) abnormal findings in the control group. Regardless of the cause, we know that the eventual pathway ends with bone death that results from inadequate perfusion.

Despite this wealth of associated conditions and known risk factors, no one factor has proven to have a direct causative effect. In fact, the ultimate development of ONFH is more likely the unfortunate nexus of multiple risk factors that individually fall short of causing osteonecrosis but that collectively tip the scales toward an intraosseous ischemic event.

We have studied the efficacy, both clinically and in the laboratory, of the free vascularized fibular graft (FVFG) for the treatment of ONFH. With the use of a canine model in which ONFH was induced with cryotherapy, we implanted into the canine femoral head core either nonvascularized bone grafts, pedicled muscular flaps, or vascularized bone grafts. The necropsy femoral head analysis at 1 year demonstrated statistically significant increased trabecular thickness only in the vascularized bone grafts.

## INDICATIONS

- Patients 40 to 50 years old with 40% or less femoral head involvement and no femoral head flattening or articular step off; must have a preserved joint space and a center-edge angle of 35 degrees or more
- Patients less than 40 years old with less than 50% femoral head involvement and 1 mm to 2 mm of articular step off; must have preserved joint space
- Patients less than 30 years old with any amount of femoral head involvement and any degree of subchondral collapse but with preserved joint space
- Pediatric patients (18 years old or younger) with any amount of femoral head involvement and any degree of subchondral collapse with mild joint space narrowing

For all patients, as adjuncts to this list of objective criteria, we include the patient's "hip health," which is determined by the degree of limp, the limitation of motion, and the degree and frequency of pain. For example, if we are equivocal about the benefit of the FVFG for a certain patient on the basis of radiographic analysis alone but discover that the patient has only mild groin pain and nearly full or full range of hip motion, we are inclined to offer the procedure. Conversely, if this same patient reports severe hip pain with limited hip motion and a severely antalgic gait, we are more likely to recommend arthroplasty for that hip.

In our hands, core decompression alone is effective only for patients who are less than 50 years old with a stage I or stage II central lesion of dense bone (not cystic) that involves less than 20% of the femoral head. If the procedure is performed for conditions outside of these parameters, we believe that core decompression may exacerbate the already compromised vascular status of the femoral head and ultimately hasten the progression of the condition and the subchondral collapse.

## CONTRAINDICATIONS

- Age of more than 50 years (although age is not an absolute contraindication, we do consider more heavily the relative merits of total hip arthroplasty for patients who are more than 50 years old)
- Unwillingness of patient to participate in lengthy rehabilitation period with restricted weight-bearing status for 3 to 6 months
- Sickle cell disease

## BRIEF HISTORY AND PHYSICAL EXAMINATION

Our examination of the patient begins with a gait analysis, and we note any limp, Trendelenburg lurch, or other abnormality. A complete neurovascular examination of the operative leg is performed. The absence of either palpable or biphasic Dopplerable pulses is investigated further with an arteriogram; however, we have only needed to obtain this study 5 times for more than 3000 cases.

Next, we examine the range of hip motion in flexion, extension, internal rotation, external rotation, abduction, and adduction. The degree of pain throughout the arc of motion is noted, and the strength of the hip musculature (i.e., the flexors and abductors) is documented in accordance with the British Medical Research Council grading system.

## IMAGING AND DIAGNOSTIC STUDIES

We use plain radiographs and a noncontrast magnetic resonance imaging study to make the diagnosis. We request an anteroposterior pelvic view and bilateral frog-leg lateral radiographs to evaluate the femoral head shape, the presence of a crescent sign, the joint space, and the degree of femoral head coverage. We rely heavily on the serpiginous border between viable and nonviable bone, which is best seen on T1 coronal magnetic resonance images, to make the definitive diagnosis of ONFH. Magnetic resonance imaging is further helpful for quantifying the necrotic bone. We have found neither nuclear medicine studies nor computed tomography scans to be helpful for making the diagnosis. However, we have on rare occasions made use of computed tomography scans postoperatively to evaluate for either subtrochanteric stress fractures or subchondral fractures in patients with otherwise unexplainable increases in hip pain. Nucleotide body scans are helpful if osteonecrosis is suspected in other joints (i.e., multiple sites).

## SURGICAL TECHNIQUE

### Overview

The procedure is performed with the patient under general anesthesia and with the adjunct of an epidural block, which remains in place for 24 to 48 hours postoperatively. The patient is placed in

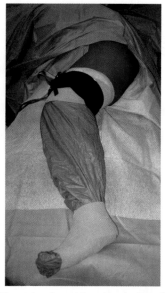

**Figure 31–1** The patient is positioned in the lateral decubitus position, and the entire lower extremity is prepared above the anterosuperior iliac spine. An impervious stocking is placed on the leg, and a tourniquet is placed over that for use during the fibular harvest. Care is taken to ensure that the tourniquet is above the superior pole of the patella to prevent peroneal nerve compression.

the lateral decubitus position and supported by a pegboard. The entire lower extremity to the level of the iliac crest proximally is prepared and draped. The leg is covered with an impervious stocking up to the mid thigh, over which a sterile tourniquet is placed just proximal to the knee; this is to be used during the fibular graft harvest (Figure 31-1). A Betadine-impregnated occlusive drape is used for both the hip and the leg. The operative procedure on the hip and the harvest of the fibular graft occur contemporaneously and, as such, require cooperation between the surgeons.

### Fibular Graft Harvest

With the use of tourniquet control, a straight, lateral, 15-cm longitudinal incision is made coincident with the natural sulcus between the lateral and posterior compartments of the leg. The incision is begun at least 10 cm distal to the fibular head, and it ends at least 10 cm proximal to the lateral malleolus. The peroneal muscles are reflected in an extraperiosteal fashion off of the lateral aspect of the fibula, working from posterior to anterior and stopping when the anterior intermuscular septum is visualized (Figure 31-2).

The anterior intermuscular septum is then divided to expose the anterior musculature, which is reflected bluntly off of the fibula. At this point, the interosseous membrane is easily visualized, and the adjacent anterior musculature, with its accompanying deep peroneal nerve and anterior tibial artery, is gently swept off of the interosseous membrane and away from the fibula. With the use of a specially designed right-angle beaver blade, the interosseous membrane is divided close to its fibular attachment along the entire length of the proposed fibular graft. The posterior intermuscular septum is then divided to expose the posterior muscles: the soleus proximally and the flexor hallucis longus distally.

### Fibular Osteotomy

Directly beneath the distal aspect of the flexor hallucis longus muscle, the distal pedicle of the peroneal vessels is identified, and malleable retractors are passed between this pedicle

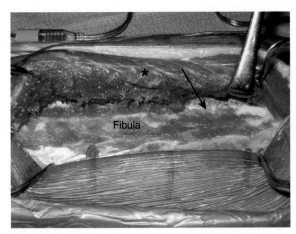

**Figure 31-2** A view of the lateral fibula, with the lateral compartment (*) reflected anteriorly. The arrow points to the anterior compartment fascia. This is divided, and then the anterior compartment is reflected to expose the underlying interosseous membrane.

and the fibula. Diligent care is critical during the placement of the retractors to ensure the protection of the pedicle during the osteotomy. After reconfirming that the planned osteotomy is at least 10 cm proximal to the distal tip of the fibula, an oscillating saw is used to cut the fibula. Irrigation during the osteotomy is vital to prevent thermal osteonecrosis. Next, the proximal pedicle is identified deep to the soleus muscle along the posterior aspect of the fibula (Figure 31-3). It is protected, and the proximal fibular osteotomy is performed in a manner similar to that of the distal osteotomy. The fibular cuts are made 15 cm apart to ensure an adequate pedicle length. It is important when performing the proximal osteotomy to identify and protect the superficial peroneal nerve, which is exposed proximally on the deep surface of the peroneus longus muscle.

After the proximal and distal fibular osteotomies are performed, a bone clamp is placed around the fibula to allow for better control and easier rotation during the delicate pedicle dissection. Starting distally, the peroneal vessels are again identified, isolated, and divided with the use of hemostatic clips. The now-free distal pedicle is attached to the distal aspect of the fibula with a hemoclip to ensure that the peroneal vessels and any nutrient branches to the bone are not avulsed from the fibula during the remainder of the harvest. The fibula and the adjoining peroneal vessels are then dissected from the surrounding

flexor hallucis longus, posterior tibialis, and soleus muscles. The fibula is elevated until it is tethered only by the proximal vascular pedicle. The tibial nerve can often be seen coursing in close proximity to the peroneal vessels at this level and should be carefully dissected away. After adequate pedicle length is established, the vessels are ligated with two large hemostatic clips and divided with scissors, and the graft is passed to a back table. The tourniquet is then deflated, the wound is copiously irrigated, and any bleeding is addressed. The leg wound is closed a short time later during the vascular anastomosis at the hip. The deep fascial layers of the leg are not closed in an effort to prevent compartment syndrome. The subcutaneous layer and the skin are closed over a drain, and the leg is wrapped in a soft, bulky dressing.

## Preparation of the Fibular Graft

On a back table, the artery and the two veins of the fibular pedicle are delineated from one another and separated with the use of microscissors and jewelers' forceps. All three vessels are then irrigated with a heparin-impregnated lactated Ringer's solution and visually inspected for any major leaks. Neither vein will fill over the entire length of the graft because of the valves, but the artery should insufflate throughout its entire course during the injection of the heparin solution. Some oozing from the attached muscle and the periosteum is anticipated and considered normal; however, we consider any leaks from the main vessels that form a stream to be major and worthy of repair with either 8-0 suture or micro hemostatic clips. Such attention to detail is imperative to minimize the risk of the patient's developing a vascular steal and thus to ensure adequate endosteal blood flow after the anastomosis. The vein with the better size match is chosen as the recipient, whereas the other vein is ligated with a hemostatic clip. The diameter of the fibula is reported to the hip surgeon to determine the endpoint for the core reaming of the hip; this is discussed in detail later in this chapter. Next, the proximal pedicle is reflected in a subperiosteal fashion from the fibula until a nutrient vessel is seen entering the cortex (Figure 31-4). The length of the pedicle at this point should be approximately 4 cm to 5 cm. The proximal fibula is then cut with an oscillating saw at the level of the most proximal nutrient vessel, with the pedicle being protected during the osteotomy. Again, copious irrigation should accompany all osteotomies to prevent thermal necrosis. After the exact length of fibula required has been determined by the preparation of the proximal femur (see Operative Procedure on the Hip Section, p. 254), this length is measured and marked on the fibular graft. The distal pedicle and a small cuff of evaginated periosteum are secured to the

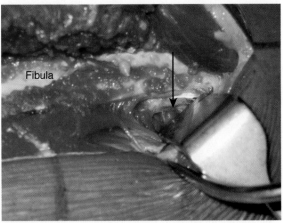

**Figure 31-3** A view of the proximal fibula just before the osteotomy, with visualization of the proximal peroneal artery and two veins (arrow).

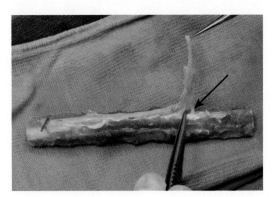

**Figure 31-4** The harvested fibula is inspected with heparinized saline for any leaks along the pedicle. The arrow is pointing to the nutrient artery, which enters the fibula approximately 15 cm distal to the head of the fibula.

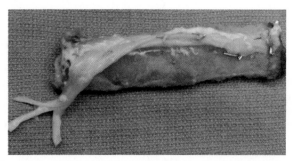

**Figure 31–5** The pedicle is secured to the end of the fibula with a 4–0 absorbable suture to prevent stripping during insertion into the femur. The pedicle extends approximately 4 cm beyond the end of the fibula.

distal extent of the fibula with a 4–0 absorbable suture to prevent the stripping of the pedicle and the periosteum during insertion into the femoral core (Figure 31-5).

## Operative Procedure on the Hip

Certain anatomic landmarks are marked to assist with the placement and design of the surgical incision (Figure 31-6). The lateral aspect of the femur is approached through an interval between the tensor fascia lata and the gluteus medius. The vastus lateralis is then encountered, and the donor vessels (i.e., the ascending branch of the lateral femoral circumflex artery and two veins) are identified as they lie between the rectus femoris and the vastus intermedius. After the vessels are identified, the origin of the vastus lateralis is reflected sharply from the vastus ridge and then in a posterior direction for approximately 5 cm. The origin of the vastus intermedius is then carefully detached with a right-angle clamp and knife from its anterior position on the proximal femur. A specially designed four-quadrant retractor is introduced to provide better visibility for the dissection of the donor vessels.

## Isolation of the Vascular Pedicle

With the vastus intermedius reflected from its origin, the falx or aponeurotic bridge that spans from the anterolateral femur to the rectus femoris can be seen anteriorly. With the use of

sponge sticks, the adjacent deep fat pad is swept away to expose the ascending branch of the lateral femoral circumflex artery and its two accompanying veins. With the use of loupe magnification, the pedicle is carefully mobilized. A tension-free anastomosis can be performed with a minimum pedicle length of 4 cm, which is obtainable if the ascending branch off of the lateral femoral circumflex artery is ligated just distal to its first bifurcation. Any small branches are cauterized or ligated with small hemostatic clips. The artery and the two veins are divided and clamped with a small hemostatic clip. The wound is irrigated with warm saline, the artery is inspected for pulsations, and the four-quadrant retractor is removed for the preparation of the proximal femur.

## Preparation of the Femoral Head

A C-arm fluoroscope is draped with a sterile sleeve and then positioned over the patient's hip region like an arch (Figure 31-7); this provides for the obtaining of anteroposterior and frog-leg lateral views of the proximal femur with relative ease. Starting no lower than the middle of the lesser trochanter and at the junction of the middle and posterior third of the lateral femur, a 3-mm guide pin is inserted under fluoroscopic control into the center of the necrotic nidus within the femoral head. Pin position must be checked on both anteroposterior and lateral views. The pin must not only be positioned within the center of the necrotic bone, but it must also be spaced appropriately between the cortices of the femoral neck to allow for the passage of a large reamer (Figure 31-8). With correct pin placement confirmed by fluoroscopy, sequential reaming ensues over the guide pin; the procedure starts with a 10-mm reamer, the reamers are then increased in size, and the increasing then stops at the measured diameter of the harvested fibula. The reaming should extend to within 3 mm to 5 mm of the femoral head subchondral plate. This portion of the reaming is best performed with the use of live fluoroscopic guidance. Necrotic bone removed during the reaming process is discarded, whereas healthy appearing bone is saved for later grafting (Figure 31-9). Additional bone is captured with a filtered suction tip (KAM Super Sucker, Anspach, Palm Beach Gardens, FL) during the reaming process, when bone slurry is expressed from the core. Bone from this process is emptied onto a surgical sponge, dried, and fashioned by the scrub nurse into rectangular "bullets" to be used later for

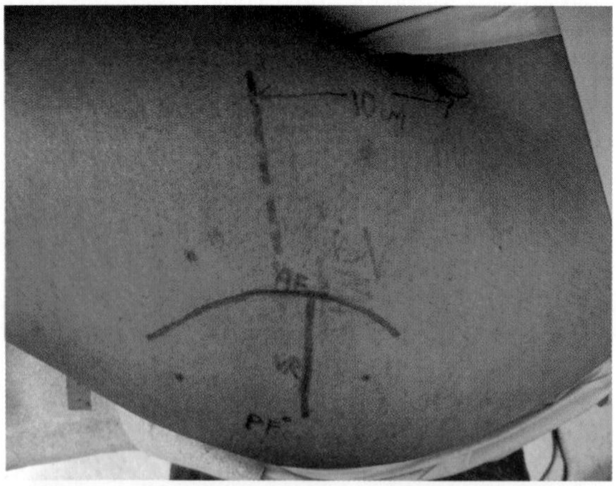

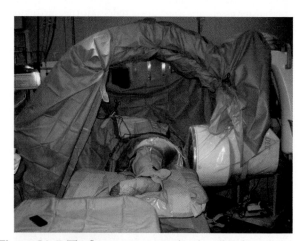

**Figure 31–6** The anterosuperior iliac spine (*ASIS*) is marked as drawn circle, and 10 cm below the ASIS is where the lateral femoral circumflex vessels predictably lie. The vastus ridge (*VR*) is marked, and a curvilinear convex anterior incision is marked, with one third of the incision above the VR and two thirds distal to it. *AF*, anterior femur; *PF*, posterior femur.

**Figure 31–7** The fluoroscopy unit is placed to allow for a cross-table anteroposterior hip view. The leg is positioned by the surgeon to obtain a frog-leg lateral view. The C-arm can be tilted (not shown here) toward the patient's head to provide the hip surgeon with additional working room.

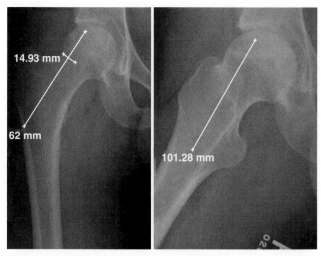

**Figure 31–8** Preoperative templating includes the placement of a line that is representative of the anticipated vector, which will allow for the correct placement of the fibula within the femoral head without violating the femoral neck.

grafting. After the final straight reamer is passed, the guide pin is removed, and a special ball-tip reamer is introduced into the femoral core. With the use of fluoroscopic control, additional necrotic bone is excavated from the femoral head to create a bulbous cavity, usually in the anterior and superior quadrants. This step is performed with a water-soluble radiographic contrast medium injected into the femoral core to assess the adequacy and amount of the necrotic bone removed (Figure 31-10, *A* and *B*).

Next, with the use of a large curette, cancellous bone is taken from the greater trochanteric region, with the use of the proximal femoral core as an access point. Some of the cancellous graft is then placed into the femoral head cavity with DeBakey forceps and impacted with the use of a custom-made cancellous bone impaction instrument. This instrument is particularly helpful for elevating the sunken subchondral floor in cases of femoral head collapse. At its inserted end, the device has several windows through which additional cancellous bone is extruded with the help of a specialized drill bit, thus filling voids in the subchondral bone (Figure 31-11). With the impactor fully inserted, the length of the fibular graft is determined by reading the circumferential markings (units in millimeters) on the impactor's side. After the cancellous bone is inserted, the bone "bullets" created from the reamings are inserted and extruded

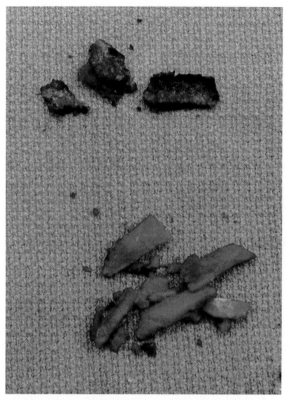

**Figure 31–9** Bone reamings from the femoral head. The top darker bone is clearly necrotic, whereas the red bone at the bottom is healthier and more viable.

likewise into the femoral head cavities. Finally, contrast material is reinjected to confirm the adequate filling of the femoral subchondral voids (Figure 31-12, *A* and *B*). The femoral head is now ready to receive the fibular graft.

### Placement of the Fibular Graft

The pedicle that courses along the fibula is placed superiorly and anteriorly, and it is usually resting in and protected by a natural fibular recess. To further protect the pedicle, the fibula is inserted along the posterior border of the femoral core, which should be capacious enough to accommodate the fibula without excessive compression of the pedicle. The graft is gently

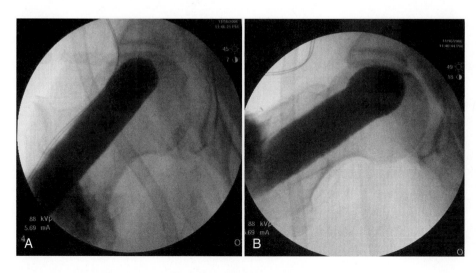

**Figure 31–10  A,** Anteroposterior and **B,** lateral intraoperative radiographs that show renograffin injected into the femoral core. These images confirm the adequacy or inadequacy of the femoral head excavation.

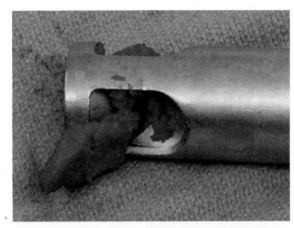

**Figure 31-11** This custom-made bone impactor is sealed at the bottom and has only three windows, one of which can be seen in this image. Note the extruded bone exiting through one of the apertures.

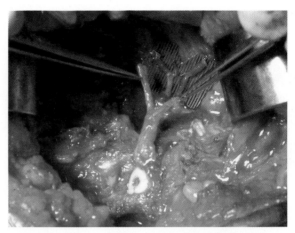

**Figure 31-13** The outer edge of the implanted fibula can be seen from the opening in the lateral femur. The jewelers forceps are holding the peroneal artery and vein just before the anastomosis. The ascending lateral femoral circumflex artery and vein can be seen in the background lying on a micro-suction mat.

advanced with the use of a bone tamp farther into the cavity of the prepared femoral head. Its final position is confirmed with fluoroscopy, and, if the surgeon is concerned, an arteriogram of the peroneal vessels can be obtained to confirm that there is no compression on the pedicle within the core. The graft is secured within the core with a 0.062 Kirschner wire that crosses both cortices of the fibula and the medial femoral cortex at the level of the lesser trochanter. The K-wire is bent, cut short, twisted posteriorly, and buried in the fibers of the gluteus medius. At this point, the fluoroscopy unit can be removed from the operative field.

### Vessel Anastomosis

The four-quadrant hip retractor is replaced to optimize the exposure of the harvested vessels (i.e., the ascending branch of the lateral femoral circumflex artery and the two veins). Attention is initially directed toward the venous anastomosis. We have continued to enjoy success with our venous anastomoses with the use of a coupling device (Microvascular Anastomotic Coupler system, Medical Companies Alliance, Homewood, AL). The device comes in sizes that range from 1.0 mm to 3.5 mm in 0.5-mm increments; however we use either the 2.5-mm or 3.0-mm coupler for the majority of cases. After this, the microscope is brought into the surgical field, a blue microsurgical suction

mat (Micromat, PMT, Chanhasen, MN) is placed as a backdrop, and the arterial anastomosis is completed with the use of an 8-0 or 9-0 black nylon monofilament suture with a 100-μm needle (Sharpoint, Pearsalls Limited, Taunton, Somerset TAI, IRY, UK) (Figure 31-13). After the anastomosis, the repair site is observed for any leaks. We will often place a small local fat graft over a minor leak, whereas larger leaks require additional suturing. Next, the exposed end of the fibular graft is observed for endosteal bleeding. Bleeding from the endosteal vessels is seen within 5 minutes of completing the anastomosis in more than 90% of cases. For those cases in which flow is absent after 5 minutes, we recommend several steps. First, we check the patient's blood pressure and core body temperature. If either or both are low, elevation will often produce adequate flow. In addition, we irrigate the medullary canal of the exposed fibula with papavarin and heparin. If this does not improve the flow, we recheck the anastomosis site for leaks and perform a patency test on both sides of the anastomosis. If flow is sluggish or absent on the femoral side of the anastomosis, we trace the artery back to its origin from the lateral femoral circumflex artery. The ascending branch can be either kinked or tethered anywhere along this course. If this is the case, the removal of the aggravating tissue (most often the vastus intermedius) will often allow for adequate flow. If poor flow is localized to the fibular pedicle side, we check the vein that was not used for the venous

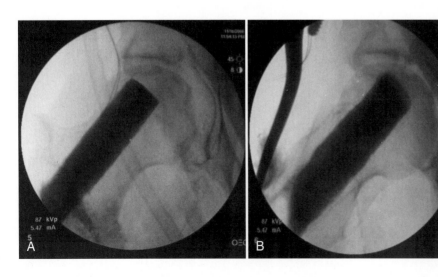

A    B

**Figure 31-12 A,** Anteroposterior and **B,** lateral intraoperative radiographs after bone grafting with renograffin. Notice how the bulbous area (see Figure 31-10) is now squared off, which demonstrates the adequate filling of the area with cancellous bone graft.

anastomosis, because often this vein can have a small leak that induces spasm throughout the vessels or that causes a vascular steal. Any leaks are repaired with either 8-0 suture or micro hemoclips. Rarely if ever does the graft have to be removed entirely for size adjustment if accurate measurements have been made during the preparation of the core and of the fibular graft. If all else fails, the anastomosis is redone, and an interpositional vein graft is used if there is tension.

The vastus lateralis and the intermedius muscles are not reattached during closure for fear of constricting the vascular pedicle. The tensor fascia lata and the iliotibial band are closed over a drain. The subcutaneous tissue and the skin are closed in the same manner as the leg wound.

### TECHNICAL PEARLS

- Ensure that the femoral core is large enough to accept the fibula without compressing the vessels; however, avoid over-reaming, because this increases the chances for notching the femoral neck.
- Harvest cancellous graft only from the greater trochanteric region.
- Premature weight bearing on the affected side can lead to femoral head collapse and fracture; this must be conveyed to the patient preoperatively.
- Remember: measure twice, cut once. A short pedicle on either the donor side or the recipient side will jeopardize the creation of a tension-free anastomosis and thus necessitate the use of a vein graft.
- An uncommon problem is the patient with an allergy to the radiographic contrast medium, which limits the ability to assess the adequacy of the reaming of the necrotic bone. In these cases, we recommend using only air, which will demonstrate—albeit less dramatically—the adequacy of the necrotic bone removal and the replacement grafting.
- Neither an excess amount of fibula nor a prominent pin should protrude laterally at the hip, because either can cause trochanteric bursitis.

## POSTOPERATIVE REHABILITATION

Postoperatively, all patients are placed on an intravenous infusion of dextran for 3 days and then transitioned to aspirin and Persantine daily, which is continued for 6 weeks. The operative drains, the Foley catheter, and the epidural catheter are removed on the second postoperative day, and physical therapy

is also initiated on that day. The average hospital stay is 3 days. Patients do not bear weight on the operative side for 6 weeks, after which time progressive weight bearing is permitted. Full weight bearing is achieved by 5 to 6 months. We recommend aquatherapy and stationary bicycling at the 6-week postoperative mark. Patients are encouraged to begin early active and passive motion of the toes and ankle, with special emphasis on the passive stretching of the great toe. The great toe is susceptible to a flexion contracture as a result of the scarring of the flexor hallucis longus muscle. Follow up radiographic and clinical examinations are performed at 3 months, 6 months, and yearly thereafter. Unrestricted activity is allowed at 1 year after surgery (Tables 31-1 and 31-2).

## COMPLICATIONS

Less than 1% of our patients have required a blood transfusion, and we have had only four infections occur during the entire duration that we have performed the procedure.

A contracture of the great toe has occurred in our series in 3% of cases. We have performed Z-lengthenings of the flexor hallucis longus in those patients whose contractures were profound enough to either impede the normal gait or cause painful pressure on the tip of the toe.

**Table 31-1 RESULTS AND OUTCOMES FOR PATIENTS WITH AVASCULAR NECROSIS OF THE FEMORAL HEAD TREATED WITH FREE VASCULARIZED FIBULAR GRAFTING**

| Type | No. of Cases | No. of Revisions |
|---|---|---|
| Idiopathic | 492 | 107 (22%) |
| Steroids | 726 | 123 (17%) |
| Alcohol | 380 | 77 (20%) |
| Trauma | 274 | 53 (17%) |
| Perthes | 25 | 2 (8%) |
| Other | 37 | 4 (11%) |
| SCFE | 32 | 1 (3%) |
| Pregnancy | 34 | 2 (6%) |

*SCFE*, Slipped capital femoral epiphysis.

**Table 31-2 COMPARATIVE REPORTS**

| Author | Title | No. of Patients | Length of Follow Up | Results |
|---|---|---|---|---|
| Zhang et al | Treatment of femoral head necrosis with free vascularized fibula grafting: a preliminary report | 48 patients (56 hips) | 16 months | 53 out of 56 femoral heads showed either no change or improvement; all patients had improved Harris Hip Scores |
| Urbaniak et al | Treatment of osteonecrosis of the femoral head with free vascularized fibular grafting. A long-term follow up study of 103 hips | 89 patients (103 hips) | 5 years | At 5 years, there was a 10% chance for conversion to arthroplasty for stage II hips and a 25% chance for hips in all other stages |
| Sotereanos et al | Free vascularized fibula grafting for the treatment of osteonecrosis of the femoral head | 65 patients (88 hips) | 3 years | Hip survival rates at 5.5 years: stages IC and IIA, 100%; stage IIB, 94%; stage IIC, 50%; stage IIIB, 80%; stage IIIC, 58%; stage IVA, 72%; and stage IVB, 58% |
| Marciniak et al | Osteonecrosis of the femoral head. A study of 101 hips treated with vascularized fibular grafting | 86 patients (101 hips) | 5 years | 61% survivorship at final follow up for all hips in veteran population |

Subtrochanteric femur fractures occur at a rate of approximately 1%. Since limiting the harvest of cancellous graft to only the greater trochanter (and not also harvesting from the lesser trochanter), our incidence of subtrochanteric fractures has decreased from 2% to 1%. The majority of these fractures occur 6 to 8 weeks postoperatively, which is typically when patients begin to feel better and place excessive weight on the leg, with a torsional force being applied (i.e., standing with weight on the leg and turning the torso).

Irritation of the lateral cutaneous branch of the superficial peroneal nerve occurs to some degree in less than 10% of patients. In the majority of these patients, the condition resolves completely by the 6-month postoperative visit.

Ankle pain is reported in up to 5% of patients, but, with few exceptions, this resolves by the 1-year postoperative mark. Uchiyama reported that ankle stability is maintained if at least 6 cm of distal fibula remains. We are careful to always leave 10 cm of distal fibula from the graft harvest.

Some patients experience trochanteric bursitis, which typically manifests between 3 and 12 months postoperatively. This seems to be related to a prominent Kirschner wire or to heterotopic bone being prominent at the trochanteric flare. The majority of patients respond to local steroid and lidocaine injections, but a select few with recalcitrant symptoms ultimately require surgery to remove the pin or the heterotopic bone.

## ANNOTATED REFERENCES AND SUGGESTED READINGS

Aldridge JM 3rd, Berend KR, Gunneson EE, Urbaniak JR. Free vascularized fibular grafting for the treatment of postcollapse osteonecrosis of the femoral head. Surgical technique. *J Bone Joint Surg Am.* 2004;86-A(suppl 1):87–101.

This article is part of a series of surgical technique guides. It describes in thorough detail the surgical steps to take when performing the free vascularized fibular graft procedure for the treatment of femoral head osteonecrosis.

Aldridge JM, Urbaniak JR. Avascular necrosis of the femoral head: role of vascularized bone grafts. *Orthop Clin North Am.* 2007;38(1):13–22.

This article presents the history, development, and results of the various techniques of vascularized bone grafting for the treatment of osteonecrosis of the femoral head. The results of treating more than 2800 patients who had femoral head osteonecrosis with the use of a vascularized fibular graft by way of an intraosseous approach are summarized, and certain pearls and pitfalls regarding the treatment of femoral head osteonecrosis with the use of a free vascularized fibular graft are highlighted.

Kawate K, Yajima H, Sugimoto K, et al. Indications for free vascularized fibular grafting for the treatment of osteonecrosis of the femoral head. *BMC Musculoskelet Disord.* 2007;8:78.

This study prospectively tracked 71 hips in 60 patients for an average of 7 years. Radiographs, Harris Hip Scores, and survivorship were evaluated. Overall survivorship for the group was 83% at 7 years. The authors delineate certain preoperative factors that portend an inferior clinical outcome.

Kim SY, Kim YG, Kim PT, Ihn JC, Cho BC, Koo KH. Vascularized compared with nonvascularized fibular grafts for large osteonecrotic lesions of the femoral head. *J Bone Joint Surg Am.* 2005;87(9):2012–2018.

This prospective case-control study compares hips treated with either a vascularized fibular graft or with a nonvascularized fibular graft, with

a mean duration of follow up of 4 years. The rates of radiographic progression and collapse were significantly lower and the mean dome depression was significantly less in the group that was treated with a vascularized fibular graft as compared with the group treated with a nonvascularized graft. The authors conclude that vascularized fibular grafting was associated with better clinical results and that it was more effective than nonvascularized fibular grafting for the prevention of collapse of the femoral head in a matched population with a Steinberg stage IIC or larger osteonecrotic lesion.

Marciniak D, Furey C, Shaffer JW. Osteonecrosis of the femoral head. A study of 101 hips treated with vascularized fibular grafting. *J Bone Joint Surg Am.* Volume 87 2005 Apr;(4):742–747.

Plakseychuk AY, Kim SY, Park BC, Varitimidis SE, Rubash HE, Sotereanos DG. Vascularized compared with nonvascularized fibular grafting for the treatment of osteonecrosis of the femoral head. *J Bone Joint Surg Am.* 2003;85-A(4):589–596.

This is a retrospective case-control study with a large number of patients that compared the clinical and radiographic results between two groups that were treated with either a vascularized fibular graft or a nonvascularized fibular graft. The results of this study strongly suggest that vascularized fibular grafting is associated with better clinical and radiographic results.

Sotereanos DG, Plakseychuk AY, Rubash HE. Free vascularized fibula grafting for the treatment of osteonecrosis of the femoral head. *Clinical Orthopaedics & Related Research.* 1997 Nov;(344):243–256.

Urbaniak JR, Coogan PF, Gunneson EB, Nunley JA. Treatment of osteonecrosis of the femoral head with free vascularized fibular grafting: a long-term follow-up study of one hundred and three hips. *J Bone Joint Surg.* 1995;77A:681–694.

This level IV study retrospectively evaluated the outcomes of 103 hips that were treated with free vascularized fibular grafting. Harris Hip Scores and SF-12 forms are the clinical measurements that were used, whereas radiographs were evaluated for changes in the femoral head and joint space. The overall success rate for all patients, regardless of their preoperative stage, was 80% at a 5-year follow up.

Urbaniak JR, Jones JP. *Osteonecrosis: etiology, diagnosis, and treatment.* AAOS publication; 1997.

This textbook is the only comprehensive text that addresses osteonecrosis of the human skeleton. All facets of the disease process are discussed in detail.

Vail TP, Urbaniak JR. Donor-site morbidity with use of vascularized autogenous fibular grafts. *J Bone Joint Surg Am.* Volume 78 1996 Feb;(2):204–211.

Zhang C, Zeng B, Xu Z, et al. Treatment of femoral head necrosis with free vascularized fibula grafting: a preliminary report. *Microsurgery.* 2005;25(4):305–309.

This retrospective study reported short-term results (16 months) for 56 hips with the diagnosis of osteonecrosis of the femoral head. All but 3 femoral heads demonstrated on radiographs to have either no change (25%) or improvement (69.6%). Harris Hip Scores improved for all patients.

**www.dukehealth.org/FVFG**

This is a thirty-page pdf file found online at Duke University. It addresses the many questions and challenges that the over 3000 patients treated by the two authors have had over the years. It is a comprehensive layman's review of the procedure.

# CHAPTER 32

# Proximal Femoral Osteotomies in Adults for Secondary Osteoarthritis: Femoral Osteotomies for Adult Deformity

*Daniël Haverkamp, Michel P. J. v/d Bekerom, and René K. Marti*

## INTRODUCTION

Many orthopedic surgeons consider intertrochanteric osteotomy a historic operation with no role to play in modern clinical practice. This is true for a number of hip conditions, such as idiopathic osteoarthritis, rheumatoid arthritis, and severe osteoarthritis in the elderly patient. However, there exist conditions in selected younger patients with which an intertrochanteric osteotomy can produce excellent and long-lasting results. For these conditions, an intertrochanteric osteotomy should be the preferred treatment.

Historically, the first surgical treatment for osteoarthritis was a resection of the femoral head as described by Girdlestone. This was a pure salvage procedure, and its main aim was to reduce pain. The techniques of tenotomies described by Voss and the earliest intertrochanteric osteotomies by McMurray may also be regarded as salvage procedures. During the development of hip surgery, the goal of treatment gradually changed. Apart from pain relief, improving function and quality of life became increasingly important. When total hip arthroplasty (THA) became feasible, the goal of joint-saving therapy changed from mere salvage to palliation. We define an osteotomy as palliative when osteoarthritic changes are too advanced to save the joint but when a replacement can successfully be delayed with the use of this procedure. In the meantime, the osteotomy may even facilitate a future total hip replacement by improving the bone stock. Former salvage types of surgeries have no further role to play in the treatment of hip disorders, because these have been superseded by THA. Müller and colleagues advanced joint-saving hip surgery by describing and defining the role of intertrochanteric osteotomies in more detail. In addition, they introduced a therapeutic type of osteotomy that can be performed if osteoarthritic changes are not too advanced and if the cause of these changes is a biomechanical factor that can be corrected. If a biomechanical factor such as impingement, a dislocating force (e.g., stress on the labrum), or a small weight-bearing area is present, an early correction of this factor can biomechanically normalize the hip joint, which could lead to the long-lasting preservation of the joint. The differentiation between palliative and therapeutic intertrochanteric osteotomies is important in clinical practice. It is evident that therapeutic osteotomies should have a place in modern clinical practice. However, this is different for palliative osteotomies for younger patients with secondary osteoarthritis. Several studies show that the survival rates for salvage osteotomies among younger patients are approximately 70% to 80% after 10 years. The disadvantage of this type of osteotomy is that the results are mostly unpredictable. We believe that palliative osteotomy for younger and well-motivated patients should be considered and that the advantages and disadvantages should be discussed with these patients.

## INDICATIONS

In the modern treatment regimens for severe osteoarthritis of the hip, THA is the treatment of choice for the elderly patient. During the past several decades, the age limit for this procedure has gradually been adjusted downward. Even so, the question remains regarding whether a THA is the best treatment for a young patient with mild (secondary) osteoarthritis. For patients with idiopathic osteoarthritis or rheumatic arthritis, no benefit from joint-saving surgery can be expected. However, for the treatment of the following indications, intertrochanteric osteotomies can provide good and long-lasting results:

- Coxa valga (antetorta)
- Mild dysplasia
- After slipped capital femoral epiphysis (SCFE)
- After Legg-Calvé-Perthes disease
- Posttraumatic deformities

Another somewhat controversial indication is avascular necrosis (AVN) of the femoral head. An intertrochanteric osteotomy that turns the necrotic defect away from the weight-bearing surface could prove to be useful and can be tried. However, the progression of the AVN and the subsequent collapse of the femoral head are unpredictable and still occur in a large portion of the patients after the osteotomy. The transtrochanteric rotational osteotomy described by Sugioka is, according to the literature, not reproducible by other orthopedic surgeons and therefore unsuitable for general practice. For osteoarthritis with femoral head deformities that presents after AVN when the AVN and the remodeling took place at a younger age, incongruence between the femoral head and the acetabulum can be present. An intertrochanteric valgus osteotomy improves the congruency, but subluxation of the femoral head occurs. In addition, an acetabular shelf plasty can successfully provide coverage for the severely deformed part of the femoral head. For AVN when remodeling is not yet complete, the deformed part of the femoral head that is turned from the acetabulum is covered by the bone graft, so it has the possibility of remodeling against the support provided by the graft.

## BRIEF HISTORY AND PHYSICAL EXAMINATION

It is normal practice to delay surgical interventions for elderly patients until complaints of pain or functional limitations are more severe and until more advanced osteoarthritic changes have occurred. To achieve optimal results, it is important to perform surgery as early as possible in patients who are suitable for intertrochanteric osteotomies, preferably after the first typical manifestation of the hip disorder.

Complaints among patients who are suitable for intertrochanteric osteotomy are not completely identical to those of older patients. In the latter case, complaints tend to occur after the cartilage has been destroyed to a large degree. Among patients who are suitable for intertrochanteric osteotomies, complaints are mostly caused by a factor such as incongruency, impingement, or stress on the acetabular labrum as a result of dysplasia. When screening these patients, the apprehension test (i.e., extension and external rotation) and the impingement test (i.e., flexion, adduction, and internal rotation) could play a role in detecting labral pathology at an early stage.

Every patient who is considered for an intertrochanteric osteotomy should be screened for suitability for the procedure and provided with information regarding the postoperative period. It should be explained to the patient that the osteotomy postpones the need for THA but does not eliminate it in all cases. Furthermore, the rehabilitation process should be explained, and the patient's motivation should be evaluated. The outcome of an osteotomy is thought to be better among well-motivated patients.

Range of motion is an important part of the preoperative screening, because it demonstrates the amount of correction that is possible without jeopardizing hip function. Clinical investigation also reveals the limitations of movement and contractures. Contractures are especially important, because they can influence the correction required when performing the osteotomy. For example, in cases of an extension deficit (flexion contracture), extension can be added to the osteotomy. The same principle is valid for external and internal rotation contractures. Often it is not the functional limitation of the hip that bothers the patient but rather the painful overload of the neighboring joints.

## IMAGING AND DIAGNOSTIC STUDIES

Functional x-rays can play an important role in the decision regarding the preferred intervention. An abduction view provides a radiologic impression of the amount of containment and the congruency that can be obtained by a varus osteotomy. An adduction and flexion x-ray does the same for a valgus or extension osteotomy. For patients with a coxa valga or mild dysplasia, it is important to make a clinical judgment regarding the amount of femoral torsion that is present. If an increased antetorsion is anticipated, then this should be verified by means of a Dunn x-ray or a computed tomography scan. In modern practice, the latter is more appropriate. For patients with suspected labral pathology, this can be verified with magnetic resonance arthrography.

## SURGICAL TECHNIQUE

Because the surgical technique and preoperative planning differ in accordance with the indication, we will discuss the standard surgical technique followed by specific additions to the basic technique, all with their specific pitfalls and considerations. In the last paragraphs, we will describe the specific considerations for each indication.

### Surgical Technique for Intertrochanteric Osteotomy

A standard lateral approach is used for all intertrochanteric osteotomies. The vastus lateralis is exposed by incising the fascia lata and reflected with Hohmann retractors to visualize the lateral femur (Figure 32-1, *A*). The vastus lateralis is sharply removed in the avascular plane from the vastus ridge. The vastus lateralis is detached from the intermuscular septum by blunt dissection, which allows for a wide inspection of the upper femur. Several perforating branches of the profunda femoral artery traverse the vastus lateralis and should be ligated correctly to avoid a postoperative hematoma; care should be taken so that the blunt dissection does not damage these vessels (see Figure 32-1, *B*). If it is necessary to inspect the hip joint, the approach can be extended proximally (i.e., the Watson-Jones approach), and the joint capsule can be opened to inspect the joint. The joint capsule is not routinely opened but rather only opened when indicated (e.g., for hump resection in a post-SCFE deformity). The linea aspera is decorticated. The seating chisel is inserted in the correct position, and the rotation is marked by placing a K-wire on each side of the planned osteotomy. Before this osteotomy is made, the seating chisel should be pulled back approximately 1 cm. An osteotomy parallel to the seating chisel is then made just proximal to the lesser trochanter (see Figure 32-1, *C*). Depending on the desired correction, a full or half wedge is removed to allow for the calculated varus–valgus or flexion–extension correction. During the osteotomy, blunt Hohmann retractors are placed around the femur to protect the femoral vessels and the femoral nerve. The definitive fixation is performed under compression with the classic AO (arbeitsgemeinschaft fur osteosynthesefragen) 90-degree or 100-degree blade plate, with different offsets that range from 10 mm to 20 mm. For cases in which extreme valgization is needed (e.g., for the treatment of femoral neck nonunions), a double-angled 120-degree or 130-degree blade plate can be used. For specific cases (e.g., intertrochanteric lengthening), a condylar plate is the preferred option. For all of our intertrochanteric osteotomies that involve the use of more or less right-angled blade plates, we performed the fixation under compression with the use of the AO compression device (see Figure 32-1, *D* and *E*). With the use of lateral compression, even open-wedge osteotomies heal without problems.

### Potential Pitfalls and Considerations for Intertrochanteric Osteotomy

Most of the described complications of intertrochanteric osteotomies can be avoided with the use of a good surgical technique. The incidence of a delayed union or nonunion can be greatly reduced with the proper use of an AO compression device. The anatomy of the intertrochanteric region is ideal for osteotomies, because the shape of this region allows for corrections in all planes while leaving large contact areas. Another advantage is the relatively good healing capacity of the metaphyseal bone.

In addition, the placement of the seating chisel or blade plate can cause problems. The occurrence of AVN caused by the osteotomy is a worry. The vascular supply of the femoral head is provided by branches of the dorsal circumflex artery, which can be damaged in the intertrochanteric fossa if the femoral neck is perforated by the seating chisel. This can be avoided with the correct placement of the seating chisel (Figure 32-2).

When flexion or extension is added to the osteotomy, the position of the femur after the osteotomy should be anticipated when planning the placement of the blade plate. For example, a seating chisel that is inserted too far anteriorly cannot be fixed properly to the femur after a flexion osteotomy (Figure 32-3).

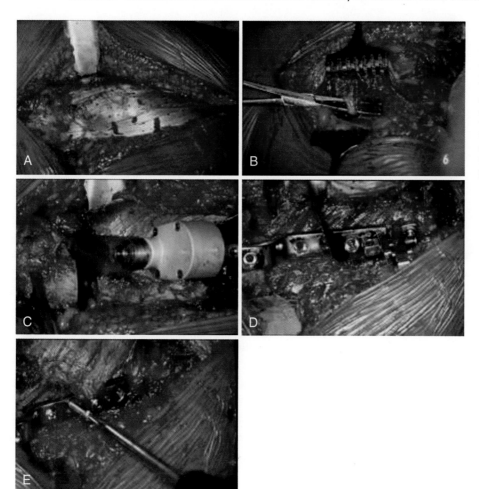

**Figure 32–1** Preoperative pictures that illustrate the surgical technique of a classic intertrochanteric osteotomy. **A,** A standard lateral approach with an exposed vastus lateralis. **B,** Perforating branch of the profunda femoral artery is visible. **C,** After inserting the seating chisel and marking the rotation, a transverse osteotomy is made. **D,** Compression of the osteotomy with an AO compression device. **E,** After compression final fixation of the blade plate is performed.

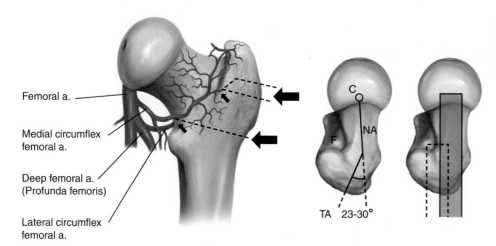

Femoral a.

Medial circumflex femoral a.

Deep femoral a. (Profunda femoris)

Lateral circumflex femoral a.

**Figure 32–2 A,** Schematic drawing of the vascular and surgical anatomy of the proximal femur. **B,** Surgical anatomy of the proximal femur with proper blade placement.

Especially after a varus osteotomy, a long-lasting Trendelenburg gait can occur as a result of the relaxation of the gluteal muscles caused by the created femoral shortening. A good varisation should show a situation in which the tip of the major trochanter is not positioned higher than the center of the femoral head. If the center of the femoral head is positioned lower than the level of the tip of the major trochanter, the Trendelenburg gait could be permanent. If it is necessary to perform so much varisation that this occurs, a distalization of the major trochanter should be considered.

## Surgical Technique for Shelf Plasty

We developed a special technique for adding superolateral bone grafts to the acetabulum in combination with an intertrochanteric osteotomy. In our clinic, 4% of all osteotomies performed involved patients with femoral head deformities and secondary osteoarthritis who required an additional shelf plasty.

For every procedure, an anterolateral approach was used that was similar to that used with a regular intertrochanteric osteotomy. The gluteal muscles are released with the use of an extracapsular

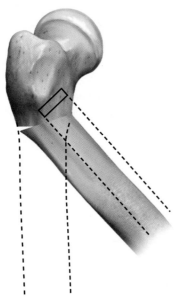

**Figure 32–3** Schematic drawing of the possible faulty placement of a blade plate in an flexion osteotomy.

osteotomy of the major trochanter. A cancellous–cortical bone graft is harvested from the ipsilateral interior iliac crest; this graft is bent into two or three blocks and predrilled for screw fixation. The joint capsule remains intact, but it is thinned on the supero-lateral side until head motion is visible. The supra-acetabular iliac bone is decorticated, and the prepared bone graft is fixated with 3.5-mm or 4.5-mm lag screws, with the patient's leg in the calculated adduction or abduction position. When the function is tested in adduction, the graft should show plastic deformity. Some cancellous bone is pressed between the thinned joint capsule and the bone graft. A temporary screw fixation of the major trochanter is performed, if necessary, in combination with a distalization procedure (Figure 32-4). We performed distalization when the tip of the major trochanter was positioned higher than the center of rotation of the femoral head after correction. An intertrochanteric osteotomy is then performed in accordance with the standard AO technique; this technique is described earlier in this chapter.

## Potential Pitfalls and Considerations for Shelf Plasty

Two major pitfalls exist when creating a shelf plasty. First, care must be taken that the joint capsule is thinned enough to avoid a too-high position of the shelf plasty. Alternatively, the joint

**Figure 32–4** Schematic drawing of the surgical technique of acetabular shelf plasty.

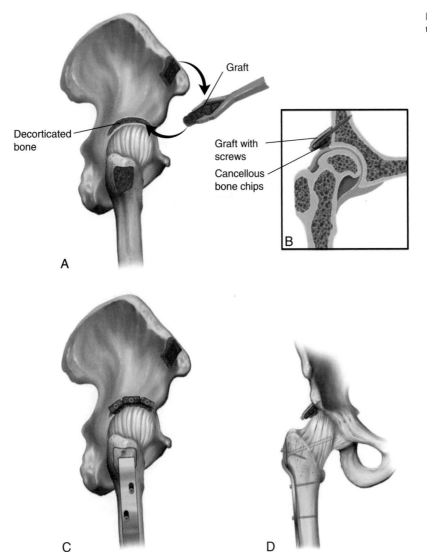

capsule should remain intact. If the joint capsule is too thick, the shelf plasty that is placed too high has no biomechanical function and is therefore useless.

The second major pitfall in our technique is a possible fracture of the major trochanter. Techniques in which the trochanter is reduced by the seating chisel cause, in our opinion, a higher risk of fracturing the trochanter, which could prove to be a disastrous complication. Temporary screw fixation can be performed quickly and safely, and it protects the patient from severe complications.

### Surgical Technique for Intertrochanteric Lengthening

In many posttraumatic cases, a shortening of the affected leg is present. In these cases, lengthening can be achieved during the intertrochanteric correction. Correction at the intertrochanteric level can also correct a malrotation, if present, at the same time that corrections are performed in the other two planes.

When an adequate correction is obtained with the use of the previously described technique for an intertrochanteric osteotomy, the blade plate is temporarily held in place by a Verbrugge clamp. A laminar bone spreader is inserted into the osteotomy and opened until the desired lengthening is achieved. The blade plate glides beneath the Verbrugge clamp, thus allowing for lengthening but maintaining the correction. Instead of a laminar bone spreader, it is also possible to use an

AO femoral distractor to achieve lengthening. Lengthening up to 3.5 cm can be safely performed without overstretching the nerves. The gap that is created at the intertrochanteric level is filled with corticocancellous bone graft from the iliac crest in combination with cancellous grafts along the decorticated linea aspera. After fixing the blade plate with 4.5-mm cortical screws, one or two of the distal screws are directed cephalad and should be fixated in the proximal fragment, thus creating extra stability (Figure 32-5).

### Potential Pitfalls and Considerations for Intertrochanteric Lengthening

When a varus osteotomy is performed in combination with lengthening, the proximal fragment should be contoured with a chisel to avoid abutment with and the eventual fracturing of the lesser trochanter.

As with all surgical interventions, preoperative planning is important. When planning lengthening in combination with other intertrochanteric corrections, the leg-length alteration created by angular correction alone should be taken into account.

Lengthening in the intertrochanteric region is a difficult procedure. Make sure that the blade plate is completely inserted during the lengthening to avoid a completely unstable situation.

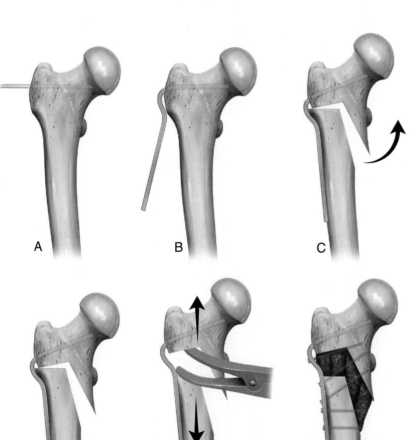

**Figure 32–5**  Schematic drawing of the surgical technique of intertrochanteric lengthening. **A,** insertion of the seating chisel in the planned correction. **B,** placement of the blade plate. **C,** Correction of osteotomy is made. **D,** Rotatonial correction is obtained if desired. **E,** Lengthening can be performed with a laminar spreader. **F,** The gap is filled with corticocancellous grafts from the iliac crest.

A   B   C

D   E   F

### Coxa Valga (Antetorta) and Dysplasia

Deformities such as coxa valga (antetorta) and acetabular dysplasia often coexist. For hips in which the main deformity is on the acetabular side, an acetabulum realigning procedure should be the first choice, and, if necessary, it can be combined with a femoral osteotomy. In these cases, there is a relatively shallow and steep acetabulum that results in a decreased contact surface between the acetabulum and the femoral head (Figure 32-6). Isolated correction of the femoral side cannot solve this problem of containment fully and will fail to eliminate the dislocation force present. Thus, the osteotomy is doomed to fail. However, with some hip deformities, the main deformity lies on the femoral side, with only a mild acetabular dysplasia; the acetabulum might be shallow but not too steep. A varus osteotomy may improve the contact area between the femoral head and the acetabulum in these types of hips and possibly eliminate the dislocating force that is present. Good and long-lasting results may occur. This will not be the case if a fixed subluxation is present, because the weight-bearing surface and the dislocating forces are not altered, thus making the expected results of an intertrochanteric osteotomy poor. The improvement of containment can be judged preoperatively from an abduction correction view. However, currently no objective measurements exist to decide whether an acetabular realigning osteotomy or an intertrochanteric osteotomy is the preferred treatment for specific patients.

The femoral antetorsion should be taken into account, because many of these patients have an increased femoral antetorsion that also needs to be corrected. A second consideration is that, after the varus osteotomy, the position of the tip of the major trochanter should not exceed the center of the femoral head to avoid a long-lasting Trendelenburg gait. If necessary, this can be addressed by performing a distalization of the major trochanter.

### Slipped Capital Femoral Epiphysis

Not all patients who suffer from SCFE develop osteoarthritis during adulthood. However, this patient population has an increased risk of developing the condition. The pathophysiology behind these arthritic changes consists of acetabulofemoral impingement that is present in an insufficient or uncorrected SCFE or in unnoticed subclinical cases. A prominent part of the anterior metaphyseal femoral neck contacts the anterior part of the acetabulum during flexion. On the basis of the cause of this disorder, a valgus or flexion osteotomy with or without resection of the hump is the best solution. Because the disorder is only present on the femoral side, there is no role for acetabular realigning procedures in these pathologic changes. Early intervention appears to produce better results for this type of

disorder. If, after the osteotomy, there is still some impingement present, the approach can be extended (i.e., the Watson-Jones approach) to perform an arthrotomy and to resect the hump with the use of osteoplasty.

### Legg-Calvé-Perthes Disease

Not all patients who suffer from Legg-Calvé-Perthes disease during childhood develop osteoarthritis during adulthood, although, in many of these patients, a deformed hip joint is present. This deformity consists mainly of a broad and flattened femoral head with a short femoral neck in the varus position. In most cases, the acetabular side is also more or less abnormal, probably as a result of an adaptation of the developing acetabulum to the deformed femoral head.

Osteoarthritic changes develop in adulthood in 50% of patients with these hip deformities. It is most likely that these arthritic changes are caused by an acetabulofemoral incongruency. The origin of this incongruency lies in the fact that the deformed femoral head does not completely fit into the acetabulum. The aim of surgical intervention should be the early correction of this incongruency. The main theory that explains the development of osteoarthritis in these hips is the hinging of the femoral head on the edge of the acetabulum. The best known is the "hinge on abduction," in which the lateral part of the femoral head hinges on the lateral part of the acetabulum. In these types of hips, a valgus extension osteotomy should be the preferred treatment to eliminate both the causative factor and the contractures that are present by realigning the leg. In hips, after Legg-Calvé-Perthes disease, in which the containment of the femoral head is not complete after osteotomy, adding an acetabular shelf plasty can produce excellent results (Figure 32-7). In some cases, valgization alone is not sufficient to restore the function of the abductors as a result of the relatively high position of the major trochanter. In these cases, a simultaneous distalization of the major trochanter is advised.

### Posttraumatic Deformities

Posttraumatic deformities can be subdivided into deformities after acetabular fractures and malunions after proximal femoral fractures. Femoral neck malunion is a rare complication. If a malunion is present, it can cause an impingement between the femoral neck and the acetabulum, which causes early osteoarthritic degeneration. An early correction is required to avoid these osteoarthritic changes. In these posttraumatic deformities, a shortening of the affected leg is often present. Correcting the malunion with an intertrochanteric osteotomy also allows for simultaneous

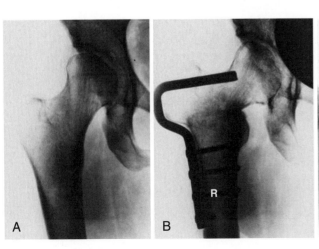
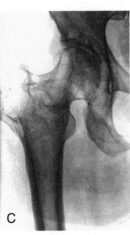

**Figure 32–6** A 35-year-old female patient with symptomatic osteoarthritis as a result of coxa valga and mild dysplasia. A varus intertrochanteric osteotomy was performed. After 21 years, this patient was still free from complaints. **A,** Preoperative x-ray. **B,** Direct postoperative x-ray. **C,** X-ray after 21 years' follow up.

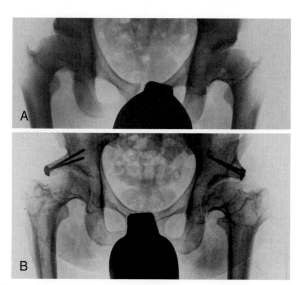

**Figure 32–7**   **A,** A 22-year-old male patient with a symptomatic hip deformity after Legg-Calvé-Perthes disease of both hips. A valgus osteotomy was performed with an acetabular roof plasty for both hips with 2 years in between. **B,** The radiographic result after 12 years is shown.

intertrochanteric lengthening. The direction of the deformity that is present in these malunions is mostly varus/extension; this means that the correction required is a valgus/flexion intertrochanteric osteotomy. The resection of the hump can be performed if partial impingement persists after the osteotomy.

Incongruency and osteoarthritis are common problems after acetabular fractures. With these fractures, cartilage damage occurs during the initial trauma, which makes the area susceptible to the development of osteoarthritis. If a malunited acetabular fracture that causes functional limitations coexists with an increased risk of the development of osteoarthritis, it seems logical to correct the acetabular side, where the deformity is located. However, these corrections are generally too complicated or even impossible. Therefore, it could be justifiable to adjust the normal femoral side to the abnormal acetabular side by aiming the largest part of the unaffected femoral head to the largest part of the unaffected acetabulum, thereby restoring normal joint motion and lowering the risk of osteoarthritic degeneration. In younger patients with more advanced osteoarthritic degeneration and in whom contractures are present, a palliative osteotomy could be considered. We have been able to document good outcomes in this patient group. This is probably the result of eliminating the contractures (i.e., realignment), and it could be caused by the biologic osteotomy effect as well.

Because of the average age of the patient with AVN, this seems like an ideal group for which to consider joint-saving surgery. This is also reflected in the large number of publications about this subject. The main thought behind intertrochanteric osteotomies in AVN is that the affected part of the femoral head is rotated away from the weight-bearing part of the joint, thus preventing collapse. This can be achieved because during intertrochanteric osteotomies corrections in all three dimensions are possible.

The literature shows no evidence of good outcomes in idiopathic AVN treated with intertrochanteric osteotomy. The benefit of intertrochanteric osteotomy is doubtful in this patient group. Most retrospective reports concern patients with atraumatic AVN, but some studies also include traumatic AVN, which demonstrates a better outcome. However, for these young patients, the outcome of intertrochanteric osteotomy remains unpredictable.

A special group of younger patients are those with a deformed femoral head after posttraumatic AVN, which is similar to a

deformity that occurs after Legg-Calvé-Perthes disease. These patients may benefit from a valgus intertrochanteric osteotomy in combination with an acetabular shelf plasty.

## TECHNICAL PEARLS

- Osteoarthritic changes are prevented by the early correction of the causative factor.
- The correction of malrotation can easily be combined with corrections in the other planes.
- Early weight bearing is allowed.
- There is a low incidence of complications.
- During the procedure, it is usually not necessary to open the joint capsule for visualization.
- After an initial osteotomy, all possibilities for future hip surgeries remain.

## POSTOPERATIVE REHABILITATION

The postoperative rehabilitation differs with the type of osteotomy performed. After a standard valgus or varus intertrochanteric osteotomy, gradual weight bearing is allowed during the first days if the wound is properly healing. During the first 6 postoperative weeks, weight bearing remains limited. An x-ray is made after 6 weeks, and, if consolidation is present, the patient is allowed to progress to full weight bearing.

Physical therapy is started and especially focused on proprioception, for which the abductors are especially important. After a varus osteotomy, a Trendelenburg gait can be present for up to a few months as a result of the relaxation of the gluteal muscles. This requires intensive physical therapy.

After osteotomy with an additional intertrochanteric lengthening, we tend to be more careful. Patients are usually kept in bed for the first 5 operative days; however, passive range-of-motion exercises are started immediately. At day 5, partial weight bearing is started until sufficient consolidation is present on the x-ray, which will then allow the patient to gradually increase to full weight bearing.

The technique of acetabular shelf plasty necessitates a different postoperative regimen. These patients are placed in a traction bed to allow for continuous traction immobilization during the first 2 weeks. During this traction period, passive range of motion is allowed, but only in flexion and extension. No rotation, abduction, or adduction is allowed to avoid excessive stress on the shelf plasty. After 2 weeks, gradual weight bearing is allowed.

## RESULTS AND OUTCOMES

The use of intertrochanteric osteotomies appears to be declining in current clinical practice. It seems that many orthopedic surgeons consider it to be a historic operation that has lost its place for the current treatment of hip disorders. This is probably the result of several retrospective studies that reported poor overall results for intertrochanteric osteotomies. However, these studies also included older patients and hips with advanced osteoarthritis. If the results from these studies are critically screened, certain hip conditions in selected patient groups can be isolated. In these isolated cases, good and long-lasting results were reported. It is important to realize this, because not all patients with osteoarthritis are identical, and it is our goal to identify those patients who could be helped by joint-preserving surgery. These patients generally seem to be younger patients with early secondary osteoarthritis caused by a correctable biomechanical factor (Table 32-1).

**Table 32-1** SUMMARY OF RESULTS IN THE RECENT LITERATURE

| Author | No. of Patients | Indication | Type of Osteotomy | Average Age (Range) | Grade of Osteoarthritis | Length of Follow Up | Survival and Conclusions |
|---|---|---|---|---|---|---|---|
| Haverkamp et al., 2006 | 276 | All | All | 45 years (16 to 79 years) | Mild to advanced | 15 to 29 years | Better results among young patients and those with mild osteoarthritis |
| Subgroup of Haverkamp, 2005 | 48 | Idiopathic | All | 57 years (34 to 79 years) | Mild to advanced | 15 to 29 years | Survival: 10 years, 50%; 15 years, 32% |
| Subgroup of Haverkamp | 166 | Dysplasia | All | 46 years (16 to 75 years) | Mild to advanced | 15 to 29 years | Survival: 10 years, 72%; 15 years, 56% |
| Subgroup of Haverkamp | 22 | Trauma | All | 37 years (17 to 68 years) | Mild to advanced | 15 to 29 years | Survival: 10 years, 91%; 15 years, 78% |
| Subgroup of Haverkamp | 14 | Slipped capital femoral epiphysis | All | 44 years (25 to 55 years) | Mild to advanced | 15 to 29 years | Survival: 10 years, 71%; 15 years, 56% |
| Subgroup of Haverkamp | 20 | Avascular necrosis | All | 38 years (16 to 60 years) | Mild to advanced | 15 to 29 years | Survival: 10 years, 60%; 15 years, 30% |
| Pecasse et al., 2004 | 15 | Legg-Calvé-Perthes disease | All | 30 years (19 to 55 years) | Mild to advanced | 4 to 25 years | 33% of patients converted after an average of 15.4 years |
| D'Souza et al., 1998 | 25 | All | All | 38 years (18 to 53 years) | Mild to advanced | 2 to 12 years | Survival: 67% after an average of 12 years |
| Perlau et al., 1996 | 16 | Idiopathic | All | 48 years (38 to 75 years) | Mild to advanced | 5 to 10 years | 44% of patients converted after an average of 6.1 years |
| Marti et al., 2001 | 10 | Osteoarthritis after acetabular fracture | All | 29 years (16 to 47 years) | Mild to advanced | 3 to 22 years | Survival: 80% after an average of 10 years |
| Perlau et al., 1996 | 18 | Dysplasia | All | 33 years (24 to 58 years) | Mild to advanced | 5 to 10 years | Survival: 79% after an average of 6.1 years |
| Toyama et al., 2000 | 67 | Dysplasia | Valgus–extension | 44 years (23 to 59 years) | Advanced | 5 to 16 years | Survival: 10 years, 79% |
| Gotoh et al., 1997 | 31 | Dysplasia | Valgus–extension | 43 years (22 to 59 years) | Advanced | 12 to 18 years | Survival: 15 years, 51% |
| Iwase et al., 1996 | 42 | Dysplasia | Varus | 25 years | Mild | 20 years | Survival: 10 years, 89%; 15 years, 87% |
| Jingushi et al., 2002 | 70 | Dysplasia | Valgus | 44 years (14 to 59 years) | Advanced | 2 to 15 years | Survival: 10 years, 82% |
| Kubo et al., 2000 | 17 | Dysplasia | Valgus–extension | 50 years (34 to 58 years) | Advanced | 10 to 14 years | 18% had good results at final follow up |
| Iwase et al., 1996 | 58 | Dysplasia | Valgus | 37 years | Moderate to advanced | 20 years | Survival: 10 years, 66%; 15 years, 38% |
| Maistrelli et al., 1990 | 277 | All | Valgus–extension | 52 years (26 to 66 years) | Mild to advanced | 11 to 15 years | 67% had perfect to good results, with better results seen among young patients with secondary osteoarthritis |

Alternatively, only a few of these studies showed survival rates that were identical or superior to those of total hip replacement and then only in selected patient groups. In a recent long-term follow up study, we demonstrated that, for specific hip disorders, intertrochanteric osteotomies can achieve good to excellent long-term results. Several recent reviews advocated the idea that intertrochanteric osteotomies should be kept in mind as a treatment option for these selected cases.

In the modern treatment regimens of osteoarthritis of the hip, THA is the treatment of choice for the elderly patient. During the past few decades, this age limit has gradually been adjusted downward. Even so, the question remains whether a THA is the best solution for a young patient with a mild secondary osteoarthritis. For patients with idiopathic osteoarthritis or rheumatic arthritis, no benefit from joint-saving surgery can be expected. However, for the treatment of coxa valga (antetorta) and dysplasia and for patients who have experienced SCFE, Legg-Calvé-Perthes disease, or traumatic deformities, intertrochanteric osteotomies can provide good and long-lasting results. Although these disorders could all be excellently treated with hip replacement, joint-saving surgery should be the treatment of choice for these young patients, because multiple revisions of the hip replacement are inevitable for patients with a life expectancy of more than 40 years.

An argument brought up by the opponents of intertrochanteric osteotomies that seems to linger is that the results of a subsequent THA after a previous osteotomy shows poorer results. Several case-control long-term follow up studies demonstrated that this idea was not true for both cemented and uncemented hip prostheses.

## COMPLICATIONS

In addition to standard postoperative complications, specific complications can occur with this procedure. The complication that is most feared with total hip replacement is deep infection. This can also occur after an osteotomy, but the result is generally less disastrous. Although this is a very difficult complication to treat, the patient's own hip joint remains intact.

Potential specific complications are AVN, nonunion, overcorrection, and undercorrection. All of these can be avoided with the use of good preoperative surgical planning and good surgical technique. Special attention should be paid to the placement of the seating chisel to avoid damage to the arterial supply of the femoral head and to avoid AVN. The occurrence of nonunion can be greatly reduced with the use of the AO compression device.

## ANNOTATED REFERENCES AND SUGGESTED READINGS

D'Souza SR, Sadiq S, New AM, Northmore-Ball MD. Proximal femoral osteotomy as the primary operation for young adults who have osteoarthrosis of the hip. *J Bone Joint Surg Am.* 1998 Oct;80(10):1428–1438.

Eijer H, Myers SR, Ganz R. Anterior femoroacetabular impingement after femoral neck fractures. *J Orthop Trauma.* 2001;15:475–481.

Describes the test of passively forcing the femoral neck against the acetabular rim in flexion, adduction, and internal rotation (Fladdir) for diagnosing anterior femoral acetabular impingement after femoral neck fractures as a cause for persisting groin pain.

Ganz R, Parvizi J, Beck M, Leunig M, Notzli H, Siebenrock KA. Femoroacetabular impingement: a cause for osteoarthritis of the hip. *Clin Orthop Relat Res.* 2003;417:112–120.

This is one of the articles that shows that femoroacetabular impingement is a cause for early osteoarthritis. Based on their large patient population who underwent a surgical hip dislocation, they showed that many of the so-called idiopathic OA were in fact caused by femoroacetabular impingement.

Girdlestone GR. Discussion on the late results of operation for chronic painful hip. *Proc R Soc Med.* 1926;19(Sect Orthop):48–49.

Gotoh E, Inao S, Okamoto T, Ando M. Valgus-extension osteotomy for advanced osteoarthritis in dysplastic hips. Results at 12 to 18 years. *J Bone Joint Surg Br.* 1997 Jul;79(4):609–615.

Haverkamp D, de Jong PT, Marti RK. Intertrochanteric osteotomies do not impair long-term outcome of subsequent cemented total hip arthroplasties. *Clin Orthop Relat Res.* 2006 Mar;444:154–160.

The common opinion that osteotomies impair the outcome of subsequent THA is proven incorrect by this long-term follow-up with matched control group.

Haverkamp D, Eijer H, Patt TW, Marti RK. Multidirectional intertrochanteric osteotomy for primary and secondary osteoarthritis—results after 15 to 29 years. *Int Orthop.* 2006 Feb;30(1):15–20.

This long-term follow up study shows which conditions and what kinds of patients are good candidates for femoral osteotomies.

Haverkamp D, Marti RK. Intertrochanteric osteotomy combined with acetabular shelfplasty in young patients with severe deformity of the femoral head and secondary osteoarthritis. A long-term follow-up study. *J Bone Joint Surg Br.* 2005;87:25–31.

This study describes the technique of valgus osteotomies in acquired femoral head deformities, combined with acetabular shelf plasty.

Iwase T, Hasegawa Y, Kawamoto K, Iwasada S, Yamada K, Iwata H. Twenty years' followup of intertrochanteric osteotomy for treatment of the dysplastic hip. *Clin Orthop Relat Res.* 1996 Oct;(331)245–255.

Jacobs MA, Hungerford DS, Krackow KA. Intertrochanteric osteotomy for avascular necrosis of the femoral head. *J Bone Joint Surg Br.* 1989;71:200–204.

The indication for intertrochanteric osteotomies in AVN is described combined with results.

Jingushi S, Sugioka Y, Noguchi Y, Miura H, Iwamoto Y. Transtrochanteric valgus osteotomy for the treatment of osteoarthritis of the hip secondary to acetabular dysplasia. *J Bone Joint Surg Br.* 2002 May;84(4):535–539.

Kubo T, Fujioka M, Yamazoe S, Ueshima K, Inoue S, Horii M, Ando K, Imai R, Hirasawa Y. Bombelli's valgus-extension osteotomy for osteoarthritis due to acetabular dysplasia: results at 10 to 14 years. *J Orthop Sci.* 2000;5(5):457–462.

Leunig M, Beck M, Dora C, Ganz R. Femoroacetabular impingement: trigger for the development of osteoarthritis. *Orthopade.* 2006;35:77–84.

In this article more evidence is provided for the theory that early OA is often caused by femoroacetabular impingement.

Maistrelli GL, Gerundini M, Fusco U, Bombelli R, Bombelli M, Avai A. Valgus-extension osteotomy for osteoarthritis of the hip. Indications and long-term results. *J Bone Joint Surg Br.* 1990 Jul;72(4):653–657.

Marti RK, Chaldecott LR, Kloen P. Intertrochanteric osteotomy for posttraumatic arthritis after acetabular fractures. *J Orthop Trauma.* 2001;15:384–393.

One of the less known indications for femoral osteotomies is described here, being posttraumatic OA after acetabular fractures.

Marti RK, ten Holder EJ, Kloen P. Lengthening osteotomy at the intertrochanteric level with simultaneous correction of angular deformities. *Int Orthop.* 2001;25:355–359.

Many posttraumatic deformities also require lengthening. The technique to combine lengthening at the intertrochanteric level, combined with other corrections, is described in the article.

**McMurray TP. Osteo-arthritis of the hip joint. 1939.** *Clin Orthop Relat Res.* **1990 Dec;261:3–10.**

**Millis MB, Kim YJ. Rationale of osteotomy and related procedures for hip preservation: a review.** *Clin Orthop.* **2002;405:108–121.**

This review nicely summarizes the indications were hip preservative surgery could give satisfactory results.

**Muller ME. Intertrochanteric osteotomy: indication, preoperative planning, technique. In: Schatzker J, ed.** *The intertrochanteric osteotomy.* **Berlin: Springer-Verlag; 1984:25–66.**

Historically the book that everyone performing osteotomies should have read.

**Pauwels F. Biomechanics of the normal and diseased hip.** *Theoretical foundation, technique and results of treatment: an atlas.* **Berlin: Springer-Verlag; 1976.**

Pauwels describes in his book the biomechanical principles behind the osteotomies, a book that every hip surgeon should have read.

**Pecasse GA, Eijer H, Haverkamp D, Marti RK. Intertrochanteric osteotomy in young adults for sequelae of Legg-Calve-Perthes' disease—a long-term follow-up.** *Int Orthop.* **2004;28:44–47.**

The special deformities in post Perthes patients, being a large aspherical femoral head with often an impingement caused by incongruency between the acetabulum and the femoral head is discussed here.

**Perlau R, Wilson MG, Poss R. Isolated proximal femoral osteotomy for treatment of residua of congenital dysplasia or idiopathic osteoarthrosis of the hip. Five- to ten-year results.** *J Bone Joint Surg Am.* **1996 Oct;78(10):1462–1467.**

**Reigstad A, Grønmark T. Osteoarthritis of the hip treated by intertrochanteric osteotomy. A long-term follow-up.** *J Bone Joint Surg Am.* **1984 Jan;66(1):1–6.**

**Santore RF, Kantor SR. Intertrochanteric femoral osteotomies for developmental and posttraumatic conditions.** *Instr Course Lect.* **2005;54:157–167.**

This instructional course lecture gives a good summary of the current knowledge.

**Sugioka Y. Transtrochanteric anterior rotational osteotomy of the femoral head in the treatment of osteonecrosis affecting the hip: a new osteotomy operation.** *Clin Orthop Relat Res.* **1978 Jan-Feb;(130):191–201.**

**Toyama H, Endo N, Sofue M, Dohmae Y, Takahashi HE. Relief from pain after Bombelli's valgus-extension osteotomy, and effectiveness of the combined shelf operation.** *J Orthop Sci.* **2000;5(2):114–123.**

**Turgeon TR, Phillips W, Kantor SR, Santor RF. The role of acetabular and femoral osteotomies in reconstructive surgery of the hip: 2005 and beyond.** *Clin Orthop Relat Res.* **2005;441;188–199.**

Besides a review and a summary of the indications, the emphasis of this article is that there is still a greater role to play for hip preservative surgery.

**Voss C. Coxarthrosis; the temporary hanging hip, a new procedure for operative treatment of painful hip in the aged and other chronic deforming diseases of the hip.** *Munch Med Wochenschr.* **1956 Jul 13;98(28):954–956.**

**Watson-Jones R, Robinson WC. Arthrodesis of the osteoarthritic hip.** *J Bone Joint Surg Br.* **1956 Feb;38-B(1):353–377.**

# CHAPTER 33

# Open Treatment for Hip Cartilage Injuries

*Michael K. Shindle, Dean G. Lorich, Robert L. Buly, and Bryan T. Kelly*

## INTRODUCTION

Articular cartilage injuries of the hip are one of the most challenging orthopedic injuries to treat, and they have received considerably less attention as compared with other joints. Before the advent of cartilage-sensitive magnetic resonance imaging, hip pain in a young patient was typically diagnosed as early arthritis, and it resulted in progressive generalized joint deterioration (e.g., osteoarthritis, rheumatoid arthritis).

Nonarthritic cartilage injuries in the hip refer to focal chondral defects on either the acetabular or femoral side of the joint. Focal chondral defects on the femoral head are relatively uncommon and may result from shear injury or the axial loading of the head within the socket. Traumatic instability from either a hip dislocation or subluxation, as occurs during high-energy contact sports or motor vehicle accidents, may result in these types of focal chondral injuries. Another mechanism of injury includes a lateral impact injury in which there is loading at the greater trochanter in association with a high-energy activity. The subcutaneous location of the greater trochanter limits its ability to absorb large forces. Thus, an impact on this area can transfer a significant amount of energy and load to the hip joint surfaces, thereby resulting in chondral lesions of the femoral head or acetabulum without associated osseous injury. In addition to trauma, other mechanisms that can cause focal chondral lesions of the femoral head include osteonecrosis, underlying bony deformity, and dysplastic conditions.

In a patient with osteonecrosis, the articular cartilage injury of the femoral head is a result of the loss of structural integrity of the subchondral bone. The degree of chondral pathology depends on the extent of the collapse of the underlying subchondral bone. The spectrum of cartilaginous lesions associated with osteonecrosis is wide and may range from mild chondromalacia to severe chondral fractures with complete collapse.

Anatomic abnormalities such as congenital hip disease (e.g., Legg-Calvé-Perthes disease, dysplasia) or slipped capital femoral epiphysis can lead to cartilage lesions of the femoral head. Acute chondrolysis may occur after slipped capital femoral epiphysis, and narrowing of the joint space may occur as early as 1 year after the acute slip injury.

The grade and character of the cartilage lesions depend on the mechanism of injury and the stage at which the lesion is detected. Lesions can be classified as shear injuries, delamination, fissuring, chondral flaps, fractures, and punch or impaction injuries. As these lesions progress to an advanced-stage degenerative condition, they often lose their specific characteristics.

Cartilage injuries on the acetabulum are more common and typically present as localized cartilage delamination defects in the anterosuperior weight-bearing zone of the acetabular rim. The cause of these defects is most commonly femoroacetabular impingement, which will be discussed in chapter 28.

## BASIC SCIENCE

The normal thickness of articular cartilage ranges from 2 mm to 5 mm, and it is determined by the contact pressures that occur across a joint. The articular cartilage of the femoral head is thickest on the central and medial surfaces, which corresponds with the loading pattern of the hip joint. The majority of the femoral head chondral surface is involved in load transfer across the joint, which makes the area particularly vulnerable to injury.

Even with minor trauma, cartilage injury may occur, and chondrocyte death has been reported to occur at 20% to 30% of strain of the articular cartilage specimens. Injured cartilage that loses it congruity by fragmentation, indentation, or a crush injury results in a loss of joint function and progressive joint deterioration. Animal models suggest that large, full-thickness osteochondral defects will undergo degenerative changes around the rim of the defect, which can progress to global joint degradation in as little as 1 year. Finite-element models of osteochondral damage have also predicted a similar progression, because compressive strains reach maximum values around the rim of a defect, and the compressive strain values increase concomitantly as the defects become larger.

## INDICATIONS

Patients with continued pain despite conservative treatment (e.g., activity modification, weight reduction, physical therapy, bracing, medications), who have imaging that is consistent with cartilage defects, and who demonstrate a positive response to an intra-articular injection are candidates for surgical intervention. Larger cartilage defects may be amenable to cartilage resurfacing procedures such as autogenous osteochondral transfer or fresh or fresh-frozen allograft femoral head transplants.

Conventional joint replacements have a long history of restoring function and relieving pain among patients with arthritis. However, primary total hip arthroplasty procedures have high rates of failure in young (i.e., less than 40 years old) and early–middle-aged (i.e., 40 to 60 years old) patients. To preserve bone stock, partial resurfacing procedures that require a minimum amount of bone removal have been developed. Devices have been developed that only require the removal of the affected area of cartilage in an attempt to maintain the natural radius of the curvature of the femoral head.

## BRIEF HISTORY AND PHYSICAL EXAMINATION

In the young patient, hip pain is often characterized by nonspecific symptoms, vague clinical findings, and normal radiographs. Common causes of groin and hip pain among young patients include hip flexor tendonitis, adductor muscle pathology, osteitis pubis, and trochanteric bursitis. However, the goal of the history and physical examination is to narrow down the differential diagnosis to intra-articular pain, extra-articular pain, or central pubic pain associated with athletic pubalgia. The intra-articular nonarthritic pathology of the hip joint includes disorders of the labrum, the iliofemoral ligament, the ligamentum teres, and the chondral surfaces of the femoral head and the acetabulum.

Patients with an intra-articular cause of hip pain may present with pain in the anterior groin, the anterior thigh, the greater trochanter, the buttock, or the medial knee. Other symptoms may include catching, clicking, locking, giving way, or restricted range of motion. Symptoms may be insidious in onset, or they may be preceded by a traumatic event.

Physical examination should include an assessment of the patient's gait and posture as well as of his or her pelvic obliquity, limb-length inequality, muscle contractures, and scoliosis. The examination of the hip begins with the palpation of specific regions, but, if the pain is truly intra-articular, palpation does not typically cause pain. The active and passive range of motion of both hips should be performed with the patient in both the seated and supine positions. Mechanical symptoms that result from intra-articular pathology can be elicited by applying an axial load while performing an internal rotation of the hip or by having the patient perform a resisted leg raise while in the supine position.

## IMAGING AND DIAGNOSTIC STUDIES

The initial workup of a patient with a suspected hip injury should include a standing anteroposterior view of the pelvis, a cross-table lateral view, and false-profile views of both hips. The main purpose of radiographs is to evaluate for the presence of femoroacetabular impingement, joint space narrowing, or acetabular dysplasia. A variety of normal radiographic indices have been described to differentiate normal from abnormal bony anatomy and include the center-edge angle, the Tönnis angle, the neck-shaft angle, the anterior offset, and the crossover sign.

With appropriate pulse sequencing, magnetic resonance imaging has become the examination of choice for the evaluation of unexplained hip pain and for noninvasively evaluating articular cartilage. Some authors have advocated the use of magnetic resonance arthrography to improve the contrast between the cartilage and the synovial fluid; however, this technique converts magnetic resonance imaging into a more invasive procedure. Noncontrast imaging with an optimized protocol can identify labral and chondral abnormalities noninvasively. At our institution, a screening examination of the whole pelvis is performed with use of coronal inversion recovery and axial proton density sequences. Detailed hip imaging is obtained with the use of a surface coil over the hip joint, with high-resolution cartilage-sensitive images acquired in three planes (sagittal, coronal, and oblique axial) with the use of fast-spin-echo pulse sequences and an intermediate echo time.

Intra-articular injections are a reliable indicator of intra-articular problems in the hip joint and should be used as an adjunct to the diagnostic workup. Significant pain relief after an intra-articular injection provides strong evidence that the patient will respond favorably to the surgical management of focal chondral lesions.

## SURGICAL TECHNIQUE

Larger cartilage defects may be amenable to cartilage resurfacing procedures such as autogenous osteochondral transfer or fresh-frozen allograft femoral head transplants. Fresh osteochondral allograft has been shown to be a successful procedure for other weight-bearing joints in both acute and nonacute settings. The success of the allograft depends on the viability of the articular cartilage and the stability of the graft–bone–host bone interface. When placed into an optimal biomechanical environment and prepared properly, the allograft can successfully incorporate into native bone and cartilage. By contrast, the use of frozen grafts may not be as optimal, because the freezing process has been shown to kill chondrocytes and to limit graft survival. The possible risks of disease transmission and graft availability are issues that are relevant to the use of this treatment strategy. An open surgical dislocation is necessary to match allograft tissue with the patient's joint surface.

### Osteochondral Autograft Transfer

Osteochondral autograft transfer is a cartilage repair technique in which an osteochondral plug is transferred from an area of less contact pressure to the full-thickness focal chondral defect. There has been limited experience with autologous osteochondral transplantation in the hip, but early results have been encouraging. The donor site for this procedure can be the ipsilateral knee or the non–weight-bearing portion of the femoral head–neck junction.

With the use of an osteochondral autograft transfer system (OATS, Arthrex, Inc., Naples, FL), a guidewire is drilled perpendicular to the central portion of the cartilage defect of the femoral head after a surgical hip dislocation has been performed as described by Ganz and colleagues (Figure 33-1). Next, an appropriately sized flat acorn reamer is carried down to the subchondral bone over the guidewire. A recipient punch guide with a diameter that is large enough to encompass the chondral defect in its entirety is selected and tapped down to the subchondral surface of the femoral head. The depth of the osteochondral plug is then measured.

The donor site should be harvested from an area of less contact pressure. At our institution, for the treatment of focal chondral injuries of the femoral head, we have used the ipsilateral knee (i.e., the superolateral aspect of the lateral femoral condyle) as the donor site. With the use of a donor punch guide of the same diameter, the guide is malleted down to the same depth as the recipient plug, and the plug is removed. The donor osteochondral plug can be press fit into the recipient site and lightly impacted with a mallet until it is continuous with the surrounding articular cartilage of the femoral head (Figure 33-2). Multiple plugs may be necessary, depending on the size of the chondral defect (Figure 33-3).

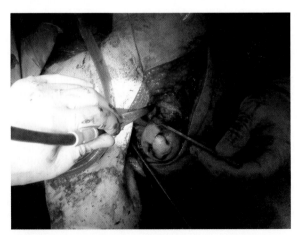

**Figure 33-1** A focal chondral defect of the femoral head after a surgical hip dislocation has been performed.

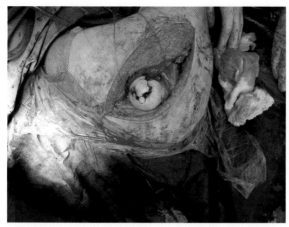

**Figure 33–2** A demonstration of the osteochondral autograft transfer system procedure with a single cylindrical core graft of articular cartilage and subchondral bone taken from non–weight-bearing regions of the knee (i.e., the donor site) and transplanted into the prepared holes within the defect (i.e., the recipient site).

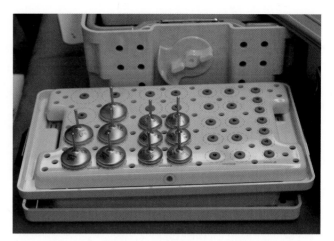

**Figure 33–4** The different articular surface caps that are available.

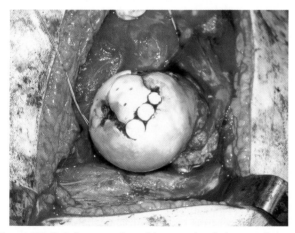

**Figure 33–3** A demonstration of the osteochondral autograft transfer system procedure, with multiple cylindrical grafts in place.

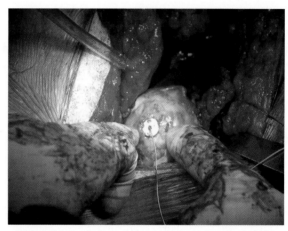

**Figure 33–5** A focal chondral defect of the femoral head has been identified and marked.

### Arthrosurface HemiCAP

The Arthrosurface HemiCAP (Arthrosurface, Inc., Franklin, MA) was designed to treat articular surface defects with an implant that can match the surface and contour of the femoral head (Figure 33-4). The device consists of a titanium fixation screw and a cap-like implant made from a cobalt chrome alloy with a central post on its underside. A surgical hip dislocation is performed as previously described by Ganz and colleagues. The diameter of the defect is measured, and a guidewire is introduced

into the middle of the defect (Figure 33-5). The fixation component is used as a central axis, and reamers are then used to map the contours of the patient's articular cartilage defect (Figure 33-6, *A* and *B*). After the surface is prepared, the articular cap implant is seated into position (Figure 33-7, *A* and *B*).

## POSTOPERATIVE REHABILITATION

As a general guideline, postoperative rehabilitation after a surgical dislocation of the hip for a partial resurfacing procedure or a chondral transplant is much lengthier as compared with an arthroscopic hip procedure. Patients are usually hospitalized for

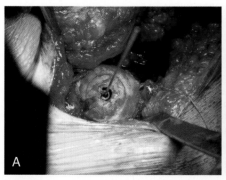

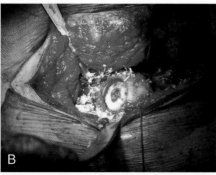

**Figures 33–6** **A** and **B**, Reamers are used to precontour the articular surface to accept the articular cap.

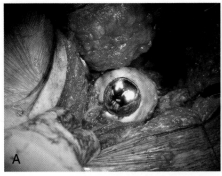
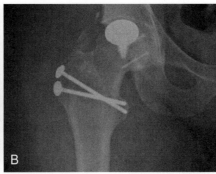

**Figures 33–7 A,** The final positioning of the arthrosurface articular component adjacent to the surrounding articular cartilage. **B,** Postoperative plain films that demonstrate the adequate positioning of the implant.

5 to 7 days, and they do not bear weight for 12 weeks to avoid the nonunion of the trochanteric flip osteotomy site. Isometric quadriceps contractions and early hip motion are encouraged. A return to full activity usually occurs between 6 and 12 months postoperatively.

TECHNICAL PEARLS

- During the surgical dislocation, meticulous dissection in combination with excellent hemostasis will decrease the incidence of heterotopic ossification. For the OATS procedure, careful surgical planning from the donor site is necessary for the more accurate recreation of the femoral head geometry. The use of precise OATS instrumentation is required.
- During the arthrosurface procedure, the center of the osteochondral lesion has to be precisely identified. The guide pin has to be inserted into the center of the osteochondral defect perfectly perpendicular to the defect; when drilling occurs, this will allow for the best restoration of the articular geometry. In addition, during the tapping portion of the procedure, sclerotic bone is commonly encountered, which may cause instrument breakage. After the screw is inserted, precise measurements need to be taken in four quadrants to allow for accurate implant selection. The largest standard-diameter prosthesis is 35 mm, so careful planning is necessary to determine whether a larger custom prosthesis is necessary.

## RESULTS AND OUTCOMES

Siguier and colleagues reported about their results with the use of the MS prosthesis (Tornier, Saint-Ismier, France) for osteonecrosis of the femoral head. Thirty-seven procedures were performed, and there was an average follow up time of 49 months. The average age of the patients was 43 years, and the preoperative Ficat classification was stage III in 26 hips, stage IV in 10 hips, and stage II in 1 hip. There were nine failed procedures that were related to the extension of the osteonecrosis. Of the 28 surviving implants, 24 patients had excellent or good hip scores according to the Merle d'Aubigné system.

## COMPLICATIONS

Although these treatments have been used clinically for more than 5 years, there is a notable absence of comparative studies and long-term outcome information. Siguier and colleagues reported about 37 partial surface replacements for osteonecrosis; there were nine failures that were mainly attributable to the extension of the osteonecrosis. The failures were treated with total hip arthroplasty. However, there were no immediate postoperative general or surgical complications.

Both procedures have complications related to the surgical hip dislocation, including the nonunion of the osteotomy site, heterotopic ossification between the gluteus minimus and the capsule, and blood clots. During the OATS procedure, complications may include a lack of incorporation of the osteochondral plugs, difficulty with restoring the normal congruity of the femoral head, and donor site pain from the superolateral aspect of the knee.

During the arthrosurface procedure, complications may include the inability to reestablish the normal congruence of the femoral head, persistent pain caused by cartilage degeneration along the acetabular side as a result of metallic irritation, the progressive collapse in the presence of osteonecrosis, and the progressive degeneration of the surrounding cartilage that leads to osteoarthritis.

## CONCLUSIONS

As a result of increased awareness and the advent of magnetic resonance imaging cartilage-sensitive pulse sequences, focal chondral injuries of the hip are becoming increasingly recognized as occult sources of hip pain that may be amenable to a variety of different surgical interventions. Focal chondral lesions of the femoral head are usually caused by direct traumatic events, whereas cartilage delamination injuries on the acetabular rim are more commonly caused by femoroacetabular impingement. Appropriate management depends on the location and size of the lesion as well as a number of patient factors, including symptoms, age, activity level, and the patient's ability to comply with postoperative rehabilitation.

The OATS and arthrosurface techniques that are discussed in this chapter are relatively new and continue to evolve. In the short term, patients have symptomatic improvement, but long-term follow up is necessary. As we develop a better understanding of the relevant disease processes, biologic solutions should be implemented in an attempt to alter the natural progression of cartilage degeneration.

## ANNOTATED REFERENCES

Byrd JW. Lateral impact injury. A source of occult hip pathology. *Clin Sports Med.* **2001;20:801–815.**

This article describes a lateral impact injury that results in an isolated traumatic chondral injury that can occur as a result of impact loading over the greater trochanter. Arthroscopy can be a valuable tool for both the assessment and management of chondral injuries.

Byrd JW, Jones KS. Diagnostic accuracy of clinical assessment, magnetic resonance imaging, magnetic resonance arthrography, and intra-articular injection in hip arthroscopy patients. *Am J Sports Med.* **2004;32:1668–1672.**

This retrospective review of 40 patients with hip pain included clinical assessment, high-resolution magnetic resonance imaging, magnetic resonance arthrography with gadolinium, intra-articular bupivacaine injection, and arthroscopy. The parameters were assessed for reliability with the use of arthroscopy for the definitive diagnosis. Response to an intra-articular injection of anesthetic was a 90%-reliable indicator of an intra-articular abnormality.

**Ganze R, Gill TJ, Gautier E, et al. Surgical dislocation of the adult hip: a technique with full access to the femoral head and acetabulum without the risk of avascular necrosis. *J Bone Joint Surg*. 2001;83B:1119–1124.**

The surgical treatment of femoroacetabular impingement focuses on improving clearance for hip motion and alleviating femoral abutment against the acetabular rim. This article describes the principles of a surgical dislocation of the hip.

**Gardner MJ, Suk M, Pearle A, Buly RL, Helfet DL, Lorich DG. Surgical dislocation of the hip for fractures of the femoral head. *J Orthop Trauma*. 2005;19:334–342.**

This article describes a surgical dislocation of the hip to provide superior visualization and fracture stabilization for the treatment of a femoral head fracture.

**Lavigne M, Parvizi J, Beck M, Siebenrock KA, Ganz R, Leunig M. Anterior femoroacetabular impingement: part I. Techniques of joint preserving surgery. *Clin Orthop Relat Res*. 2004;418:61–66.**

This article reviews open surgical treatment options for cam and pincer impingement.

**Shindle MK, Foo LF, Kelly BT, et al. Magnetic resonance imaging of cartilage in the athlete: current techniques and spectrum of disease. *J Bone Joint Surg Am*. 2006;88:27–46.**

This article reviews the basic science of articular cartilage and reviews different pulse sequences and terminology related to cartilage-sensitive magnetic resonance imaging.

**Shindle MK, Ranawat AS, Kelly BT. Diagnosis and management of traumatic and atraumatic hip instability in the athletic patient. *Clin Sports Med*. 2006;25:309–326.**

Hip instability can be considered either traumatic or atraumatic in nature. The spectrum of hip instability ranges from subluxation to dislocation with or without concomitant injuries. This review article discusses the treatment algorithm for traumatic instability.

**Siguier M, Judet T, Siguier T, Charnley G, Brumpt B, Yugue I. Preliminary results of partial surface replacement of the femoral head in osteonecrosis. *J Arthroplasty*. 1999;14:45–51.**

This study reported the initial results of the use of partial surface replacement for osteonecrosis of the femoral head. Twenty-five patients with prostheses were followed for a mean of 43 months. Overall, 78.9% of patients who retained the component had excellent or good hip scores according to the Merle d'Aubigné system, and there were six failures that led to total hip arthroplasty.

**Siguier T, Siguier M, Judet T, Charnley G, Brumpt B. Partial resurfacing arthroplasty of the femoral head in avascular necrosis. Methods, indications, and results. *CORR*. 2001; 386:85–92.**

This study reports about the results of the use of a partial surface replacement for the treatment of osteonecrosis of the femoral head. Thirty-seven patients were followed for a mean of 49 months. Overall, 85.7% of patients who retained the component had excellent or good hip scores according to the Merle d'Aubigné system, and there were nine failures that led to total hip arthroplasty.

# CHAPTER 34

# Anterior Hueter Approach for Hip Resurfacing in the Arthritic Patient

*Benoit Benoit and Paul E. Beaulé*

## INTRODUCTION

Metal-on-metal hip resurfacing arthroplasty has re-emerged as a viable alternative to traditional total hip arthroplasty for selected patients. Improvements in design technology and in the metallurgy of metal-on-metal bearings have helped solve many of the problems associated with the first generation of metal-on-polyethylene hip resurfacing, such as massive bone loss with cemented acetabular components and high wear rates associated with larger femoral head sizes. Current hip resurfacing systems make use of a hybrid design, with a press-fit acetabular component and a cemented femoral component. Early and midterm results have been favorable and comparable with traditional total hip arthroplasty, although femoral neck fractures continue to be a concern, with osteonecrosis as a leading cause.

The most commonly used approach for hip resurfacing is the posterior approach. This is an extensile approach that provides excellent visualization of the acetabulum as well as of the posterosuperior femoral head–neck junction. However, it has been well documented that the blood flow to the femoral head is compromised, thus putting the area at risk for an osteonecrotic event. Other approaches that are currently being used are the direct lateral approach, surgical dislocation as described by Ganz, and the anterior Hueter approach, each of which preserves the extraosseous blood supply to the femoral head. Since 2006, we have adopted the anterior Hueter approach with the use of an orthopedic traction table, because it represents the only true internervous surgical approach to the hip, with excellent preservation of the soft-tissue envelope.

## INDICATIONS

- Young patients
  - Men less than 65 years old
  - Women less than 55 years old
- High activity level
- Likely to require a revision procedure later in life
- Extra-articular deformity of the proximal femur that makes the insertion of a traditional hip stem difficult

## RELATIVE CONTRAINDICATIONS

- Leg-length discrepancy of more than 2 cm
- Severe deformity of the proximal femur: a high-riding greater trochanter with a short femoral neck
- Surface Arthroplasty Risk Index of more than 3
- Inflammatory arthropathies
- Women of childbearing age
- Known metal hypersensitivity

## ABSOLUTE CONTRAINDICATIONS

- Compromised renal function
- Atrophic femoral head

## CLINICAL HISTORY

The clinical history of advanced hip arthritis is straightforward, especially for younger patients with no other source of distracting pain (e.g., back pain). Intra-articular hip pain is typically reproducible and felt in the groin area with activity.

## PHYSICAL EXAMINATION

The goal of the physical examination is to confirm the clinical history. Pain in the groin area should be reproduced by passively moving the hip joint, which is usually limited with regard to flexion and internal rotation. If the patient has no groin pain with flexion, adduction, and internal rotation, other causes (e.g., back, extra-articular hip pathology) must be sought. True and functional leg-length discrepancies should be carefully assessed.

## IMAGING AND DIAGNOSTIC STUDIES

Our hip series for evaluating the patient with osteoarthritis of the hip includes a supine anteroposterior pelvic view that is centered on the hips and that shows the proximal femur down to the diaphysis as well as cross-table lateral views, Dunn views, or both (Figure 34-1). These two radiographs are scrutinized to analyze for structural abnormalities (e.g., insufficient femoral head–neck offset), the integrity of the joint space, and periarticular bone. In the rare case of a patient with radiographic osteoarthritis of the hip joint without a typical clinical history or physical examination, we perform an intra-articular anesthetic injection to determine whether the patient's symptoms are a result of the radiographic hip degeneration.

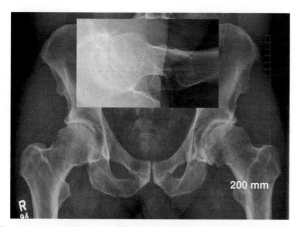

**Figure 34–1** A 42-year-old patient with advanced left hip osteoarthritis. The inset is a cross-table lateral view that assesses the femoral head–neck offset.

## SURGICAL TECHNIQUE

Although the anterior Hueter approach can be performed without a special surgical table, our main experience is with the use of a specialty orthopedic traction table (Figure 34-2). We do not exclude patients on the basis of body mass index or underlying deformity.

### Patient Positioning (Figure 34-3)

The patient is placed supine on the operative table. The operative leg is placed into a leg-holding device that allows for controlled positioning in three dimensions during surgery. The leg is not draped free but rather attached to the foot holder to allow for traction, internal and external rotation, flexion, extension, abduction, and adduction. Slight internal rotation of the operative leg allows for the better surface delimitation of the interval between the tensor of the fascia lata and the sartorius. The contralateral lower limb is set in 15 degrees of internal rotation and in neutral flexion, extension, abduction, and adduction; it is also placed under tension to serve as a radiographic control for the operated side.

### Exposure

The incision is placed 1 cm to 2 cm posterolateral and 2 cm distal to the anterosuperior iliac spine. The incision is extended distally and posterolaterally toward a line that connects to the

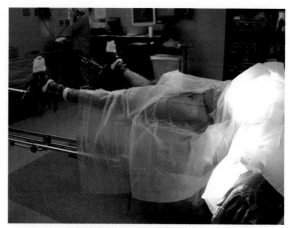

**Figure 34–3** The patient in the supine position. The incision is centered at the tip of the greater trochanter; it is 2 cm to 3 cm longer than the incision that is used when performing a total hip replacement.

fibular head for a total of 6 cm to 10 cm. The subcutaneous tissue is divided with the use of electrocautery until the aponeurosis of the tensor of the fascia lata is identified. The latter is incised longitudinally with a No. 10 blade, with all muscle fibers preserved. Blunt finger dissection is then performed between the medial aspect of the muscle belly (which can sometimes be bipennate) and the aponeurosis. At this point, retractors are placed in between the muscle and its sheath to expose the rectus femoris and the fat that overlies the hip capsule. With the use of electrocautery, this fat is removed to expose the capsule. After incising the fascia over the rectus femoris, blunt dissection is performed to expose the lateral circumflex vessels, which are then ligated and cut. These vessels can bleed briskly, and they deserve attention. Some of the lateral aspects of the rectus femoris and the iliocapsularis muscle can be elevated to maximize the exposure of the hip capsule. It is recommended to release the reflected head of the rectus femoris to facilitate the exposure of the acetabulum. At this point, the capsulotomy is performed with the use of electrocautery from inferomedial to superolateral, and a second transverse capsular incision is made from inferomedial to lateral, leaving a laterally based capsular flap attached to the proximal femur. In some cases, it is preferable to excise the lateral capsular flap to facilitate the delivery of the proximal femur (Figure 34-4). A large cobra retractor is then placed around the proximal femur to retract the tensor muscle laterally, and a blunt Hohmann retractor is placed at the inferomedial femoral neck.

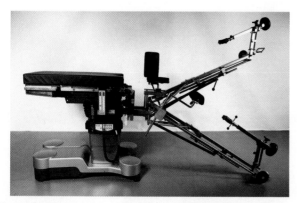

**Figure 34–2** An orthopedic traction table (Delacroix Device, Maquet-Dynamed, Paris, France) used for anterior-approach total hip arthroplasty. Note the capacity to extend the operated limb with the patient in the supine position.

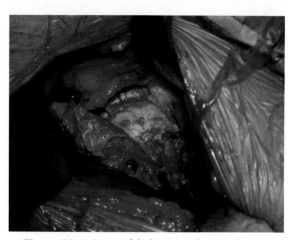

**Figure 34–4** A view of the hip joint after capsulotomy.

## Hip Dislocation

Slight traction is applied to the foot to create a gap between the head and the acetabulum. Curved Mayo scissors are used to sacrifice the round ligament. A large Weber spoon is then inserted into the hip joint, and the traction is released. The hip is then externally rotated and dislocated by levering the Weber spoon on the anterior rim of the acetabulum. The unscrubbed assistant only provides assistance by permitting the external rotation of the limb without exerting any torque. Great care has to be taken with osteoporotic patients to not fracture the tibia or the ankle with forced external rotation at the foot. To prevent this, the scrubbed surgical assistant can help with dislocation by grasping the femoral condyles and applying additional rotation, thereby decreasing the torque applied to the distal extremity. After the head has been dislocated, 90 degrees of external rotation is obtained by tensioning the medial capsule. Curved Mayo scissors are used to complete the almost circumferential capsulotomy to allow for easy external rotation up to 180 degrees. In addition, the fascia of the tensor can be further released distally to facilitate the retraction of the tensor muscle.

## Femoral Head Preparation

A femoral neck elevator is placed medially on the neck and held by a scrubbed surgical assistant on the opposite side of the patient. A large cobra retractor is placed to gently retract the tensor of the fascia lata laterally. A pointed Hohmann retractor is applied superiorly under the greater trochanter, and the leg is then brought into extension without any traction. The leg is then further externally rotated to 180 degrees. In large male patients, it may be necessary to release the anterior portion of the tensor muscle off of the iliac crest. The femoral head is then sized with the use of femoral head gauges (Figure 34-5). A smooth pin is advanced through the femoral head and into the middle of the femoral neck in about 5 degrees to 10 degrees of valgus relative to the native femoral neck shaft angle, which usually ends up being about 140 degrees (Figure 34-6). A spin-around gauge that corresponds with the femoral implant size is used to ensure the clearance of the femoral head–neck junction. The gauge should hug the inferomedial neck and clear the anterior aspect of the neck. Proximal femur preparation can follow, with the reamers chosen in accordance with preoperative templating and intraoperative findings. We usually recommend starting at least one size

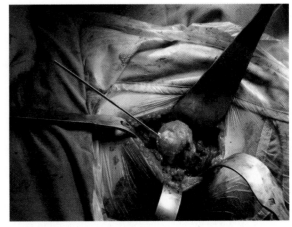

**Figure 34–6** A smooth pin positioned in the middle of the femoral neck or in a slight valgus orientation of 5 degrees to 10 degrees. The proper visualization of the superior head–neck junction may be difficult, but ensuring that the component will be along the inferomedial neck will avoid notching.

larger than the planned size and completing the first cylindrical reaming with osteotomes to provide overall better visualization for the final preparation. The final sequence of femoral head preparation will then vary from one manufacturer to another in terms of stem hole and chamber head (Figure 34-7). It is extremely important to ensure that the trial component can seat fully on the prepared femoral head; marking the endpoint where it should go may be useful.

## Acetabular Preparation

After the femoral head has been reamed definitively, the acetabulum is prepared in accordance with the size chosen on the femoral side. The retractors are taken out, no traction is applied, the rotation is freed up, and the leg is brought into neutral flexion and extension, which leaves the proximal femur to fall posterior to the socket. A long, pointed Hohmann retractor is first placed on the anteromedial lip of the acetabulum to retract the medial soft tissues away, and a second one is placed posteriorly, with the tip on the mid-posterior rim (Figure 34-8). A long knife is then used to debride the socket, and osteophytes are removed with a curved

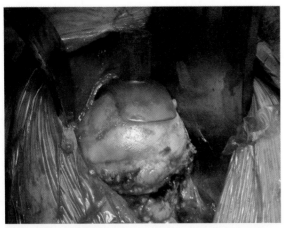

**Figure 34–5** The sizing of the femoral head with the use of a spherometer gauge (Wright Medical Technology, Memphis, TN) allows for the confirmation of the templating as well as the assessment of the head–neck offset anteriorly.

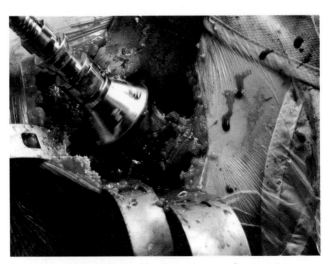

**Figure 34–7** Femoral head reaming according to sizing.

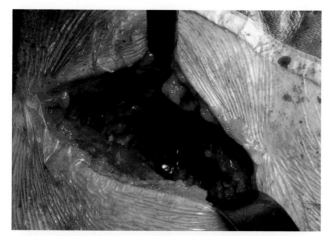

**Figure 34–8** Acetabular view after femur preparation. Performing a medial capsulotomy is critical to ensure proper visualization.

osteotome. Reaming commences with the use of tools that are three sizes smaller than those required for the planned definitive component. Offset reamer handles are critical. The reamers are usually brought in from a superior direction, slightly levering on the femoral neck. Attention is paid to maximize the bony contact between the reamers (Figure 34-9) and the bone, because most resurfacing shells do not have screw holes to supplement a poor press-fit fixation. To prevent soft-tissue damage, we suggest manually inserting and removing each reamer into and from the socket and to attach and detach the reamers to power in situ.

## Acetabular Cup Insertion

The tendency is to place the cup in a too-anteverted and vertical position because of soft-tissue interference with the cup inserter. Image intensification or intraoperative x-rays help to ensure proper component positioning. Cup positioning can be assessed by finger palpating the rim to see how closely it matches the see-through gauge. In the coronal plane (i.e., the acetabular component abduction angle), the guide rod should be parallel to a line drawn between the two anterosuperior iliac spines.

Acetabular version is then judged from the patient's longitudinal axis. After proper impaction, component stability is tested with a punch applied manually all around the cup's periphery to detect any movement. Any remaining overhanging osteophytes can be removed at this point with a curved osteotome to prevent impingement. We often leave some overhanging acetabular rim to minimize the irritation of the iliopsoas tendon. We aim for a cup abduction angle of 45 degrees, with 20 degrees of anteversion (Figure 34-10).

## Femoral Component Implantation

As described previously, the leg is carefully repositioned in extension and in 180 degrees of external rotation with a medially placed femoral neck elevator and a laterally placed large cobra retractor. The reverse Trendelenburg position can further facilitate proximal femur exposure. The femoral head is cleaned with pulsatile irrigation and dried with a metallic suction tip inserted into the stem hole. If areas of the head remain sclerotic, a size 3.5 drill bit is used create small drill holes for cement macroindentation. The cement is applied to all of the reamed femoral neck in a doughy state (i.e., after 3 to 4 minutes). If the cement is too liquid, overpenetration can occur, which will potentially create necrotic areas in the bone. The partially cement-filled femoral component is then impacted on the femoral neck to remove any excess cement. The hip is then carefully reduced with gentle traction and leg flexion. The hip joint is gently irrigated during the curing phase to minimize thermal necrosis. After cement hardening, the hip is examined under direct visualization for any soft-tissue interposition or subluxation. If a bony bump is present anterolaterally on the neck, it can be burred off to prevent impingement.

## Final Assessment and Closure

We routinely perform an intraoperative anteroposterior pelvic radiograph to confirm proper implant positioning before closure. Hip stability and impingement can be assessed by performing external rotation for anterior stability and by removing the boot from the leg holder and bringing the hip into flexion, internal rotation, and adduction to test posterior stability; however, this is usually not an issue.

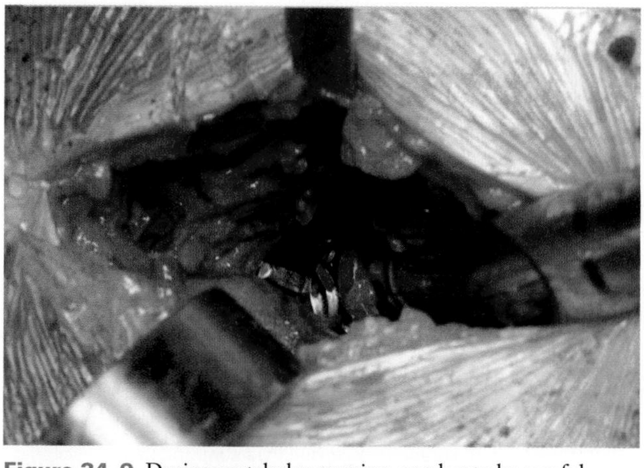

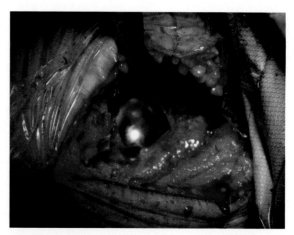

**Figure 34–10** Acetabular cup impaction to ensure the proper version and cup abduction angle. The version is referenced off of the floor and the abduction angle, with the guide being parallel to a line that joins the two anterosuperior iliac spines.

**Figure 34–9** During acetabular reaming, one has to be careful to not have the reamer handle being pushed anteriorly by the femoral neck, which could compromise the anterior wall.

## POSTOPERATIVE REHABILITATION

Patients typically leave the hospital on postoperative day 2. We let patients perform 50% weight bearing with crutches for 4 weeks to allow for femoral neck remodelling. In bilateral cases, we ask the patients to walk with the aid of a walker for the same period of time. Venous thromboembolism prophylaxis is given for 4 weeks. Transfer to a rehabilitation center is rarely necessary in the population of patients who have undergone resurfacing unless there are social issues. Outpatient physiotherapy is not prescribed routinely, because it has been shown to have no effect at 3 months postoperatively. We see every patient for follow up appointments at 6 weeks, 6 months, and then annually thereafter.

## CLINICAL RESULTS

To date, we have performed about 80 hip resurfacing procedures with the use of the anterior Hueter approach and an orthopedic traction table. Four patients have undergone bilateral procedures in the same setting. The mean age of the group is 48 years (range, 29 to 62 years) with the majority (more than 80%) being male (Figure 34-11). In terms of implant positioning, there was a tendency to have more acetabular components in the range of 45 degrees to 55 degrees of abduction, although none of the components was placed in more than 55 degrees of abduction. The femoral component has a tendency toward a slight valgus orientation and an anterior translation. Distally extending the skin incision for 1 cm or 2 cm can help to prevent the conflict between the cup impactor. The anterior translation of the femoral component is probably related to the more difficult access to the posterior femoral neck that occurs with the Hueter approach. Although we are still early in our experience, patients so far have demonstrated excellent recovery with minimal pain.

## COMPLICATIONS

We have noted that the majority of patients do complain of paresthesias of the anterolateral thigh as a result of injury of the lateral femoral cutaneous nerve. There have been no infections or deep venous thromboses in this group. No femoral neck fractures occurred in any patient in this study, and no complications were related to the orthopedic traction table. We have had one

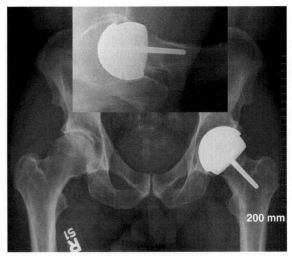

**Figure 34–11**  Postoperative radiography that demonstrates the optimal implant positioning of metal-on-metal hip resurfacing. (*Conserve Plus, Wright Medical Technology, Memphis, TN.*)

revision of an acetabular component as a result of an initial loss of fixation at 4 weeks. The patient was revised to a thick-shell acetabular component and maintained as a hip resurfacing.

## CONCLUSION

Despite the increasing popularity of resurfacing, most published reports are from implant designers or leading experts in hip resurfacing arthroplasty (Table 34-1). Further long-term studies of this implant as well as reports from independent centers and national registries will help to support generalized use in the orthopedic community. Early published results appear to indicate that hip resurfacing arthroplasty is a viable alternative to total hip arthroplasty for the young active adult. In terms of surgical approach selection, we would urge surgeons to start using the approach that they are most at ease with and to consider the anterior Hueter approach as a strong alternative to preserve femoral head vascularity and to facilitate recovery.

**Table 34–1** RESULTS SUMMARY OF HIP RESURFACING WITH NEW-GENERATION METAL-ON-METAL IMPLANTS

| Study | No. of Hips | Year | Male/ Female | Average Age | Average Weight | Survivorship | Pertinent Finding |
|---|---|---|---|---|---|---|---|
| Daniel et al | 446 | 2004 | 302/82 | 55 years | 81.8 kg | 99.8% at 3.3 years | One revision for ON |
| Treacy et al | 144 | 2005 | 107/37 | 52.1 years | N/A | 98% at 5 years | Two revisions for infection and one for neck fracture |
| Amstutz et al | 400 | 2004 | 259/96 | 48.2 years | 83.2 kg | 94.4% at 4 years | 14 revisions: 7 for femoral component loosening, 3 for fracture of the femoral neck, 1 for early acetabular pelvic protrusion, 1 for component mismatch, 1 for recurrent subluxation, and 1 for infection |
| Back et al | 230 | 2005 | 150/80 | 52.1 years | 80.62 kg | 99.14% at 3 years | One revision for cup loosening |
| DeSmet et al | 252 | 2005 | 176/76 | 49.7 years | 81.9 kg | 98.8% at 2.8 years | Mean follow up: 3 years; 3 failures: 1 neck fracture, 1 infection, 1 case of osteonecrosis of the femoral head |
| McMinn | 232 | 2005 | 147/61 | 53.3 years | Average body mass index: 25.9 | N/A | All surgeries performed via a minimally invasive posterior approach; this resulted in a shorter hospital stay, the same surgical time, less pain, faster recovery, and better cosmesis |

*ON*, osteonecrosis.

## ANNOTATED REFERENCES AND SUGGESTED READINGS

Amstutz HC, Beaulé PE, Dorey FJ, Le Duff MJ, Campbell PA, Gruen TA. **Metal-on-metal hybrid surface arthroplasty: two- to six-year follow-up study.** *J Bone Joint Surg Am.* 2004;86:28–39.

The metal-on-metal hybrid surface arthroplasty is easily revised to a standard femoral component if necessary.

Amstutz HC, Grigoris P, Dorey FJ. **Evolution and future of surface replacement of the hip.** *J Orthop Sci.* 1998;3:169–186.

The background research and better understanding of implant failure would suggest that hip resurfacing technology has now developed beyond that of an experimental procedure. Only long-term results and experience with this technology in the wider orthopedic community will give the answer as to whether the results will be durable or if hip resurfacing will simply become a bone-conserving intervention prior to conventional total hip replacement.

Back DL, Dalziel R, Young D, Shimmin A. **Early results of primary Birmingham hip resurfacings. An independent prospective study of the first 230 hips.** *J Bone Joint Surg.* 2005;87B(3):324–329.

Beaulé, PE, Campbell, P, Lu, Z, et al. **Vascularity of the arthritic femoral head and hip resurfacing.** *JBone Joint Surg* 2006;88A:85–96.

Beaulé PE, Dorey FJ, LeDuff MJ, Gruen T, Amstutz HC. **Risk factors affecting outcome of metal on metal surface arthroplasty of the hip.** *Clin Orthop.* 2004;418(418):87–93.

With surface arthroplasty risk index greater than 3 the relative risk of early problems is 12 times greater than if surface risk arthroplasty index is less or equal to 3.

Beaulé PE. **Surface arthroplasty of the hip: a review and current indications.** *Semin Arthroplasty.* 2005;16(1):70–76.

The understanding, diagnosis, and treatment of arthritic hip disease in young patients are rapidly evolving. A variety of new and refined surgical techniques are now being utilized worldwide, and continued progress in this realm of orthopedics is inevitable.

Buechel F, Drucker D, Jasty M, Jiranek W, Harris WH. **Osteolysis around uncemented acetabular components of cobalt-chrome surface replacement hip arthroplasty.** *Clin Orthop.* 1994;298:202–211.

Ten cases of major osteolysis were identified in patients with hemispherical cobalt chrome acetabular components of cementless resurfacing total hip prostheses at follow-up examinations ranging from 2 to 5 years.

Daniel J, Pynsent PB, McMinn DJ. **Metal-on-metal resurfacing arthroplasty of the hip in patients under the age of 55 years with osteoarthritis.** *J Bone Joint Surg Br.* 2004;86:177–184.

The extremely low rate of failure in spite of the resumption of high-level occupational and leisure activities provides early evidence of the suitability of this procedure for young and active patients with arthritis.

DeSmet KA. **Belgian experience with metal-on-metal surface arthoplasty.** *Orthop Clin North Am.* 2005;36:203–213.

In most cases, patients returned to a high functional level with no restrictions in their physical activity and were highly satisfied. Future refinements in surgical technique and instruments will make this procedure more accessible and reproducible for the surgeon.

Eastaugh-Waring SJ, Seenath S, Learmonth DS, Learmonth ID. **The practical limitations of resurfacing hip arthroplasty.** *J Arthroplasty.* 2006;21:18–22.

Reasons for unsuitability included collapse and/or cystic degeneration of the femoral head.

Howie D, Cornish B, Vernon-Roberts B. **Resurfacing hip arthroplasty. Classification of loosening and the role of prosthetic wear particle.** *Clin Orthop Rel Res.* 1990;255:144–159.

A clinical perspective is provided by the inclusion of the authors' recent observations of retrieval analyses of joint replacement implant wear and the tissue response to polyethylene in humans.

Kabo J, Gebhard J, Loren G, Amstutz H. **In vivo wear of polyethylene acetabular components.** *J Bone Joint Surg.* 1993;75B:254–258.

The volumetric wear rates were greatest for the surface-replacement components and for conventional components and were found to increase in a linear manner with component diameter.

McMinn DJ, Daniel J, Pynsent PB, Pradhan C. **Mini-incision resurfacing arthroplasty of hip trough the posterior approach.** *Clin Orthop Relat Res.* 2005;441:91–98.

Although the mini incision is indeed appealing, it has a steep learning curve. In the early phase of the learning curve, care should be taken to avoid suboptimal component placement, which has the potential to affect long-term outcome adversely.

Siguier T, Siguier M, Brumpt B. **Mini-incision anterior approach does not increase dislocation rate: a study of 1037 total hip replacements.** *Clin Orthop Rel Res.* 2004;426:164–173.

The mini-incision approach allows for adequate positioning of the two prosthetic components. Preserving the muscular potential also may contribute to dynamic stabilization of the hip.

Treacy RB, McBryde CW, Pynsent PB. **Birmingham hip resurfacing arthroplasty. A minimum follow-up of five years.** *J Bone Joint Surg Br.* 2005;87B(2):167–170.

This study confirms that hip resurfacing using a metal-on-metal bearing of known provenance can provide a solution in the medium term for the younger more active adult who requires surgical intervention for hip disease.

Treuting RJ, Waldman D, Hooten J, Schmalzried TP, Barrack RL. **Prohibitive failure rate of the total articular replacement arthoplasty at five to ten years.** *Am J Orthop.* 1997;26(2):114–118.

Seventy-five percent of the AOA attendees thought that surgical care is deficient, indicating a need for improved medical management in these patients.

# CHAPTER 35

# Total Hip Arthroplasty in the Young Active Patient With Arthritis

*Aditya V. Maheshwari, Amar S. Ranawat, and Chitranjan S. Ranawat*

## INTRODUCTION

The treatment of disabling hip pain as a result of degenerative joint disease in the young patient has many surgical options, the least palatable of which has traditionally been total hip arthroplasty (THA). The innate desire of the orthopedic surgeon to preserve the native hip joint in this population has led to the successful development of a variety of procedures, such as hip arthroscopy, surgical dislocation, and hip resurfacing. At the same time, the evolving technology and long-term success of THA have engendered increased confidence in the durability of this procedure and led to expanded indications.

Although indicating a young patient for THA is always disheartening, the good news is that patients can usually expect excellent pain relief and a high level of performance in a reproducible and predictable manner. Long-term results are tempered by wear-induced failures, which are a function of the increased number of loading cycles as a result of increased activity levels (Table 35-1) and increased life expectancies (Table 35-2). This data shows that there is a higher risk of failure in a younger patient during the subsequent 15 years after THA.

Sir John Charnley articulated this problem well: "The challenge comes when patients between 45 and 50 years of age are to be considered for the operation, because then every advance in technical detail must be used if there is to be a reasonable chance of 20 or more years of trouble free activity."

This chapter will discuss the inherent challenges involved when performing a THA in a young patient.

## INFORMED CONSENT

The process of obtaining informed consent from a young patient is, not unexpectedly, detailed and laborious. Multiple family members are frequently involved. Many questions will be asked, and tensions will usually be high. Quite often, the discussion is focused on the different alternative bearings and fixation options that are currently available. At the present time, the greatest challenge may be offering a balanced view of the risks and benefits of hip resurfacing. A detailed comparison of hip resurfacing with THA is beyond the scope of this chapter.

## INDICATIONS

Although young age was a relative contraindication during earlier days, the current indications for THA in young patients do not differ significantly from those of older patients. From 1969 to 1971, of the 2000 consecutive patients who underwent THA at the Mayo Clinic, only 187 (9.3%) were less than 50 years old. In the United Kingdom, this figure was even less than 1% (93 out of 10,469). According to a survey by Mancuso and colleagues in 1996, only 17% of surgeons were willing to perform a THA in young patients. However, with increased success, predictability, and experience with THA, the indications have been broadening. Although pain remains the primary indication for surgery, disability and reduced function associated with a painful and stiff hip are increasingly seen as indications for THA. The diagnosis pattern of the young arthritic hip is usually secondary arthritis caused by dysplasia, avascular necrosis, impingement, epiphysiolysis/Perthes disease, slipped capital femoral epiphysis, inflammatory conditions, or trauma.

## HISTORY AND PHYSICAL EXAMINATION

The patient history determines the source of the patient's symptoms, with the understanding that a wide spectrum of musculoskeletal and nonmusculoskeletal diseases can present with a chief complaint of hip pain. Detailed questioning is performed to clarify the character, location, duration, and severity of the symptoms; the resultant functional disability; and the realistic expectations of the patient. Concurrent spine pathology, ipsilateral knee disease, and a history of inflammatory arthritis should be investigated. A history of childhood or adolescent hip disease, previous hip surgery, hip trauma, risk factors for avascular necrosis, and current medical problems and medications should also be determined.

The physical examination includes the patient's general condition and body habitus. In general, large, muscular males are more likely to have difficulty with exposure than are obese patients. The posture and gait pattern are observed. Hip abductor function is assessed with the use of the Trendelenburg test and side-lying abduction strength testing. Functional and real limb-length discrepancy should be distinguished and quantified. While assessing the range of motion, it is important to steady the pelvis to appreciate the endpoint and the forced motion of the pelvis through the hip. The impingement test is

**Table 35–1** AGE AND ACTIVITY AFTER TOTAL HIP ARTHROPLASTY AND TOTAL KNEE ARTHROPLASTY (TKA)

| Age | Average No. of Steps per Day | Cycles per Year | *P* Value |
|---|---|---|---|
| Less than 60 years | 5933 | 1,082,773 | .02 |
| 60 years or more | 4434 | 809,205 | |

From Zahiri CA, Schmalzried TP, Szuszczewicz ES, Amstutz HC. Assessing activity in joint replacement patients. *J Arthroplasty.* 1998;13(8):890–895.

**Table 35–2** 15-YEAR SURVIVAL OF PATIENTS WITH TOTAL HIP ARTHROPLASTIES

| Age at Surgery | Percentage of Patients Still Alive | Percentage of Arthroplasties Still in Place |
|---|---|---|
| 45 years | 96% | 77% |
| 65 years | 72% | 92% |

From Berry DJ, Harmsen WS, Cabanela ME, Morrey BF. Twenty-five-year survivorship of two thousand consecutive primary Charnley total hip replacements: factors affecting survivorship of acetabular and femoral components. *J Bone Joint Surg Am.* 2002;84-A:171–177.

a very useful and sensitive test for any intra-articular pathology, and the McCarthy test can indicate labral pathology. It is also important is to evaluate the previous surgical interventions as well as the current neurovascular status of the limb.

## IMAGING AND DIAGNOSTIC STUDIES

We prefer to routinely obtain five radiographs for preoperative evaluation:
1) a low anteroposterior view of the pelvis with the proximal one third of the femur;
2) an anteroposterior view of the affected hip;
3) a false-profile view of the hip;
4) an anteroposterior view of the lumbosacral spine; and
5) a lateral view of the lumbosacral spine.

It is important to obtain the anteroposterior view of the pelvis with the hips internally rotated about 10 degrees to 15 degrees to calculate the offset accurately. Specific parameters to be assessed include the lateral center-edge angle, the anterior center-edge angle, the acetabular inclination and version, the sphericity of the femoral head, the head–neck offset, the alignment and morphology of the proximal femur, and the height of the greater trochanter. Adjunctive imaging studies are sometimes needed to evaluate and define the cause of symptoms; these include computed tomography scanning and magnetic resonance imaging. Sometimes a scanogram may be needed if the limb-length discrepancy is the result of extra-articular causes distally in the extremity (e.g., healed fractures in the distal femur or tibia).

## PREOPERATIVE TEMPLATING

Because these patients are usually healthy, the most important issue is usually preoperative planning. Careful consideration must be given to proximal femoral and acetabular deformities to

ensure the availability of modular implants. Preoperative radiographs are important when planning the type and the size of the prosthesis and when making decisions about the position and orientation of the components with the aim of restoring the biomechanics of the hip in terms of the center of rotation, the offset, and the limb length. In addition, the distance from the top of the lesser trochanter to the center of the femoral head is also measured, and every attempt is made to match this length with that of the normal side during surgery. It is crucial to consider the effect of magnification during these measurements.

The next step is to template the implants. In cases of unilateral hip disease, the goal is to match the opposite leg in terms of limb length and offset. Thus, the templating should be performed on the normal side, provided that the socket would reproduce the normal hip center. A template is made of the acetabulum for the approximate component size and position and to find out its effect on the center of rotation. The acetabular template is placed just lateral to the lateral edge of the teardrop at an angle of 40 degrees to 45 degrees. Ideally, the cup should be completely covered by bone, and it should span the distance between the teardrop and the superolateral margin of the acetabulum. In most cases, this will restore the anatomic center of rotation. Templating of the femoral canal is performed to determine the type and size of the component to be selected, its position relative to the lesser trochanter, the level of the neck osteotomy, and the selection of the head length to reproduce both leg length and femoral offset. The component size that best accomplishes this is chosen. All of the preoperative sizes for which templates have been made should be noted and correlated with the operative findings.

## ANESTHESIA AND SURGICAL TECHNIQUE

We prefer hypotensive regional anesthesia in the form of a single spinal shot. Regional anesthesia has shown advantages with respect to blood loss, deep vein thrombosis, postoperative pain management, and rehabilitation. We usually supplement the anesthesia with 1000 IU of intravenous heparin during femoral preparation to minimize the risk of deep vein thrombosis.

Patient positioning and its assessment before patient preparation and draping are crucial. The relative position of the knees and feet with symmetric flexion of the hips and knees can provide an idea about the starting leg-length relationship. Usually the superior side when the patient is in the lateral position would appear to be slightly shorter because of the adduction. Moreover, correct patient positioning is extremely important if external acetabular guides are used.

The choice of approach and the implant used are subjective and often geographic. Most surgeons in North America prefer cementless fixation, whereas cemented fixation is still popular in Europe. We use a posterolateral approach with the patient in a lateral position. We prefer a tapered wedge, a proximally hydroxyapatite (HA)-coated non-cemented femoral stem, and an HA-coated non-cemented acetabular cup. The choice of bearing surface is often discussed at length with the patient; in our practice, it is most often ceramic on highly cross-linked polyethylene or metal on metal. Ceramic-on-ceramic articulations have fallen out of favor in our practice as a result of their tendency to squeak.

We prepare the acetabulum first; some surgeons who use computer navigation prefer to prepare the femur first to have an idea of the femoral anteversion and to then adjust the combined anteversion on the acetabular side. In many cases, 1 mm to 2 mm of acetabular over-reaming is necessary to compensate for the hard bone associated with younger, healthier patients. This technique is helpful for avoiding acetabular insertional rim fractures and the incomplete seating of the component.

Uncemented femoral preparation is also critical for the young patient, because it can be complicated by fracture, subsidence, or leg-length discrepancy. We use a burr to open up the posterolateral neck and to remove the overhanging tro-chanteric bone. This not only avoids varus position and calcar fracture, but it also prevents tip contact with the posterior femoral cortex. "Touch, feel, and pitch" change are learned skills of broaching that come with experience. Once again, we recommend overbroaching to ensure the proper fit and seating of the tapered wedge component. The use of selective distal broaching may be necessary if the diaphyseal fit is too tight.

For the assessment of limb-length discrepancy, we prefer the method described by Ranawat and colleagues. This technique involves the use of the posterior approach. After the initial dissection and release of the short external rotators, the inferior capsule is incised at the 6-o'clock position to expose the posteroinferior lip of the acetabulum. A %₁₆-inch Steinmann pin is inserted into the posterior infracotyloid groove (Figure 35-1, A through C); this represents the bony groove inferior to the posteroinferior lip of the acetabulum. The pin is placed initially at an angle of approximately 60 degrees until it touches the ischium, and it is then made vertical and allowed to slide along the bone into the infracotyloid groove. The pin is kept vertical and viewed end-on from above, and then a mark is made on the greater trochanter before hip dislocation (see Figure 35-1, B). The hip is then dislocated. The center of the femoral head is marked with electrocautery, and the distance between the center and the lesser trochanter is noted and compared with the calculation made during the preoperative planning (Figure 35-2, A). The neck resection is now completed in accordance with preoperative templating.

After bone preparation and the placement of the trial implants, the offset and the distance from the center of the head to the lesser trochanter are assessed (see Figure 35-2, B). After

reduction, the component position is assessed with the use of the combined anteversion test (Figure 35-3, A and B). This test measures the angle of internal rotation required for the femoral head to be coplanar with the face of the acetabulum with 10 degrees of flexion and 10 degrees of adduction. Normally, the angle is between 35 degrees and 45 degrees of internal rotation for women and between 25 degrees and 35 degrees for men.

Assuming that the components are in the proper position, attention is turned to the soft-tissue envelope. The tightness of the tensor fascia lata is assessed by direct palpation and the Ober test. The tightness of the anterior capsule is evaluated by keeping the patient's leg in full extension and externally rotating the hip. The posterior border of the greater trochanter should be within one fingerbreadth of the ischial tuberosity without impinging. The "shuck test" can be used to determine overall laxity. In general, more than half of the femoral head should not disengage from the liner with direct axial traction. The "drop-kick test" is a maneuver with which the hip is held in extension while the knee is concomitantly flexed to 90 degrees. If the extremity has been overlengthened, the extensor mechanism becomes excessively taut; this may manifest as a passive swing of the knee into extension as the leg is released.

It should be emphasized that all of these soft-tissue tension tests are subjective and depend on the muscle relaxation at that point in the operation, the amount of effective force applied to distract the joint, the muscularity and habitus of the patient, and the extent of soft-tissue release that occurred during surgery. Moreover, because these tests provide an assessment of stability, they may sometimes encourage increased neck lengths, which leads to potential limb lengthening. Thus, these tests should be used in conjunction with

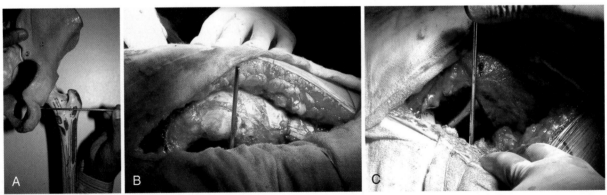

**Figure 35–1** The Ranawat and colleagues method of intraoperative assessment of limb-length discrepancy. **A,** A schematic representation of the placement of the Steinmann pin in the posterior infracotyloid groove in a bone model. **B,** During surgery and before the hip is dislocated, the pin is initially placed at an angle of approximately 60 degrees until it touches the ischium. It is then made vertical and allowed to slide along the bone into the infracotyloid groove. With the pin kept vertical and viewed end-on from above, a mark is made on the greater trochanter before the hip is dislocated. **C,** After the trial reduction, the Steinmann pin is reinserted, with the pin and the leg kept in the same position. The difference in the leg length is measured by noting whether the point on the trochanter has moved up or down, which indicates shortening or lengthening, respectively.

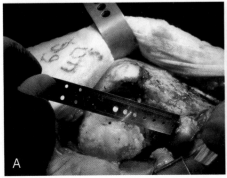
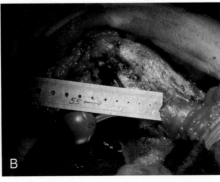

**Figure 35–2 A,** The center of the femoral head is marked with electrocautery before neck osteotomy, and the distance between the center and the lesser trochanter is noted. **B,** After the placement of the trial implants, the distance from the center of the head to the lesser trochanter is again reassessed and correlated with the preoperative plan. A symmetric relationship among the head, the greater trochanter, and the lesser trochanter usually implies satisfactory implant positioning.

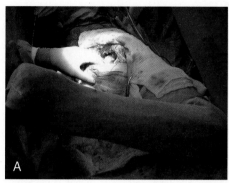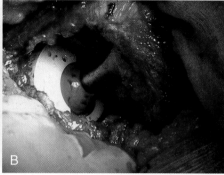

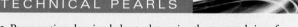

**Figure 35–3** After trial reduction, the component position is assessed with the use of the combined anteversion test. This test measures **A,** the amount of internal rotation required for the femoral head to be **B,** coplanar with the face of the acetabulum, with about 10 degrees of flexion and 10 degrees of adduction at the hip.

each other along with the preoperative template to determine the appropriate construct. After an adequate soft-tissue balance is achieved around the hip, the Steinmann pin is reinserted, with the pin and the patient's leg kept in the same position (see Figure 35-1, *C*). The difference in the leg length is measured by noting whether the point on the trochanter has moved up or down, which is indicative of shortening or lengthening, respectively. If lengthening of the limb (especially of more than 2 cm) is anticipated, the sciatic nerve must be palpated to determine whether it is excessively taut before the length that has been gained is accepted.

### TECHNICAL PEARLS

- Preoperative planning helps to determine the type and size of the prosthesis and aids in the positioning of the components with the aim of restoring the biomechanics of the hip in terms of the center of rotation, the offset, and the limb length.
- Although preference should be given to non-modular components, occasionally preoperative deformities demand modular prostheses.
- Exposure of the hip can be more difficult in the young patient as a result of robust musculature. Larger incisions are sometimes necessary.
- Bone quality is generally excellent in the young patient. As a result, the preparation of the bone often requires over-reaming and over-broaching to prevent fractures or "hanging up."
- Although long-term studies are still needed, alternate bearings should be considered for these patients to minimize wear.
- Perioperative education is important, because these patients may have different expectations than their older counterparts.
- Postoperative pain management may be the most important determinant of patient satisfaction and subsequent function.
- Most younger patients should limit their early rehabilitation and focus on allowing the healing process to run its course.

## PAIN MANAGEMENT AND REHABILITATION

Changes in pain management have probably had the greatest impact on patients' recovery after THA. Improved pain control means that patients are more satisfied and comfortable and thus more willing to participate in physical therapy. We prefer a multimodal approach that emphasizes patient education and preemptive analgesia and that avoids the use of parenteral narcotics. This approach is designed to limit the patient's sensitization to pain and thus reduces the overall analgesic requirement. At our institution, patients receive 400 mg of celecoxib, 20 mg of extended-release oxycodone, 40 mg of pantoprazole, and 5 mg of warfarin in the preoperative holding area.

A local periarticular injection has been shown to have a significant effect on the reduction of immediate postoperative pain. We perform two such injections: 1) one before the final reduction in the anterior capsule, the iliopsoas tendon, and the insertion site; and 2) one after the final reduction in the abductors, the fascia lata, the gluteus maximus and its insertion, the posterior capsule, the short external rotators, and the synovium (Table 35-3).

Postoperatively, the patients are managed with around-the-clock pain medications, which consist of a combination of acetaminophen, celecoxib, ketorolac, and oral narcotics. The use of a parenteral narcotic is discouraged. The anticoagulation consists of warfarin with a therapeutic international normalized ratio level of 1.5 to 2, along with in-bed exercises, foot pumps, and rapid mobilization. A routine Doppler scan is performed on the second postoperative day; if it is negative, the patient is put on aspirin for the next 6 weeks, depending on individual medical comorbidities. In-bed exercises are begun the same day, and patients are mobilized to ambulate on the first postoperative day, with weight bearing as tolerated; these patients are usually discharged by postoperative day 3. They start with a walker and then graduate to two crutches, then one crutch, and then a cane. The patients are instructed to walk every day, gradually increasing their distance to a goal of 1 mile. Most of these patients can walk without support, pain, or limp at 4 to 6 weeks.

### Table 35–3 RANAWAT ORTHOPEDIC CENTER COCKTAIL

| Medication | Strength/Dose | Amount |
|---|---|---|
| **First Injection** | | |
| Bupivacaine | 0.5% (200 mg to 400 mg) | 24 ml |
| Morphine sulfate | 8 mg | 0.8 ml |
| Epinephrine (1:1000) | 300 μg | 0.3 ml |
| Methylprednisolone acetate | 40 mg | 1 ml |
| Cefuroxime | 750 mg | 10 ml (reconstituted in normal saline) |
| Sodium chloride | 0.9% | 22 ml |
| **Second Injection** | | |
| Bupivacaine | 0.5% | 20 ml |
| Sodium chloride | 0.9% | 20 ml |

A clonidine transdermal patch is applied in the operating department (100 μg/24 hours). No steroid is given to diabetic, immunocompromised, elderly, or revision patients. Vancomycin is used if the patient is allergic to penicillin.

From Parvataneni HK, Ranawat AS, Ranawat CS. The use of local periarticular injections in the management of postoperative pain after total hip and knee replacement: a multimodal approach. *Instr Course Lect.* 2007;56:125–131.

## COMPLICATIONS

Apart from the general complications of THA, young, active patients are more prone to dislocation, periprosthetic fracture, implant breakage, wear, osteolysis, and aseptic loosening. In a study by Kerboull and colleagues, the mean wear rate was $0.12 \pm 0.21$ mm per year; a wear rate of more than 0.1 mm per year was found to be predictive of implant loosening. A high level of participation in sports is associated with at least a two-fold increase in the polyethylene wear rate after 10 years. Implant loosening and instability may be the most common indications for reoperation.

## SPORTS AND TOTAL HIP ARTHROPLASTY

Preoperative athletic activity is an important factor to consider when recommending athletic activity after THA. Patients who have achieved high levels of skill in athletics have the best chance of safely resuming these activities; patients who have not participated in specific sports or recreational activities are less likely to achieve high skill levels after THA. Moreover, the latter group may have an increased risk of injury while participating in a new activity after THA.

Participation in sports after a THA is a subjective question. Surgeons have a duty to educate their patients regarding the risk of athletic activity after THA. The most significant risk is accelerated wear, but loosening and traumatic complications may also occur.

Generally, high-contact, high-impact activities are discouraged after THA. Current recommendations are shown in Table 35-4. Improving function is an increasing indication for THA, and we believe that athletic activity is important to many of our patients. We prefer to educate our patients regarding the risks associated with athletic activity rather than to directly discourage the practice. Some patients accept this risk, whereas others choose to avoid sports.

## RESULTS AND OUTCOMES

The results of THA in the young patient require careful evaluation. The factors to be considered are the length of follow up, the definition of failure (e.g., any revision, aseptic loosening, septic revision, radiographic loosening), the method of obtaining fixation, the underlying diagnosis, and the bearing surface. Diagnosis (e.g., osteoarthritis as compared with rheumatoid arthritis, avascular necrosis as compared with osteoarthritis), male sex, accelerated wear, and varus position of the femur have been linked to the decreased survival of the prosthesis. According to the National Institute for Health and Clinical Excellence, with the use of the most recently available evidence of clinical effectiveness, the best prosthesis (when considering long-term viability as the determinant) should demonstrate a survival rate of more than 90% at 10 years. Although there are not many studies among young patients that fulfill the National Institute for Health and Clinical Excellence criteria, certain trends are evident (Table 35-5).

The results of non-cemented THA will always lag behind those of cemented THA in terms of follow up duration for historic reasons. The long-term results of cemented THA and the mid- to long-term results of uncemented fixation are shown in Table 35-5. Early reports of disappointing clinical results of cemented THA in young patients caused concern and prompted some authors to recommend alternative procedures. Dorr and colleagues found revision rates of 12% at 4.5 years, 33% at 9.2 years, and 67% at 16.2 years. However, recent reports have been more encouraging, with long-term survival rates of 65% to 88% (see Table 35-5). Better survival outcomes have been reported for the femoral stem as compared with the acetabular cup.

Uncemented fixation is growing in popularity, especially for younger patients in most parts of the world. Modern uncemented stems have also shown a good survival rate of 90% to 100% at 10 to 15 years (see Table 35-5). However, the weak link with either type of fixation is the acetabular side: aseptic loosening with cemented components and wear and osteolysis with

**Table 35–4** CONSENSUS GUIDELINES FOR THE RETURN TO ACTIVITY AS RECOMMENDED BY THE MEMBERS OF THE HIP SOCIETY AND THE ASSOCIATION OF HIP AND KNEE SURGEONS

| Allow | Allow With Experience | Do Not Allow | Undecided |
|---|---|---|---|
| Bowling | Cross-country skiing | Baseball | Martial arts |
| Dancing (ballroom, jazz, and square) | Downhill skiing | Contact sports (football, soccer, and basketball) | Singles tennis |
| Doubles tennis | Ice skating | High-impact aerobics | |
| Elliptical | Pilates | Jogging | |
| Golf | Rollerblading | Racquetball | |
| Hiking | Weightlifting | Snowboarding | |
| Low-impact aerobics | | Softball | |
| Road cycling | | Squash | |
| Rowing | | | |
| Speed walking | | | |
| Stair climbing | | | |
| Stationary cycling | | | |
| Stationary skiing | | | |
| Swimming | | | |
| Treadmill walking | | | |
| Walking | | | |
| Weight machines | | | |

Seventy-one percent of Hip Society and 59% of the Association of Hip and Knee Surgeons recommend a return to sports 3 to 6 months after a total hip arthroplasty.
From Klein GR, Levine BR, Hozack WJ, Strauss EJ, D'Antonio JA, Macaulay W, Di Cesare PE. Return to athletic activity after total hip arthroplasty. Consensus guidelines based on a survey of the Hip Society and American Association of Hip and Knee Surgeons. *J Arthroplasty.* 2007 Feb;22(2):171–175.

**Table 35–5** RESULTS OF TOTAL HIP ARTHROPLASTY AMONG YOUNG PATIENTS

| Study | No. of Arthroplasties (No. of Patients) | Mean Age (Range) | Mean Length of Follow Up (Range) | Acetabular Type | Femoral Type | Aseptic Acetabular Survival | Aseptic Femoral Survival | Overall Survival |
|---|---|---|---|---|---|---|---|---|
| **Cemented (with a minimum of 15 years of follow up)** | | | | | | | | |
| Sochart and Porter, 1998 | 83 (55) | 24.9 years (17 to 29 years) | 20 years (5 to 30 years) | Cemented Charnley | Cemented Charnley | 68% at 25 years | 73% at 25 years | 65% at 25 years |
| Kerboull et al, 2004 | 52 (45) | Less than 50 years | More than 20 years | Cemented; all PE | Cemented Charnley-Marcel Kerboull | 93.6% | 95.8% | 85.4% |
| Neumann et al, 1996 | 188 (165) | 34 to 55 years | 18 years (15 to 21 years) | Cemented Charnley | Cemented Charnley | | | 88.3% at 20 years |
| Keener et al, 2003 | 57 (42) | 42 years (18 to 49 years) | 26 years (25 to 30 years) | Cemented Charnley | Cemented Charnley | 66% | 87% | 69% |
| Devitt et al, 1997 | 110 (77) | 42.2 years (16 to 49 years) | 16 to 25 years | Cemented Charnley | Cemented Charnley | 84% at 20 years | 79% at 20 years | 75% at 20 years |
| Berry et al, 2002 | 43 | Less than 40 years | More than 25 years | Cemented Charnley | Cemented Charnley | 73.7% | 82.4% | 63.7% |
| Berry et al, 2002 | 144 | 40 to 49 years | More than 25 years | Cemented Charnley | Cemented Charnley | 80.7% | 82.6% | 62% |
| **Uncemented/Hybrid/Reverse Hybrid (with a minimum of 5 years of follow up)** | | | | | | | | |
| Singh et al, 2004 | 38 (33) | 42 years (22 to 49 years) | 10 years (5 to 14 years) | 37% cemented JRI PE, 63% JRI CSF HAC coated | JRI Furlong HAC | 90.5% at 12 years for cemented and 96% at 10 years for uncemented | 100% at 12 years | 90.5% at 12 years |
| Callaghan et al, 1997 | 45 (37) | 41 years (26 to 49 years) | 8.2 years (5 to 10 years) | HG1 and Osteonics | Cemented Iowa | 100% | 82% | 82% |
| Kim et al, 2002 | 64 (55) | 43.4 years (21 to 50 years) | 9.4 years (8 to 10 years) | Duraloc | Cemented Elite Plus or Elite | 100% | 100% | 98% (1 case was revised as a result of infection) |
| Bizot et al, 2004 | 71 (62) | 46 years (21.3 to 54.8 years) | 6 to 11 years | Ceraver-Osteal | Ceraver-Osteal | 98.3% | 100% | 93.7% |
| Besette et al, 2003 | 16 (12) | 16.5 years (10 to 20 years) | 13.6 years (10 to 25 years) | Cemented/uncemented/hybrid | Cemented/uncemented/hybrid | 67% | 93% | 67% |
| **Uncemented (with a minimum of 5 years of follow up)** | | | | | | | | |
| McAuley et al, 2004* | 561 (488) | 40 years (16 to 50 years) | 7 years (0 to 19 years) | Multiple, but all porous coated | Multiple, but all porous coated | 60% at 15 years if PE exchange is excluded | 96% at 15 years | 60% at 15 years (86% if PE exchange is excluded) |
| Kearns et al, 2006 | 299 (221) | 41 years (18 to 50 years) | 8.4 years (5 to 15 years) | Multiple, but all porous coated | Multiple | 52.5% at 15 years | 96.8% at 15 years | 46.8% at 15 years |

*Continued*

**Table 35-5** RESULTS OF TOTAL HIP ARTHROPLASTY AMONG YOUNG PATIENTS—CONT'D

| Study | No. of Arthroplasties (No. of Patients) | Mean Age (Range) | Mean Length of Follow Up (Range) | Acetabular Type | Femoral Type | Aseptic Acetabular Survival | Aseptic Femoral Survival | Overall Survival |
|---|---|---|---|---|---|---|---|---|
| Kim et al, 2003 | 118 (80) | 46.8 years (21 to 49 years) | 9.8 years (8 to 11 years) | Duraloc | Profile | 100% | 100% | 99% (1 case was revised as a result of recurrent dislocation) |
| Kim et al, 2004 | 70 (62) | 37 years (17 to 49 years) | 7 years (5 to 9 years) | Standard Ti modular shell (Sulzer) with Metasul | CLS | 100% | 100% | 98.6% (1 case had a liner exchange) |
| Migaud et al, 2004 | 39 (30) | 39.8 years (23 to 49 years) | 5.7 years (5 to 6.7 years) | Armor-Impacted Ti-6Al-7Nb with Metasul | Alloclassic Zweymuller | 100% | 100% | 100% |
| Migaud et al, 2004 | 39 (32) | 40.5 years (15 to 50 years) | 5.7 years (4.8 to 7.5 years) | HG | ABG1 | | | 97% |
| D'Antonio et al, 1997 | 155 (142) | 38.4 years (16 to 49 years) | 6.8 years (5 to 8 years) | Various | Omnifit | 90% | 100% | |
| Capello et al, 2003 | 152 (133) | 39 years (16 to 49 years) | 10 to 14 years | | Omnifit | 89% | 99.1% | |
| Archibeck et al, 2006 | 100 (91) | 39 years (14 to 50 years) | 9 years (5 to 13 years) | HPGII or Trilogy | Multilock | 97.1% | 100% | 87.5% |
| Eskelinen et al, 2006 | 5607 | Less than 55 years | More than 5 years | Multiple | Multiple | 94% for Biomet Universal and 95% for HGII at 13 years | 90% at 10 years | Less than 80% (except for HGII) |
| Crowther and Lachiewicz, 2002 | 71 (56) | 37 years (22 to 49 years) | 11 years (9 to 14 years) | HGI | HG and CDH Precoat (1) | 100% at 10 years for metal shell | 93% | 90% |

*Although the minimum follow up time in this study was 0 years, this article has been included, because it raises several important concerns and provides an excellent review of the literature regarding total hip arthroplasty among young patients.
Additional information on implants can be found in the Expert Consult website.

uncemented modular components. In a study of uncemented THA by McAuley and colleagues, the overall survival rate dipped dramatically from 89% at 10 years to 60% at 15 years. However, if liner exchange was excluded, the survival rate at 15 years was 83.3%. In a report from the Finnish registry about 4661 primary THA cases in young patients who were followed up for 0 years to 22 years, modern uncemented stems and cups fared better than cemented ones in term of aseptic loosening. However, when all revisions were considered (including liner exchange), the survival of uncemented cups was no better than that of all polyethylene (PE) cemented cups. Because of this, alternate options should be considered. Three possible solutions include a reverse hybrid construct, an uncemented cup with improved liner congruence and diminished wear (i.e., a highly cross-linked PE), or a hard-on-hard articulation (Table 35-6).

## SUMMARY

As disheartening as it is to replace a young person's hip, both the surgeon and the patient should take solace in the likelihood of excellent pain relief and restoration of function. Uncemented fixation and alternative bearings offer hope for a THA that could last 30 years or more.

Technically, exposure is often more difficult as a result of a more robust musculature, and it usually requires longer incisions. Bone preparation may require over-reaming and over-broaching to optimize fixation and avoid complications.

More research is needed to evaluate the long-term results of THA for the young patient, especially with newer designs and materials. However, our current understanding supports the notion that these patients may experience earlier failure and an increased need for reoperation as compared with older patients.

**Table 35-6** BEARING COMBINATIONS FOR TOTAL HIP ARTHROPLASTY AMONG YOUNG PATIENTS

| Bearing Surface | Advantages | Disadvantages |
| --- | --- | --- |
| Highly cross-linked polyethylene | Improved wear properties, no systemic toxicity, multiple liner options (e.g., elevated rim), lower cost | Compromise with other material properties, increased bioactivity of wear particles |
| Metal on metal | Higher wear resistance, allows for bigger diameters | Increased ion levels with concerns for carcinogenesis, delayed hypersensitivity, position sensitive |
| Ceramic on ceramic | Highest wear and corrosion resistance, no systemic toxicity | Position sensitive, fracture risk, liner chipping, increased synovitis, stripe wear, squeaking, difficult revision if Morse taper is damaged, higher cost |

Metal-on-polyethylene and ceramic-on-polyethylene bearing surfaces may combine some of the advantages of each, but they demonstrate higher wear than metal-on-metal or ceramic-on-ceramic bearing surfaces.
The use of newer combinations (e.g., ceramic-on-metal) requires further research. In preliminary studies, theses combinations have shown lower wear, absence of stripe wear, and lower metal ions.
From Williams S, Schepers A, Isaac G, Hardaker C, Ingham E, van der Jagt D, Breckon A, Fisher J. The 2007 Otto Aufranc Award. Ceramic-on-metal hip arthroplasties: a comparative in vitro and in vivo study. *Clin Orthop Relat Res.* 2007;465:23-32; Heisel C, Silva M, Schmalzried TP. Bearing surface options for total hip replacement in young patients. *Instr Course Lect.* 2004;53:49-65; and Fisher J, Jin Z, Tipper J, Stone M, Ingham E. Tribology of alternative bearings. *Clin Orthop Relat Res.* 2006;453:25-34.

## ANNOTATED REFERENCES AND SUGGESTED READINGS

Archibeck MJ, Surdam JW, Schultz Jr SC, Junick DW, White RE. Cementless total hip arthroplasty in patients 50 years or younger. *J Arthroplasty.* 2006;21:476-483.

Berry DJ, Harmsen WS, Cabanela ME, Morrey BF. Twenty-five-year survivorship of two thousand consecutive primary Charnley total hip replacements: factors affecting survivorship of acetabular and femoral components. *J Bone Joint Surg Am.* 2002;84-A:171-177.

Bessette BJ, Fassier F, Tanzer M, Brooks CE. Total hip arthroplasty in patients younger than 21 years: a minimum, 10-year follow-up. *Can J Surg.* 2003;46:257-262.

Bizot P, Hannouche D, Nizard R, Witvoet J, Sedel L. Hybrid alumina total hip arthroplasty using a press-fit metal-backed socket in patients younger than 55 years. A six- to 11-year evaluation. *J Bone Joint Surg Br.* 2004;86:190-194.

Callaghan JJ, Forest EE, Sporer SM, Goetz DD, Johnston RC. Total hip arthroplasty in the young adult. *Clin Orthop Relat Res.* 1997;344:257-262.

Capello WN, D'Antonio JA, Feinberg JR, Manley MT. Ten-year results with hydroxyapatite-coated total hip femoral components in patients less than fifty years old. A concise follow-up of a previous report. *J Bone Joint Surg Am.* 2003;85:885-889.

Charles MN, Bourne RB, Davey JR, Greenwald AS, Morrey BF, Rorabeck CH. Soft-tissue balancing of the hip: the role of femoral offset restoration. *Instr Course Lect.* 2005;54:131-141.

This article provides an overview of the rationale, the biomechanical principles, and the clinical implications associated with the soft-tissue balancing of the hip. It also outlines various strategies to restore adequate soft-tissue balance along with limb-length equalization.

Charley J. Low friction arthroplasty of the hip. *In Theory and practice.* New York: Springer Verlag; 1981.

This is a classic textbook by Sir John Charnley, one of the most remarkable innovators of his generation. Charnley should be remember by posterity for his low friction arthroplasty, the surgery that revolutionized the treatment of hip diseases.

Clohisy JC, Keeney JA, Schoenecker PL. Preliminary assessment and treatment guidelines for hip disorders in young adults. *Clin Orthop Relat Res.* 2005;441:168-179.

In a young patient with hip disease, optimal clinical results depend on the combination of careful patient selection and the successful application of the appropriate surgical procedure. This article outlines the general guidelines for the assessment and treatment of hip pain among young adults.

Crowther JD, Lachiewicz PF. Survival and polyethylene wear of porous-coated acetabular components in patients less than fifty years old: results at nine to fourteen years. *J Bone Joint Surg Am*. 2002;84:729–735.

D'Antonio JA, Capello WN, Manley MT, Feinberg J. Hydroxyapatite coated implants. Total hip arthroplasty in the young patient and patients with avascular necrosis. *Clin Orthop Relat Res*. 1997;344:124–138.

Devitt A, O'Sullivan T, Quinlan W. 16- to 25-year follow-up study of cemented arthroplasty of the hip in patients aged 50 years or younger. *J Arthroplasty*. 1997 Aug;12(5):479–489.

Dorey FJ. Survivorship analysis of surgical treatment of the hip in young patients. *Clin Orthop Relat Res*. 2004;418:23–28.

This article emphasizes the methods of the survival analysis of the surgical treatment of the hip among young patients. It discusses the need for more sophisticated instruments that measure patient activity and for statistical procedures that are necessary for the proper presentation and interpretation of data that involve young patients.

Dorr LD. *Hip arthroplasty. Minimally invasive techniques and computer navigation*. Philadelphia, PA: Saunders Elsevier; 2006.

Dorr LD, Kane 3rd TJ, Conaty JP. Long-term results of cemented total hip arthroplasty in patients 45 years old or younger. A 16-year follow-up study. *J Arthroplasty*. 1994;9(5):453–456.

Eggli S, Pisan M, Müller ME. The value of preoperative planning for total hip arthroplasty. *J Bone Joint Surg Br*. 1998;80(3):382–390.

Eskelinen A, Remes V, Helenius I, Pulkkinen P, Nevalainen J, Paavolainen P. Total hip arthroplasty for primary osteoarthrosis in younger patients in the Finnish arthroplasty register. 4,661 primary replacements followed for 0–22 years. *Acta Orthop*. 2005;76(1):28–41.

Eskelinen A, Remes V, Helenius I, Pulkkinen P, Nevalainen J, Paavolainen P. Uncemented total hip arthroplasty for primary osteoarthritis in young patients: a mid to long-term follow-up study from the Finnish Arthroplasty Register. *Acta Orthop*. 2006;77(1):57–70.

Furnes O, Lie SA, Espehaug B, Vollset SE, Engesaeter LB, Havelin LI. Hip disease and the prognosis of total hip replacements. A review of 53,698 primary total hip replacements reported to the Norwegian Arthroplasty Register 1987–99. *J Bone Joint Surg Br*. 2001;83(4):579–586.

Ganz R, Parvizi J, Beck M, Leunig M, Nötzli H, Siebenrock KA. Femoroacetabular impingement: a cause for osteoarthritis of the hip. *Clin Orthop Relat Res*. 2003;(417):112–120.

Geschwend N, Frei T, Morscher E, Nigg B, Loehr J. Alpine and cross-country skiing after total hip replacement: 2 cohorts of 50 patients each, one active, the other inactive in skiing, followed for 5–10 years. *Acta Orthop Scand*. 2000;71(3):243–249.

Hardidge AJ, Hooper J, McMahon S. Current attitudes to total hip replacement in younger patients: a comparison of two nations. *ANZ J Surg*. 2003;73(5):280–283.

This comparative article—just as the article by Tennent and colleagues—demonstrates how the choice of prosthesis and fixation is different among Australian surgeons as compared with UK surgeons. The roles of papers, peers, personal experiences, patient assessments, budgets, institutions, theories, fashions, and differences in autonomy and advertising have been proposed as the reasons for these differences.

Healy WL, Iorio R, Lemos MJ. Athletic activity after joint replacement. *Am J Sports Med*. 2001;29(3):377–388.

Jäger M, Endres S, Wilke A. Total hip replacement in childhood, adolescence and young patients: a review of the literature. *Z Orthop Ihre Grenzgeb*. 2004;142(2):194–212.

This excellent review of the literature that addresses THA in young patients concludes that cementless fixation with THA is a sufficient technique for total hip replacement for young patients. There are few data available in the literature that deal with the outcome of one implant type within a defined clinical picture.

Kearns SR, Jamal B, Rorabeck CH, Bourne RB. Factors affecting survival of uncemented total hip arthroplasty in patients 50 years or younger. *Clin Orthop Relat Res*. 2006;453:103–109.

Keener JD, Callaghan JJ, Goetz DD, Pederson DR, Sullivan PM, Johnston RC. Twenty-five-year results after Charnley total hip arthroplasty in patients less than fifty years old: a concise follow-up of a previous report. *J Bone Joint Surg Am*. 2003;85:1066–1072.

Kerboull L, Hamadouche M, Courpied JP, Kerboull M. Long-term results of Charnley-Kerboull hip arthroplasty in patients younger than 50 years. *Clin Orthop Relat Res*. 2004;(418):112–118.

Kim YH, Kook HK, Kim JS. Total hip replacement with a cementless acetabular component and a cemented femoral component in patients younger than fifty years of age. *J Bone Joint Surg Am*. 2002;84:770–774.

Kim SY, Kyung HS, Ihn JC, Cho MR, Koo KH, Kim CY. Cementless Metasul metal-on-metal total hip arthroplasty in patients less than fifty years old. *J Bone Joint Surg Am*. 2004;86:2475–2481.

Kim YH, Oh SH, Kim JS. Primary total hip arthroplasty with a second-generation cementless total hip prosthesis in patients younger than fifty years of age. *J Bone Joint Surg Am*. 2003;85:109–114.

Lucas DH, Scott RD. The Ranawat sign. A specific maneuver to assess component positioning in total hip arthroplasty. *J Orthop Tech*. 1994;2:59–61.

Maheshwari AV, Malik A, Dorr LD. Impingement of the native hip joint. *J Bone Joint Surg Am*. 2007;89(11):2508–2518.

Impingement may be one of the most common causes of idiopathic arthritis among young patients. This article reviews the pathophysiology involved, and it elaborates on the basis of clinicoradiologic diagnosis as well as the various treatment options and their results.

Malik A, Maheshwari A, Dorr LD. Impingement with total hip replacement. *J Bone Joint Surg Am*. 2007;89(8):1832–1842.

Although the true incidence of impingement after THA is unknown, it is a significant contributor to the failure of THA, especially among young and active patients. This article reviews the various causes and possible solutions.

Mancuso CA, Ranawat CS, Esdaile JM, Johanson NA, Charlson ME. Indications for total hip and total knee arthroplasties. Results of orthopaedic surveys. *J Arthroplasty*. 1996;11(1):34–46.

McAuley JP, Szuszczewicz ES, Young A, Engh CA, Sr. Total hip arthroplasty in patients 50 years and younger. *Clin Orthop Relat Res*. 2004;(418):119–125.

McCarthy JC, Busconi B. The role of hip arthroscopy in the diagnosis and treatment of hip disease. *Orthopedics*. 1995;18(8):753–756.

Migaud H, Jobin A, Chantelot C, Giraud F, Laffargue P, Duquennoy A. Cementless metal-on-metal hip arthroplasty in patients less than 50 years of age: comparison with a matched control group using ceramic-on-polyethylene after a minimum 5-year follow-up. *J Arthroplasty*. 2004;19(8 Suppl 3):23–28.

National Institute for Health and Clinical Excellence (NICE). *Guidance on the selection of the prosthesis for primary hip replacement*. 2003. London www.nice.org.uk.

Neumann L, Freund KG, Sørensen KH. Total hip arthroplasty with the Charnley prosthesis in patients fifty-five years old and less. Fifteen to twenty-one-year results. *J Bone Joint Surg Am*. 1996;78:73–79.

Parvataneni HK, Ranawat AS, Ranawat CS. The use of local periarticular injections in the management of postoperative pain after total hip and knee replacement: a multimodal approach. *Instr Course Lect*. 2007;56:125–131.

Parvizi J, Campfield A, Clohisy JC, Rothman RH, Mont MA. Management of arthritis of the hip in the young adult. *J Bone Joint Surg Br*. 2006;88(10):1279–1285.

This article reviews the contemporary status of the cause, diagnosis, and treatment of arthritis of the hip in the young adult.

Ranawat CS, Rao RR, Rodriguez JA, Bhende HS. Correction of limb-length inequality during total hip arthroplasty. *J Arthroplasty*. 2001;16(6):715–720.

Ranawat CS, Rodriguez JA. Functional leg-length inequality following total hip arthroplasty. *J Arthroplasty*. 1997;12(4):359–364.

Schreurs BW, Gardeniers JW. Factors affecting survival of uncemented total hip arthroplasty in patients 50 years or younger. *Clin Orthop Relat Res*. 2006;453:103–109.

This study retrospectively reviewed 299 uncemented THAs among young patients and looked at the various factors that affect survival.

Schreurs BW, Gardeniers JW. Total hip arthroplasty for primary osteoarthrosis in younger patients in the Finnish arthroplasty register. *Acta Orthop*. 2005;76(4):604–605. Author reply 605–607.

Second letter to the editor concerning: Total hip arthroplasty for primary osteoarthrosis in younger patients in the Finnish arthroplasty register," by Eskelinen et al and correspondence. *Acta Orthop*. 2005;76:28–41, 604–607. *Acta Orthop*. 2006;77(2):337–338; author reply 338–341.

These series of letters from the Finnish registry raise several important things to consider with regard to THA in young patients.

Singh S, Trikha SP, Edge AJ. Hydroxyapatite ceramic-coated femoral stems in young patients. A prospective ten-year study. *J Bone Joint Surg Br*. 2004;86:1118–1123.

Sochart DH, Porter ML. Long-term results of cemented Charnley low-friction arthroplasty in patients aged less than 30 years. *J Arthroplasty*. 1998;13(2):123–131.

Tennent TD, Goddard NJ. Current attitudes to total hip replacement in the younger patient: results of a national survey. *Ann R Coll Surg Engl*. 2000;82(1):33–38.

This article demonstrates the geographic variation with regard to the use of the fixation method for THA in young patients. Surgeons in the United Kingdom still appear to prefer a cemented fixation.

CHAPTER **36**

# Proximal Femoral Osteotomy in the Skeletally Immature Patient With Deformity

*Perry L. Schoenecker, Margaret M. Rich, and Ryan M. Nunley*

## INTRODUCTION

Osteotomies of the proximal femur are frequently performed as part of the treatment of deformities of the hip joint in the skeletally immature patient. The severity of the deformity and the complexity of the surgical procedure necessary to obtain a satisfactory clinical outcome are quite variable. In the young child, a redirectional proximal femoral (intertrochanteric) osteotomy can be effective for the treatment of residual developmental hip dysplasia. The surgical approach and the osteotomy technique are straightforward. By contrast, the correction of a complex deformity that results from a slipped capital femoral epiphysis in a large adolescent patient can be very technically challenging. This may require a comprehensive reconstructive approach that includes multiplane proximal femoral osteotomy and osteochondroplasty and that makes use of an extensive surgical approach. Fixation must be secure enough to maintain correction until the osteotomy heals to ensure a satisfactory outcome. In this chapter, indications and techniques of commonly performed proximal femoral osteotomies in both children and adolescents will be presented.

## BASIC SCIENCE

A varus-producing proximal femoral varus osteotomy (PFO) that creates a neck shaft angle of 100 degrees to 110 degrees is indicated to correct coxa valga for the treatment of hip dysplasia in the young child. The secondary remodeling of the neck shaft angle to near normal (i.e., 130 degrees) is anticipated, as is the overgrowth of the femur, which results in a limb-length inequality (i.e., long on the operated side).

When correcting valgus deformities with a varus-producing osteotomy, the osteotomy and the point of correction are typically distal to the site of deformity (i.e., the head–neck junction). Consequently, undesirable medial deviation of the mechanical axis of the lower extremity can occur. To minimize this occurrence, the distal fragment may be displaced medially to maintain the passage of the lower-extremity mechanical axis through the center of the knee joint. Similarly, when performing a valgus-producing PFO to correct coxa vara, fixation that displaces the distal fragment medially may result in the lateral deviation of the lower-extremity mechanical axis, which potentiates a genu valgum deformity. This can be prevented by ensuring that the distal fragment is translated and fixed lateral to the proximal fragment. When correcting varus or valgus deformities in older children or adolescents with the use of a PFO, the distal fragment should be aligned with the piriformis fossa; this will facilitate the passage of the stem of the femoral prosthesis if a total hip replacement becomes necessary later in life. This is particularly important when a PFO is used to correct a severe deformity that results from a chronic slipped capital femoral epiphysis (SCFE) in which the correction is intertrochanteric and distal to the site of the deformity in the physis.

Valgus-producing osteotomies typically lengthen the lower extremity, whereas varus osteotomies shorten the extremity. Abductor length also changes in relation to the position of the greater trochanter. When correcting varus deformities with a proximal valgus osteotomy, the tip of the trochanter—which is cartilaginous in younger patients and bony in older patients—should be at the level of the center of the femoral head. This may not be possible if the femoral neck is very short. In older children, the distal transfer of the greater trochanter can be performed to accomplish this. Similarly, when performing a varus osteotomy, the resulting location of the tip of the trochanter varies with the underlying pathology and the amount of varus introduced. The tip of the greater trochanter may be normally located so that it is level with the center of the head after the correction of coxa valga or proximal to the center of the head after PFO for containment treatment of Legg-Calvé-Perthes disease. In the former situation, the tip of the trochanter was below the center of the head because of an increased neck shaft angle in a valgus deformity; in the latter situation, the neck shaft angle was normal before the osteotomy, so the varus PFO raises the level of the greater trochanter.

Nonunion after osteotomy of the proximal femur in children is very unlikely. Those with underlying neuromuscular disorders (e.g., static encephalopathy, myelodysplasia) may have delayed healing, which can lead to a loss of correction. Among older children (i.e., those who are more than 10 years old), adequate rigid fixation is essential to ensure healing without a loss of correction. However, there are limitations to the stability of a blade plate and osteotomy construct that may compromise healing. This is more likely after an osteotomy that is performed to correct a very severe deformity, such as SCFE in a large adolescent, in which case it may be difficult to establish adequate contact of the osteotomy fragments and provide sufficient deformity correction. Morbid obesity (i.e., a body mass index of more than 40) is a frequent risk factor for patients with severe SCFE, particularly in North America. Deformity may persist at any age in a child as a result of undercorrection. Deformity may also recur because of unpredictable growth patterns, particularly among young children.

Knowledge of the vascular supply to the proximal femur is important to avoid avascular necrosis as a complication. The medial femoral circumflex artery takes its origin from the deep femoral artery. It passes just medial to the proximal femur at the level of the iliopsoas tendon and then courses posteriorly to its entry into the proximal posterior lateral femoral neck. Injury to this vessel is possible when performing an intertrochanteric osteotomy if there is excessive medial penetration with either a saw or osteotome. Similarly, the terminal branches of the medial circumflex vessel can be injured at the base of the femoral neck while performing a femoral neck osteotomy or an osteotomy of the greater trochanter.

## INDICATIONS

There are numerous indications for performing PFO in young children, preadolescents, and adolescents:

- Young children
  1. Developmental dysplasia of the hip (DDH)
     - Shortening to facilitate open reduction
     - Varus with or without rotation to treat persistent dysplasia (i.e., coxa valga and subluxation)
  2. Coxa valga, subluxation, or both as a result of neuromuscular disease
     - Varus, shortening, and rotation
  3. Congenital (developmental) coxa vara (i.e., Hilgenreiner/epiphyseal angle of more than 60 degrees, progressive varus, or both)
     - Valgus and rotation
  4. Coxa vara as a result of avascular necrosis (a complication of DDH treatment or hip sepsis)
     - Valgus and flexion
- Preadolescents
  1. Residual or recurrent hip dysplasia (DDH or neuromuscular)
     - Varus or valgus may include pelvic osteotomy
  2. Containment treatment for Legg-Calvé-Perthes disease
     - Varus with or without rotation
  3. Coxa vara as a result of avascular necrosis
     - Valgus
  4. Coxa valga as a result of avascular necrosis
     - Varus (may include pelvic osteotomy)
  5. Rotational abnormality (i.e., excess version)
     - Rotational
- Adolescents
  1. Residual varus after PFO for containment of Legg-Calvé-Perthes disease
     - Valgus to increase motion
  2. Residual or recurrent hip dysplasia
     - Varus or valgus (may include pelvic osteotomy)
  3. Chronic deformity as a result of SCFE
     - Flexion and rotation with or without valgus

## BRIEF HISTORY AND PHYSICAL EXAMINATION

The history and physical examination findings of patients who are candidates for a PFO vary with the etiology of the underlying hip pathology. A growing child with hip dysplasia usually has no complaints and presents with minimal if any abnormalities during the examination. A limp is often not noted, and the range of motion may be normal. The decision to perform a PFO is based solely on persistent abnormal radiographic findings. The history of prior treatment for DDH, however, may be important to explain the proximal femoral deformity that occurs as a result of avascular necrosis. Limb-length inequality should be taken into consideration when performing a PFO (i.e., varus shortens, valgus lengthens); this may influence the need for temporary shoe lifts or later limb-length equalization. Patients with coxa vara often limp because of limb shortening or abductor weakness, which produces a Trendelenburg gait. These patients tend to walk with an external rotation deformity. Children with Legg-Calvé-Perthes disease have a history of intermittent limp and pain that may be anterior hip pain or referred pain in the distal thigh. The adolescent patient who presents with a proximal femoral deformity as a result of an SCFE will have a history of noted functional hip joint disability as well as intermittent pain that is often in the distal thigh and reported as knee pain. These patients walk with an externally rotated lower-extremity deformity and often sit with limited hip flexion and abduction. When symptomatic, these patients present for evaluation complaining of hip pain, particularly with activities that require flexibility. Adolescent patients who are being considered for a PFO may present with morbid obesity. Anesthetic consultation may be indicated for patients with a history of sleep apnea, a body mass index of more than 40, or both. The families of children with excessive version express concern about the appearance of their gait as well as their clumsiness.

## IMAGING AND DIAGNOSTICS

Appropriate imaging of the pelvis, hip joint, and proximal femur is essential during preoperative planning to ensure a satisfactory outcome after osteotomy treatment of hip joint pathology. The initial radiographic evaluation should include both standing anteroposterior and supine frog-leg lateral views. Any pelvic tilt and associated limb-length discrepancy (LLD) should be noted. When planning for the osteotomy, it may be helpful to repeat the standing pelvic x-ray and to note the lift necessary to balance the pelvis. Functional radiographs with the hip in variable combinations of flexion and extension, abduction and adduction, and internal and external rotation can be helpful when determining the best position for optimal hip joint congruity and developing the strategy for the performance of the osteotomy. The potential effect of a varus osteotomy to redirect the femoral head into the acetabulum can be assessed with the use of a Von Rosen view (i.e., a supine anteroposterior view with the hips in flexion, abduction, and internal rotation). By contrast, a supine x-ray with the hip adducted can demonstrate the potential effect of a proximal femoral valgus osteotomy. Sagittal plane deformities—such as those seen with DDH, Legg-Calvé-Perthes disease, and coxa valga—can readily be seen on the frog-leg lateral views. To better identify the pathology with an severe deformity such as the posterior tilt of the epiphysis seen with an SCFE, a cross-table lateral view with the hip in 15 degrees of internal rotation should also be obtained. On occasion, it may be helpful to obtain a computed tomography scan for a more detailed image of the pathologic anatomy. The use of three-dimensional reconstruction is helpful for addressing complex femoroacetabular deformities. Whether a three-dimensional computed tomography scan would provide a better understanding of the bony deformity that could optimize the outcome of surgical treatment must be weighed against the increased radiation exposure for the patient. Alternatively, magnetic resonance imaging can be used to further define the proximal femoral and hip joint morphology and to facilitate the planning of the optimal surgical strategy.

## SURGICAL TECHNIQUE

Although the indications and ages of patients who are candidates for PFO are quite variable, the surgical anatomy and the basic technique for performing a PFO are quite similar. In both young and older children, PFOs are typically performed with the patient in the supine position on a radiolucent table. The patient is positioned so that the involved hip and thigh are close to the edge of the table and the operating surgeon. A soft bump (lift) is placed under the operative hip. For the smaller child, a rolled sheet is positioned against the opposite side of the patient to minimize the patient's sliding away from the surgeon during the procedure. The ipsilateral lower torso and leg are prepped down to the ankle. A stockinet covers the extremity from the toes to the mid thigh. Drapes are secured and sealed to the skin with an adhesive barrier material. The lateral approach is used for most PFOs.

## Surgical Technique for the Lateral Approach to the Proximal Femur

The lateral surgical approach is similar for all age groups. A straight lateral incision that extends from the tip of the trochanter to a point several centimeters distal to the greater trochanter is used for exposure. The length of the incision varies with the size of the implant to be used for fixation and with the size of the child. Sharp dissection is carried down to the fascia lata with the scalpel and electrocautery. The skin and subcutaneous tissue are elevated together off of the fascia lata for a few centimeters in both the anterior and posterior directions. The fascia lata is divided in line with the skin incision. Just deep to the fascia lata lies the fascia of the vastus lateralis, which is longitudinally incised directly over the vastus lateralis muscle.

With lateral traction on the posterior edge of the vastus lateralis fascia and counter (medial) traction on the vastus lateralis muscle mass, the electrocautery is used to mobilize and reflect the vastus muscle from lateral to medial off of the lateral intermuscular septum. Care is taken to avoid dissecting through the septum and into the posterior muscle compartment of the thigh. Proximally, the vastus release extends anteriorly over the shaft of the femur. The lateral-to-medial reflection of the vastus lateralis muscle mass is completed from proximal to distal. Within the distal vastus muscle, care should be taken to identify and coagulate the vessels that distally perforate through the lateral intermuscular septum from the posterior to the anterior compartment.

As the vastus lateralis is retracted medially, the periosteum of the femur is visualized. The lateral periosteum is incised, and the femur is subperiosteally exposed just distal to the lesser trochanter. A curved retractor is carefully placed subperiosteally around the anterior shaft of the femur. Posteriorly, the periosteum and the soft tissues are more securely attached to the bone; they are best elevated off of the bone with the electrocautery and the elevator. With blunt dissection, the subperiosteal exposure can be extended distally. With an adequate exposure, the femur should be visible and accessible from the proximal aspect of the greater trochanter to a point distal to the lesser trochanter, which is sufficient for the application of the fixation plate (Box 36-1).

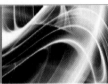

### BOX 36-1 TECHNICAL PEARL: LATERAL APPROACH TO THE PROXIMAL FEMUR

● Avoid incising the vastus lateralis fascia too posteriorly; such an incision may make it more difficult to repair this fascia during closure.

## Surgical Technique for Correcting Proximal Femoral Valgus Deformity in Young Children

For children who are less than 5 years old, a small fragment, a semi-tubular straight plate, a Wagner forked plate (Aesculap, San Francisco, CA), or a small blade plate (Synthes, Paoli, PA) can be used for fixation. The appropriate implant is temporarily inserted into the incision to assess the adequacy of the exposure. If necessary, the skin and fascial incisions are extended distally to facilitate the insertion of the plate. C-arm imaging is used to confirm the optimum position of hip abduction, flexion, and internal rotation needed to reduce or satisfactorily position the femoral head into the acetabulum. A four- or five-hole small-fragment straight semi-tubular plate is the best choice for a femoral shortening osteotomy in conjunction with the open reduction of a developmentally dislocated hip. The anterior iliofemoral approach and open reduction are performed first through an oblique incision that parallels the lateral edge of the iliac crest. For the shortening osteotomy, the lateral proximal femur is approached as previously described. The osteotomy (Figure 36-1) is performed just distal to the lesser trochanter. The plate is placed just distal to the inferior edge of the greater trochanter physis as assessed with the C-arm. The plate is provisionally fixed by inserting a screw in the most proximal screw hole. A drill hole is also made in the bone that corresponds with the second most proximal hole. The proximal screw is loosened, and the plate is rotated anteriorly. The femoral osteotomy is performed just distal to the predrilled second proximal hole.

With the femoral head reduced, the amount of fragment overlap is directly measured; it is typically 1 cm to 2 cm. This determines how much shortening is required. A second osteotomy that is parallel to the first is completed. The fragments are reduced and fixed to each other with the correction of excess anteversion as appropriate. The femoral head is reduced, and the position and stability are assessed. If additional shortening or a change in the rotational alignment is needed, the distal screws are removed, the distal fragment is further shortened or rotated, and the plate is reapplied with the use of new holes.

A Wagner forked plate works well for younger, smaller patients as fixation if angular correction is desired beyond shortening or rotation, as in a varus osteotomy to correct coxa valga associated with residual DDH or with static encephalopathy. If the Wagner plate is to be used, a smooth K-wire is inserted just proximal to the intended site of plate insertion (Figure 36-2). The K-wire is inserted from lateral to medial and placed superiorly in the neck on the anteroposterior view to provide enough space for the subsequent insertion of the Wagner plate. It is centered in the femoral neck on the lateral view. Subperiosteal retractors are circumferentially placed around the femur to protect the soft tissues. A femoral osteotomy is performed at the midpoint of the lesser trochanter, and this is confirmed with

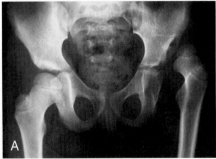
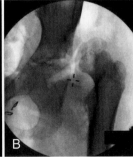
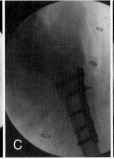
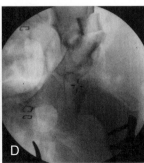

**Figure 36–1 A,** Anteroposterior pelvic radiograph of a 6-year-old girl that shows dislocation of the left hip (developmental dysplasia of the hip) with proximal displacement of the femur. Anteroposterior intraoperative C-arm radiographs, **B,** before and, **C,** after the open reduction of the left femoral head into the true acetabulum facilitated by a 2.5-cm proximal femoral shortening osteotomy fixated with a five-hole semi-tubular small fragment plate and, **D,** after left pelvic (Pemberton-type) osteotomy.

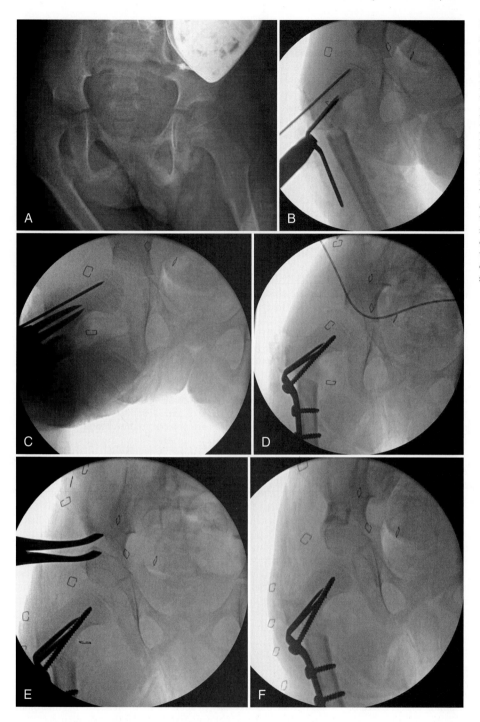

**Figure 36–2 A,** Anteroposterior radiograph of the pelvis of a 6-year-old boy with hip dysplasia (subluxation, coxa valga, and acetabular deficiency as a result of static encephalopathy). **B,** A guide pin has been inserted into the femoral neck. The osteotomy was performed at the lower half of the lesser trochanter, and a Wagner forked plate was introduced. **C,** Lateral C-arm image confirming the placement of the forked plate. **D,** An anteroposterior radiograph that shows the proximal femoral osteotomy fixated with a Wagner plate and noted acetabular dysplasia. **E,** Anteroposterior radiograph that shows a laminar spreader opening a periacetabular (Pemberton-type) osteotomy. **F,** Final C-arm image after the insertion of a bone graft that was obtained as the femur was intentionally shortened during a femoral osteotomy.

the use of C-arm imaging. The femur is transversely cut with an oscillating power saw under direct vision. After completing the osteotomy, consideration should be given to shortening the distal fragment 1 cm to 2 cm, because growth stimulation and secondary limb-length discrepancy often occur in these young patients. A Wagner forked plate of appropriate size is inserted into the proximal femoral fragment with the use of the previously inserted K-wire as a guide. The forked tips of the plate are inserted through the distal lateral cortex and carefully advanced medially and proximally into the femoral neck; the correct position is confirmed with the C-arm. After the prongs of the plate are fully inserted, the distal femoral fragment is reduced and secured to the proximal fragment with a self-centering bone-holding clamp. When performing a varus-producing osteotomy,

the distal fragment should be slightly medialized relative to the proximal fragment. The proportion of medialization will vary slightly, depending on the entry point of the plate in the proximal fragment. Excessive medialization can produce an unstable construct as a result of a loss of contact between the fragments.

The reduction of the femoral head in the acetabulum and the neck shaft angle is assessed with the use of C-arm imaging. If necessary, the varus/valgus alignment can be adjusted by removing the bone-reduction clamp and bending the side plate in situ. In small children (i.e., those less than 3 years old) a varus neck shaft angle of 105 degrees to 110 degrees will typically remodel into an acceptable neck shaft angle at maturity. Obtaining an excessive neck shaft angle (i.e., more than 90 degrees) is undesirable. Remodeling occurs slowly, and a near-normal neck shaft angle may never be achieved. A neck shaft angle of 110 degrees to 115 degrees is used in older children, who have less remodeling potential. The rotational alignment of the two fragments is adjusted to help optimize the reduction of the femoral head into the acetabulum. By doing so, excess external rotation of the distal fragment should be avoided, because this may lead to an out-toeing gait. It may be desirable to slightly extend the distal fragment to create flexion of the proximal fragment, which provides anterior femoral head coverage by the acetabulum in the weight-bearing position. The extension of the distal fragment is achieved by tilting the plate posteriorly as the prongs are inserted into the proximal fragment.

The hip range of motion should be assessed, with flexion and extension, abduction and adduction, and internal and external rotation being noted; passive abduction should be at least 30 degrees. If passive hip abduction motion is limited by an adductor muscle contracture, which is likely with neuromuscular hip dysplasia, an adductor tenotomy may be indicated; this is typically performed at the beginning of the surgical procedure. Hip rotation motion should be assessed, and external and internal rotation should be approximately equal. After a satisfactory reduction of the fragments is achieved, the plate is secured to the distal femur with two bicortical screws. The most proximal hole on the plate should be filled with one long screw directed into the femoral neck to securely engage the proximal fragment.

The final neck shaft angle, the plate fixation, and the hip reduction should be evaluated using the C-arm. A deep suction drain is placed, and the wound is closed in separate fascial layers. For young children (i.e., those less than 6 years old), a 1½ hip spica cast holding the thigh in a slightly abducted and flexed position is applied for 5 to 6 weeks (Box 36-2).

### Surgical Technique for Correcting Femoral Valgus Deformity in Older Children, Preadolescents, and Adolescents

Among 5- to 12-year-old children, the varus osteotomy is usually secured with an intermediate 90-degree angled blade plate with a 10-mm offset and a 35- to 40-mm blade length (Synthes, Paoli, PA). The correction needed in this patient population is determined from functional radiographic images, noting the position of flexion, abduction, and internal rotation that optimally reduces the femoral head into the acetabulum. Alternatively, recently developed relatively low-profile locking plates of appropriate size for children (Synthes, Paoli, PA) have become available. The locking plate provides secure fixation, and, during insertion, it allows for some adjustment with regard to the degree of correction that can be obtained. The locking plate technique can be particularly advantageous when performing osteotomies on bones with relative osteomalacia. To insert a blade plate, a channel that corresponds with the size of the blade must be cut into the bone.

A special chisel is used to cut the channel from lateral to medial in the proximal femur. The chisel insertion site must be proximal enough in the proximal femur so that there will be sufficient femoral neck length to allow for the insertion of the entire blade (i.e., approximately 35 mm to 40 mm). The desired direction of the proximal and distal site of chisel entry into the proximal fragment is determined with the use of both of the K-wires as reference points as well as with C-arm imaging. With the use of a 90-degree template, the first reference wire is placed in a lateral to medial direction perpendicular to the shaft of the proximal diaphysis. While monitoring with a C-arm that provides anteroposterior and lateral views, the second wire is inserted proximal to the first wire into the femoral neck. This wire will serve as a directional guide for subsequent chisel placement. The chisel is advanced into the proximal femur parallel to the proximally placed guide pin to a depth equal to the length of the blade selected with the use of preoperative templating. The chisel insertion is carefully monitored with frequent anteroposterior and lateral C-arm images. If increased anterior coverage of the femoral head is desired, this can be accomplished by tilting the chisel posteriorly in the sagittal plane. When the blade plate is inserted into the posteriorly angulated chisel slot, the side plate will be extended. After the completion of the osteotomy and the reduction of the proximal and distal fragments to the blade plate, desired flexion will occur at the osteotomy site. The proximal fragment will be tilted posteriorly into the acetabulum, which will result in an improvement in the anterior coverage of the femoral head.

With the use of C-arm guidance, an osteotomy site is selected approximately 1.5 cm to 2 cm distal to the chisel channel. Subperiosteal retractors are placed circumferentially around the osteotomy site to protect the soft tissues, including the medial circumflex artery, from injury. A transverse intertrochanteric osteotomy is performed with a power saw, and the distal fragment is mobilized. The chisel is removed from the proximal fragment, and the blade plate is inserted. C-arm imaging is used to ensure that the blade is advanced into the same channel developed by the chisel. Next, the distal femoral fragment is reduced to the side plate and secured with a bone-reduction clamp. C-arm imaging is used to evaluate the neck shaft angle, to assess the adequacy of the varus correction, and to ensure that the femoral head will be optimally seated within the acetabulum. If less varus is desired, the 90-degree blade plate can be exchanged for a 100-degree blade plate. Alternatively, the blade plate can be removed and the side plate bent with plate benders to increase or decrease the blade-plate angle and to achieve the appropriate varus/valgus correction. Rotational correction can be adjusted by rotating the distal fragment as needed. Minor changes in flexion and extension (i.e., 10 degrees or less) can be obtained by altering the anterior and posterior angulation of the distal femoral fragment as it is secured on the side plate. This adjustment is limited by the necessity of achieving the bicortical fixation of all three distal screws that are used to secure the side plate.

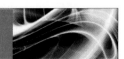

### BOX 36-2 TECHNICAL PEARLS: CORRECTING PROXIMAL FEMORAL VALGUS DEFORMITY IN YOUNG CHILDREN

- The osteotomy is performed with care taken to avoid medial soft-tissue penetration and injury to the medial circumflex vessels. Subperiosteal retractors are placed circumferentially around the osteotomy site to protect the soft tissues, including the medial circumflex artery, from injury.
- The appropriate medialization of the distal fragment can be best accomplished by obliquely excising the distal lateral edge of cortical bone from the proximal fragment before the insertion of the plate into the proximal fragment. The tips of the Wagner plate

are inserted into the proximal fragment at the site of the oblique bone excision.
- To ensure optimal fixation, the proximal fixation screw should be relatively long and extend through the center of the femoral neck to a point medial to the tip of the Wagner plate (but not through the growth plate). This should be a fully threaded cortical screw. If a partially threaded cancellous screw is used, it often breaks during attempted removal after osteotomy healing.

After the optimal correction has been achieved, the side plate is secured to the distal fragment with three bicortical screws with the use of the standard compression plating technique. After osteotomy fixation, hip range of motion is assessed to ensure that adequate flexion and extension, abduction and adduction, and approximately equal internal and external rotation have been obtained. Final C-arm images are taken to assess that both an appropriate redirection of the proximal femur and a stable osteotomy construct have been achieved (Figure 36-3). If the PFO is performed in conjunction with a pelvic osteotomy for the treatment of residual DDH, the pelvic osteotomy is performed first, followed by the PFO. If these procedures are performed in conjunction with a pelvic osteotomy to treat severe neuromuscular hip dysplasia, the PFO and any accompanying soft-tissue releases are done first, followed by the pelvic osteotomy. A deep suction drain is inserted into the fascial layers. The fascia of the vastus lateralis and the tensor fascia lata are repaired separately.

Fixation achieved with a blade-plate construct is typically rigid enough to maintain osteotomy correction without the need for supplemental spica casting. Despite this, we still recommend applying a 1½ hip spica cast for children 7 years old or younger to ensure patient comfort and to assist with transfers. For children who are 7 to 10 years old who are being treated for residual hip dysplasia, a removable abduction foam pillow can be used as an alternative to hip spica casting. Patients are allowed to be up with crutches and to have touch-down weight bearing on the involved extremity if they can comply with limited weight bearing. Patients who are undergoing proximal femoral varus osteotomy for the treatment of Legg-Calvé-Perthes disease benefit from abduction cast splinting (i.e., a bilateral cylinder cast connected with an abducting bar) to ensure femoral head containment during the acute stages of the healing of the osteotomy.

A proximal femoral varus-producing osteotomy is similarly performed for both preadolescents and adolescents. The same lateral approach and subperiosteal femoral exposure as described previously are used. The osteotomy site is typically located just proximal to the lesser trochanter in the intertrochanteric region. The osteotomy is fixated with either an adolescent-size (i.e., 90-degree angled, 40-mm blade length, and 10-mm offset) or an adult-size (i.e., 90-degree angled, 40-mm blade plate, and 10-mm offset) blade plate (Synthes, Paoli, PA). The radiographically monitored techniques for chisel and plate insertion are the same as those that were previously described. However, it is often considerably more difficult to insert both the chisel and the blade plate into the relatively denser bone of the adolescent. The chisel is gradually driven into the femur to a depth that is equal to the length of the blade plate that has been selected during preoperative planning (Figure 36-4).

Postoperatively, older patients are mobilized with protective weight bearing equal to the weight of the lower extremity for 6 weeks. When early bone consolidation callus formation appears on plain radiographs, progressive weight bearing is allowed. Most patients can perform full weight bearing without crutch protection by 8 to 10 weeks. Elective hardware removal is advised before excessive lateral bone overgrowth (Box 36-3).

## Surgical Technique for Correcting Proximal Femoral Varus Deformity

Valgus osteotomy of the proximal femur in younger patients is indicated for the treatment of varus deformities of the proximal femur. Clinical problems that are commonly treated with a proximal femoral valgus-producing osteotomy include congenital (developmental) coxa vara, growth disturbance from

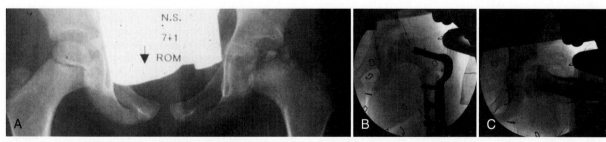

**Figure 36-3 A,** Anteroposterior bilateral hip radiograph of a 7-year-old child with evolving Legg-Calvé-Perthes disease of the left hip. **B** and **C,** Anteroposterior and lateral intraoperative C-arm radiographs of the left hip after a varus proximal femoral osteotomy fixated with a 100-degree adolescent-size blade plate.

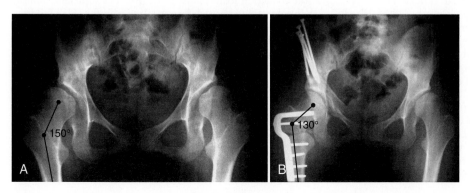

**Figure 36–4 A,** Anteroposterior pelvic radiograph of a 15-year-old girl with hip dysplasia: acetabular dysplasia, coxa valga (i.e., a neck shaft angle of 150 degrees), and subluxation. **B,** Anteroposterior pelvic radiograph 5 weeks after combined Bernese periacetabular and proximal femoral varus osteotomies. The latter was fixated with a 90-degree adult-size blade plate. The neck shaft angle was restored to 130 degrees.

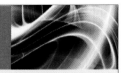

## BOX 36-3 TECHNICAL PEARLS: CORRECTING FEMORAL VALGUS DEFORMITY IN OLDER CHILDREN, PREADOLESCENTS, AND ADOLESCENTS

- The amount of varus achieved is directly determined by the attitude (i.e., the proximal-to-distal inclination) of the cutting chisel as it is inserted in a lateral-to-medial direction. If a 90-degree plate is to be used and, for example, 20 degrees of varus correction is desired, then the proximal K-wire is inserted and angulated approximately 20 degrees more vertical in reference to the distal K-wire.
- The initial insertion of the cutting chisel through the lateral cortex can be facilitated by making two or three parallel drill holes with a 3.2-mm drill bit in the lateral cortex and connecting them with a small, straight osteotome before inserting the chisel.
- A competent closure is essential when performing a varus-producing osteotomy. Care should be taken to ensure that the fascial layers are securely reapproximated over the greater trochanter and the shoulder of the blade plate to minimize the

- potential for subsequent chronic incisional discomfort/pain over these relatively prominent structures.
- The chisel or the subsequent blade plate may become incarcerated in the dense bone of the proximal femur of the adolescent patient. To minimize this occurrence, it is helpful to extract and reinsert the chisel before encountering marked resistance during insertion.
- When correcting coxa valga, medialization of the distal fragment is necessary to align the medullary canal with the piriformis fossa of the proximal fragment. This can be achieved by further impacting the nail into the proximal fragment to achieve more medialization. Alternatively, a blade plate with a shorter blade or a blade plate with a greater offset can be used. If less medialization is necessary, the blade plate can be slightly extracted, or a blade plate with a longer blade can be used.

avascular necrosis associated with previous treatment for DDH, and residual varus after a proximal femoral varus-producing osteotomy for Legg-Calvé-Perthes disease. Patients with coxa vara have limited hip abduction and more external rotation than internal rotation. The goals of a valgus-producing osteotomy are to increase the neck shaft angle, and to improve hip mechanics by increasing hip abduction and normalizing the abductor function that reduces gait deviations. Preoperatively, the desired correction can be determined from functional radiographic images with the hip in adduction and internal rotation.

A proximal femoral valgus osteotomy is performed through the same lateral approach as previously described for performing a varus osteotomy. The proximal femoral valgus osteotomy in young children is fixated with an intermediate blade plate that is 130-degree angled with a 35-mm to 45-mm blade length and a three- or four-hole side plate (Synthes, Paoli, PA). K-wires are inserted under C-arm guidance and used as a reference when inserting the chisel. To accomplish this, the first K-wire is inserted perpendicular into the proximal femoral diaphysis from a lateral to medial direction, which simulates the position of a side plate parallel to the shaft of the femur after the blade is inserted. A second and more proximal guidewire is placed into the proximal femoral neck at an angle predetermined with the use of preoperative templates to obtain the desired varus deformity correction.

Next, the bone-cutting chisel is inserted into the proximal fragment parallel to the second, proximal K-wire. With the use of C-arm guidance, the cutting chisel is advanced into the femoral neck to a depth that is equal to the length of the blade on the preselected blade plate. Later, after the osteotomy has been completed and the 130-degree blade plate has been inserted and fixed to the distal fragment, a 30-degree valgus correction will have been achieved. If flexion or extension correction is also desirable, the chisel should be tilted either anteriorly or posteriorly; anterior tilt flexes the distal fragment and functionally increases hip joint flexion, thus potentially decreasing anterior head coverage. Similarly, if the chisel is tilted posteriorly, the distal fragment is extended, which in turn increases femoral head coverage during weight bearing.

When using the 130-degree blade plate to fix a valgus osteotomy, it is desirable and possible to remove the chisel and insert the blade plate before the osteotomy is performed. When it is positioned in valgus, the blade plate will not be in the way of the performance of the osteotomy. The osteotomy is performed at the intertrochanteric area with the power saw. Subperiosteal retractors are placed

circumferentially around the osteotomy site to protect the soft tissues, including the medial circumflex artery, from injury.

When the osteotomy is complete, the distal fragment is mobilized and secured to the side plate with a bone clamp. If additional lengthening of the extremity is not desired, then one or both osteotomy fragments should be appropriately shortened to avoid the overlengthening of the extremity. After the blade plate has been inserted, a more normal neck shaft angle will be noted when the varus deformity is corrected as assessed with the C-arm (Figure 36-5). If necessary, it is possible to alter the relative degree of varus and valgus by changing to a different angle blade plate or bending the blade plate with a plate bender. Passive hip abduction will be notably increased. Patients with the coxa vara deformity often have inherent shortening of the adductor muscles. If after the correction of the varus deformity it appears that the shortening of the adductor muscle is limiting passive abduction, an adductor tenotomy should be performed, typically of the adductor longus tendon. Internal and external hip rotation is assessed. It may be necessary to internally rotate the distal fragment to correct an out-toeing gait deformity. The medial and lateral relationship of the two fragments is assessed. The fixation screws are inserted into the distal fragment with the use of a compression technique. Final C-arm images are taken to confirm that the desired correction has been achieved.

A suction drain is placed deep to the vastus lateralis muscle; it exits through the skin proximally and laterally. The fascial layers (i.e., the vastus lateralis fascia and the fascia lata) are securely closed in separate layers, and the subcutaneous tissue and skin are closed. To protect the osteotomy and to minimize discomfort in a young child (i.e., those 6 years old or younger), a spica cast or an abduction cast is used for 5 to 6 weeks. Alternatively, for older children (i.e., those 6 years old and older), the use of a soft abduction foam pillow often provides sufficient comfort when correcting a varus deformity. Typically, for older children, protective early weight bearing is permitted. Healing readily occurs without a loss of correction in these patients.

Very severe varus deformities can occur among younger children as a result of either congenital (developmental) coxa vara or coxa vara that occurs as a result of the treatment of DDH. The trochanter in these patients is often very high riding, the femoral neck is shortened, and the neck shaft angle is less than 90 degrees. When correcting this severe deformity, consideration must be given to restoring a more normal neck shaft angle, distal and lateral repositioning of the greater trochanter, and restoring a more normal femoral neck length. Both Wagner and Morscher have used a three-part osteotomy when attempting to correct all

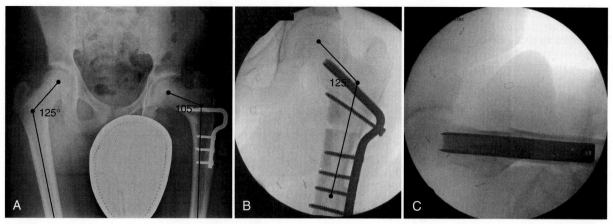

**Figure 36–5  A,** Anteroposterior bilateral hip radiograph of a 13-year-old adolescent after a varus osteotomy for the containment treatment of Legg-Calvé-Perthes disease at the age of 9 years. Residual pathologic varus deformity persists. The neck shaft angles of the proximal femurs are 105 degrees on the left and 125 degrees on the right. **B,** Anteroposterior and, **C,** lateral intraoperative C-arm radiographs of the left proximal femur after a valgus osteotomy fixated with a 120-degree adult-size blade plate. The neck shaft angle has been restored to 125 degrees. Note that the center of the medullary canal of the distal fragment is aligned with the piriformis fossa.

aspects of this often severe deformity. When performing either of these two relatively complex femoral osteotomies, the surgeon should be aware of the circulatory pathways of the medial femoral circumflex artery as it courses into the femoral capital epiphysis. There is an inherent risk of injury to the critical terminal branches of the medial circumflex artery as well as a risk for the subsequent occurrence of femoral capital epiphysis avascular necrosis that occurs with any osteotomy that cuts through the lateral femoral base of the trochanter or the femoral neck. Similarly, Cech and colleagues reported about the use of a two-part osteotomy to obtain correction, specifically of the typically severe coxa vara deformity that can occur after marked growth disturbance associated with the closed treatment of DDH. The 100-degree blade plate is inserted directly through the lateral aspect of the trochanter, and the osteotomy cut is a two-part triangle that is centered along the newly elongated inferior neck of the proximal femur. This osteotomy is theoretically less likely to injure the circulation of the proximal femur than the Wagner and Morscher osteotomies. When correcting relatively severe coxa vara deformities with any of the previously described valgus osteotomies, the trochanter is moved distally. This places the abductor muscles under increased tension, and a relative abductor contracture may be noted intraoperatively. With time, the functional abduction muscle tightness will resolve (Box 36-4).

## Surgical Technique for Proximal Femoral Osteotomy for Slipped Capital Femoral Epiphysis

A proximal femoral osteotomy is frequently performed to correct the chronic and often severe proximal femoral deformity that results from an SCFE. The slip deformity is characterized by the posterior displacement of the epiphysis on the metaphysis. This exposed femoral neck impinges on the anterior acetabulum during flexion. Patients with this condition present with some of the most challenging of all problems related to joint-preservation surgery. The surgical approach that is necessary to correct complex SCFE deformities often includes both a proximal femoral redirectional osteotomy and a femoral head–neck osteochondroplasty. The proximal femoral redirectional osteotomy flexes and internally rotates the distal fragment (i.e., the lower extremity) relative to the displaced epiphysis. The proximal femur osteochondroplasty further reduces or eliminates anterolateral cam hip joint impingement. The surgical correction of the slip deformity with PFO and osteochondroplasty is indicated for healed slip deformities and chronic stable deformities; it is not indicated for slip deformities that are unstable.

The two current surgical techniques that provide the comprehensive correction of an SCFE deformity include the anterolateral (Watson-Jones) approach and the more recently described

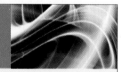

## BOX 36–4  TECHNICAL PEARLS: CORRECTING PROXIMAL FEMORAL VARUS DEFORMITY

- The proximal K-wire will be the guide for the frontal plane direction of both the chisel cut and the blade plate insertion. The degree of correction is determined by the relative frontal plane alignment of the two wires. If a 130-degree angled blade plate is to be used and, for example, 30 degrees of valgus correction is desired, then the proximal K-wire is inserted and angulated approximately 10 degrees more vertical in reference to the distal K-wire.
- Performing a varus-correcting osteotomy proximal to the lesser trochanter allows for correction close to the center of the deformity, which is typically the head–neck junction. However, because of this, the osteotomy is proximal to the insertion of the psoas, which may make it more difficult to eventually abduct the distal fragment. Performing the osteotomy distal to the insertion of the psoas tendon attachment will make it easier to abduct the

distal fragment relative to the proximal fragment. However, the lesser trochanter may become relatively prominent and potentially impinge on the lateral pelvis during hip adduction.
- A valgus osteotomy of the proximal femur will variably lengthen the extremity, which may be desirable. However, soft-tissue tension may make it difficult to readily correct the varus deformity as the fragments are reduced to the blade plate. Shortening the distal fragment will facilitate the redirection of the fragments.
- When performing a valgus osteotomy, excessive medialization of the distal fragment can adversely shift the mechanical axis of the lower extremity laterally in the knee joint, thus potentiating a valgus thrust. To avoid this, if less medialization is needed when reducing the fragments to one another, either do not seat the blade completely or select a blade plate with a longer blade.

surgical hip dislocation. The extensive reconstructive procedures that are needed to adequately correct this deformity can be facilitated with a surgical hip dislocation. In North America, many patients with SCFE deformity have associated morbid obesity. For those patients with severe obesity, the surgical correction of a problematic slip deformity should be deferred until the patient has achieved an appropriate weight loss.

The anterolateral (Watson-Jones) hip approach provides sufficient exposure for performing a proximal intertrochanteric femoral osteotomy, a capsulotomy, and an anterolateral osteochondroplasty. The patient is positioned supine with a bump under the ipsilateral buttock. The incision starts at a point approximately 4 cm to 5 cm posterior and 3 cm distal to the anterosuperior iliac spine, extends to and then gradually curves anteriorly around the posterior edge of greater trochanter, and extending distally for several centimeters parallel with the shaft of the femur. The skin and the subcutaneous tissue are reflected together to anteriorly and posteriorly expose the fascia lata. Distal to the trochanter, the fascia lata is incised in a longitudinal direction parallel to the shaft of the femur. This is extended proximally across the greater trochanter, along the posterior edge of the gluteus maximus muscle. The posterior border of the tensor is separated from the anterior border of the gluteus medius muscle. The surgeon should further develop this interval proximally, being careful to avoid injury to the branches of the superior gluteal nerve, which courses in an anteromedial direction and innervates the tensor fascia lata muscle.

Deep to the anterior border of the gluteus medius, the greater trochanter and the anterolateral base of the femoral neck can be identified. Just distal to the anterolateral base of the femoral neck are the origins of the vastus lateralis and the vastus intermedius muscles. The vastus fascia is longitudinally incised in line with the femur, and the vastus muscle is reflected off of the lateral intramuscular septum in a proximal-to-distal and lateral-to-medial direction. The reflection of the vastus lateralis is extended proximally and medially to include the vastus intermedius muscle, which completes the exposure of the base of the proximal femur.

Starting laterally at the base of the neck, the hip capsule is exposed medially up to the anterolateral edge of the acetabulum. Narrow, deep-type retractors are helpful for exposing the capsule. An arthrotomy is made in the direction of the femoral neck; care should be taken when incising the capsule proximally to avoid cutting the labrum. Further exposure of the femoral neck is achieved by proximally extending the capsulotomy medially and laterally. After the labrum has been visualized, the anterior rim of the acetabulum can be palpated. A cobra-type retractor is inserted on the anterolateral acetabulum rim and placed around the medial femoral neck to optimize the exposure. This type of retractor should not be placed around the superior/posterior femoral neck because of the risk of injury to the terminal branches of the medial femoral circumflex artery as it enters the posterior lateral femoral neck. The normal bony anatomy will be distorted by a prominent anterolateral metaphyseal bump of bone. The size of the prominence varies with the severity of the slip. If the slipped epiphysis had previously been stabilized, the screw heads may protrude on the anterior neck of the femur. The epiphysis, which has been displaced posteriorly on the metaphysis, will not be visible at this time. The screws should be removed if the physis is closed. If the physis is still open and the slip has not been previously stabilized with screw fixation, then consideration should be given to inserting a 6.5-mm cannulated screw into the epiphysis before performing the redirectional osteotomy.

The intertrochanteric osteotomy can be fixed with either a 120-degree or a 90-degree angled blade plate. The 120-degree blade plate is inserted through the lateral cortex of the femur beginning at the level of the greater trochanter and is directed proximally into the femoral neck, whereas the 90-degree blade plate is inserted through the lateral femoral cortex and transversely across the proximal femur at the base of the femoral neck and is perpendicular to the femoral shaft (Figure 36-6).

The exact slope of the chisel channel that is used to cut the channel in the proximal femur is determined with the use of two K-wires for reference. The first reference K-wire is placed perpendicular to the proximal lateral femoral cortex under C-arm guidance. If the 120-degree angled blade plate is used, the second wire is inserted from lateral to medial into the femoral neck but sloping 30 degrees proximally. If the 90-degree blade plate is to be inserted, the second wire is inserted into the proximal femur parallel to the first K-wire and just proximal to the desired entry site of the blade plate in a lateral-to-medial direction.

Whichever blade plate is to be used (i.e., 120 degree or 90 degree), the chisel is inserted just distal and parallel to the proximal reference K-wire. To facilitate the insertion of the chisel, three parallel drill holes are made at the preselected chisel entry site. On the sagittal plane, the chisel entry site must be anteriorly inclined equal to the degree of desired correction of the pathologically posteriorly angulated epiphysis; the amount of correction may be as much as 60 degrees. Accordingly, the parallel drills are similarly inclined proximal to distal in the anteroposterior plane. The cutting chisel is inserted with critical C-arm guidance; two views made at 90 degrees to each other are essential (these are typically anteroposterior and frog-leg lateral views). The chisel is slowly advanced into the proximal femur medially to a depth that equals the length of the blade of the blade plate that has been selected.

The intertrochanteric osteotomy is performed just proximal to the lesser trochanter with a power saw at a site that is 2 cm or less distal to the blade plate insertion.

When performing the osteotomy, subperiosteal retractors are placed circumferentially around the osteotomy to protect the soft tissues, most importantly, the medial circumflex artery, from injury. After the completion of the osteotomy, the soft tissues are further stripped from the proximal aspect of the distal fragment, which allows the fragment to be flexed and reduced to the blade plate; the blade plate is in a flexed position and securely fixed in the proximal fragment. The distal fragment is firmly secured to the blade plate with a bone clamp. As the hip is carefully extended, the previously posteriorly displaced epiphysis will reduce anteriorly back into the acetabulum. The preliminary reduction is assessed with the C-arm.

The varus deformity noted on the preoperative anteroposterior x-ray is more apparent than real as a result of the external rotation of the posteriorly displaced or tilted epiphysis. If the condition does not appear to have been corrected, which is uncommon, additional varus correction can be achieved by exchanging the 120-degree blade plate for a 130-degree blade plate or by exchanging the 90-degree blade plate for a 100-degree blade plate. More medialization of the distal fragment can be achieved by driving the 120-degree blade plate farther into the femoral neck or by using a blade plate with a shorter blade. When using the 90-degree blade plate, further medialization can be achieved by driving the nail more medially or, more likely, by exchanging the 10-mm offset blade plate for a 15-mm offset 90-degree blade plate. More lateralization is achieved with either the 120-degree or the 90-degree blade plate by partially extracting the previously placed blade plate or exchanging it with a blade plate with a longer blade. Optimal positioning of the femoral shaft relative to the head aligns the piriformis fossa with the medullary canal of the distal fragment. A long cortical screw is used to fix the proximal fragment to the blade plate. Next, two screws are inserted in a compression mode to secure the distal fragment to the side plate. The bone clamp is removed, and the range of hip motion is assessed. Passive flexion and abduction motion should be notably improved with the

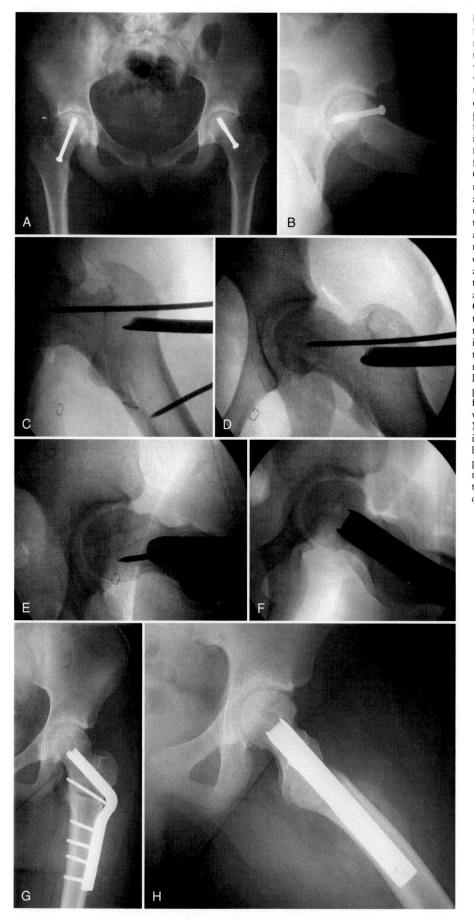

**Figure 36–6  A,** Anteroposterior pelvic radiograph of a 14-year-old girl with a previous in situ pinning of bilateral slipped capital femoral epiphyses; she walks with an external rotation deformity which is greater on the left side than on the right. **B,** Frog-leg lateral radiograph of the left hip that demonstrates the posterior tilt of the femoral head and femoroacetabular impingement. There is noted anterolateral hip pain with flexion and obligatory external rotation in flexion. **C,** Anteroposterior intraoperative C-arm radiographs that show the screw removal, the insertion of reference wires, and the initial chisel placement to be used for cutting a tract for inserting the blade plate. **D,** Anteroposterior and, **E,** lateral intraoperative C-arm radiographs that show the advancement of the chisel. Note the large bony ridge along the anterolateral proximal femur that pathologically impinges on the acetabulum. **F,** Lateral intraoperative C-arm radiographs after the fixation of the flexion osteotomy (i.e., the posterior tilt of the femoral head as seen in image **B** has been corrected) and after the large anterolateral bump has been resected. **G,** Anteroposterior and, **H,** lateral radiographs of the left hip 6 weeks postoperatively showing proximal femoral flexion and rotational osteotomy fixated with a 120-degree adult-size blade plate. Note that the center of the femoral shaft is aligned with the piriformis fossa on both views. Also note the resection of a previously existing anterolateral head–neck bony "bump" (as seen in image **D**); the hip now flexes to 95 degrees with 15 degrees of internal rotation in flexion.

hip flexed 45 degrees. Internal rotation should be equal to external rotation. The reduction is assessed with the C-arm and the final two screws are inserted.

Despite the flexion-correcting osteotomy, a prominent anterolateral metaphyseal bump may still impinge on the acetabulum during hip flexion and internal rotation in flexion and abduction. This abnormal bony prominence can also be visualized radiographically on the frog-leg lateral view. Through this anterolateral approach, it is possible to perform an osteochondroplasty to excise the bony prominence for an approximately 100-degree to 110-degree arc at the head–neck junction. After the completion of the osteochondroplasty, the range of hip motion is assessed. The goal is to achieve equal internal and external rotation as measured with the hip in approximately 45 degrees of flexion, 90 degrees or more of flexion, 15 degrees of internal rotation in 90 degrees of flexion, and more than 30 degrees of abduction. The capsule is loosely reapproximated. A deep drain is placed and brought out laterally through the soft tissue. The vastus lateralis and the intermedius fascia are reapproximated. If the anterior edge of the gluteus medius tendon was incised during the exposure, it should be securely repaired with a heavy permanent suture. The fascia lata and the gluteus maximus fascia are approximated with No. 1 interrupted absorbable suture. The subcutaneous and skin tissues are closed.

Patients ambulate on postoperative day 1 or 2, as previously described. Large corrections have often been made at the osteotomy site. Weight bearing should not be progressed until there is radiologic evidence of progressive consolidation, which may take several weeks. With this approach, bone overgrowth on the implant often occurs. Implant removal is advised within 1 to 1.5 years (Box 36-5).

## POSTOPERATIVE REHABILITATION

Rehabilitation after PFO for younger patients is quite variable. For very young children and those with neuromuscular or DDH-associated hip dysplasia, postoperative immobilization in a spica cast precludes any immediate rehabilitation. After the spica cast is removed, children are appropriately mobilized. Range-of-motion exercises are initiated, and ambulation is resumed as the osteotomy consolidates. Younger children may require the use of a wheelchair or walker rather than crutches

in order to limit weight bearing. If secure intraoperative fixation is achieved (i.e., with a blade or a locking plate) after a PFO in an older child, a postoperative spica cast is often not required. These patients are allowed to perform touch-down weight bearing equivalent to the weight of the involved lower extremity. Children who undergo varus osteotomies for the treatment of acute Legg-Calvé-Perthes disease often have variably restricted abduction. To ensure that the femoral head is contained, both hips are immobilized in a broomstick abduction cast for 4 to 5 weeks during the immediate postoperative period. Older patients, such as those undergoing PFO for the correction of a rotation deformity or a deformity that resulted from SCFE, should be mobilized as soon as possible after surgery. Long-term strengthening exercises for the abductor muscles are emphasized. Limb-length inequalities are accommodated with appropriate lifts for patients of all ages.

## COMPLICATIONS

Most of the complications and problems that occur after PFO are related to failure to obtain adequate bony correction or failure of fixation. With a loss of fixation, the healing of the osteotomy may occur in suboptimal alignment, which may result in a failure to achieve the desired deformity correction. Similarly, delayed healing or even nonunion can occur. In the younger child, the Wagner plate is very versatile for achieving the stabilization of an intertrochanteric osteotomy when attempting combined corrections (e.g., varus or valgus, rotation and flexion or extension). However, the inherent relative flexibility of the Wagner implant may provide for only relatively limited osteotomy stability during the immediate postoperative period. A loss of fixation, delayed union or nonunion, and a resulting loss of the optimal correction of the deformity can and do occur.

A blade plate or a locking plate provides for relatively optimal inherent osteotomy stability. However, complications and problems when performing osteotomies with more rigid implants in older and larger children do occur. Inadequate planning, suboptimal osteotomy technique, and relatively weak bone strength are factors that potentiate the problems of achieving less-than-satisfactory intraoperative deformity correction and of the loss of both fixation and correction postoperatively.

---

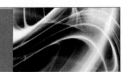

### BOX 36-5 TECHNICAL PEARLS: PROXIMAL FEMORAL OSTEOTOMY FOR SLIPPED CAPITAL FEMORAL EPIPHYSIS

- Incise the fascia lata distally where the plane between it and the underlying vastus lateralis fascia is easily developed. Extend the fascial incision proximally across the greater trochanter, along the posterior edge of the tensor fascia lata muscle, and anterior to the adjacent edge of the gluteus maximus muscle. Separate the posterior border of the tensor from the anterior border of the gluteus medius muscle deep to the tensor.
- If necessary, the exposure can be augmented by making a small transverse incision through the most anterior edge of the gluteus medius tendon just proximal to its attachment to the greater trochanter. However, this must be repaired at the end of the procedure.
- Although the 90-degree blade plate is easier to insert, relatively greater fixation can be achieved with the 120-degree blade plate. However, to insert the 120-degree blade plate, the femoral neck must be wide enough to allow for the full insertion of the blade. For younger and smaller patients, this may not be possible.

- It is usually possible to remove the chisel and insert the blade plate before the osteotomy is performed. After the blade is inserted into the anteriorly inclined chisel channel, the plate will be anteriorly flexed and not in the way of the performance of the osteotomy.
- When performing an intertrochanteric osteotomy to correct an SCFE deformity, the osteotomy is performed several centimeters distal to the site of deformity (i.e., the proximal epiphyseal metaphyseal junction of the physis). Therefore, the distal fragment should be translated anteriorly on the proximal fragment. The medullary canal of the distal fragment is aligned with the piriformis fossa of the proximal fragment on both the anteroposterior and lateral C-arm images. The reduction is made "end to side" rather than "end to end." This will minimize the establishment of a permanent zigzag deformity in the medullary canal of the proximal femur; it is relatively easier to do with the 120-degree blade plate.

Intraoperative technique is important to avoid specific neurovascular complications. The medial femoral circumflex artery courses medially across the psoas tendon at the level of the hip joint. In younger patients, avascular necrosis of the femoral head has been reported, presumably as a result of direct injury during the performance of a PFO. When approaching the proximal femur, a subperiosteal plane of dissection should be used to expose the medial cortex; curved subperiosteal retractors serve to protect the medial soft tissues when completing the osteotomy with an oscillating saw. Similarly, when exposing the posterior proximal femoral cortex, there is a potential for injury to the adjacent sciatic nerve, which courses proximal to distal just posterior to the femur. Injury to the sciatic nerve can be minimized with the use of a subperiosteal approach; this necessitates elevating the firm attachment of the gluteus maximus muscle from the proximal surface of the femur.

When performing a varus osteotomy to correct valgus, the proximal lateral greater trochanter and the lateral shoulder of the 90-degree blade plate become relatively more prominent. Later, after the healing of the osteotomy, relatively incompetent soft-tissue coverage over this variably prominent blade plate and greater trochanter can potentiate chronic lateral proximal thigh discomfort. To minimize this potential for discomfort, it is essential to achieve competent soft-tissue closure. Both the vastus lateralis fascia and the fascia lata should be separately and securely approximated.

## ANNOTATED REFERENCES AND SUGGESTED READINGS

Abraham E, Gonzalez MH, Pratap S, Amirouche F, Atluri P, Simon P. Clinical implications of anatomic wear characteristics in slipped capital femoral epiphysis and primary osteoarthritis. *J Pediatr Orthop.* 2007;27:788–795.

Axer A. Subtrochanteric osteotomy in the treatment of Perthes' disease. *J Bone Joint Surg.* 1965;47B:489.

Bucholz RW, Ogden JA. Patterns of ischemic necrosis of the proximal femur in nonoperatively treated congenital hip disease. In: *The Hip. Proceeding of the sixth open scientific meeting of the Hip Society.* St. Louis: CV Mosby; 1978:44–63.

Cech O, Vavra J, Zidka M. Management of ischemic deformity after the treatment of developmental dsyplasia of the hip. *J Pediatr Orthop.* 2005;25:687–694.

Description of the technique used for intertrochanteric valgus osteotomy of the proximal femur with simultaneous fusion of the greater trochanteric epiphysis, femoral neck lengthening, and fixation of the osteotomy with a 120-degree blade plate.

Crawford AH. The role of osteotomy in the treatment of slipped capital femoral epiphysis. In: Barr SJ, ed. *Instructional course lectures.* Park Ridge: American Academy of Orthopaedic Surgeons; 1989:273–279.

Good overview of the purpose and types of different proximal femoral osteotomies that have been described to treat slipped capital femoral epiphysis. They found that the results of trochanteric osteotomies are not as good as the neck osteotomies, but there is a lower rate of AVN in osteotomies performed in the trochanteric region than in the neck region.

Diab M, Hresko MT, Millis MB. Intertrochanteric versus subcapital osteotomy in slipped capital femoral epiphysis. *Clin Orthop Relat Res.* 2004;(427):204–212.

Compared intertrochanteric and subcapital osteotomies for SCFE and found that a flexion intertrochanteric osteotomy was more effective in restoring proximal femoral anatomy and had a lower reoperation rate. Describes the technique of using a 90-degree blade plate for osteotomy fixation.

Galpin RD, Roach JW, Wenger DR, Herring JA, Birch JG. One-stage treatment of congenital dislocation of the hip in older children, including femoral shortening. *J Bone Joint Surg Am.* 1989;71(5):734–741.

Description of the surgical technique for femoral shortening osteotomy in the treatment of DDH of children over 2 years old.

Ganz R, Gill TJ, Gautier E, Ganz K, Krugel N, Berlemann U. Surgical dislocation of the adult hip a technique with full access to the femoral head and acetabulum without the risk of avascular necrosis. *J Bone Joint Surg.* 2001;83B:1119–1124.

Classic article describing the technique for surgical dislocation of the hip and the vascular anatomy that must be preserved.

Gautier E, Ganz K, Krugel N, Gill T, Ganz R. Anatomy of the medial femoral circumflex artery and its surgical implications. *J Bone Joint Surg Br.* 2000;82(5):679–683.

The classic article describing the vascular anatomy of the proximal femur and how to avoid injuring the medial femoral circumflex artery when performing a proximal femoral osteotomy.

Gordon JE, Capelli AM, Delgado ED, Schoenecker PL. Pemberton pelvic osteotomy and varus rotational osteotomy in the treatment of acetabular dysplasia in patients who have static encephalopathy. *J Bone Joint Surg.* 1996;78A:1863–1871.

Reviews the results and surgical technique of varus rotational osteotomy in the neuromuscular patient with hip dysplasia. Recommends a femoral shortening osteotomy at the time of varus rational osteotomy if unable to achieve a minimum of 45 degrees of abduction following adductor tenotomies.

Gordon JE, Hughes MS, Shepherd K, Szymanski DA, Schoenecker PL, Parker L, Uong EC. Obstructive sleep apnoea syndrome in morbidly obese children with tibia vara. *J Bone Joint Surg.* 2006;88B:100–103.

Kalamchi A, MacEwen GD. Avascular necrosis following treatment of congenital dislocation of the hip. *J Bone Joint Surg Am.* 1980;62(6):876–888.

Describes the pattern of AVN in the femoral head following treatment for DDH.

Karadimas JE, Holloway GM, Waugh W. Growth of the proximal femur after varus-derotation osteotomy in the treatment of congenital dislocation of the hip. *Clin Orthop Relat Res.* 1982;(162):61–68.

Describes the remodeling that occurs over time following proximal femoral osteotomy in children with hip dysplasia. The best outcome was when the neck-shaft angle measured 100 to 110 degrees immediately after osteotomy.

Kasser JR, Bowen JR, MacEwen GD. Varus derotation osteotomy in the treatment of persistent dysplasia in congenital dislocation of the hip. *J Bone Joint Surg.* 1985;67A:195–202.

Description of the indications, limitations, and surgical technique for varus derotational osteotomy in patients with persistent DDH. Best results are found in patients less than 4 years old at the time of osteotomy and acetabular development continues to improve until the age of 8.

Leunig M, Casillas MM, Hamlet M, Hersche O, Notzli H, Slongo T, Ganz R. Slipped capital femoral epiphysis: early mechanical damage to the acetabular cartilage by a prominent femoral metaphysis. *Acta Orthop Scand.* 2000;71:370–375.

Good description of the spectrum femoral head–neck deformity found in slipped capital femoral epiphysis and reviews the mechanical impingement that can trigger early damage to the labrum and articular cartilage resulting in early hip arthrosis.

Leunig M, Slongo T, Kleinschmidt M, Ganz R. Subcapital correction osteotomy in slipped capital femoral epiphysis by means of surgical hip dislocation. *Oper Orthop Trauma.* 2007;19:389–410.

Detailed description of the pathoanatomy of the proximal femur and the technique used for surgical dislocations of the hip in conjunction with subcapital osteotomy in the treatment of slipped capital femoral epiphysis.

**McNerney NP, Mubarak SJ, Wenger DR.** One-stage correction of the dysplastic hip in cerebral palsy with the San Diego acetabuloplasty: results and complications. *J Pediatr Orthop.* 2000;20:93–103.

Reviews the results and surgical technique of varus rotational osteotomy in the neuromuscular patient with hip dysplasia. Avoid creating excessive varus that can weaken the patient's abductors, predispose the osteopenic bone to fall progressively into varus, and hinder hip abduction. Recommends a 90-degree blade plate to secure the femoral osteotomy. They had an 8% rate of AVN of the femoral head, which was attributed to disruption of blood supply during soft-tissue lengthening (especially iliopsoas), blade plate insertion, or excessive pressure on the femoral head due to inadequate femoral shortening or aggressive acetabuloplasty.

**Morscher E.** Osteotomy to lengthen the femur neck with distal adjustment of the trochanter major in coxa vara after hip dislocation. *Orthopade.* 1988;17:485.

**Oh CW, Guille JT, Kumar SJ, Lipton GE, MacEwen GD.** Operative treatment for type II avascular necrosis in developmental dysplasia of the hip. *Clin Orthop Relat Res.* 2005;(434):86–91.

Good summary of using a varus osteotomy to correct coxa valga resulting from secondary AVN following previous childhood treatments for hip dysplasia.

**Paley DR.** Hip joint considerations. In: Paley DR, Herzenberg JE, eds. *Principles of deformity correction.* Berlin: Springer-Verlag; 2002:650–653.

**Schoenecker PL, Anderson DJ, Capelli AM.** The acetabular response to proximal femoral varus rotational osteotomy. Results after failure of post-reduction abduction splinting in patients who had congenital dislocation of the hip. *J Bone Joint Surg.* 1995;77A:990–997.

Summary of the technique for femoral varus rotational osteotomy in the treatment of DDH indicates improvement of the acetabular index in the majority of hips. Results suggest proximal femoral osteotomy is best reserved for patients under the age of 4.

**Schoenecker PL, Strecker WB.** Congenital dislocation of the hip in children. Comparison of the effects of femoral shortening and of skeletal traction in treatment. *J Bone Joint Surg.* 1984;66A:21–27.

Description of the surgical technique for femoral shortening osteotomy in the treatment of DDH. Acetabular remodeling occurs after femoral osteotomy and may not require pelvic osteotomy if concentric hip reduction is achieved.

**Spencer S, Millis MB, Kim Y-J.** Early results of treatment of hip impingement syndrome in slipped capital femoral epiphysis and pistol grip deformity of the femoral head-neck junction using the surgical dislocation technique. *J Pediatr Orthop.* 2006;26:281–285.

**Tonnis D.** Femoral osteotomies to improve the hip joint. In: Tonnis D, ed. *Congenital dysplasia and dislocation of the hip in children and adults.* Berlin: Springer-Verlag; 1987:336–355.

**Wagner H, ed.** The hip: Proceedings of the 4th open scientific meeting of the hip society. St. Louis: CV Mosby; 1976.

**Weiner SD, Weiner DS, Riley PM.** Pitfalls in treatment of Legg-Calve-Perthes disease using proximal femoral varus osteotomy. *J Pediatr Orthop.* 1991;11(1):20–24.

Femoral varus osteotomy to contain the femoral head in LCP disease should avoid varus <105 degrees and consideration should be given to performing a greater trochanteric epiphysiodesis at the time of varus osteotomy.

**Whiteside LA, Schoenecker PL.** Combined valgus derotation osteotomy and cervical osteoplasty for severely slipped capital femoral epiphysis: mechanical analysis and report preliminary results using compression screw fixation and early weight bearing. *Clin Orthop Rel Res.* 1978;132:88–97.

Very early description of the pathoanatomy of the metaphyseal prominence found with slipped capital epiphysis. Description of the surgical technique used for cervical osteotomy and the importance of excising the prominence at the time of intertrochanteric valgus derotational osteotomy.

# CHAPTER 37

# Pediatric Pelvic Osteotomies and Shelf Procedures

*Teresa M. Ferguson and Stuart L. Weinstein*

## INTRODUCTION

The goal of the treatment of a child with developmental dysplasia of the hip is to attain a radiographically confirmed normal hip at maturity to hopefully prevent degenerative joint disease. Residual acetabular dysplasia, with or without hip subluxation, will lead to degenerative joint disease. Studies of the causes of degenerative joint disease of the hip estimate that 20% to 50% of cases may be attributed to acetabular dysplasia or hip subluxation, especially among females. The correction of residual acetabular dysplasia theoretically provides for a better weight-bearing surface for the femoral head, restores normal biomechanics of the hip, reduces contact pressures, and increases the longevity of the hip. Biomechanical studies have shown that the onset of joint degeneration correlates with both the magnitude and duration of exposure to contact stresses above 2 MPa.

## BASIC SCIENCE

The normal growth and development of the hip joint require a genetically determined balance of growth of the acetabular and triradiate cartilages in conjunction with a well-located femoral head. By the eleventh week of intrauterine life, the hip joint is fully formed. Several factors come into play to allow for the normal development of the acetabulum. The main stimulus for the concave shape of the acetabulum is the presence and maintenance of a reduced spheric femoral head. There must also be normal interstitial and appositional growth within the acetabular cartilage as well as periosteal new bone formation in the adjacent bones of the pelvis. At puberty, the development of three secondary centers of ossification serves to further enhance the depth of the acetabulum. The os acetabulum is the epiphysis of the pubis, and it forms the anterior wall of the acetabulum. The acetabular epiphysis is the epiphysis of the ilium, and it forms the superior edge of the acetabulum. The ischial epiphysis also contributes to normal growth.

In a child with developmental hip dysplasia, some aspects of normal growth and development are altered. The femoral head is the key stimulus for acetabular development, so it must be reduced as soon as possible. If the reduction is maintained, it will provide the stimulus for acetabular development, and there is the potential for the recovery and resumption of normal growth and development. The capacity for the acetabular cartilage to resume normal growth depends on its intrinsic growth potential and on whether it was damaged by the subluxated or dislocated femoral head, by various attempts at reduction, or by surgery. After the age of 4 years, the potential for the restoration of normal anatomy is markedly decreased.

## INDICATIONS

- The failure of the progression of normal acetabular development after the reduction of developmental hip dysplasia
- Residual acetabular dysplasia in a growing child
- Symptomatic dysplasia in a mature adolescent with mild to no hip arthrosis

## HISTORY AND PHYSICAL EXAMINATION

Children with residual dysplasia are most often asymptomatic. Early complaints may be of vague discomfort with activity; complaints of more severe pain may indicate the presence of degenerative changes in the hip. Catching, locking, or giving way may be indicative of labral pathology. Sharp groin pain, especially with hip flexion, may suggest acetabular impingement.

The physical examination should include an assessment of the hip's range of motion, joint contractures, motor strength (specifically of the abductor), limb alignment, limb-length discrepancy, and gait pattern. Physical findings are usually normal, even among patients with severe dysplasia. With significant symptoms, however, a limp or an abductor lurch may be evident. Pelvic obliquity is assessed by palpating the posterior iliac crests while the patient is standing. Patients with acetabular impingement may have decreased motion or pain with the provocative maneuvers of hip flexion and internal rotation.

## IMAGING STUDIES

The evaluation of dysplasia can be accomplished in most cases with the use of plain radiographs. Essential views include a standing anteroposterior pelvic view and a frog-leg lateral view. The anteroposterior view allows for the evaluation of the Shenton line; a broken Shenton line indicates subluxation of the hip. The acetabular sourcil (which is French for "eyebrow") is usually a smooth curve of uniform thickness. In dysplastic hips, the sourcil is thicker laterally, which indicates a focal loading of the joint; it may also fail to completely "turn down" at its peripheral extent. On the anteroposterior view, measures of the acetabular index, the center-edge angle of Wiberg, and the acetabular angle of Sharp can also be made. The abduction and internal rotation view can be used to assess the true femoral neck–shaft angle and to simulate the amount of coverage possible with proximal femoral derotation osteotomy. The false-profile view is a true lateral view of the acetabulum, and it allows for the assessment of the anterior coverage of the femoral head. Three-dimensional computed tomography scans may provide increased information regarding the shape and orientation of the acetabulum and of the fit of the femoral head within it. Magnetic resonance imaging may be useful to evaluate any underlying labral pathology.

## SURGICAL TECHNIQUES

Treatment options are divided into three groups: rotational osteotomies, volume-reducing osteotomies, and salvage procedures.

### Rotational Osteotomies

Rotational osteotomies attain femoral head coverage by cutting one to three of the pelvic bones, with the acetabulum being rotated on the intact structures. These osteotomies cover the femoral head with acetabular cartilage, and they intuitively are the first choice for femoral head coverage procedures. They all require a concentrically reduced femoral head.

The innominate osteotomy of Salter is the most widely used of the rotational osteotomies for the pediatric population. It divides the ilium just above the acetabulum, which allows the acetabulum to be rotated through the symphysis pubis. Neither the contour nor the volume of the acetabulum is changed. This procedure can obtain 20 degrees of improvement in the center-edge angle and 10 degrees of improvement in the acetabular index.

The patient is placed in the supine position with a sandbag under the ipsilateral thorax, and the affected limb is draped free. Adductor contracture is released with a subcutaneous or open tenotomy. Incision and exposure are provided via a Smith-Peterson approach to the hip. A so-called bikini incision starts 2 cm distal to the center of the iliac crest, extends 1 cm distal to the anterosuperior iliac spine, and ends below the middle of the inguinal ligament. The interval between the tensor fascia latae and the sartorius is developed to expose the rectus femoris and the anteroinferior iliac spine. The iliac apophysis is incised down to bone along the iliac crest from the posterior end of the skin incision to the anteroinferior iliac spine. The lateral portion of the apophysis and the periosteum of the outer table are carefully stripped in a continuous sheet to the lateral edge of the acetabulum and posteriorly to the greater sciatic notch; this space is then packed. Adhesions of the joint capsule to the lateral aspect of the ilium can be freed with a periosteal elevator. The medial half of the apophysis and the periosteum of the inner wall are carefully stripped in a continuous sheet to expose the sciatic notch. Care is taken to remain subperiosteal to avoid injury to the sciatic nerve and the superior gluteal artery. The tendinous portion of the iliopsoas is exposed on its deep surface at the level of the pelvic brim and rolled over to visualize the musculotendinous junction. A scissors is passed between the tendon and the musculotendinous junction, and the tendon is cut sharply with a scalpel. The tip of a curved forceps is passed subperiosteally from the medial side and through the sciatic notch to grasp the end of the Gigli saw. The index finger of the opposite hand is used to guide the forceps. The skin and the soft tissues are retracted widely. The osteotomy extends in a straight line from the sciatic notch to the anteroinferior iliac spine, with care taken to remain at right angles to the vertical axis of the ilium. The hands are kept far apart, and continuous tension is placed on each end of the saw to keep it from binding (Figure 37-1). A triangular-shaped bone graft is then taken from the iliac crest with large bone cutters. (A saw may be used in older children.) The base of the graft extends from the anterosuperior iliac spine to the anteroinferior iliac spine. A towel clip is placed on each fragment. The proximal fragment should only be steadied. The towel clip on the distal fragment should be placed well posterior to avoid fracture. The distal fragment is then rotated downward and forward in line with the ilium, which opens the osteotomy anterolaterally. Avoid the posterior or medial displacement of the distal fragment. If the hip capsule has not been opened, the leg can be used to attain the desired correction by placing it in a figure-four position. Downward pressure on the knee as the heel is moved toward the child's chin produces the desired rotation. The wedge-shaped bone graft is then inserted into the osteotomy site, and the traction is

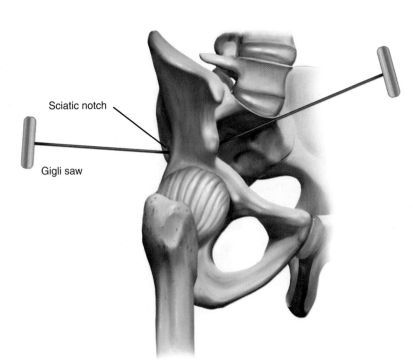

Sciatic notch

Gigli saw

**Figure 37–1**  The inner and outer tables of the ilium are exposed. The periosteum is elevated carefully from the sciatic notch with a curved periosteal elevator, such as a Crego elevator. A right-angled forceps is passed medial to lateral while the finger of the other hand is used to push the periosteum down and away from the sciatic notch on the outer table. A Gigli saw is grasped in the forceps and pulled through the sciatic notch. Retractors are placed in the sciatic notch on each side of the ilium to provide wide retraction and to protect the soft tissues. The osteotomy is performed with the Gigli saw, which emerges at or just above the anterior inferior iliac spine. While using the Gigli saw, the hands should be spread as far apart as possible. Constant tension should be kept on each end of the Gigli saw, because it has a tendency to bind. The bone graft that is used to hold the osteotomy site open is taken from the anterior iliac crest. This can be done with bone-biting forceps in young children, but it is facilitated by the use of a power saw in older children. At this point, it is imperative to perform an intramuscular tenotomy of the iliopsoas as decribed for the anterior approach to the congenitally dislocated hip.

released from the distal fragment. The posterior aspect of the osteotomy should remain closed. Two heavy, threaded K-wires are inserted across the osteotomy site, through the graft, and into the distal segment that lies medial and posterior to the acetabulum (Figure 37-2). Care is taken to avoid penetrating the hip joint. The hip is carefully moved so that crepitus can be heard and felt for; this may indicate that a pin has penetrated the joint. The two halves of the iliac apophysis are sutured together. The K-wires are cut so that their ends lie in subcutaneous fat. A drain is usually not necessary if only an innominate osteotomy has been performed. The wound is then closed. A 1½ hip spica cast is applied with the hip in slight abduction, flexion, and internal rotation and with the knee in flexion. In older, reliable children, three-point partial weight bearing with crutches may be permitted with no immobilization.

Osteotomies in which all three pelvic bones (e.g., Steel, Tönnis, Carlioz) are cut offer greater rotational advantages. The Ganz periacetabular osteotomy may be performed for patients with a closed triradiate cartilage. This procedure is discussed in detail in Chapter 26, and it will not be discussed here. Variations of the triple osteotomy exist for patients with open triradiate cartilage.

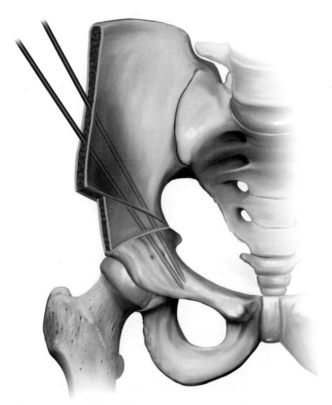

**Figure 37–2**  Although the graft should be secure, it is not secure enough at this point to be left alone without fixation. Smooth or thin wires should not be used. Two heavy threaded Kirchner wires should be used and passed from the proximal fragment into the distal fragment. In the distal fragment, these should lie medial and posterior to the acetabulum; this determines their starting point in the proximal fragment. There is a danger of passing one of the wires into the hip joint when the capsule has not been opened, as may occur during the treatment of acetabular dysplasia. This danger and the fact that properly placed pins appear on the postoperative radiograph to be penetrating the hip joint make it imperative that the surgeon has a good grasp of the pelvic anatomy and that he or she carefully moves the hip to feel and listen for crepitus. After this, the wound is closed. A drain is usually not necessary when only an innominate osteotomy has been performed.

## Volume-Reducing Osteotomies

Volume-reducing osteotomies involve the use of incomplete cuts and hinge on different aspects of the triradiate cartilage; thus, these procedures are limited to patients with open triradiate cartilage.

The Pemberton osteotomy addresses a size "mismatch" between the acetabulum and the femoral head. By hinging on the posterior limb of the triradiate cartilage, the shape of the acetabulum can be changed to provide improved coverage for the femoral head.

The patient is positioned supine, with a bump placed under the involved hip. Exposure is via a Smith-Peterson approach to the hip. Just as with the Salter osteotomy, the iliac apophysis is split, and both the inner and outer tables of the ilium are exposed subperiosteally. Exposure is carried out to the sciatic notch, and the rectus insertion is left alone. Although it was not recommended by Pemberton in his original article, the division of the psoas tendon (as in the Salter osteotomy) may facilitate correction. Two flat-blade retractors are inserted into the sciatic notch on either side of the ilium. The osteotomy is performed with a narrow curved osteotome through the outer table, starting 1 cm above the anteroinferior iliac spine and extending posteriorly, keeping 1 cm to 1.5 cm from the attachment of the hip capsule. Because the osteotomy is carried posteriorly and then inferiorly through the outer table, it will disappear into the soft-tissue attachments behind the capsule. Visualization can be facilitated by the rotation of the retractor in the sciatic notch. Care must be taken to avoid cutting into the sciatic notch. Direct the osteotomy to the ilioischial limb of the triradiate cartilage. With the use of the same osteotome, a corresponding cut is made on the inner table. As with the outer table, avoid cutting into the sciatic notch. The plane of the osteotomy may be adjusted on the basis of the type of coverage that is necessary. A more transverse cut will provide more anterior coverage, whereas a laterally inclined osteotomy will provide more lateral coverage. After both cortices of the ilium have been cut, a wide curved osteotomy is used to connect the two cuts. As the osteotome proceeds posteriorly, it will become apparent that it cannot make the sharp turn inferiorly into the posterior column. A special Pemberton right-angled curved osteotome is used to complete this cut into the triradiate cartilage (Figure 37-3). A small lamina spreader can hold the osteotomy apart and facilitate this cut. The acetabulum can now be directed into the desired position. A groove is cut into each surface of the osteotomy with a narrow gouge or curette. A triangular wedge of bone is removed from the anterior iliac crest and placed in the osteotomy site (Figure 37-4). Because the graft will be recessed in the osteotomy site, the graft should be larger than the gap created by the osteotomy. This osteotomy is quite secure, and it does not require additional fixation. The iliac apophysis is reapproximated, and the wound is closed. The patient is placed in a 1½ hip spica cast.

The San Diego acetabuloplasty was developed to address the problems with dislocated hips in children with spastic cerebral palsy. Specifically, these issues are an elongated acetabulum and a superolateral acetabular deficiency. As with other acetabuloplasties, soft-tissue releases, open reduction, and femoral osteotomy may also be performed in conjunction with this procedure.

The patient is positioned supine, with a bump placed under the involved hip. Exposure is via a Smith-Peterson approach to the hip. Unlike the previously described procedures, only the outer table of the ilium is exposed subperiosteally. Exposure is carried out to the sciatic notch. The iliac apophysis is not split but instead elevated as a unit. A 1.5-cm-wide straight osteotome is used to make an osteotomy 0.5 cm to 1 cm above the edge of the acetabulum on a line drawn from the anteroinferior iliac spine to the sciatic notch. A preliminary notch is made at the extreme ends of the intended osteotomy, at the sciatic notch and the anteroinferior iliac spine, to prevent inadvertent fracture.

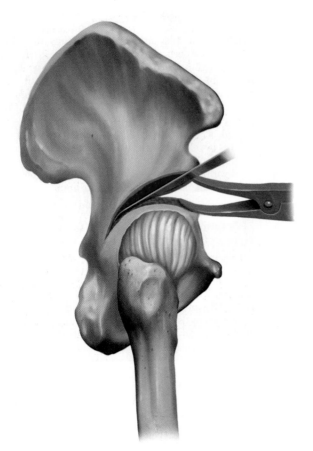

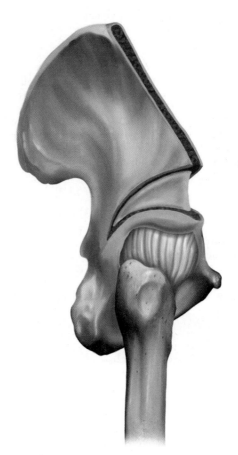

**Figure 37–3** After the inner and outer cortices of the ilium are divided as far as can be seen, a wider curved osteotome is used to connect these two cuts. As the osteotome proceeds posteriorly, it becomes apparent that it is not able to make the sharp turn inferiorly to avoid cutting into the sciatic notch. At this point, an osteotome with a right-angled curve (available via special order from Zimmer Co., Warsaw, IN) is inserted into the osteotomy. This can be made easier by prying down on the acetabular roof with an osteotome and then inserting a small lamina spreader to hold the osteotomy apart. The special osteotome is used to complete the cut into the triradiate cartilage. It is not possible to see the tip of the osteotome as it completes the osteotomy. It is not necessary and usually not possible to see the triradiate cartilage unless the acetabulum is levered down excessively. When the osteotomy is complete, the acetabular roof can be levered down into the desired position and held there with a lamina spreader.

**Figure 37–4** Grooves are prepared in the cancellous surface on each side of the osteotomy to provide the secure fixation of the bone graft. This can be done with a curette. A triangular wedge of bone is cut from the anterior iliac crest. It should be larger than the gap that it is designed to span, because it will be recessed into the cancellous bone. When in place, the bone graft should be secure and stable; this can be verified by attempting to dislodge the graft. The wound is then closed in a routine manner.

## Salvage Procedures

These procedures are usually reserved for hips that lack significant femoral head coverage because of an inability to acquire such coverage with articular cartilage by other osteotomies (i.e., rotational or volume reducing). These procedures place bone over the hip joint capsule on the uncovered portion of the femoral head. However, there are data that document the good long-term results of these procedures.

The medial displacement osteotomy of Chiari consists of the construction of a congruent shelf above the femoral head. It is primarily indicated for older patients with painful subluxated hips. The concentric reduction of the hip is not a prerequisite. This procedure medializes the hip joint, thereby reducing the forces. However, it is unable to provide much anterior coverage, and it may cause a prolonged limp by shortening the abductor lever arm.

Position the patient supine, with a bump placed under the involved hip. Exposure is via a Smith-Peterson approach. As with the Salter osteotomy, the inner and outer tables of the ilium are exposed. The superior aspect of the hip capsule needs to be well exposed anteroposteriorly to facilitate the correct placement of the osteotomy. A guidewire should be drilled lateral to medial, with a 10-degree to 15-degree cephalad incline just above the acetabular roof. The osteotomy should be between the capsular

The lateral cortex is cut, but the medial wall is kept intact; this will allow the fragment to bend freely. A 2-cm-wide curved osteotome is used to deepen the osteotomy in a medial and caudal direction behind the acetabulum to the horizontal limb of the triradiate cartilage (Figure 37-5). The osteotome should be directed halfway between the medial wall of the ilium and the medial wall of the acetabulum; this can be monitored with image intensification. Bicortical bone graft is obtained from the anterosuperior iliac spine and shaped into three or four small triangles with a base of 1 cm. The osteotomy site is opened with an osteotome or a lamina spreader. The grafts are placed into the osteotomy site, with the largest graft placed in the area in which maximum coverage is needed (Figure 37-6). This osteotomy is stable and does not require further fixation. The wound is closed. A 1½ hip spica cast is placed on the patient, with the hip in 45 degrees of flexion and 30 degrees of abduction.

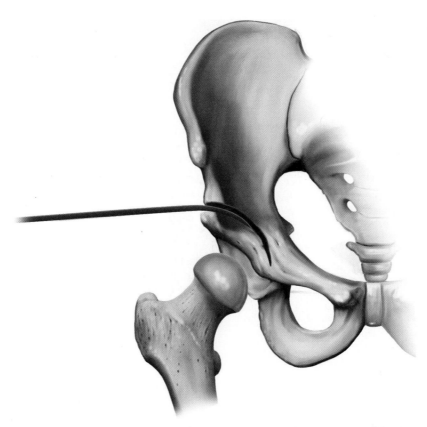

**Figure 37–5**   With the use of a combination of straight and curved osteotomes, the osteotomy is deepened by heading medially and caudally behind the acetabulum. This cut must proceed between the medial wall of the ilium and the medial wall of the acetabulum; this can be monitored with an image intensifier. Mubarak and colleagues describe the osteotomy as going to—but not through—the triradiate cartilage. In our experience, the osteotomy does not have to be carried to the triradiate cartilage, as illustrated here. In the soft bone of the usual child with paralytic hip disease, there is sufficient mobility without the use of the triradiate cartilage; in fact, the osteotomy can be used in some cases in which the triradiate cartilage has closed. Next, a Kerrison rongeur is used to remove the cortex anteriorly and posteriorly as it extends around to the medial iliac wall. This is essential to allow the fragment to bend freely. In contradistinction to the Dega osteotomy, which involves the cutting of a considerable portion of the medial iliac cortex, these two areas that are removed with the Kerrison rongeur are the only cuts made into the medial wall.

insertion and the reflected rectus head, it should head in a curvilinear fashion along the capsular insertion, and it should end anteriorly under the anteroinferior iliac spine and posteriorly in the sciatic notch (Figure 37-7). Pass a Gigli saw through the sciatic notch (i.e., like the initiation of the Salter osteotomy) to score the anterior cortex of the sciatic notch to ensure that the osteotomy fractures through that point in the notch. The lateral cortex is cut first, and this is followed by the medial cortex. Ensure that there are no posterior tethers. The distal fragment is displaced medially by abducting the leg. Further displacement can be achieved by placing direct pressure over the greater trochanter. After the desired displacement is achieved, fixation is obtained with two or three screws or large threaded Steinmann pins. Coverage can be augmented anteriorly by obtaining corticocancellous bone from the inner table of the ilium and placing it in the osteotomy site before fixation (Figure 37-8). Additional cancellous bone graft is added and held in place by the periosteum when the wound is closed.

Several variations of the shelf procedure exist. The goals of this procedure are to increase the load-bearing area of the hip and to increase the stability of the hip. The procedure is indicated for patients with asymmetric incongruity in whom redirectional osteotomies would not be appropriate.

The patient is positioned supine, with a bump placed under the involved hip. Exposure is via a Smith-Peterson approach.

Only the outer table of the ilium is exposed subperiosteally. The reflected head of the rectus femoris is sectioned at the junction of the conjoint tendon; it is reflected to expose the entire hip capsule, and it will be used to secure the bone graft. The location of the slot should be at the edge of the acetabulum; the correct location can be verified with image intensification. When the correct location is identified, a $\frac{5}{32}$-inch drill or a burr is used to make a series of 1-cm-deep holes that incline 20 degrees cephalad at the edge of the acetabulum (Figure 37-9). A narrow rongeur or burr is used to connect the holes and to produce a slot; the floor of the slot should be the subchondral bone of the acetabulum. Corticocancellous and cancellous strips of bone graft are obtained from the outer table of the ilium. The cancellous grafts are cut into 1-cm-wide strips that are long enough to provide adequate lateral femoral head coverage. They are placed in the slot so that they extend out over the capsule. A second layer of cancellous strips is placed perpendicular to the first layer (Figure 37-10). Extending the graft too anterior or lateral may result in impingement, so this should be avoided. The reflected head of the rectus is sutured back to the conjoint tendon, which holds the grafts in place. The remaining bone is cut into small pieces and placed over the graft. The wound is closed, and the patient's hip is placed in a 1½ hip spica cast in 20 degrees of flexion and 15 degrees of abduction.

TECHNICAL PEARLS

**Salter Osteotomy**

- The iliopsoas must always be sectioned at the pelvic brim.
- The towel clip that is used to grasp the proximal fragment must never be used to manipulate the ilium but only to stabilize the ilium.
- As the osteotomy is opened, it is important that the posterior aspect of the osteotomy remain closed.

**Pemberton Osteotomy**

- Direct visualization of the osteotomy in the posterior column is important.
- Cobra retractors can facilitate the visualization of the posterior column by providing gentle rotation in the sciatic notch.
- A cervical spreader and various sizes of cervical bone tamps can be used to hold the osteotomy open while the curved osteotomes and the Pemberton osteotome are used to completely cut back to the triradiate cartilage.
- The more coverage that is needed laterally, the steeper should be the angle between the lateral and medial iliac wing cuts.

**San Diego Acetabuloplasty**

- Both cortices of the anterior aspect of the sciatic notch and the anteroinferior iliac spine should be notched with a Kerrison rongeur to control the fracture of the ilium that will be created by the osteotomes.
- Cervical lamina spreaders or various sizes of cervical bone tamps are useful to hold the osteotomy open until the bone grafts can be placed.

**Chiari Osteotomy**

- The osteotomy can be cut by a series of osteotomes by leaving one in place as the next one is placed at the appropriate angle directly anterior or posterior to the first index osteotome.
- If the procedure is performed on a fracture table, it may be facilitated by moving the patient's hip into abduction after the osteotomy is complete; this will facilitate the medial displacement.
- An anterior bone graft must be placed before internal fixation of the fragments.

**Shelf Procedure**

- Avoid stripping the periosteum too far down the ilium to avoid damage to the groove of Ranvier.
- Fluoroscopic visualization of a scalpel blade wrapper cut to simulate the bone graft shape and placed into the acetabular slot and over the femoral head will serve as a template for the shaping of the harvest bone graft.

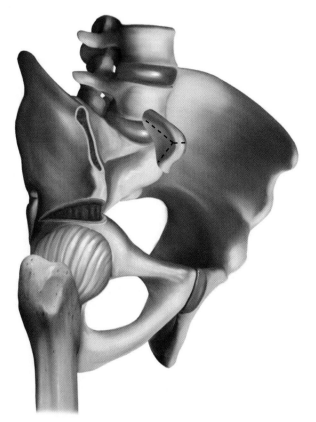

**Figure 37–6**  A piece of the ilium in the region of the anterosuperior iliac spine is removed, and three tricortical triangular pieces of bone are fashioned. These are wedged securely into the osteotomy site, which is held open with a lamina spreader. The amount of correction and where it occurs vary slightly with the size of the grafts and the site of placement of the largest and smallest grafts. The largest graft is usually placed anteriorly. It has generally been difficult to attempt to get more posterior coverage by placing the largest graft posteriorly. The amount of coverage should be verified, and the surgeon should be certain that the grafts are secure. No internal fixation is necessary. The wound is then closed.

## POSTOPERATIVE REHABILITATION

Patients treated with a Salter osteotomy have the spica cast removed after 6 weeks. At that time, the K-wires may be removed with the patient under local or general anesthetic. The patient is allowed to progress from protected to full weight bearing over the next 4 to 6 weeks.

Patients treated with a Pemberton osteotomy have the spica cast removed after 6 to 8 weeks. They too then progress from protected to full weight bearing over the next 4 to 6 weeks. Older children who were not in a cast may now begin to progressively wean themselves from the crutches over the next several weeks and to continue to strengthen their hip musculature.

Patients treated with a San Diego acetabuloplasty have the spica cast removed at 6 weeks postoperatively and progress from protected to full weight bearing over the course of 4 to 6 weeks.

Chiari osteotomies performed in young children are protected with a hip spica cast for 6 weeks. At that time, the cast is removed, and the patient progresses from protected to full weight bearing over the course of 4 to 6 weeks. Crutches are maintained until radiographic evidence of healing is seen and any abductor weakness is corrected.

Patients treated with a shelf procedure are placed in a single-leg hip spica cast for 6 weeks. Reliable patients may begin partial weight bearing for 4 weeks and then subsequently progress to full weight bearing. Less reliable patients should be not be allowed to walk and instead kept in a chair until graft incorporation is seen on radiographs. Graft incorporation usually requires a minimum of 4 months.

## RESULTS AND OUTCOMES

See Table 37-1.

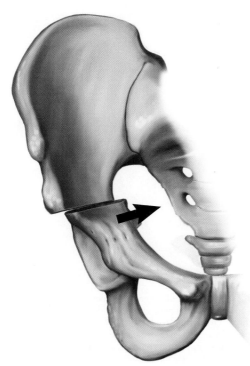

**Figure 37–7**   The placement of the osteotomy is crucial to the success of the operation. If it is too high, it does not provide coverage for the hip; if it is too low, there is not a sufficient capsule between the femoral head and the ilium. Therefore, it is important that the superior aspect of the hip capsule be well exposed anteroposteriorly. In addition, it is necessary to know where the roof of the acetabulum lies. This may be difficult in many subluxated hips because of a markedly thickened capsule. In some cases, it may be necessary to thin this capsule. Conceptualizing how the distal fragment is displaced medially in relation to the proximal fragment (despite the fact that the pelvic ring is divided in only one place) is important to the understanding of the osteotomy. The displacement occurs as the distal fragment rotates on the symphysis pubis; this is the reason why the direction of the osteotomy is important for obtaining "displacement." Proceeding lateral to medial, the osteotomy should incline cephalad by about 10 degrees. This permits the inferior fragment that contains the hip joint to displace medially.

These two crucial points—the location of the acetabular roof and the direction of the osteotomy—can be verified by drilling a small guidewire or by driving an osteotome lateral to medial in the estimated direction of the osteotomy at the proposed site of the osteotomy while viewing this with a radiograph or an image intensifier. The osteotomy should incline cephalad 10 degrees to 15 degrees from lateral to medial to facilitate the displacement (or, more correctly, the rotation).

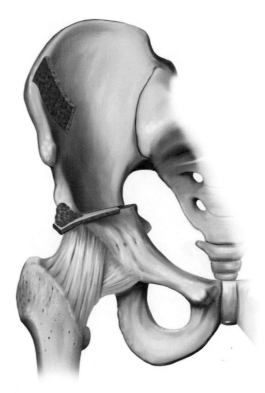

**Figure 37–8**   As mentioned previously, it is often necessary to augment the coverage obtained with the Chiari osteotomy. This is especially true anteriorly, where the ilium is thin. An excellent method for accomplishing this coverage has been described. An appropriately sized piece of corticocancellous bone is removed from the inner table of the ilium and then placed in the osteotomy site before fixation. The screws or pins that are used for fixation will then transfix this graft. Additional cancellous bone graft is added over this graft and held in place by the periosteum and the muscles when the wound is closed.

## COMPLICATIONS

Wound infection rates of 1% to 8% have been reported. Several reports of injury to the lateral femoral cutaneous nerve can be found in the literature, with rates that vary from 0.5% to 48%. Chiari and shelf procedures involve a high incidence of postoperative limp, with results that have ranged from 44% to 87%. However, in many of these cases, patients had a limp preoperatively. Other concerns with pelvic osteotomies include a change in the pelvic shape and its effects on future childbirth. Chiari, Salter, and triple osteotomies all have the potential—although it is a rare occurrence—to alter the pelvic shape; the possible need for Caesarean section delivery with future pregnancies should be discussed preoperatively.

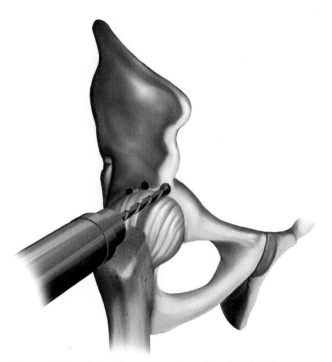

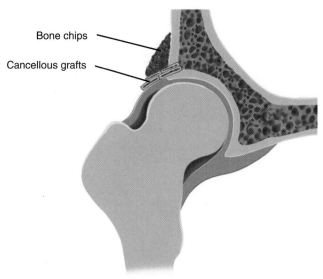

**Figure 37–10** The cancellous grafts are cut into strips that are 1 cm wide and of appropriate length to provide the desired amount of lateral coverage. These are placed into the slot so that they extend out over the capsule. A second layer of cancellous strips are placed at 90 degrees to the first layer of strips of graft. The grafts must not extend too far laterally or anteriorly in the quest for spectacular radiographic coverage of the hip, because this could lead to a loss of motion as a result of impingement.

**Figure 37–9** During the exposure, the reflected head of the rectus tendon should be identified, dissected free of the capsule, and divided somewhere between its mid portion and its junction with the conjoined tendon; this procedure is used to secure the grafts in place. The most important part of the surgery is identifying the correct location for the slot: it should be placed at the exact acetabular edge. The surgeon must determine whether this is the true or false acetabulum; this is done by determining which of the two affords greater stability and congruity. The acetabulum is identified by creating a small incision in the capsule or by inserting a probe. In the subluxated and dysplastic hip, the capsule is usually thickened and adherent to the ilium, which may cause the surgeon to place the slot and therefore the graft too high. The correct location should be verified radiographically by placing a guide pin into the ilium at the presumed acetabular edge. In some cases, it may necessary to thin the capsule to permit the graft to be placed in the proper location. After the correct location is verified, a ⁵⁄₃₂-inch drill bit is used to make a series of holes at the edge of the acetabulum. These holes should be drilled to a depth of about 1 cm, and they should incline about 20 degrees, as illustrated. They should extend far enough anteriorly and posteriorly to provide the necessary coverage.

**Table 37-1** OUTCOMES

| Osteotomy | Study | Title | No. of Patients/Hips | Patient Age | Median Length of Follow Up | Results |
|---|---|---|---|---|---|---|
| Salter | Salter et al, 1974 | The first 15 years' personal experience with innominate osteotomy in the treatment of congenital dislocation of the hip | 140 patients | | 15 years | Patients between the ages of 18 months and 4 years had 93.6% good or excellent results<br><br>Patients between the ages of 4 and 10 years had 56.7% good or excellent results |
| | Barrett et al, 1986 | The effectiveness of the Salter innominate osteotomy in the treatment of congenital dislocation of the hip | 68 hips | 18 months to 11 years | 8 years | Radiographically, 74% of patients had good or excellent results<br><br>Clinically, 51% of patients had good or excellent results<br><br>Patients between the ages of 18 months and 4 years had better results |

**Table 37-1** OUTCOMES—CONT'D

| Osteotomy | Study | Title | No. of Patients/Hips | Patient Age | Median Length of Follow Up | Results |
|---|---|---|---|---|---|---|
| | Ito et al, 2001 | Middle-term results of Salter innominate osteotomy | 35 hips | 4 years | 16.5 years | Radiographically, 74% of patients had good or excellent results<br><br>Clinically, 74% of patients had good or excellent results<br><br>Acetabular index improved from 34 degrees preoperatively to 18 degrees at the final follow up<br><br>Center-edge angle improved from –0.5 degrees preoperatively to 25 degrees at final follow up |
| | Bohm et al, 2002 | Salter innominate osteotomy for the treatment of developmental dysplasia of the hip in children | 73 hips | 4 years | 30 years | With revision as the endpoint, there was 90% survivorship at 35 years (7% had undergone THA)<br><br>Acetabular index improved from 32 degrees preoperatively to 11 degrees at final follow up |
| | Thomas et al, 2007 | Outcome at forty-five years after open reduction and innominate osteotomy for late-presenting developmental dislocation of the hip | 80 hips | 4 years | 45 years | With THA as the endpoint, there was 99% survivorship at 30 years<br><br>86% survivorship at 40 years<br><br>54% survivorship at 45 years<br><br>At the final follow up, the acetabular index was 32 degrees, and the center-edge angle was 40 degrees |
| Pemberton | Pemberton, 1965 | Pericapsular osteotomy of the ilium for treatment of congenital subluxation and dislocation of the hip | 91 patients | | 5 years | Patients who were less than 4 years old had 100% good results<br><br>Patients between the ages of 4 and 7 years had 83% good results<br><br>Patients between the ages of 7 and 12 years had 57% good results |
| | Faciszewski et al, 1993 | Pemberton osteotomy for residual acetabular dysplasia in children who have congenital dislocation of the hip | 52 hips | 4 years | 10 years | 81% had radiographically normal hips<br><br>Acetabular index improved from 33 degrees preoperatively to 11 degrees at final follow up<br><br>Center-edge angle improved from 3 degrees preoperatively to 35 degrees at final follow up |
| | Wada et al, 2003 | Pemberton osteotomy for developmental dysplasia of the hip in older children | 17 hips | 9 years | 9 years | Radiographically, 76% had good or excellent results<br><br>Clinically, 82% had good or excellent results<br><br>Sharp acetabular angle improved from 57 degrees preoperatively to 44 degrees at final follow up<br><br>Center-edge angle improved from 2 degrees preoperatively to 24 degrees at final follow up |
| San Diego | Mubarak et al, 1992 | One-stage correction of the spastic dislocated hip. Use of pericapsular acetabuloplasty to improve coverage. | 18 hips | 8 years | 6 years | 94% of patients were pain free<br><br>Acetabular index improved from 30 degrees preoperatively to 14 degrees at final follow up<br><br>Center-edge angle improved from –29 degrees preoperatively to 33 degrees at final follow up |
| | McNerney et al, 2000 | One-stage correction of the dysplastic hip in cerebral palsy with the San Diego acetabuloplasty: results and complications in 104 hips | 104 hips | 8 years | 6 years | Acetabular index improved from 26 degrees preoperatively to 11 degrees at final follow up |

*(Continued)*

**Table 37-1** OUTCOMES—CONT'D

| Osteotomy | Study | Title | No. of Patients/Hips | Patient Age | Median Length of Follow Up | Results |
|---|---|---|---|---|---|---|
| Chiari | Chiari, 1974 | Medial displacement osteotomy of the pelvis | 200 hips | Less than 16 years | 2 to 18 years | 66% of patients had good or excellent results |
| | Calvert et al, 1987 | The Chiari pelvic osteotomy: a review of long-term results | 49 hips | 19 years | 14 years | 57% of patients were pain free |
| | | | | | | 16% of patients had mild pain with no functional deficit |
| | | | | | | Center-edge angle improved from −2 degrees preoperatively to 28 degrees at final follow up |
| | | | | | | 25 of 38 women had children: 16 of 25 had vaginal deliveries, whereas 9 of 25 had Caesarean section deliveries |
| | Windhager et al, 1991 | Chiari osteotomy for congenital dislocation and subluxation of the hip: results after 20 to 34 years follow up | 236 hips | 14 years | 24 years | Clinically, 51% had good or excellent results |
| | | | | | | 8% converted to THA and 0.8% converted to arthrodesis an average of 15 years after the index procedure |
| | Rozkydal et al, 2003 | Chiari pelvic osteotomy in the management of developmental hip dysplasia: a long term follow up | 130 hips | 29 years | 22 years | 50% of patients were satisfied |
| | | | | | | 38% converted to THA an average of 12 years after the index procedure |
| | | | | | | Conversion to THA occurred at an average age of 33 years |
| | | | | | | No conversion had occurred at an average age of 24 years |
| Shelf | Love et al, 1980 | A long-term review of shelf arthroplasty | 45 hips | 12 years | 11 years | 73% had good or excellent results |
| | | | | | | 3 patients converted to THA, 1 patient converted to arthrodesis |
| | Summers et al, 1988 | The shelf operation in the management of late presentation of congenital hip dysplasia | 27 hips | 14 years | 16 years | 63% had good results |
| | | | | | | 33% failure rate, with an average time to failure of 9 years |
| | | | | | | 2 patients converted to THA, 1 patient converted to hemiarthroplasty |
| | | | | | | Center-edge angle improved from −28 degrees preoperatively to 63 degrees at final follow up |
| | Staheli et al, 1992 | Slotted acetabular augmentation in childhood and adolescence | 108 hips | 11 years | 5 years | 83% had good or excellent results |
| | | | | | | Center-edge angle improved from 0.5 degrees preoperatively to 59 degrees at final follow up |
| | Nishimatsu et al, 2002 | The modified Spitzy shelf operation for patients with dysplasia of the hip | 119 hips | 25 years | 23 years | If the patient was less than 25 years old at the time of surgery, 84% had good results |
| | | | | | | If the patient was more than 25 years old at the time of surgery, 50% had good results |
| | | | | | | Revisions occurred in 0.9%; 9 patients converted to THA, 2 patients converted to hemiarthroplasty |

*THA,* Total hip arthroplasty.

## ANNOTATED REFERENCES AND SUGGESTED READINGS

Barrett WP, Staheli LT, Chew DE. The effectiveness of the Salter innominate osteotomy in the treatment of congenital dislocation of the hip. *J Bone Joint Surg*. 1986;68:79–87.

Bohm P, Brzuske A. Salter innominate osteotomy for the treatment of developmental dysplasia of the hip in children: results of seventy-three consecutive osteotomies after twenty-six to thirty-five years of follow-up. *J Bone Joint Surg*: 2002; 84-A:178–186.

Calvert PT, August AC, Albert JS, et al. The Chiari pelvic osteotomy. A review of the long-term results. *J Bone Joint Surg Br*. 1987;69:551–555.

Chiari K. Medial displacement osteotomy of the pelvis. *Clin Orthop*. 1974;98:55–71.

Chiari describes his technique and provides data from his first 200 cases. He reports 66% satisfactory results with these first 200 cases, with a minimum of 2 years of follow up. The author notes that advanced arthritis was present preoperatively in the cases that went on to be unsuccessful.

Faciszewski T, Kiefer GN, Coleman SS. Pemberton osteotomy for residual acetabular dysplasia in children who have congenital dislocation of the hip. *J Bone Joint Surg*. 1993;75:643–649.

Gillingham BL, Sanchez AA, Wenger DR. Pelvic osteotomies for the treatment of hip dysplasia in children and young adults. *J Am Acad Orthop Surg*. 1999;7:325–337.

This review article summarizes the causes, the evaluation, and the treatment principles of acetabular dysplasia. The authors provide an algorithm to help guide treatment, and they discuss various treatment options.

Hadley NA. The effects of contact pressure elevations and aseptic necrosis on the long-term outcome of congenital hip dislocation. *J Orthop Res*. 1990;8:504–513.

Eighty-four patients with unilateral congenital hip dislocations were treated with closed reduction and followed for an average of 29 years. Articular contact stress was computed and correlated with long-term radiographic degenerative changes. A time pressure product of more than 10 MPa (i.e., years of pressure exposure of more than 2 MPa) yielded unsatisfactory outcomes in 90.4% of hips, whereas less than 10 MPa yielded unsatisfactory outcomes in 80.4% of hips.

Harris NG. Acetabular growth potential in congenital dislocation of the hip and some factors upon which it may depend. *Clin Orthop*. 1976;119:99–106.

Sixty-six patients (79 hips) with congenital hip dislocations and a minimum age of 8 years at follow were followed for a mean of 10 years after reduction of the hip. A satisfactory acetabulum was attained in 44 hips (mean age of congruity, 33 months), and an unsatisfactory acetabulum was attained in 30 hips (mean age of congruity, 48 months). The author concluded that 4 years is the critical age for attaining a congruous reduction to produce a normal or only mildly dysplastic acetabulum.

Ito H, Ooura H, Kobayashi M, et al. Middle-term results of Salter innominate osteotomy. *Clin Orthop*. 2001;387:156–164.

Love BR, Stevens PM, Williams PF. A long-term review of shelf arthroplasty. *J Bone Joint Surg Br*. 1980;62:321–325.

McNerney NP, Mubarak SJ, Wenger DR. One-stage correction of the dysplastic hip in cerebral palsy with the San Diego acetabuloplasty: results and complications in 104 hips. *J Pediatr Orthop*. 2000;20:93–103.

Morrissy RT, Weinstein SL. *Atlas of pediatric orthopaedic surgery*. 4th ed. Philadelphia: Lippincott Williams & Wilkins; 2006.

This book provides instructions regarding surgical techniques for a number of pediatric pelvic osteotomies.

Mubarak SJ, Valencia FG, Wenger DR. One-stage correction of the spastic dislocated hip. Use of pericapsular acetabuloplasty to improve coverage. *J Bone Joint Surg*. 1992;74:1347–1357.

Eleven children (18 hips) between the ages of 5 and 16 years with spastic cerebral palsy and subluxation or dislocation of the hip underwent single-stage soft-tissue releases, open reduction, femoral shortening varus-derotation osteotomy, and a novel pericapsular acetabuloplasty. At a mean follow up of 6 years and 10 months, 17 of the 18 hips were pain free and anatomically reduced. The acetabular index improved from 30 degrees to 14 degrees, and the center-edge angle improved from –29 degrees to 33 degrees at the latest follow up.

Nishimatsu H, Iida H, Kawanabe K, et al. The modified Spitzy shelf operation for patients with dysplasia of the hip. A 24-year follow-up study. *J Bone Joint Surg Br*. 2002;84:647–652.

Pemberton PA. Pericapsular osteotomy of the ilium for treatment of congenital subluxation and dislocation of the hip. *J Bone Joint Surg*. 1965;47:65–86.

This is Pemberton's original description of his novel osteotomy, which was designed to address the apparent size mismatch between the acetabulum and the femoral head. He presents data from 8 years and 91 patients (115 hips), with a mean follow-up time of 5 years. Better outcomes were seen among younger patients (i.e., 7 years old or younger).

Ponsetti IV. Growth and development of the acetabulum in the normal child. *J Bone Joint Surg*. 1978;60:575–585.

Postmortem studies of 13 children were carried out to describe the anatomy and histology of the growth of the normal acetabulum. The architecture of the triradiate cartilage and of the secondary centers of ossification that contribute to the growth of the acetabulum are described in detail.

Rozkydal Z, Kovanda M. Chiari pelvic osteotomy in the management of developmental hip dysplasia: a long term follow-up. *Bratisl Lek Listy*. 2003;104:7–13.

Salter RB. Innominate osteotomy in the treatment of congenital dislocation and subluxation of the hip. *J Bone Joint Surg Br*. 1961;43B:518–539.

This is Salter's original description of his novel osteotomy, which was designed to maintain the reduction of the congenitally dislocated or subluxated hip in functional positions. The technique is described in detail, and the author provides the early results of 18 patients (25 hips) with 1 to 3 years of follow up.

Salter RB, Dubos JP. The first fifteen year's personal experience with innominate osteotomy in the treatment of congenital dislocation and subluxation of the hip. *Clin Orthop*. 1974;98:72–103.

Staheli LT. Chew DE. Slotted acetabular augmentation in childhood and adolescence. *J Pediatr Orthop*. 1992;12:569–580.

Ninety-eight patients (108 hips) with mean age of 11 years and 8 months underwent slotted acetabular augmentation. The procedure was initially described by the author in 1981. In addition to reporting 5-year follow-up data, the author provides indications for the procedure as well as considerations for other procedures with which it may be combined.

Summers BN, Turner A, Wynn-Jones CH. The shelf operation in the management of late presentation of congenital hip dysplasia. *J Bone Joint Surg Br*. 1988;70B:63–68.

Twenty-four patients (27 hips) with congenital hip dysplasia and a mean age of 14 years underwent shelf procedures. At a mean follow up of 16 years, 18 hips had good results. Of the 9 hips with poor results, 6 underwent further surgery (2 total hip arthroplasties, 1 hemiarthroplasty, 1 revision shelf procedure, and 2 femoral osteotomies), with an average time to failure of 9 years.

**Thomas SR, Wedge JH, Salter RB. Outcome at forty-five years after open reduction and innominate osteotomy for late-presenting developmental dislocation of the hip.** *J Bone Joint Surg.* **2007;89:2341–2350.**

Sixty patients (80 hips) between the ages of 18 months and 5 years underwent Salter innominate osteotomy and were followed for a mean of 45 years. With the use of Kaplan-Meier survival analysis and total hip arthroplasty as the endpoint, 30-year survival rates were 99%, and 40-year survival rates were 85%. By 45 years, survival rates dropped off to 54%.

**Wada A, Fujii T, Takamura K, et al. Pemberton osteotomy for developmental dysplasia of the hip in older children.** *J Pediatr Orthop.* **2003;23:508–513.**

**Weinstein SL. Natural history of congenital hip dislocation (CDH) and hip dysplasia.** *Clin Orthop.* **1987;225:62–76.**

This review article discusses the natural history of complete congenital hip dislocation, congenital subluxation, and acetabular dysplasia in the absence of subluxation.

**Weinstein SL, Mubarak SJ, Wenger DR. Developmental hip dysplasia and dislocation: part I.** *Instr Course Lect.* **2004; 53:523–530.**

This review article addresses the normal growth and development of the hip, pathoanatomy, and the management of developmental hip dysplasia and dislocation.

**Windhager R, Pongracz N, Schonecker W, et al. Chiari osteotomy for congenital dislocation and subluxation of the hip: results after 20 to 34 years follow-up.** *J Bone Joint Surg Br.* **1991;73B:890–895.**

Two hundred thirty-six hips (more than 90% of which were treated with Chiari procedures) with congenital dislocation and subluxation underwent Chiari osteotomies when the affected patients were a mean of 14 years old. At a mean follow-up time of 24 years, 51% of the hips had good or excellent results. Twenty-one hips (8.8%) underwent reoperation after an average of 15 years. Patients with an older age at the time of operation or with preoperative osteoarthritis had poorer results.

# CHAPTER 38

# Surgical Treatment for Athletic Pubalgia ("Sports Hernia")

*William C. Meyers, David Kahan, Octavia Devon, and Marcia A. Horner*

## INTRODUCTION

The proverb "one size does not fit all" definitely applies to the surgical treatment of athletic pubalgia ("sports hernia"). These are a variety of very specific injuries and one operation is not appropriate for all patients with these conditions. The most important thing is to dismiss the concept of hernia and to instead think in terms of the applicable anatomy and the likely pathophysiology of the injuries. Therefore, an accurate diagnosis must take into account a wide differential diagnosis. When a specific diagnosis is established, then one must consider the best operation for that particular patient. The term *sports hernia* conveys two large assumptions that are inaccurate: 1) that the cause of these sets of injuries has something to do with the presence of occult hernias; and 2) that these injuries can be lumped together into one entity and therefore be treated in a similar fashion.

## BASIC SCIENCE

When treating these injuries, a detailed understanding of the musculoskeletal and visceral anatomy of the pelvis is necessary. One must also appreciate the physiologic concept that the pubic symphysis is a functional joint. The pubis is the center of normal symmetric motion—flexion, extension, abduction, adduction, and rotation—with naturally opposing groups of muscles and other soft tissues. We have described the musculoskeletal anatomy and the concept of the pubic joint in several publications.

Briefly, the musculoskeletal anatomic considerations are as follows. Consider mainly the anterior pelvis, excluding the spine, and then consider the anatomy inside and outside of the hip joint. It is easiest to think of the hip joint as a ball-and-socket joint that is relatively independent of the musculature outside of the socket. From the standpoint of anatomic proximity, it also seems logical to think that some interplay must occur between the hip joint and the pelvic musculature around it. If so, then injury to the adjacent musculature might also negatively affect the hip joint or vice versa, and primary and compensatory forces likely play important roles in the pathogeneses of these two types of injuries.

The hip is a synovial joint that is comprised of the femoral head and the acetabulum of the pelvis. The hip, which is also known as the acetabulofemoral joint, connects the lower limb to the axial skeleton. Both joint surfaces are covered in hyaline cartilage, and the acetabulum also has a fibrocartilaginous rim called the *labrum* that firmly holds the femoral head in place.

In addition, the joint is encased in a fibrous capsule and stabilized by three ligaments: the iliofemoral ligament, the pubofemoral ligament, and the ischiofemoral ligament. The ligamentum teres, which is located at the femoral head, also serves to support joint integrity.

The pubic musculature outside of the hip joint consists of a vast set of muscles and soft tissues. The anterior pelvis includes multiple structures (excluding the hip, sacrum, and spine) such as the lower abdominal soft tissues; both sides of the pubic symphysis; and multiple thigh and pelvic adductors, abductors, flexors, extendors, and rotators. We think in terms of three compartments of muscles or other attachments that provide ligamentous-type support (Figure 38-1). The anterior compartment consists mainly of the abdominal muscles, including the sartorius, the anterior attachment of the psoas, portions of the quadriceps, and some complex interdigitations with fibers from the thighs and the medial and posterior pelvis. The posterior compartment consists primarily of the hamstrings, a portion of the adductor magnus, several key nerves, and an artery. The medial compartment consists of the most important thigh components, which include the three adductors that attach to the symphysis, the gracilis, the obturator externus, and several other structures.

The muscular attachments provide different types of either central or strap supports, depending on their medial or lateral locations, insertions, or origins. For example, a combination of the rectus femoris and the obturator externus is particularly important for place kicking, and the adductor longus and magnus are particularly important as push-off muscles for pitching. We can think in terms of four groups of muscles: adductors, abdominal flexors, thigh flexors, and internal or external rotators. The most important adductors are the adductor longus, the adductor brevis, and the pectineus. The adductor magnus and gracilis usually play minor roles in pelvic stabilization. The rectus abdominis and, to a lesser degree, the obliques and the transversalis comprise the more superior or anterior flexors, and the psoas major and minor combine with other thigh flexors as key inferior or posterior flexors of the pubic joint. The rotators consist primarily of the obturator externus and internus and the quadrator femoris, although other muscles also play roles in rotation. One should not forget the importance of some of the back muscles, particularly the large transversus, which play important roles in both rehabilitation after injury and in performance in general.

Lastly, in addition to musculoskeletal tissue, one must take into account the solid and hollow viscera organs in the pelvis. These include the small and large intestine, the rectum, the genitourinary system, the gynecologic system, and some important

Anterior view

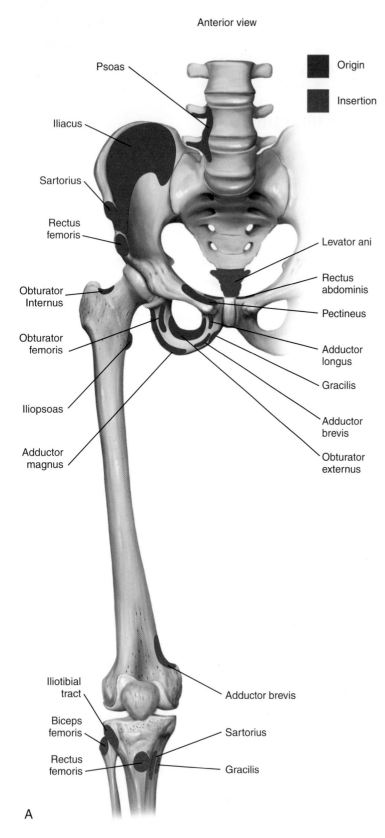

Origin

Insertion

Psoas

Iliacus

Sartorius

Rectus
femoris

Obturator
Internus

Obturator
femoris

Iliopsoas

Adductor
magnus

Levator ani

Rectus
abdominis

Pectineus

Adductor
longus

Gracilis

Adductor
brevis

Obturator
externus

Iliotibial
tract

Biceps
femoris

Rectus
femoris

Adductor brevis

Sartorius

Gracilis

A

**Figure 38–1  A,** Anterior view of muscle origins and insertions. Note that all adductors originate in the pubic ramus, and also note the relatively anterior location of insertion of the psoas tendon onto the lesser trochanter. **B,** Anterior view. **C,** Lateral view. *From: Meyers WC, Yoo E, Devon O, et al.,: Understanding "sports hernia" (athletic pubalgia): the anatomic and pathophysiologic basis for abdominal and groin pain in athletes.* Oper Tech Sport Med. *Elsevier, 15:4, pp 165-177, October 2007.*

Coronal  Sagittal  **Figure 38–1** cont'd

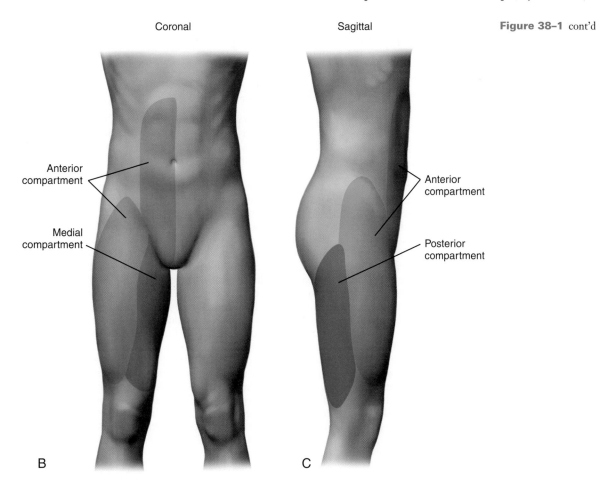

Anterior compartment

Medial compartment

Anterior compartment

Posterior compartment

B

C

blood vessels. Any of these systems can be involved in patients who present with sports hernia. The causes of pelvic pain can be many, and accurate diagnosis can be confusing. To make matters even more complex, visceral diseases can produce symptoms during exertion. Therefore, during the evaluation of the athlete or nonathlete with any type of pelvic pain, one needs to strongly consider possible visceral causes. Thus, one has three main things to consider as part of the differential diagnosis: 1) hip problems; 2) nonhip musculoskeletal problems; and 3) visceral problems. Remember, we are excluding the spine as part of this anatomy, because it rarely causes problems in this area.

## INDICATIONS

- Persistent pain with identified specific pathology amenable to repair, release, or other procedure
- Persistent pain with the previously mentioned identifiers that limits performance in an athlete who depends on sports as a way of life
- Persistent pain with either of the previously mentioned identifiers that greatly diminishes that patient's quality of life

## HISTORY AND PHYSICAL EXAMINATION

A careful history must take into account all of the previously mentioned systems and anatomy. One must remember that pelvic pain has a wide differential diagnosis and that these patients, who are for the most part young, can have pain from a wide variety of sources. For example, Crohn's disease and endometriosis have mimicked musculoskeletal disorders, and they have initially presented with exertion-related pelvic pain. In addition, we have picked up a wide variety of malignancies, benign tumors, and unusual other problems involving the gastrointestinal, genitourinary, and gynecologic systems. More recently, now that trainers and team physicians are recognizing these problems earlier, we have also seen appendicitis as a primary cause of acute exertion-related pelvic pain in athletes.

One must also consider the historic differentiators between intra-articular hip problems and problems that involve the soft tissues outside of the hip. These can be tricky, particularly considering that there is considerable overlap among these symptoms. For the hip, one usually looks for pain with simple changes in posture that often involve minimal exertion. There can be a continuous nature to the pain, particularly after activity. Any inflammatory process (e.g., pubic osteitis) can cause the pain to have a continuous nature, but injuries to the soft-tissue structures outside of the hip joint usually cause pain with extremes of activity that is often reproducible with the same maneuvers.

During the physical examination, one looks primarily for pain with resistive maneuvers versus pain with passive range of motion of the hip. Each of the soft-tissue structures outside of the hip can be tested with specific physical tests. For example, one can easily differentiate among the three adductors that insert on the pubic symphysis, and one can also test individually for the adductor magnus, the rectus femoris, the sartorius, the iliopsoas, the gracilis, and other structures. Tenderness should immediately alert the observer to the possibility of an intraperitoneal problem. Hip examination is often particularly important for these patients. The examination should be thorough and consider all of the potential musculoskeletal and nonmusculoskeletal causes of pain; it definitely includes the examination of the abdomen and the chest as well as the scrutiny of the regional lymph nodes and the vascular system. This examination may even include rectal and gynecologic examinations.

## IMAGING AND OTHER DIAGNOSTIC TOOLS

During the past 2 to 3 years, imaging and the proper interpretation of that imaging have gained increasing importance. The most important advances have been in magnetic resonance imaging and magnetic resonance arthrography with Sensorcaine. A magnetic resonance image of the pelvis details the soft-tissue structures that attach to and cross the pubic symphysis. We can now identify with about 91% specificity the soft-tissue injuries that occur outside of the hip. This accuracy of interpretation is directly related to improvement in the techniques and an improved understanding of the anatomy and pathophysiology. Things that were documented in these patients as "nonspecific findings" in the past have turned out, in fact, to have specific correlations with the pathology.

With magnetic resonance arthrography of the hip with an anesthetic, a combination of a gadolinium injection and a Sensorcaine/lidocaine mixture is injected into the hip joint to determine whether signs or symptoms go away after the injection. When performed properly, this test can be very important for differentiating between hip and nonhip musculoskeletal problems. One must also appreciate that hip and nonhip problems can occur together. We see simultaneous injury (i.e., intra-articular hip injury and athletic pubalgia) in as many as 10% of athletes.

Other anesthetic blocks are also used to help determine the site of the pain. Psoas injections can be useful. Although one must understand that simply blocking certain nerves usually leads to a relatively nonspecific diagnosis, nerve injections can be useful for differentiating lateral pelvic musculature problems from intrinsic hip injury. We see many patients with persistent or new pain after an attempt at conventional hernia repair for athletic pubalgia. The differential diagnosis often includes pain related to mesh or nerve entrapment. In these cases, ilioinguinal, iliohypogastric, and genitofemoral blocks may be considered.

Other imaging that we commonly use is abdominal and pelvic computed tomography. This can be particularly helpful for identifying certain visceral problems, abscesses, and tumors. For many gastrointestinal problems, endoscopy and contrast imaging are often more helpful. However, these are rarely helpful for the diagnosis of most musculoskeletal disorders of the pelvis. Abdominal, pelvic, or lower-extremity computed tomography scanning may be better tests than magnetic resonance imaging for suspected soft-tissue neoplasms. In addition, bone scans may be helpful for identifying osteitis that involves the pubic bone or other bones of the pelvis, and these scans may occasionally be useful for addressing the possibility of metastatic disease as the cause of the pelvic pain. For example, we have had several cases of patients with prostate cancer for which this test was useful. In general, magnetic resonance imaging of the pelvis is more useful than bone scan for osteitis as well as for most of the other considerations in the differential diagnosis.

We rarely use ultrasound as a modality for diagnosing most of the problems of athletic pubalgia. Ultrasound can sometimes be helpful for identifying hematomas or soft-tissue avulsions. This modality can occasionally be helpful for women to identify other sources of pathology. If one is using this test routinely for identifying abdominal or pelvic hernias, then one misunderstands the basic considerations involved in these injuries.

## SURGICAL TECHNIQUE

Because of the complexity of the anatomy of this region of the body, one should readily appreciate that many injuries may occur here. Therefore, a wide variety of operations and combinations of procedures apply, depending on the proper identification of the primary injury and any compensatory injuries. In a recent review, we identified 19 clear categories of injuries, and we applied 26 different procedures and 121 different combinations of procedures.

The specific identification of the primary and secondary injuries as well as of the possibility of an associated hip injury provides a guideline for the correction of the problem. First, consider the principal soft-tissue structures that attach to and help stabilize the pelvis. Table 38-1 lists many of these. In general, for males, the more medial structures play greater roles. For women, the lateral structures come more into play. This may be the result of differences in anatomic structure (Figure 38-2). The forces applied to the pubis by these structures are important to consider, and they vary considerably. Note the subtle differences that are schematically represented in the anterior and medial views in Figures 38-3 and 38-4. For each force, there are structures that apply parallel counterforces. In the fresh cadaver laboratory, one can cut certain structures and cause dramatic increases in pressure within other structures or compartments. Such changes in forces likely account for much of what we see clinically in terms of primary and compensatory injuries. The compensatory problems likely result from the "over pulling" of the attachments related to the loss of counterforces and increased pressures within muscles or compartments. Clinically and on a magnetic resonance image, one often finds acute or chronic reactions in the various tissues. These reactions probably represent avulsion, scarring, or tightness within the various compartments involved. Figures 38-5 through 38-8 provide more anatomic direction.

Next, consider the wide variety of musculoskeletal problems that can occur as a result of the disruption of these forces. Table 38-2 lists a number of them that were determined by a recent review of our data. There are still a variety of other problems that are not listed here. The table also summarizes the general approach for the correction of these problems. Initial treatment is usually nonsurgical, and some of these problems can be adequately treated this way. However, when the nonoperative approach does not work, surgery is indicated.

It is important to recognize that these procedures require a combination of the tightening and loosening of various structures, depending on the primary and secondary problems. Mesh for the most part is not necessary. "Tightening" usually means that some specifically placed sutures are used to create more stability in the region where the primary injury occurred. "Loosening" or "releasing" usually refers to decreasing the pressure in a compartment, usually via a specific episiotomy. For the most part, all intact muscle fibers are left intact. However, if an intracompartmental scar is identified, this should be released. When we talk in terms of release operations, we are usually talking about a focal decompression of a particular muscle or part of a muscle, like the treatment of a compartment syndrome. The muscle usually remains intact. The muscles that attach to the pubis or the cartilaginous plate usually attach separately from the investing epimysium. In most cases, we aim to keep as much normal muscle intact as possible.

**Table 38-1** MUSCLES THAT ATTACH TO AND STABILIZE THE PELVIS

| Muscle | Origin | Insertion | Main Actions |
|---|---|---|---|
| Rectus abdominis | Pubic symphysis, pubic crest, and aponeurotic plate | Xiphoid process, costal cartilage, and ribs | Flexes trunk; compresses abdominal viscera; opposes adductors, rotators, and extendors |
| Adductor longus | Pubic symphysis, pubic crest, and aponeurotic plate | Middle third of linea aspera of femur | Adducts thigh; flexes lower extremity |
| Adductor brevis | Pubic symphysis and inferior ramus | Pectineal line and proximal linea aspera of femur | Adducts thigh; flexes thigh and lower extremity |
| Pectineus | Symphysis and superior ramus | Pectineal line of femur just inferior to lesser trochanter | Adducts and flexes thigh and lower extremity; assists with medial rotation of thigh |
| Gracilis | Body and inferior ramus of pubis | Superior part of medial surface of tibia | Adducts thigh; flexes lower extremity; assists with medial rotation |
| Adductor magnus | Two parts: 1) adductor from inferior pubic ramus and ischium; 2) hamstring from ischial tuberosity | Adductor to gluteal tuberosity, linea aspera, and medial supracondylar line; hamstring to adductor tubercle of femur | Adducts, flexes, and extends thigh |
| Obturator externus | Margins of obturator foramen and obturator membrane | Trochanteric fossa of femur | Medially (internally) rotates thigh; assists with stabilizing head of femur in acetabulum |
| Obturator internus | Pelvic surfaces of ilium and ischium, obturator membrane | Greater trochanter of femur | Laterally (externally) rotates thigh; assists with stabilizing head of femur in acetabulum |
| Psoas major | Sides of T12-L5 vertebrae and discs, transverse processes of all lumbar vertebrae | Lesser trochanter of femur | Acts conjointly in flexing thigh at hip joint and stabilizing joint |
| Psoas minor | Sides of T12-L5 vertebrae and discs | Pectineal line and iliopectineal eminence via iliopectineal arch | Acts conjointly with psoas major |
| Quadratus femoris | Ischial tuberosity | Intertrochanteric crest of femur | Laterally rotates thigh; assists with femoral head stabilization |
| Levator ani (pubococcygeus, puborectalis, and iliococcygeus) | Body of pubis, tendinous arch of obturator fascia, and ischial spine | Perineal body, coccyx, anococcygeal ligament, walls of prostate or vagina, rectum, and anal canal | Helps support pelvic viscera; opposes increases in abdominal pressure |
| Semimembranosus | Ischial tuberosity | Medial condyle of tibia | Extends thigh; flexes lower extremity with knee flexed; extends trunk |
| Biceps femoris | Long head from ischial tuberosity; short head from linea aspera of femur | Head of fibula | Extends thigh; flexes lower extremity and rotates it laterally with knee flexed |
| Rectus femoris | Reflected head from superior acetabulum; straight head from anteroinferior iliac spine | Patella | Flexes thigh and assists with stabilization of pubic joint in females |
| Sartorius | Anteroinferior iliac spine | Proximal medial tibia | Flexes, adducts, and laterally rotates thigh |

TECHNICAL PEARLS

- Athletic pubalgia is not one entity, and these injuries are not hernias.
- One needs to understand the anatomy and likely pathophysiology involved in these injuries. The concept of the "pubic joint" is particularly important.
- Accurately identify the primary and secondary injuries, and base the operation on a combination of the correction of the primary problem and the relief of pain from the compensatory problems with the use of tightening and releasing procedures.
- Intra-articular hip problems and athletic pubalgia injuries coexist in up to 10% of athletes.

## POSTOPERATIVE REHABILITATION

Recovery time varies according to the specific injury and the procedure performed. The repair associated with the shortest time might be called a *minimal repair*, which involves a specific tightening and a slight reinforcement of the specifically identified afflicted area, possibly in combination with the nerve division of afflicted branches. Athletes with minimal injury and minimal repair may be able to return to activity within days of surgery. However, the downside of the minimal repair of a minimal injury is the possibility of early recurrence as a result of the undertreatment of pelvic instability. We have had to perform revision surgery on a

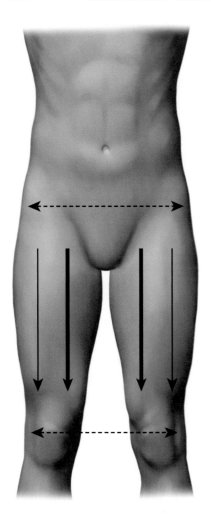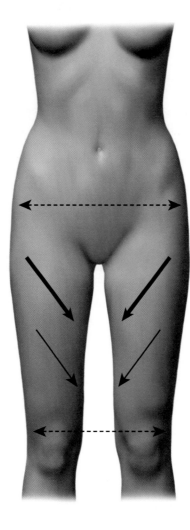

**Figure 38–2** Basic differences in the male and female anatomy that relate to the pubic joint and injury. Note the differences in width between the pelves and knees of the two genders. These differences suggest a different distribution of forces during extremes of exertion. For example, more lateral forces emanate from the female pelvis, and more acutely angled forces are transmitted to the female knees during landing. *From: Meyers WC, Yoo E, Devon O, et al.: Understanding "sports hernia" (athletic pubalgia): the anatomic and pathophysiologic basis for abdominal and groin pain in athletes.* Oper Tech Sport Med. *Elsevier; 15:4, pp 165-177, October 2007.*

number of such patients. The patient needs to understand the increased risk of revision surgery if he or she chooses this in-season approach. However, in selected patients, return to full play by 3 weeks after the procedure is possible. So far, early return in general has not been associated with an early recurrence of injury. It is interesting to note that such an aggressive protocol does seem to work despite the relatively limited time allowed for wound healing.

Alternatively, more extensive repairs require the longest recovery times. An example of one of these is the reattachment of multiple avulsions, such as the entire rectus abdominis in combination with the entire pubic–adductor complex, which is common among bull riders. In such cases, a full return to performance may not occur for several months. Patients with severe osteitis pubis are less predictable in terms of returning to full play without experiencing a recurrence. Other variables that affect both the timing of surgery and the duration of postoperative rehabilitation include the following: the timing of the injury (i.e., within a season or between seasons); contractual considerations; injury complexity; concomitant hip injury; performance with the injury; the specific sport and the player's position; and team standings.

Briefly, the most important parts of postoperative rehabilitation are an aggressive return to activity, the avoidance of movements that cause pain, and massage and other mechanical means of reducing scar bands. We have some specific sport rehabilitation programs, and we modify these protocols on the basis of the specific injury and repair. For long-term rehabilitation and

the prevention of further pelvic injury, we strongly recommend certain core stability programs.

## RESULTS

In general, 95% to 96% of athletes can expect to return to sports participation (Table 38-3). The most important endpoints are at 1 and 2 years after surgery. Success rates vary according to multiple factors, such as the site and severity of the injury, concomitant hip injury, and whether the patient is an athlete or a nonathlete. Recurrence rates are about 0.4%, but new involvement of the contralateral side can be as high as 4%. Return to play by 3 months should occur in approximately 90% of patients. Nonathletes and patients without a clear primary injury going into surgery will have a success rate of between 50% and 90%, depending on the specific problem. Workers compensation injuries are less predictable than other injuries with regard to the reporting of successful operations.

## COMPLICATIONS

Potential operative sequelae that can occur include incisional infection, hematoma, bothersome insensitivity of the skin, penile venous thrombosis, late reaction to sutures, and anesthetic complications. Fortunately, long-term undesirable sequelae have been rare.

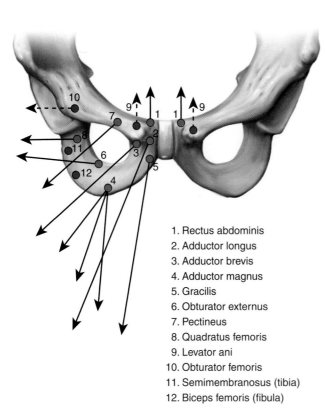

**Figure 38–3** Anterior view of the pubic ramus with a schematic depiction of the many forces that act on the pubic joint. *From: Meyers WC, Greenleaf R, Saad A: Anatomic basis for evaluation of abdominal and groin pain in athletes. Oper Tech Sports Med. Elsevier, 13:1, pp 55-61, 2005.*

1. Rectus abdominis
2. Adductor longus
3. Adductor brevis
4. Adductor magnus
5. Gracilis
6. Obturator externus
7. Pectineus
8. Quadratus femoris
9. Levator ani
10. Obturator femoris
11. Semimembranosus (tibia)
12. Biceps femoris (fibula)

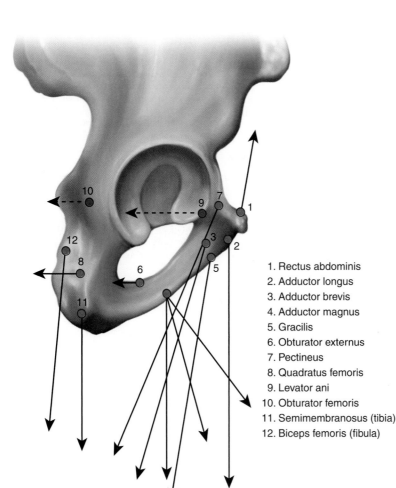

**Figure 38–4** Medial view of the pelvis that depicts the direction of the forces that act on the pelvis and that influence pelvic tilt. *From: Meyers WC, Greenleaf R, Saad A: Anatomic basis for evaluation of abdominal and groin pain in athletes. Oper Tech Sports Med. Elsevier, 13:1, pp 55-61, 2005.*

1. Rectus abdominis
2. Adductor longus
3. Adductor brevis
4. Adductor magnus
5. Gracilis
6. Obturator externus
7. Pectineus
8. Quadratus femoris
9. Levator ani
10. Obturator femoris
11. Semimembranosus (tibia)
12. Biceps femoris (fibula)

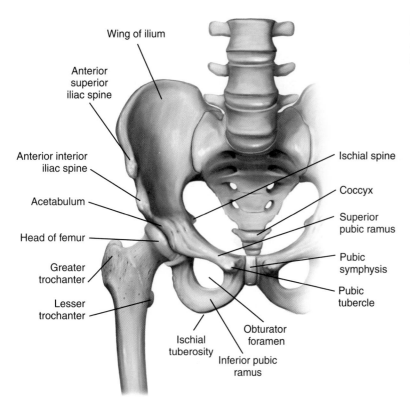

**Figure 38–5** Anterior view of the bony anatomy and the proximal femur. *From: Meyers WC, Greenleaf R, Saad A: Anatomic basis for evaluation of abdominal and groin pain in athletes.* Oper Tech Sports Med. *Elsevier, 13:1, pp 55-61, 2005.*

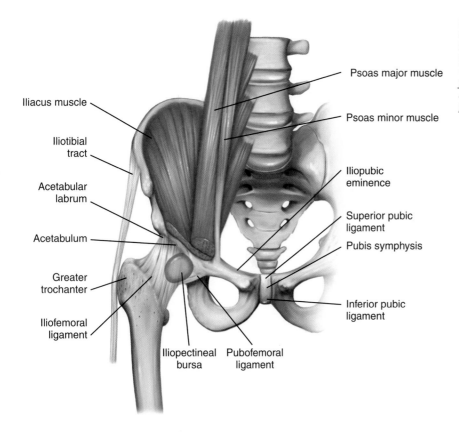

**Figure 38–6** The ligamentous anatomy of the pelvis and the proximal femur. The iliopsoas muscle tendon, which inserts on the lesser trochanter, is cut. *From: Meyers WC, Greenleaf R, Saad A: Anatomic basis for evaluation of abdominal and groin pain in athletes.* Oper Tech Sports Med. *Elsevier, 13:1, pp 55-61, 2005.*

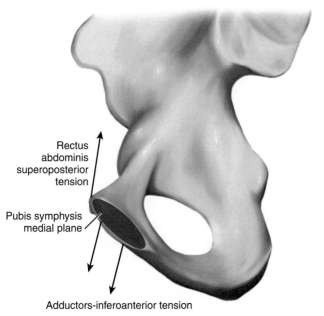

**Figure 38–7** Cross-sectional view through the pubis symphysis that shows the main opposing forces that act on the pubic joint. *From: Meyers WC, Greenleaf R, Saad A: Anatomic basis for evaluation of abdominal and groin pain in athletes.* Oper Tech Sports Med. *Elsevier, 13:1, pp 55-61, 2005.*

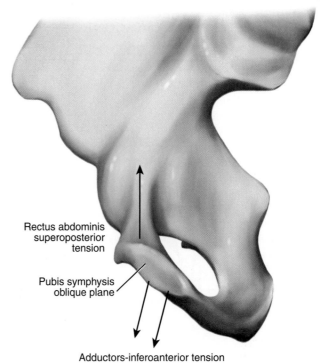

**Figure 38–8** Oblique view of the pubis symphysis that shows the direction of the opposing forces exerted on the pubic joint by the rectus abdominis and the adductors. *From: Meyers WC, Greenleaf R, Saad A: Anatomic basis for evaluation of abdominal and groin pain in athletes.* Oper Tech Sports Med. *Elsevier, 13:1, pp 55-61, 2005.*

### Table 38–2 MORE FREQUENT CLINICAL ENTITIES AND POSSIBLY INDICATED PROCEDURES FOR ATHLETIC PUBALGIA

| Structure/Clinical Syndrome | Relative Incidence | Defect | Possibly Indicated Procedure |
|---|---|---|---|
| Unilateral RA injury with isolated specific AD injury | 15% | T and CS | Repair and release |
| Unilateral RA injury with multiple AD injuries | 14% | T and CS | Repair and releases |
| Unilateral RA injury without significant compensatory injury | 16% | T | Repair |
| Bilateral RA injury without significant compensatory injury | 9% | T | Repairs |
| Bilateral RA injury with unilateral AD injury | 8% | T and CS | Repairs and release |
| Bilateral RA injury with bilateral AD injury | 14% | T and CS | Repairs and releases |
| Unilateral or bilateral RA injury with other significant compensatory injury | 16% | T and CS | Repair and releases |
| Pure unilateral AD injury | 17% | Usually CS | Usually release |
| Pure bilateral AD injury | 8% | Usually CS | Usually releases |
| AD longus involvement | 36% | Mainly CS | Usually release |
| AD brevis involvement | 18% | Mainly CS | Usually release |
| Pectineus involvement | 28% | Mainly CS | Usually release |
| Severe secondary osteitis | 11% | T, CS, edema, and inflammation | Usually repairs and releases |
| Iliopsoas variant | 9% | Impingement and bursitis | Release |
| Baseball pitcher/hockey goalie syndrome | 9% | AD muscle belly tear and CS | Release |
| Spigelian variant | 3% | T | Repair |
| High RA variant | 1% | T | Repair |
| Female variant | 4% | Medial disruption with lateral thigh compensation | Repair and release(s) |

*Continued*

**Table 38–2** MORE FREQUENT CLINICAL ENTITIES AND POSSIBLY INDICATED PROCEDURES FOR ATHLETIC PUBALGIA—CONT'D

| Structure/Clinical Syndrome | Relative Incidence | Defect | Possibly Indicated Procedure |
|---|---|---|---|
| Round ligament variant | 1% | Inflammation with T | Excision and repair |
| Dancers' variants | <1% | Usually obturator externus or internus T | Release(s) |
| Rower's rib syndromes | <1% | Subluxation | Excision and mesh |
| Avulsions (grade 3 injuries) | 2% | Usually acute T | Release(s) or repair |
| AD and RA calcification syndromes | 1% | Usually chronic avulsion | Excision and release |
| Midline RA variant | 1% | T and muscle separation | Repair and mesh |
| Anterior ischial tuberosity variant | 1% | Posterior perineal inflammation and often gracilis or hamstring T | Release |
| AD contractures | 1% | Often associated with hip pathology | Release and hip repair |
| Rectus femoris variant | 4% | Usually impingement | Release |
| Obturator externus variant | 1% | T | Release |
| Sartorius involvement | 3% | CS or impingement | Release |

*RA*, Rectus abdominis; *AD*, adductor; *T*, tear(s); *CS*, compartment syndrome(s).
These data include information about some of the patients reported in Meyers WC, McKechnie A, Philippon MJ, et al. Experience with "sports hernia" spanning two decades. Presented at the 2008 meeting of the American Surgical Association. *Ann Surg*, Oct 2008, 248:4, p. 656-665.

**Table 38–3** RESULTS OF STUDIES WITH ADEQUATE LONG-TERM FOLLOW UP

| Study | No. of Patients | Procedure | Results |
|---|---|---|---|
| Meyers, 2000 | 279 | Pelvic floor repairs and adductor releases | 94.6% and 95.3% success rates among athletes during two time periods with 3.9 years overall mean follow up time |
| Meyers, 2008 | 8490 | Multiple procedures | 95.3% of athletes able to return to play within 3 months of surgery; further analysis of patients with 1-year minimum follow up showed success rates that varied from 83% to 98%; concomitant hip problems accounted for the majority of patients with persistent problems, but in most such cases pain resolved after hip surgery |

## ANNOTATED REFERENCES AND SUGGESTED READINGS

Albers SL, Spritzer CE, Garrett WE, Meyers WC. MRI findings in athletes with pubalgia. *Skeletal Radiol.* 2006;30:270–277.

Gilmore OJA. Gilmore's groin: ten years of experience of groin disruption—a previously unsolved problem in sportsmen. *Sport Med Soft Tissue Trauma.* 1991;3:12–14.

About the same time that we did, Dr. Gilmore recognized that there were nonhernia problems that afflicted athletes. He provided a new name for the set of syndromes.

McKechnie A, Celebrini R. *Hard core strength.* Vancouver, BC. Available at http://www.p2soccer.com/Content/Main%20pages/Resource%20Centre.asp.

Meyers WC, Foley DP, Garrett WE, et al. Management of severe lower abdominal or inguinal pain in high-performance athletes. *Am J Sports Med.* 200;28:2–8.

Meyers WC, Greenleaf R, Saad A. Anatomic basis for evaluation of abdominal and groin pain in athletes. *Oper Tech Sports Med.* 2005;13(1):55–61.

Meyers WC, McKechnie A, Philippon MJ, et al. Experience with "sports hernia" spanning two decades. Presented at the 2008 meeting of the American Surgical Association. *Ann Surg.* Oct 2008;248:(4):656–665.

Meyers WC, Szalai L, Potter N, et al. Extraarticular sources of hip pain. In: Byrd JWT, ed. *Operative hip arthroscopy.* Vol 5. 2nd ed. New York: Springer; 2005:86–97.

Meyers WC, Yoo EY, Devon ON, et al. Understanding "sports hernia" (athletic pubalgia): the anatomic and pathophysiologic basis for abdominal and groin pain in athletes. *Oper Tech Sports Med.* 2007;15:165–177.

Nesovic, Treatise on maladies of the pubic symphysis (privately published monograph).

Omar IM, Zoga AC, Meyers WC, et al. Athletic pubalgia and the "sports hernia": optimal MR imaging technique and pictorial review of MR findings. Scientific exhibit. *Proceedings of the Radiologic Society of North America,* Cum Laude Award winner 2006. *Radiographics.* 28:1415–1438, 2008.

**Swan KG, Wolcott M. The athletic hernia; a systematic review.** *Clin Orthop Rel Res.* **2006;455:78–87.**

This review describes well the tremendous confusion in the literature regarding this set of problems, the large number of different descriptions of these entities, and the numerous reports that do not include adequate follow up.

**Taylor DC, Meyers WC, Moylan JA, et al. Abdominal musculature abnormalities as a cause of groin pain in athletes.** *Am J Sports Med.* **1991;19:239–242.**

This was our first article about these entities. We saw that these were not hernias, and we were initially very selective with regard to the patients on which we chose to operate. The term *athletic pubalgia* originated with this paper.

**Zoga AC, Kavanaugh EC, Meyers WC, et al. MRI of the rectus abdominis/adductor aponeurosis: findings in the "sports hernia." In: Scientific paper presentation,** *Proceedings of the American Roentgen Ray Society.* **2007.**

**Zoga AC, Kavanaugh EC, Meyers WC, et al. MRI findings in athletic pubalgia and the "sports hernia."** *Radiol.* **2008;247:(3): 797–807.**

# Index

Note: Page numbers followed by *b* indicate boxes; *f* indicate figures and *t* indicate tables.